POLIO WARS

Polio Wars

SISTER ELIZABETH KENNY AND THE GOLDEN
AGE OF AMERICAN MEDICINE

Naomi Rogers

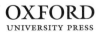

OXFORD
UNIVERSITY PRESS

OXFORD
UNIVERSITY PRESS

Oxford University Press is a department of the University of Oxford.
It furthers the University's objective of excellence in research, scholarship,
and education by publishing worldwide.

Oxford   New York
Auckland   Cape Town   Dar es Salaam   Hong Kong   Karachi
Kuala Lumpur   Madrid   Melbourne   Mexico City   Nairobi
New Delhi   Shanghai   Taipei   Toronto

With offices in
Argentina   Austria   Brazil   Chile   Czech Republic   France   Greece
Guatemala   Hungary   Italy   Japan   Poland   Portugal   Singapore
South Korea   Switzerland   Thailand   Turkey   Ukraine   Vietnam

Oxford is a registered trademark of Oxford University Press in the UK and
certain other countries.

Published in the United States of America by
Oxford University Press
198 Madison Avenue, New York, NY 10016

© Oxford University Press 2014

Library of Congress Cataloging-in-Publication Data
Rogers, Naomi, 1958–
Polio wars: Sister Elizabeth Kenny and the golden age of American medicine/Naomi Rogers.
    p. ; cm.
Includes bibliographical references.
ISBN 978–0–19–538059–0 (hardback: alk. paper)—ISBN 978–0–19–970146–9 (updf ebook)—
ISBN 978–0–19–933413–1 (epub ebook)
I. Title.
[DNLM: 1. Kenny, Elizabeth, 1886–1952.   2. Nurses—Australia—Biography.
3. Poliomyelitis—history—Australia. WZ 100]
RA644.P9
614.5′49—dc23   2013011373

9 8 7 6 5 4 3 2 1
Printed in the United States of America
on acid-free paper

For Nat, Dory,
and JH

Contents

Introduction

⌒⌒———————————————————————————————————————

STANDING ON MY bookshelf is a coin container in an outrageous bright orange that was popular in the 1940s. Under white letters urging me to "Sock Polio" are 3 figures: a toddler in a loin cloth standing awkwardly but steadily; singer Bing Crosby, with a pipe and a jaunty hat; and a white-haired woman in a black dress and pearls, her hands reaching up toward the child with a look of intense pride. "Please Give to the Sister Elizabeth Kenny Foundation," the container pleads. Crosby was the national chairman of the foundation's 1945 appeal, but who was Sister Kenny? When this can was passed down the aisle at movie theaters, no one in America needed to ask. She was so familiar and iconic a figure that Holly Golightly in *Breakfast at Tiffany's* declared that she would not testify against a friend, "not if they can prove he doped Sister Kenny."[1]

Sister Elizabeth Kenny, an Australian nurse, came to the United States in 1940 to seek medical approval for her new methods of treating patients paralyzed by polio. ("Sister" was a British designation for senior nurse, not a religious title.) Despite the skepticism and even hostility of American physicians, she succeeded. With the sometimes grudging support of the National Foundation for Infantile Paralysis (NFIP), a polio philanthropy committed to funding patient care, research, and professional training, her methods were made standard polio care by the mid-1940s. Kenny became one of the most prominent women of her era: the subject of a Hollywood movie *Sister Kenny* (RKO 1946) starring Rosalind Russell; an expert witness at Congressional hearings on the founding of the National Science Foundation; and in 1952, not long before her death, chosen in a Gallup poll as America's most admired woman, outranking former first lady Eleanor Roosevelt. Yet by the mid-1950s she was almost forgotten. Crosby's 1953 autobiography *Call Me Lucky* never mentioned her.[2]

Kenny's was a life of passionate outrage. She spent years defending her work, inspiring her patients, and attacking prejudice. She knew how to stir up controversy and how to play medical politics using the media, the public, and politicians. Challenging established medical knowledge on its weak points and inconsistencies, Kenny was a quick study, adopting insights pointed out by her critics and making them integral to her work. Her feisty style mocked the deference nurses were expected to show physicians but she could also make fun of herself as a middle-aged woman. With what was called her Irish humor she thanked one group of doctors who greeted her at an airport carrying roses, telling them it was gratifying to receive flowers from doctors while she was "still here to smell them."[3]

This book tells the story of Sister Kenny and the Kenny method. Kenny's battles with American medical professionals illuminate the medical politics that lay at the heart of American medicine, even during its Golden Age. After her struggles with government bureaucrats and medical professionals in Australia Kenny was neither shocked nor fazed by the need to pull strings and gain influential allies in order to alter clinical care in the United States. Polio was a high-profile disease, and responsibility for its prevention and treatment rested on diverse authorities: local and state health officials and the U.S. Public Health Service; individual physicians, nurses, and physical therapists; civic and charity groups that ran hospitals and "crippled children's homes," did surveys, and set up services for families with disabled members; and the NFIP, which supported its activities through an annual national fundraising campaign known as the March of Dimes and numerous regional campaigns organized by its local and state chapters. Kenny's heated battles with the NFIP and organized medicine captured the public imagination. Standing outside the elite scientific community, she sought to gain its respect through clinical and laboratory confirmation of her theories of polio. Simultaneously, however, she resented being held to standards of scientific rigor that she suspected were imposed more strictly on her because she was a woman and a nurse and because she dared to question the expertise of male orthopedic surgeons.

This book also focuses on the limber, healthy child patient featured on the 1945 container. Here is a dramatic, if sentimentalized, depiction of the results of a special kind of clinical care, yet the container does not show any doctor, hospital bed, syringe, or other symbol of medical science. For the American public the most powerful omission may have been the familiar picture of a polio patient: the crying child in a hospital bed with arms or legs in plaster casts; the fearful child waiting for an orthopedic operation; or the "recovered" child discharged with crutches or braces, all images typical in March of Dimes campaigns. On this "Sock Polio" container, health has been achieved in another way, through compassion and care based on a distinctive understanding of the body shared by Kenny and her staff but not by other professionals.

In an era when nurses were seen as the recipients of medical science rather than its designers, Kenny knew that her claims to a new understanding of polio were controversial before their content was even known. At first she presented herself as a supplicant to scientists, seeking their assistance to explain the meaning of the new symptoms she had identified and the reasons her methods worked. Her 1941 textbook had the temperate title *Treatment of Infantile Paralysis in the Acute Stage.* But as the Institute prospered and Kenny was feted as a savior, she began to argue that her work embodied a new concept of polio drawn from a close reading of the body. Polio, she said, was not solely a neurological disease but also a disease of muscles and "peripheral structures." By the time Kenny published her 1943 textbook *The Kenny Concept of Infantile Paralysis* she had begun to argue that it was impossible to teach anyone to treat the symptoms she had identified if they did not understand her concept of the disease. Indeed, she frequently added, the prognosis for a patient treated without this new knowledge would always be far poorer than for a patient treated by professionals who fully understood the Kenny concept of polio.

Kenny knew to speak of "improvement" rather than "cure," but she often did exaggerate her results. As early as the 1930s she learned the power of the press and the importance of a good story. She was accused by her critics of being a publicity hound, of practicing mistaken and perhaps even harmful methods, and of making unrealistic promises to disabled patients and their families. At times she boasted of her distance from the medical establishment; at other times she made much of her medical allies. She found strong public support when she attacked the elitism of the medical profession in both Australia and North America, but she also sought out and relied on the financial and social assistance from the elite in business and society. She said she chose to follow only "orthodox" physicians, but her clinical practice and its values drew on alternative attitudes toward medical science, toward the disabled, and toward chronic care. Her patients as well as the nurses and physical therapists she trained to become Kenny technicians were central to the functioning of her work. Her students saw her life as one of struggle and sacrifice, a story that was central to the image she projected and one they frequently retold as a way to keep their own spirits up as they battled for clinical autonomy and professional respect from skeptical peers and medical supervisors.

Her critics denigrated her work by drawing on their understanding of medical history, technical innovation, and gender relations. Yet many professionals were frustrated that neither the techniques of modern medical science nor an appeal to medical history enabled them to attack Kenny effectively. Indeed Kenny's experiences illuminate a side of American medical politics in which claims of nonpartisanship by philanthropies failed and where political and social allegiances defined who was on a hospital's medical staff, where a patient was cared for, and which patient was seen as suitable for orthopedic surgery and which for home care. In this world, as polio patients ruefully learned, wheelchairs were expensive, ramps nonexistent, and schools and workplaces inaccessible. The lived experience of polio paralysis meant social discrimination as well as physical disability.

The process of therapeutic change has a disturbingly messy history, as medical historian Erwin Ackerknecht pointed out long ago.[4] At the dawn of the twentieth century, despite emerging laboratory-trained experts preaching rationality and caution, Americans continued to seek out therapeutic panaceas: in the 1920s goat glands for enhanced male virility and in the 1930s sulfa drugs to cure all kinds of infections and vitamins to treat and prevent newly identified "deficiency" diseases. But how could professionals decide what worked and when to change their practice? And how did they know who to trust? Drugs and surgical techniques were concrete, discrete interventions that appeared to have clear effects on the body and could be tested against a placebo in a medical trial. But other clinical methods were more amorphous, resisting any simple test.

Moreover, the popular and professional understanding of scientific innovation was profoundly gendered. The slow, careful procedures of physical therapy were mostly carried out by women; innovation in science through animal experiments or the study of human tissues and body fluids was something so dramatic and transformative that it was the province of male professionals. A clinical trial was also a gendered project, since it involved "masculine" strength for clinicians to withhold a therapy despite their humane feelings for individual patients. Although there was much discussion about the importance of such trials to assess Kenny's methods, no clinical trial of her work was ever undertaken. Her methods were widely accepted, reflecting popular and professional enthusiasm rather than rational, measured assessment. And once her methods were taken up, as Kenny had hoped, no one wanted to use the old methods.

A NEW DISEASE

Polio is a common, contagious viral infection that has been endemic around the world for many centuries. The earliest records of a disease resembling polio were found in ancient Egypt. Until the late nineteenth century the virus rarely caused paralytic symptoms as most infants were protected from infection by maternal antibodies and young children usually experienced only mild symptoms that were often mistaken for a gastrointestinal attack or influenza. As levels of sanitation improved, children were protected from infection until they were older and more vulnerable. Children exposed to the virus after the age of 2 or 3 years were more likely to develop paralysis as the virus traveled from the intestines to the central nervous system. In the late 1890s polio outbreaks appeared first in Scandinavia and then in other industrialized Western countries including the United States. In 1909 the virus was identified as a "filterable agent," smaller than a bacterium, but it could not be seen through a microscope until the electron microscope was developed in the late 1930s. Patients without clear paralytic symptoms were often given spinal taps, mainly to establish that the patient did not have meningitis or another similar disease.[5] Today, despite the existence of effective vaccines, polio remains both endemic and epidemic in countries with inadequate sanitation, nutrition, and medical resources. Today there is a consensus that the polio virus is spread by contaminated fecal matter, but until the early 1950s there were many theories about how the disease spread and just how contagious it was.

Working with children paralyzed during polio outbreaks in the 1910s, Boston surgeons Robert Lovett and Arthur Legg and physical therapists Wilhemine Wright and Janet Merrill developed therapies based on the concept of rest and the enforced straightening of limbs. The improper use of muscles, they argued, would cause deformities and therefore patients, especially children whose movements could not easily be controlled, had to be strictly confined to positions that would keep their bodies straight. Often this involved casts and splints, followed by braces and corsets. As polio was considered infectious new patients were confined for 3 to 6 weeks in an infectious disease hospital or a general hospital's isolation ward. In polio's early or acute stage no massage or exercises were used for expert opinion held, in the words of nurse Jesse Stevenson, that "deformities develop even more quickly when the muscles are sensitive."[6] During the next "convalescent" stage, which could range from several months to 2 years, patients stayed in general wards or crippled children's homes, usually restrained in casts and splints. After weeks or months, patients were sent home and given exercises and perhaps also heat or electrical therapies, sometimes under the direction of a physical therapist. As there were few of these professionals outside of specialized rehabilitation institutions, however, more often exercises were explained to the patient's mother when the patient was discharged. The patient was told to continue to wear the braces and use the crutches and to return for a follow-up examination, which usually involved testing individual muscles for strength and range of motion. When underused muscles withered and limbs grew unevenly, and after physicians determined that no further recovery of muscle strength could be expected, they prescribed orthopedic surgery such as muscle transplantation.[7] "Probably no other one disease requires so many different types of operations for its satisfactory treatment," reflected one orthopedist in the 1920s.[8] On rare occasions critics warned that immobilization, while important, could lead to "vasomotor and trophic disturbances in the affected extremities" as well as "circulatory interference."[9] Only much later did polio experts admit that many orthopedic surgeons got "terrible results." In 1955, an orthopedist recalled with horror 24 patients in the 1930s who were placed in casts and splints, some for as long as 2 years, while he and other specialists waited "for their muscles to recover."[10]

Muscle testing, codified by Lovett and Legg, was the major technology used by physical therapists to show patients and other professionals improvement in muscle strength and power, and to assess the necessity for orthopedic surgery. It was based on 2 techniques: muscle positioning and muscle movement. In muscle positioning the body parts not being tested had to be held as firm and stable as possible as the therapist applied pressure (or "resistance") to the muscle or muscle group in order to estimate its strength based on the amount of pressure applied and the amount of strength required to hold the test position. The therapist had to understand the intricate workings of muscles and muscle groups to be able to detect any substitution movements used by the patient (consciously or unconsciously) to compensate for muscle weakness. To assess a muscle's range of motion and flexibility, a part was moved through a specified arc of motion and in a specified direction. These tests were used to seek a pattern of muscle weakness, for the degree of functional strength was believed to bear a definite relationship to the extent and degree of pathology, including the site of the nerve lesion. Such tests required a detailed understanding of anatomy and muscle function to be able to achieve an accurate grading of muscle strength and motion.[11] Their accuracy depended on the skill and judgment of each individual physical therapist. Indeed, testing could also be used to assess the efficacy of therapies; thus, Lovett used the muscle test to indicate the danger of excessive "massage and therapeutic exercise."[12] Further, while muscle testing demanded that the therapist understand intricate muscle anatomy and physiology, it did not assume any such knowledge for the patient. Indeed these tests tended to point out muscle weakness and inability, rather than strength and functionality.

In the early 1920s a few orthopedic surgeons developed other treatments. Los Angeles orthopedist Charles Lowman turned a former fish pond on the grounds of the Orthopedic Hospital-School into a modern therapeutic pool, shortened the long watchful waiting period typical for early polio cases, and began to allow patients into the pool using muscle reeducation under water as early as a week after the quarantine period. These techniques Lowman believed helped to keep "the channels of communication open between the central nervous system and the muscle."[13] The experience of Franklin Roosevelt in the 1920s inspired a surge of optimism around hydrotherapy. Roosevelt, a wealthy lawyer who had been nominated for the vice presidency by the Democratic Party, was paralyzed by polio in 1921 at the age of 39 years. In his search for therapies that would enable him to walk again he traveled to Warm Springs, then a run-down resort in rural Georgia, to try out its heated mineral springs. He was sufficiently impressed by this treatment to purchase the resort and develop it into a polio rehabilitation center. By 1928 when he was elected governor of New York he was known as the man who had battled and conquered his paralysis, a story that, although not really true, was even more crucial during his successful campaign for the presidency in 1932.[14]

During the 1930s polio care took a conservative turn. Physicians learned not to expect much improvement in their patients' muscles and were suspicious of those who claimed success.[15] Orthopedic surgeons George Bennett and Robert Johnson and physical therapists Henry and Florence Kendall at the Baltimore Children's Hospital-School were disheartened to see that some of their patients recovered "to normal with little or no treatment" while others remained "hopelessly crippled even though given the best care." "No one is justified in making an early prognosis," they concluded, for "it is impossible to determine the outcome."[16] The Kendalls were also convinced that patients were harmed by "frequent, improper handling, and over-treatment." Concerned about muscles that lost their natural reflexes through overstretching they relied on frames, casts, splints, and very mild exercises, rejected underwater exercises, and suggested that some patients might benefit from "complete rest in the bed for several years."[17] By the early 1940s, muscle exercises were still part of polio care, but there was a consensus that underwater exercises had been overemphasized. Even at Warm Springs, according to its chief surgeon, only a quarter of his patients exercised in the center's thermal pools.[18]

Tracing the relationship between polio's clinical symptoms and the pathology of the virus was difficult. Theories to explain the paralysis of muscles abounded, but the standard pathological concept reinforced a faith in immobilization. The polio virus was believed to create lesions in the brain and spinal cord, severing connections between muscles and nerves; a paralyzed limb, therefore, could be expected to regain only limited movement. As physicians saw polio as a neurological disease, they warned that any active movements could exacerbate these lesions and that muscle exercises should not be used until at least 8 weeks after a patient's fever had subsided, suggesting that the lesions had healed.[19] Reflecting the profound stigma around physical disability and their own skepticism about recovery, physicians used splinting to keep the patient's body looking straight and "normal" rather than focusing on functionality.[20] Although plaster splints and casts were often painful, clinicians considered them crucial in order to spare patients "the mental and physical pain of a hideous deformity," as one orthopedic nurse noted.[21]

The most challenging part of polio therapy was the enforced period of rest through immobilization. To ensure that this therapeutic regime was followed hospitals had to rely on the efforts of trained graduate nurses. Indeed, argued one nursing textbook, "the entire success of the treatment depends upon the loyalty of the nurse in maintaining the position effected by splinting."[22] To dramatize how "a few seconds of nonsupport may do serious harm" orthopedic nurse Jessie Stevenson pointed out that "the nurse would be horrified at the thought of maintaining sterile technic in the operation room for *only part of the time*." Even when muscle stimulation was allowed, she noted, it must be practiced "very gently" and by a professional who knew "the origin, insertion and action of all the important muscles."[23] Given the lack of such professionals, however, in practice immobilizing therapy frequently meant therapeutic neglect.

KENNY AS POLIO CLINICIAN

Elizabeth Kenny gained attention because her work dealt with a high profile disease and filled the therapeutic vacuum that surrounded it. Polio epidemics in the 1930s grew more serious and more frequent. Although the disease remained a relatively minor cause of morbidity and mortality, parents saw it as a major threat to their children's health. Polio left family doctors at a terrifying loss: epidemics could not be predicted or controlled; paralyzed patients sometimes recovered mobility, but often remained disabled in a world unfriendly to the disabled; and until the mid-1950s there was no vaccine to prevent it.

Kenny provocatively promised ambitious results. Her goal was fully recovered movement. She transformed standard polio therapies—especially splinting and surgery—into symbols of a failed and even harmful clinical program. Her therapies, especially her hot packs and muscle exercises, were based on distinctive ideas about polio as not solely a neurological disease but also one that affected muscles and skin. At first she talked about clinical signs (physical manifestations visible to the outside eye) that had been ignored and left untreated by polio experts, but gradually she came to see them as crucial symptoms (experiences of the patient) that provided evidence for a rethinking of polio's pathology and physiology.[24] Her challenge to existing concepts of polio attracted patients and families as it embodied a different style of clinical practice: optimistic, energetic, patient-centered care.

In describing the experience of polio as she saw it Kenny relied on 3 crucial terms: *spasm* (a muscle in pain and contracting), *alienation* (a "physiologic block" that prevented "the proper transmission of a nerve impulse from the central nervous system to a contractible or nonparalyzed muscle"), and *incoordination* (the "loss of ability to use muscles in proper relationship to one another").[25] The language she used was strange to physicians' ears. The only term familiar to many orthopedic surgeons and physical therapists was spasm: a spastic muscle was well known in a variety of neuromuscular conditions, especially cerebral palsy.[26] But Kenny's definition made polio's spasm unfamiliar, especially when she linked it to her system of treatment. Using a distinctive understanding of polio's clinical picture and her own techniques, her methods, she claimed, would help to restore normal function to a patient's muscles "to the fullest extent possible."[27]

Immobilization, Kenny argued, had many dangers; most crucially, it prevented the treatment of the symptoms she had identified. It also interfered with the nutrition of skin, tissue, and muscles and diminished the volume of nerve impulses through the nervous system "along the afferent and efferent paths," as well as interfering with "the normal function of the subconscious mind" and giving patients "an adverse psychological outlook." Yet immobilization was "the paramount principle upon which the orthodox system is founded" and, according to the Kendalls, the main treatment for polio was "rest in a well-protected position." The orthodox system was therefore based on principles that were the exact opposite of her system, especially in its view of how muscles were affected by the polio virus and how to ameliorate paralysis. In orthodox polio care affected muscles were not seen as spastic but flaccid, and were depicted as hanging loosely "like a hammock between their two points of attachment." Paralysis was believed to be caused by healthy muscles stretching these weaker ones. But in Kenny's view, muscles in spasm were in fact the central cause of paralysis.[28]

According to Kenny, her methods treated properly identified symptoms correctly and therefore had far better clinical results. Spasm was the main reason that patients with polio experienced pain and paralysis. The *affected* muscles in polio were not those that could not move but their antagonists that were in a state of painful contraction or spasm that rendered the opposing muscles unable to move. Muscle spasm in polio could be distinguished from other kinds of shortened or contracted muscles for it did not relax under deep general anesthesia.[29] To treat spasm she used what became known as hot packs or Kenny packs: soft, wool cloths immersed in boiling water, put through a wringer, and wrapped around the belly of the muscle in spasm, followed by protective coverings of oiled silk or rubber sheeting and then a dry cloth or towel. After around 15 minutes the hot packs cooled but they remained in place for about 2 hours on the principle that alternating heat and cooling would aid circulation and improve the "vitality" of the body's tissues.[30] If spasm was not treated, she warned, muscles would become "toneless, flat, shortened and narrowed."[31]

Alienation was the term Kenny used to explain other muscles that appeared to be paralyzed. These muscles were, she argued, alienated from the "conscious voluntary mind." Unlike physicians' usually pessimistic prognosis, she argued that in most cases the "nerve pathways" were not destroyed but divorced from the voluntary "motor center." On occasion, she conceded, there were some permanently paralyzed muscles, but alienated muscles could be identified by their ability to exhibit a slight amount of "tonus," that is the tendon of the muscle would appear after the attendant had flexed the appropriate joint several times.[32] Because of the pain associated with spasm and because the opposing alienated muscle was stretched beyond its normal resting place, patients lost awareness of this muscle, causing it to be "drop[ped] from the patient's consciousness and become alienated or divorced from voluntary action." The attendant's job was to reestablish the "normal brain pathways" through careful passive muscle movements during which the body was kept in a normal alignment, and the patient was told to relax and think of nothing so as to conserve "nervous energy."[33] These movements were intended to stimulate both the muscle and the neural pathway. As it was crucial to keep the muscles "at their normal length between their points of origin and insertion," she emphasized her attendants' detailed knowledge of muscle anatomy and physiology and the importance of giving the patient a fundamental knowledge of muscle function as well.[34] To counter an alienated flexion of the forearm, for example, the attendant bent the patient's arm and placed the patient's elbow in the palm of her hand, supporting the patient's forearm with her hand. To help the patient gain "mental awareness," the attendant asked the patient to visualize the point of attachment of the brachial muscle, then passively flexed the forearm, telling the patient not to make any physical effort. The attendant also watched the patient closely to see that no effort was made in any other muscle group. After the attendant had passively flexed the forearm 3 times and felt "that the brain path has been restored, the patient is required to put forth a physical effort at the end of the session." This effort must be "concentrated, both mentally and physically, to the group from which a movement is expected to occur."[35] If left untreated alienated muscles could become paralyzed from disuse and lead to permanent paralysis and deformity.[36]

To explain the awkward ways that patients initially began to use their limbs and other body parts—which Kenny termed "spasmodic"—she developed the concept of incoordination. Polio, she argued, had disorganized the "normal physiological activity of the nervous system." This disruption of "the natural rhythmic and cooperative action of associated muscles" persisted after spasm had been released.[37] The attendant needed a detailed understanding of "the harmonious action of the [muscle] groups working in sympathy" and how to apply "measures...to insure perfect harmony in all muscles." The attendant also needed to be careful that the patient did not begin to use other muscles instead, for muscle substitution, Kenny warned, could make incoordination permanent.[38] To reestablish connections "between the patient's mind and the more peripheral parts of his body" Kenny technicians held muscles using special "grips" or hand positions. Indeed, Kenny argued that a patient's mental effort to produce a muscular contraction could often be felt by an attendant's hand before the contraction actually occurred.[39] The aim of this careful muscle reeducation was "to get the patient to picture everything in terms of normal function" and thereby counter the "disorganization" that had "occurred at the lesion which interferes with the co-ordination of movements."[40] While Kenny rejected standard hydrotherapy she did urge the use of warm baths and alternating cold sprays and warm douches as adjuncts to muscle reeducation to assist in the reestablishment of consciousness of the body's peripheral structures. These techniques would provide "afferent stimuli" that would keep the paralyzed body part in the patient's consciousness.[41]

Although Kenny rejected standard protective devices such as casts, frames, and splints she did protect her patients' muscles. Her patients would lay on a firm mattress supported by bed boards and a foot board so that their heels and toes were not on the mattress. When necessary she used a small rolled towel under or on either side of the knees; she never used anything that would seem like a splint that might "interfere with the proprioceptive reflexes" and with "the patient's feeling of normalcy."[42]

Most of the therapies she used were drawn from the standard therapeutic repertoire for dealing with pain, sensitivity, and paralysis. Heat therapies were known to be helpful in "relieving and relaxing the sensitive extremities," although physicians disagreed whether heated cloths and hot baths worked better than dry heat in lamps or diathermy (electrically induced heat).[43] Before the 1940s some physicians used intermittent hot packs to increase circulation and maintain muscle nutrition but most agreed that the most important thing was to prevent deformity and relieve pain through the use of splints and casts.[44]

Patients in the early stages of polio were frequently misdiagnosed. Kenny believed that her trained clinical eye worked better than any other standard diagnostic tool. Indeed she suggested that the use of spinal taps was usually unnecessary and just added to a patient's pain. She firmly rejected standard muscle testing as likely to increase pain and produce inaccurate results, which would then lead to pessimistic prognoses. Testing muscles on patients in the acute stage of polio was particularly dangerous as it undermined the principles of her methods. Until spasm had been treated the patient was not allowed to attempt to use any muscles for "the only effective treatment...for the brain path" must be given "to counteract mental alienation."[45]

Kenny alienated health professionals by her arrogant confidence in herself, her abrasive clinical teaching style, and her clear disdain for those who, as she characterized them in her 1943 autobiography, "have eyes but they see not." She engaged in public debates with leading figures in American medicine and health philanthropy, including Morris Fishbein, general secretary of the American Medical Association (AMA), and Basil O'Connor, head of the NFIP. Despite her dismissive manner, however, Kenny recognized the high status of physicians in American society and wanted to be taken seriously by them. And however unorthodox her ideas may have appeared, she was certainly never antiscience. She consistently tried to use the tools and vocabulary of modern experimental science to try to gain the respect of the medical establishment.

More controversially she claimed that the efficacy of her work and her own clinical observations had led to a distinctive understanding of polio as not a neurotropic disease (a disease in which the virus infects nerve cells) but a systemic disease (one that affects a number of organs and tissues). It is possible that the debate over this theory influenced the work of American virologists who discovered in the early 1950s that the polio virus was spread throughout the body by the blood. Most elite physicians and scientists, however, were not convinced by the kinds of evidence she used or the authority she claimed; and her popularity with the American public further alienated scientists already sceptical of medical populism.

Kenny never married, choosing the single life typical of ambitious women professionals in the early and mid-twentieth century. The Hollywood movie based on her autobiography portrayed Kenny as being forced to choose between her work and a fiancé, a story that was probably false.[46] In any case hers was an unusual career: crossing boundaries, breaching professional and social mores, a nurse claiming the authority of a scientist, a discoverer, a healer, and a celebrity. Kenny was able to carve out (at times with a rather blunt knife) a path for herself that led to fame, autonomy, and professional respect throughout much of the Western world. Challenging the mostly male world of virologists, orthopedic surgeons, epidemiologists, and pediatricians meant using her height (5' 10"), her Australian-Irish humor, her age (a number that diminished over time), and, outside Australia, her identity as an exotic. It meant adopting a distinctive, feminine public persona. Dressed in dramatic hats and corsages, Kenny used her title "Sister," ignoring its religious significance for many Americans, and presented herself as a mixture of Florence Nightingale and Marie Curie. She was a distinctive kind of celebrity who combined clinical skills and abrasive wit with demands for public expressions of loyalty. In the eyes of most orthodox physicians and scientists, her attitude to medical expertise and scientific evidence marked her as an outsider, despite her efforts to enter the medical mainstream. But it is through her refusal to be so easily categorized and dismissed that we can start to understand some of the boundaries of medical orthodoxy in this period.

Kenny sought to straddle the gendered medical culture of her time and to gain respect as both a hands-on therapist and a scientific discoverer. She presented an alternative paradigm of the body and by extension of patient autonomy. At a time when doctors rarely explained what they were doing or why and nurses were often close-mouthed and harried with the sense that the patient's foremost responsibility was obedience to medical direction, Kenny's emphasis was on explaining what was happening and arguing that the patient's active participation—physically and mentally—played a crucial role in the healing process. Her therapy demanded that patients understand the names of muscles and the reasons behind correct muscle movements, for, she said, "in the last analysis, it is the patient who must reopen the nerve path between mind and affected muscle."[47]

Her notions of science were equally provocative. She was convinced that scientific theory had to be based on clinical evidence, even for an understanding of invisible microbes. Thus, she believed that the empirical evidence embodied in her patients' recovery proved her therapy worked, and saw scientific investigation as a way of demonstrating the physiological processes underlying its efficacy. Kenny's suspicion of clinical trials and her emphasis on understanding disease in the living body rather than through tissue pathology convinced her detractors that she lacked an appreciation of true, strong, masculine science whose proponents were not swayed by weaker emotions of caring and empathy.

Kenny's efforts to transform polio care and polio theory brought to the forefront the competing claims for authority by physicians and unorthodox practitioners and exposed the dynamics among patients, families, communities, and medical experts. She interrogated themes of respectability, expertise, objectivity, and insight into the workings of the human body in sickness and health. Physicians and scientists in the mid-twentieth century claimed public respect and a rarefied command of medical science. But Kenny's success in presenting herself as a clinical investigator able to debate clinicians and scientists demonstrated that such claims were not as stable or as widely established as members of elite research institutions and academic medical centers wanted the public to believe.

Part One of this book examines the strategies Kenny used to establish herself as a polio expert first in Minneapolis (the city that became her American base for the following decade) and then across the nation. It discusses the way in which the battle between Kenny and the experts became a gendered struggle, not only male doctors against a female nurse, but also a masculinized version of medical authority challenged by a female clinician claiming expertise in both patient care and medical theory. And it explores the way in which Kenny's work was enhanced by her emerging reputation as a celebrity and as an author.

Part Two examines the clinical, political, intellectual, and cultural challenges posed by Kenny's work and her concept of polio at the height of the polio wars. Kenny sought to redefine the healthy disabled body by making functionality more important than combating visible disability. She redefined the meaning of pain in polio treatment from an accepted adjunct of treatment to a symptom of something wrong. Her work countered a widespread therapeutic nihilism around polio care, and her methods demanded active patient involvement. This radical approach was adopted enthusiastically by many of her patients. These chapters explore how the voices of Kenny's patients and their families became increasingly central in shaping both clinical care and a new populist "Kenny movement," which defined itself against the medical establishment, exemplified by the AMA and the NFIP, and how Kenny's cause provided a national forum for the public to express long-standing frustration with unresponsive physicians and hospitals, autocratic public officials, the dismissal of strong women, the neglect of chronic disease, and the enforced orthodoxy of medical care. Hollywood embraced Kenny's story as the basis for an RKO movie that dramatized the story of a beautiful, unblemished heroine who heals the "crippled" and understands polio better than the doctors. True to Hollywood conventions Kenny's character must reject love for the altruistic goal of saving the world's children while fighting professional prejudice every step of the way.

This section also discusses how Kenny's claims complicated the debate over what constituted scientific proof in medicine, how her theory that the polio virus was not restricted to the central nervous system but directly affected muscles and "peripheral structures" filled a large hole in the physiology and pathology of muscle function, and

how new ideas in polio virology in the late 1940s undermining the old neurotropic concept of polio began to make her theory sound less fantastical.

Part Three examines the medical politics of polio in the early Cold War years, at a time
when the Kenny Foundation—now with its own donation containers—was a significant
competitor to the NFIP and set its sights on funding not only Kenny care and the training of Kenny technicians but also an alternative research establishment, epitomized by
the work of Columbia University virologist Claus Jungeblut. It discusses the new kind
of legitimacy Kenny garnered when in 1948 she was invited to Washington, D.C. as an
expert witness at hearings on the proposed National Science Foundation, and describes
the complicated medical politics of these hearings, as well as the way in which polio
became part of the global health politics of the early Cold War and how Kenny promoted
her work internationally. Finally, it describes how Kenny's name and work began to fade
from public and scientific consciousness in the mid-1950s with the discovery of a polio
vaccine and a new conservative domestic ideology that fashioned women as the wives of
(male) scientists or as nurses who aimed not for professional respect but for physician
husbands. And it notes the brief reappearance of her story in the 1980s with the emergence of Post-Polio Syndrome.

Kenny died at the age of 72, frustrated that her work had not achieved the scientific
acclaim she so desired. But the changes in clinical practice she initiated and sought to
direct were nonetheless profound.

NOTES

1. Truman Capote *Breakfast at Tiffany's: A Short Novel and Three Stories* (New York: Random
House, 1958), 103.

2. Bing Crosby as told to Pete Martin *Call Me Lucky* (New York: Simon & Schuster, 1953).
Ruth Prigozy and Walter Raubicheck eds. *Going My Way: Bing Crosby and America Culture*
(Rochester: University of Rochester Press, 2007) also fails to refer to Crosby's involvement
with Kenny or the Kenny Foundation.

3. Victor Cohn "Sister Kenny…Back in the Battle Again" *Minneapolis Sunday Tribune*
March 26 1950.

4. Erwin Ackerknecht *Therapeutics from the Primitives to the 20th Century* (New York: Hafner
Press, 1973); Charles E. Rosenberg "Erwin H. Ackerknecht, Social Medicine, and the History
of Medicine" *Bulletin of the History of Medicine* (Fall 2007) 81: 511–532.

5. On polio's early history see John R. Paul *A History of Poliomyelitis* (New Haven: Yale
University Press, 1971); Naomi Rogers *Dirt and Disease: Polio before FDR* (New Brunswick,
NJ: Rutgers University Press, 1992).

6. Jessie L. Stevenson "After-Care of Infantile Paralysis" *American Journal of Nursing* (1925)
25: 730–732.

7. Robert W. Lovett *The Treatment of Infantile Paralysis* (Philadelphia: P. Blakiston's Son &
Co., 1917); Arthur T. Legg and J. B. Merrill *Physical Therapy in Infantile Paralysis* (Hagerstown,
MD: W. F. Prior Co., 1932); Frank R. Ober "Physical Therapy in Infantile Paralysis" *JAMA*
(January 1 1938) 110: 45–46.

8. Fred H. Albee "The Orthopedic Treatment of Infantile Paralysis" *Bulletin of the New York
Academy of Medicine* (September 1926) 2: 463.

9. Richard Kovacs "The After-Care of Poliomyelitis: Electricity in the After-Care of Poliomyelitis" *American Journal of Nursing* (1932) 32: 2.

10. [Cohn interview with] Robert Bingham, May 19 1955, Victor Cohn Papers in Elizabeth Kenny Papers, Minnesota Historical Society, St Paul (hereafter MHS-K).

11. Donald A. Neumann "Polio: Its Impact on the People of the United States and the Emerging Profession of Physical Therapy" *Journal of Orthopaedic and Sports Physical Therapy* (2004) 34: 479–492; Lovett *The Treatment of Infantile Paralysis*; Henry O. Kendall and Florence P. Kendall *Muscles: Testing and Function* (Baltimore: Williams & Wilkins Co., 1949).

12. Robert W. Lovett "Orthopedic Problems in the After-Treatment of Infantile Paralysis" *Journal of Bone and Joint Surgery* (1917) 2: 690.

13. Charles L. Lowman "The After-Care of Poliomyelitis: Physiotherapy in the Water" *American Journal of Nursing* (1932) 32: 8–10; see also C. L. Lowman "Underwater Gymnastics" *JAMA* (October 10 1931) 97: 1074–1076; William H. Park "Epidemic Poliomyelitis or Infantile Paralysis" *Scientific Monthly* (September 1931) 33: 261–264.

14. On Roosevelt and Warm Springs see Hugh Gregory Gallagher *FDR's Splendid Deception* (New York: Dodd, Mead, 1985); Davis W. Houck and Amos Kiewe *FDR's Body Politics: The Rhetoric of Disability* (College Station: Texas A&M University Press, 2003); Theo Lippman, Jr. *The Squire of Warm Springs: F.D.R. in Georgia 1924–1945* (Chicago: Playboy Press, 1977); Turnley Walker *Roosevelt and the Warm Springs Story* (New York: A. A. Wyn, 1953); Amy L. Fairchild "The Polio Narratives: Dialogues with FDR" *Bulletin of the History of Medicine* (2001) 75: 488–534.

15. For a brief survey of changes in polio treatment between the 1910s and early 1940s see Richard Kovacs ed. *The 1942 Year Book of Physical Therapy* (Chicago: Year Book Publishers, 1942), 273–275; Daniel J. Wilson *Living with Polio: The Epidemic and Its Survivors* (Chicago: University of Chicago Press, 2005).

16. Henry O. Kendall "Some Interesting Observations About the After Care of Infantile Paralysis Patients" *Journal of Exceptional Children* (1937) 3: 107–112; G. E. Bennett, M. C. Cobey, and H. O. Kendall "Molded Plaster Shells for Rest and Protection Treatment of Infantile Paralysis" *JAMA* (October 2 1937) 109: 1120–1121.

17. Kendall "Some Interesting Observations About the After Care of Infantile Paralysis Patients," 107–112; Henry Otis Kendall and Florence P. Kendall *Care During the Recovery Period in Paralytic Poliomyelitis* (Washington, DC: Government Printing Office, 1938, rev. 1939, Public Health Service Bulletin No. 242); see also John G. Kuhns et al. "Sixty-Sixth Report of Progress in Orthopedic Surgery" *Archives of Surgery* (1938) 37: 336–337.

18. Frank H. Krusen *Physical Medicine: The Employment of Physical Agents for Diagnosis and Therapy* (Philadelphia and London: W. B. Saunders, 1941), 594–595.

19. Polio frequently appeared in textbooks under "Diseases of the Nervous System"; see Heinrich F. Wolf *Textbook of Physical Therapy* (New York: D. Appleton-Century, 1933); see also W. Russell Brain *Diseases of the Nervous System* (London: Oxford University Press [1933], 3rd ed. 1948), 454–464. For the argument that polio patients needed both immobilization and rest see Lovett *The Treatment of Infantile Paralysis*; Robert Jones and Robert Williamson Lovett *Orthopaedic Surgery* (New York: William Wood and Company, 1929); Krusen *Physical Medicine*, 592–593.

20. Ober "Physical Therapy in Infantile Paralysis," 45–46; "Infantile Paralysis" *American Journal of Nursing* (1931) 31: 1142; Legg and Merrill *Physical Therapy in Infantile Paralysis*.

21. Stevenson "After-Care of Infantile Paralysis," 729.

22. Evelyn C. Pearce *A Textbook of Orthopaedic Nursing* (New York: G.P. Putnam's Sons, 1930), 40–41.

23. Jessie L. Stevenson *The Nursing Care of Patients with Infantile Paralysis* (New York: National Foundation for Infantile Paralysis, 1940), 12–13, 25, 35; Stevenson "After-Care of Infantile Paralysis," 730–732.

24. Her major textbooks were Kenny *Infantile Paralysis and Cerebral Diplegia: Methods Used for the Restoration of Function* (Sydney: Angus and Robertson, 1937); Kenny *Treatment of Infantile Paralysis in the Acute Stage* (Minneapolis: Bruce Publishing Co., 1941); John F. Pohl and Kenny *The Kenny Concept of Infantile Paralysis and Its Treatment* (Minneapolis: Bruce Publishing Co., 1943); and Kenny *Physical Medicine: The Science of Dermo-Neuro-Muscular Therapy as Applied to Infantile Paralysis* (Minneapolis: Bruce Publishing Co., 1946).

25. Philip Moen Stimson "Minimizing the After Effects of Acute Poliomyelitis" *JAMA* (July 25 1942) 119: 990; see also Kenny *Treatment of Infantile Paralysis*.

26. See, for example, Michael S. Burman "Curare Therapy for the Release of Muscle Spasm and Rigidity in Spastic Paralysis and Dystonia Musculorum Deformans" *Journal of Bone and Joint Surgery* (1938) 20: 754–756.

27. Kenny *Treatment of Infantile Paralysis*, 25.

28. Kenny *Treatment of Infantile Paralysis*, 16–22, 38–39.

29. Pohl and Kenny *The Kenny Concept of Infantile Paralysis*, 48.

30. Pohl and Kenny, *The Kenny Concept of Infantile Paralysis*, 117–118; Kenny *Treatment of Infantile Paralysis*, 214. Hot packs were initially made in a complex system involving a small galvanized iron wash tub filled with boiling water mounted on a frame so it could be rolled from bed to bed, with a hand wringer on one side. Later hot pack machines were standardized, and the material for hot packs was Munsingwear, produced by a Minnesota company.

31. Kenny *Treatment of Infantile Paralysis*, 109.

32. Pohl and Kenny *The Kenny Concept of Infantile Paralysis*, 51–54, 133.

33. Kenny *Treatment of Infantile Paralysis*, 39–40; Pohl and Kenny *The Kenny Concept of Infantile Paralysis*, 51–54, 77, 136, 139.

34. Kenny *Treatment of Infantile Paralysis*, 109; Pohl and Kenny *The Kenny Concept of Infantile Paralysis*, 152.

35. Kenny *Treatment of Infantile Paralysis*, 157; photograph on 158.

36. Kenny *Treatment of Infantile Paralysis*, 40, 115.

37. Pohl and Kenny *The Kenny Concept of Infantile Paralysis*, 51, 55.

38. Kenny *Treatment of Infantile Paralysis*, 134–137; Pohl and Kenny *The Kenny Concept of Infantile Paralysis*, 56.

39. Pohl and Kenny *The Kenny Concept of Infantile Paralysis*, 147, 151, 185.

40. Kenny to Dear Dr. Pye, August 18 1939, Home Secretary's Office, Special Batches, Kenny Clinics, 1938–1940, A/31752, Queensland State Archives, Brisbane (hereafter QSA).

41. Pohl and Kenny *The Kenny Concept of Infantile Paralysis*, 303–313. She had used these techniques since the 1930s; see Kenny *Treatment of Infantile Paralysis*, 81.

42. Alice Lou Plastridge "Report of Observation of Work of Sister Elizabeth Kenny in Minneapolis, Minnesota, January 1941" [read to Georgia Chapter of American Physiotherapy Association on February 14 1941, at Warm Springs], Florence Kendall Collection, Silver Springs, Maryland, 3. For a similar description see Wallace H. Cole and Miland E. Knapp "The Kenny Treatment of Infantile Paralysis: A Preliminary Report" *JAMA* (June 7 1941) 116: 2579–2580.

43. Ober "Physical Therapy in Infantile Paralysis," 45–46; Wolf *Textbook of Physical Therapy*, 239–241; William Joseph Mane Alois Maloney *Locomotor Ataxia (Tabes Dorsalis): An Introduction to the Study and Treatment of Nervous Diseases, for Students and Practitioners* (New York: D. Appleton & Company, 1918), 147.

44. Carmelita Calderwood "Nursing Care in Poliomyelitis" *American Journal of Nursing* (1940) 40: 629; Krusen *Physical Medicine*, 592; Stevenson *The Nursing Care of Patients with Infantile Paralysis*, 22.

45. Kenny *Treatment of Infantile Paralysis*, 232.

46. Victor Cohn *Sister Kenny: The Woman Who Challenged the Doctors* (Minneapolis: University of Minnesota Press, 1975), 34–36.

47. Kenny quoted in Marvin L. Kline "The Most Unforgettable Character I've Ever Met" *Reader's Digest* (August 1959) 75: 205.

FURTHER READING

For discussions of medical practice see Rima Apple *Vitamania: Vitamins in American Culture* (New Brunswick, NJ: Rutgers University Press, 1996); Barbara Clow *Negotiating Disease: Power and Cancer Care, 1900–1950* (Montreal/Kingston: McGill-Queen's University Press, 2001); Christopher Crenner *Private Practice in the Early Twentieth Century Medical Office of Dr. Richard Cabot* (Baltimore: Johns Hopkins University Press, 2005); Christopher Lawrence ed. *Medical Theories, Surgical Practice: Studies in the History of Surgery* (New York: Routledge, 1992); John E. Lesch *The First Miracle Drugs: How the Sulfa Drugs Transformed Medicine* (New York: Oxford University Press, 2007); Martin Pernick *A Calculus of Suffering: Pain, Professionalism, and Anesthesia in Nineteenth-Century America* (New York: Columbia University Press, 1985); John Pickstone *Ways of Knowing: A New History of Science, Technology and Medicine* (Chicago: Chicago University Press, 2001); Anson Rabinbach *The Human Motor: Energy, Fatigue, and the Origins of Modernity* (New York: Basic Books, 1990); Morris J. Vogel and Charles E. Rosenberg eds. *The Therapeutic Revolution: Essays in the Social History of American Medicine* (Philadelphia: University of Pennsylvania Press, 1979); John Harley Warner *Against the Spirit of System: The French Impulse in Nineteenth-Century American Medicine* (Princeton: Princeton University Press, 1998); John Harley Warner *The Therapeutic Perspective: Medical Practice, Knowledge, and Identity in America, 1820–1885* (Cambridge, MA: Harvard University Press, 1986); Elizabeth Watkins *The Estrogen Elixir: A History of Hormone. Replacement Therapy in America* (Baltimore, MD: Johns Hopkins University Press, 2007).

Acknowledgments

IN DECEMBER 1992 I traveled to the Minnesota Historical Society to look at its Eliza-beth Kenny Collection for the first time. I also contacted Richard Owen, a rehabilitation specialist and polio survivor who had been treated by Kenny as a child, and Margaret Opdahl Ernst, Kenny's first American secretary, who invited me to attend the fiftieth reunion of the Kenny Institute. At the celebration I was asked to interview former Kenny patients, most of them in their sixties and seventies, as they sat in front of a camera and talked eagerly about their lives. Being treated at the Institute with Kenny in charge of their therapy was for them an intense experience, made even more significant by their growing disabilities as the result of Post-Polio Syndrome. Polio had defined their child-hood, had been conquered to a lesser or larger extent, and was now returning to redefine their senior years. Kenny herself—her height and bearing, her Australian accent and idio-syncrasies, and most of all her techniques—had left an indelible mark. For them clinical care was not a question of intellectual debates or professional boundaries but the fabric of their lives. These impressions have stayed with me through years of research and writing.

This book has been sidetracked many times. Since that first visit to Minnesota I got married, had 2 children, completed another book and various articles, got a position at Yale, and recovered from 2 serious illnesses. I also discovered that Kenny research can be endless. This project, I now recognize, is simply my assessment of polio care and Kenny's American years. There have been other books on Kenny and on polio; there will surely be more.

I want to acknowledge with gratitude the efforts of librarians and archivists at various locations: in Minneapolis/St. Paul, the Minnesota Historical Society and the University of Minnesota's Archives and Special Collections; in Philadelphia, the American

Philosophical Society; in White Plains, New York, the March of Dimes Archives; in New York City, the New York Academy of Medicine's main library and Rare Book Room, and Cornell University's Medical Center Archives at the New York-Presbyterian Hospital; in Rochester, New York, the archives at the University of Rochester; in Hyde Park, New York, the Franklin Delano Roosevelt Presidential Library and Museum's archives; in Albany, New York, the New York State Archives; in Baltimore, Maryland, the Alan Chesney Medical Archives of Johns Hopkins University and the Maryland Historical Society; in Chicago, the University of Chicago Special Collections Research Center; in Washington, D.C., the National Academy of Sciences; in Beverly Hills, California, the Margaret Herrick Library of the Academy of Motion Picture Arts and Sciences; in Winnipeg, Manitoba, the Province Archives of Manitoba; in Ottawa, Ontario, the Library and Archives Canada; in Quoiba, Tasmania, John Wilson's personal archives; in Brisbane, Queensland, the John Oxley State Library of Queensland; and in St. Lucia, Queensland, the Fryer Library and Special Collections at the University of Queensland. At Yale I am surrounded by a profusion of scholarly riches that I was able to sample with the help of librarians and archivists at Yale's Harvey Cushing/John Hay Whitney Medical Library and the Sterling Memorial Library. Ramona Moore and Ewa Lech at Yale's Section of the History of Medicine patiently provided logistical and practical aid and I am especially grateful for their support. Melissa Grafe and Florence Gillich graciously helped me through the tangle of image permissions and reproductions. I have also benefited from the organizational efforts of many research assistants including Ashley McGuire Ferrara, Catherine Gliwa, Natalie Holmes, Amber Levinson, Catherine Ly, Robyn Schaffer, Amanda Tjemsland, and Allison Walker. David Rose encouraged and guided me through the March of Dimes Archives, and Meg Hyre gave me thoughtful editorial assistance. My ability to travel to archives and to write has benefited from grants from the Australian Research Council, the Santa Fe Art Institute, the Minnesota Historical Society, and the National Library of Medicine.

I have met and corresponded with many people who remembered Kenny and the polio wars of the 1940s, including physicians, nurses, physical therapists, patients, and family members. Conversations with Mary Kenny McCracken and Stuart McCracken at their home in Caloundra, Queensland, allowed me to recapture some of the experiences of the 5 years that Mary spent as Kenny's companion in Minnesota. Florence Kendall spent 2 days talking with me and letting me read some of her personal papers; Mary Pohl recalled the alliance between Kenny and her father John Pohl; Margaret Ernst shared documents and memories with me as well as Kenny materials collected by Chris Sharpe; and Victor Cohn provided materials from his visits to Australia in the 1950s that are now at the Minnesota Historical Society. Sadly a number of my informants are no longer alive, including 2 other people unable to celebrate the publication of this book: Barbara Seaman, a friend and mentor, and Gina Feldberg, who was my loving confidant.

Colleagues and friends have been encouraging and patient. Janet Golden and Susan Smith read an early draft and offered wise comments. My fellow historians at Yale have offered me advice and critique as have the graduate student members of the Frederick L. Holmes Workshop. My wonderful wide community of medical historians gave me intellectual and physical sustenance. I especially thank Emily Abel, Rima Apple, Charlotte Borst, Ted Brown, David Cantor, Pat D'Antonio, Nadav Davidovitch, Brian Dolan, Jackie Duffin, Julie Fairman, Jennifer Gunn, James Hanley, Bert Hansen, Kerry Highley, Robert Johnston, Esyllt Jones, Suzanne Junod, Wendy Kline, Judy Leavitt, Sue Lederer, Janet

MacCalman, Ellen More, Dorothy Porter, Leslie Reagan, Susan Reverby, Corrine Sutter, John Thearle, Janet Tighe, Nancy Tomes, and Daniel Wilson. Debbie Doroshow read and edited parts of the book with verve and ruthlessness; Kennie Lyman provided extraordinary help in cutting, shaping, and tightening; and Cindy Connelly and Liz Watkins have been crucial sources of insight, guidance, and encouragement. In Melbourne my mother June Factor has been a caring critic; Joanne Aslanis Maguire, Juliette Borenstein, and Greg Chambers reminded me about the joys and trials of ordinary life. In New Haven Nancy Johnson provided glasses of wine and calming conversation; Darcy Chase gave me the gift of time by helping to care and cook for my family.

This project has long been part of my children's lives and when they were toddlers my husband taught them to say "Not Sister Kenny." Nat and Dory have not made working easier but they always made it worthwhile. As a fellow historian John Harley Warner has shared my delight in archival finds and my struggles in writing and editing. He provided sustenance and comfort and knew when to back off. I dedicate this book to him and to my children.

List of Archives

California:
— Sister Kenny Collection, Margaret Herrick Library Special Collections, Academy of Motion Picture Arts and Sciences, Beverly Hills.

Connecticut:
— John Enders Papers, Yale University Library Manuscripts and Archives, New Haven.
— John Rodman Paul Papers, Yale University Library Manuscripts and Archives, New Haven.

Illinois:
— Morris Fishbein Collection, Joseph Regenstein Library, University of Chicago Special Collections Research Center, Chicago.

Maryland:
— George E. Bennett Papers, Alan Mason Chesney Medical Archives, Johns Hopkins University, Baltimore.
— David Bodian Papers, Alan Chesney Medical Archives, Johns Hopkins University, Baltimore.
— Florence Kendall [private] Collection, Silver Springs, Maryland.
— George L. Radcliffe Papers, Maryland Historical Society, Baltimore.

Massachusetts:
— W. Lloyd Aycock Papers, Francis A. Countway Library of Medicine, Harvard Medical Library, Boston.

Minnesota:
— James Henry Papers, Minnesota Historical Society, St Paul.
— Hubert H. Humphrey Papers, Minnesota Historical Society, St Paul.

— Walter H. Judd Papers, Minnesota Historical Society, St Paul.

— Elizabeth Kenny Papers, Minnesota Historical Society, St Paul.

— Jay Arthur Myers Papers, University of Minnesota Archives and Special Collections, Minneapolis.

— Minnesota Poliomyelitis Research Committee, University of Minnesota Archives and Special Collections, Minneapolis.

— Presidents Papers, University of Minnesota Archives and Special Collections, Minneapolis.

— University Relations: Medical School 1950–1952, University of Minnesota Archives and Special Collections, Minneapolis.

— Maurice Visscher Papers, University of Minnesota Archives and Special Collections, Minneapolis.

New York:

— Rare Book and Manuscript Collection, New York Academy of Medicine, New York City.

— Philip Stimson Papers, Medical Center Archives, New York-Presbyterian/Weill Cornell, New York.

— Public Relations Records, March of Dimes Archives, White Plains.

— Government Relations (Foreign) Argentina, March of Dimes Archives, White Plains.

— Alan Valentine Papers, Rush Rhees Library, University of Rochester, Rochester.

— Archives at the University of Rochester, Rochester.

— President's Papers, Office Files 5188, Franklin Delano Roosevelt Presidential Library and Museum Archives, Hyde Park.

— President's Papers, Presidential Personal Files 4885 (1939–1945), Franklin Delano Roosevelt Presidential Library and Museum Archives, Hyde Park.

— Record Group III-2K, OMR, Series: Medical Interest, Rockefeller Archive Center, Tarrytown.

— Basil O'Connor Papers, Manuscripts and Special Collections, New York State Archives, Albany.

Pennsylvania:

— Thomas Rivers Papers, American Philosophical Society, Philadelphia.

Washington D.C.:

— Claus Washington Jungblut Papers, National Library of Medicine.

— National Research Council, General, Medical Sciences, 1944, National Academy of Sciences.

— Record Group 102, Children's Bureau Central File, 1941–1944, 4-5-16-1, Infantile Paralysis, National Archives.

Australia: Queensland:

— Charles Chuter Papers, John Oxley Library, State Library of Queensland, Brisbane.

— Home Secretary's Office, Special Batches, Kenny Clinics 1941–1949, A/31753, Queensland State Archives, Brisbane.

— Elizabeth Kenny Collection, Fryer Library and Special Collections, University of Queensland, St Lucia.

Australia: Tasmania:

— John R. Wilson [private] Collection, Quoiba, Tasmania.

Australia: ACT:

— Series A-1928, 802/17/Section, 3, Australian Archives, ACT Regional Office.

— Secretary, Prime Minister's Department [A.S. Brown], #707/9/A, Series A462, Australian Archives, ACT Regional Office.

Canada: Ottawa:

— "Conference On Poliomyelitis, December 3,4, & 5 1945, Minneapolis, Minnesota," Record Group 29, vol. 201, file 311-P11-15, National Archive Centre, the Library and Archives Canada.

Canada: Manitoba:

— Children's Hospital of Winnipeg MG 10B33, Box 7, Province Archives of Manitoba, Winnipeg.

PART ONE

1

A Bush Nurse in America

⌒

ELIZABETH KENNY INTENDED to visit 2 places in America: New York City, the headquarters of the National Foundation for Infantile Paralysis (NFIP), and Rochester, Minnesota, the site of the world famous Mayo Clinic. In April 1940, after traveling almost a month by boat from Australia and by train across the United States, 59-year-old Kenny and her 23-year-old ward Mary Stewart Kenny arrived in New York. The daughter of Irish-Australians from rural Australia and trained as a bush nurse, Kenny had come to the United States with a bold plan. She was determined to gain a hearing from American experts in order to explain her methods of treating patients with polio, and then, she hoped, physicians everywhere would adopt them.

Armed with a letter of introduction from William Forgan Smith, the Labor Party premier of her home state of Queensland, to Basil O'Connor, the NFIP's director, Kenny was eager "to meet this gentleman and outline my ideas."[1] When she called, however, O'Connor's secretary explained that the NFIP director was in Warm Springs with the President but that he had received word of her coming from Forgan Smith and was looking forward to her visit.[2] Reminded in this way of O'Connor's connections (President Franklin Roosevelt was his former law partner) and his dominant position in the field of polio care (Warm Springs was the nation's foremost polio rehabilitation center), Kenny and Mary faced the delay (an international symbol of the powerful) and waited for his return.

While in New York, Kenny contacted Kristian Hansson, the physician in charge of physical therapy at the Hospital for the Ruptured and Crippled, a charity orthopedic hospital. A few months earlier Hansson, a graduate of Cornell's medical school with training in Swedish physical therapy, had published an article on the treatment of polio in the *Journal of the American Medical Association* (*JAMA*), which Kenny had read closely before her trip across the Pacific.[3] Hansson invited her to his department where she met "several very alert and capable-looking men." Such physicians were, Kenny was pleased to discover, different from those she had encountered in London a few years before whose eyes had held "the superciliousness...of the home-born Britisher toward the 'colonial.'" At this first meeting at a New York City hospital she left feeling hopeful about a new, more welcoming medical outlook.[4] Kenny hoped to escape attitudes that demeaned her as a woman, a nurse, and an Australian. She also hoped that her Irish background and rural upbringing, which had placed her in a subordinate category in Australian society, would not matter in the United States. And, here, her hopes were probably realized. As Australian diplomat Richard Casey noted in 1940, "the American people know very little about Australia" and "except on the Pacific coast they think very little about Australia."[5]

In appearance and manner Kenny was not easily dismissed. She was "large in every dimension," recalled Marvin Kline, who had first met her when he was a member of the city council of Minneapolis. Her hat had "an incredibly wide brim and a plume of flowers blooming from a broad bend around the crown," which though "quite out of style...only added to her dignity."[6] Tall, dressed formally although oddly to American eyes, this nurse was clearly a respectable older woman aware of proper genteel conduct. And having come of age during the last decades of the Victorian era, Kenny understood respectability in starkly gendered terms: in public ladies were prim and restrained, expecting courtesy and respect from gentlemen. But she also had a tough and pragmatic side. Proud of her physical strength, she later mocked the mores of her childhood days when girls were told "it was vulgar to be healthy, ladylike to be delicate."[7] And she demanded more than respect for a foreign lady visitor; she wanted professional support for her work.

KENNY IN AUSTRALIA

In Kenny's youth, a few middle-class British women, inspired by the example of Florence Nightingale, trained in elite hospital nursing schools such as St Thomas's and left England to set up Nightingale-like nursing schools in Sydney and Melbourne. Australian working-class women who sought professional autonomy kept far from such hierarchical urban hospitals, working instead as bush nurses. Most, including Kenny, were trained through informal apprenticeship. Australian bush nursing, like rural nursing in North America, was physically demanding work, requiring confidence, ingenuity, and technical skills. Bush nurses were usually the sole health providers for families living many miles apart, and they tended to work with rather than for physicians.

Born in 1880, the fifth child of 9, Elizabeth Kenny spent most of her early life among agricultural and grazing communities in northeastern Australia. Her father Michael Kenny, an Irish immigrant, worked as a transient farmhand, and the family moved many times in rural New South Wales and then in southern Queensland. The children had a few years of formal schooling but relied on their mother Mary Moore to teach them at home. Living in small towns and with few resources Kenny's sisters all chose to marry local farmers; but Kenny was dissatisfied with domesticity. She worked briefly as a music teacher and a broker selling farmers' produce, but was especially interested in caring for the sick. As a young girl after breaking her wrist she stayed with surgeon Anneas McDonnell and his family in Toowoomba and studied anatomy and physiology informally with him. She then used her knowledge to help her frail younger brother improve his physique by teaching him to "isolate the principal muscles of his body by voluntary contraction."[8]

In 1911 with money from her successful produce selling venture, Kenny set up a small clinic in Nobby, about a hundred miles west of Brisbane, and became a bush nurse. She reveled in this professional independence, gaining skill and respect as she worked in the sparsely populated Darling Downs in southern Queensland delivering babies, setting bones, and healing wounds. It was in the bush that Kenny first developed her methods of treating polio. She had never seen the disease before. She found that applying heated wool cloths and gently, carefully exercising muscles relieved her patients' pain and muscle tightness. Continuing these exercises after the pain and sensitivity were gone helped patients to strengthen weakened muscles and, Kenny came to believe, to reconnect pathways between the nerves and the muscles and thus ameliorate their paralysis.[9] She began to specialize in the care of the physically disabled, especially patients whose doctors had said they would never improve, and soon her clinic was primarily for their care.

In the early twentieth century polio outbreaks were a new phenomenon. Away from the city, rural patients frequently depended on idiosyncratic methods practiced by a doctor, nurse, or family member. In urban institutions there was an effort to standardize polio care. Patients with paralysis were first isolated in separate wards until their fever subsided and they were deemed noncontagious. As polio's early symptoms were frequently confused with other diseases such as tubercular meningitis some physicians recommended a spinal tap. Even after the polio virus was identified in 1909 it was not visible in an ordinary microscope, so analyzing spinal fluid was more often a search to rule out other possible infections. Polio paralysis was believed to be caused by nerve cells damaged by an inflammation of the central nervous system, so doctors recommended strict bed rest and immobilization. Especially for children who were restless casts were used to restrain movement. Patients were immobilized sometimes for many months in what was seen as "physiological rest." Children's limbs became flabby (flaccid) and wasted, and, with casts that restricted growth, both bones and muscles tended to atrophy. Patents were offered massage, baths, exercises, and sometimes electrical treatment to try to regain muscle strength but usually in gloomy institutions with limited nursing staff and a sense of prognostic pessimism. After 18 months of treatment patients were considered unlikely to improve and were fitted for braces and/or crutches, and told to anticipate tendon transfers and other orthopedic interventions involving hospitalization after a year or so.

Until the late 1930s Kenny saw mainly patients who had had this kind of polio care, sometimes years earlier. She took the casts, stomach corsets, and other apparatus off her patients and encouraged them to move their long-neglected stiff muscles. She used a variety of rehabilitative methods, including hot- and cold-water sprays, muscle exercises, and an unusual technique she called "manual vibration" in which her arm vibrated as she tried to stimulate a patient's unused muscles and thereby, she believed, reconnect the muscle to its corresponding neuron. Unlike most physical therapy recipients, her patients played an active role in their rehabilitation, learning to understand the function of individual muscles. Kenny began to wonder whether her methods might be even more effective applied to patients in polio's acute early stages. She also came to believe that the standard polio therapies were not only unhelpful but actually harmful.

Kenny gained nursing experience outside the Queensland bush with the outbreak of the Great War. Although she was initially ineligible for the Nursing Service as she had not attended nursing school and had no nursing certificate, she was able to join the Australian Army's Medical Corps based on her clinical experience and a letter of reference from a respected senior professional (probably Anneas McDonnell). Despite lacking the formal education usually required for such an honor, she received her title "Sister" (the British and Australian term for senior nurse and the Army equivalent of First Lieutenant) when she worked as an army nurse on troop ships bringing wounded Australian soldiers home from the battles of Europe.[10] Nursing soldiers while traveling under the threat of enemy submarines was rough and dangerous work, but it reinforced Kenny's love of adventure and willingness to take risks. She had closed her clinic before joining the army, but after the war she continued to work as a nurse, taking on individual disabled private patients and caring from them in their homes. In the 1920s, after her widowed mother Mary Moore Kenny moved to a small house in Nobby, Kenny, concerned about her mother's declining health, adopted Lucy Lily Stewart, a 9-year-old girl from Brisbane, and renamed her Mary Kenny.[11] In 1926 Kenny designed a new kind of stretcher she called the Sylvia stretcher for carrying patients across rough terrain. Royalties from the stretcher along with her war pension gave her some financial stability.[12]

A NEW AUSTRALIAN NIGHTINGALE?

Kenny's challenge to standard polio care would probably have remained the work of a little-known rural nurse if polio had not become a growing problem in North America and Western Europe, a disease whose "very name strikes terror to the heart of parents," as one American physician dramatically phrased it in 1930.[13] Hope flared briefly during the late 1930s with the testing of a polio vaccine and a preventive nasal spray, both supported by the President's Birthday Ball Commission (the antecedent of the NFIP), but one led to 11 deaths and the other caused children to temporarily lose their sense of smell and did not prevent paralysis.[14] Kenny's methods captured public and professional attention just as Australian medical journals were filled with disappointing news about these latest American polio therapies.[15] By the 1930s Kenny had become a national figure, featured in newspapers and popular magazines as "a new Florence Nightingale" whose discovery of new methods of treating polio made her "as well known as Brisbane's Town Hall."[16] Formal and imposing in photographs she wore her grey hair in a bob with a string of pearls around her neck.[17]

The 1920s and 1930s were also a period when Queensland's government became a force for medical progress in opposition to the professional establishment. Queensland's Labor Party began to establish a nascent health and welfare system. After abolishing the state's upper house in 1922, Labor politicians began to address many of the state's health and welfare problems, expanding the state funding of hospitals and adding an additional subsidy based on profits from Queensland's Golden Casket, a government-run lottery whose revenues helped finance the state's public hospitals.[18] With the new oversight of regional hospital boards the power structure of most state-funded hospitals shifted away from specialist consultants who tended to give priority to their private practices and preferred hospital directors to be young, inexperienced, and easily controlled physicians.

Now Queensland hospital directors were trained medical administrators who sought efficient and progressive hospital policies and were empowered to employ full-time, salaried medical staff.[19]

Prominent among Kenny's political friends was Charles Chuter, a powerful civil servant. In the 1930s despite fierce attacks from the Queensland medical elite Chuter was appointed undersecretary of the new Department of Health and Home Affairs. Like Edward (Ned) Hanlon who headed this department, Chuter was sympathetic to Kenny's complaints that doctors did not know what they were talking about when they defended standard polio care.[20]

In 1933 Chuter arranged for Kenny to give a special demonstration of her work at the Brisbane General Hospital.[21] It was a turning point for Kenny, a moment she returned to many times—and it was a disaster. Brisbane orthopedist Harold Crawford and most of the other physicians present dismissed her as an "ignorant, uncouth bush nurse," especially when she tried to explain how to "stimulate a dormant muscle by manual vibration" or claimed that she had cured patients who had polio and cerebral palsy. There was silence when Kenny said boldly that she did not believe in casts, splints, or immobilization; and when she pointed to a groove in the back of the neck of a 9-year-old boy as a sign of impending paralysis the audience responded with "disgusted looks and then jeering laughter."[22] As Crawford, who was head of the Queensland branch of the Australian medical association as well as president of the state's physical therapy society, pointed out, Kenny was not a trained masseur (physical therapist) and therefore was not "registered" to carry out this kind of therapy. In his view she did not seem to understand the intricacies of muscle exercises and even those of her therapies that were based on familiar methods were used "in a wrong or even harmful manner." Indeed he feared some of the "severe and forcible" movements she advocated might fracture a limb or even "increase paralysis."[23] Under Crawford's guidance the Queensland branch of the Australian Massage Association later sought to bar her trained nurses from hospital positions on the grounds that muscle education should be the province of a formally trained physical therapist, not someone trained for a few months by an idiosyncratic bush nurse.[24]

Nonetheless Chuter was able to persuade Ned Hanlon to have the state government pay for a clinic to be managed by Kenny.[25] The clinic, in which Kenny had already been working, was based in a hotel's refurbished ground floor in Townsville, a port centered around northern Queensland's agricultural and mining industries, about 800 miles north of Brisbane. The government clinic opened in 1934 as a trial to see if Kenny's work was sound and could be taught to other nurses. Kenny made sure the walls were painted in a soothing blue, and that both the surroundings and her nurse-trainees were "gentle and encouraging" to ensure there were no "suggestions of future helplessness."[26] The clinic was supervised by local physicians including James Guinane, a surgeon who was the son of the hotel's owner. Although Kenny was supposed to restrict her care to 17 patients who were to be assessed by medical supervisors she refused to turn away other disabled patients who began to arrive in "all sorts of vehicles from swanky motor cars to broken-down spring carts."[27] Like other medical observers Guinane noticed that Kenny was a quick study, learning from comments by visiting physicians. Yet, also like other physicians, he found her at times "quite fanatical."[28] Still he began to prepare a textbook with her, published in 1937 as *Infantile Paralysis and Cerebral Diplegia*, its title reflecting her interest in treating patients with cerebral palsy as well as polio. The text argued that

specially trained attendants could help to restore "functional power to apparently paralysed muscles" and counter the "deleterious effect of immobilization" with every exercise
"guided by the attendant, and mentally controlled by the patient."[29]

Kenny's teaching skills were less easy to assess. Her relations with the Brisbane nurses
sent to work with her in the Townsville clinic were at times stormy and difficult. She
found it hard to teach the manual vibration technique and no longer emphasized it. The
nurses disliked her use of nonstandard terminology and her tendency to alter methods depending on the improvement of the patient.[30] Dissatisfied with what she saw as
the nurses' resistance to her methods and limited understanding of physiology Kenny
warned them that "their nursing training with its tendency to stereotype information
acted as a bar to their adaptability" and that it would probably take at least a year to alter
their unfortunate "fixation" of orthodox ideas about polio.[31]

The Queensland government chose Raphael Cilento, the state's director-general of
health, as the official assessor of Kenny's Townsville clinic. A medical graduate from the
University of Adelaide and with public health experience in Queensland's tropical north,
Cilento shared the Labor Party's belief in a centralized health policy to expand the public's
access to hospitals and clinics.[32] In a series of reports to the state minister of health he
came to decry both her techniques and her understanding of disability care. He became
convinced that her results were "merely suggestion" and due largely to the impression of
"her dominant personality upon each case." Nor did he believe Kenny was a good teacher
as her methods could not "be taught with ease to anyone." After Kenny had left for a few
months, he noted, one patient experienced "partial retrogression," which only strengthened his case that positive results were due entirely to her personality.[33] In 1935 he began
to attack her claims of originality, suggesting publicly that the work of Boston physical
therapist Wilhemine Wright was "very similar" to hers. Later he claimed that he had lent
Kenny Wright's muscle training pamphlet, which she then returned to him with passages
marked in pencil and turned into her method.[34]

Outraged by Cilento's suggestion that she had secretly copied another's work Kenny
told local reporters that that "even if Dr. [sic] Wright's ideas were the same as hers, the
question was whether he [sic] or others would have satisfactory methods of putting
them into effect."[35] While she had initially admitted that her methods were not new,
Cilento's remarks led her to defend her work more fiercely, including its originality.[36] The
Townsville clinic, she declared provocatively, aware that this public debate would reach
the ears of her government sponsors, was being funded "not to test her method, but to
train students in that method."[37]

Although she was still careful to have physicians supervise her patients, Kenny began
to claim clinical authority distinct from that of an ordinary nurse or physical therapist.
She saw herself as a supervisor of nurses, teaching a new method of treatment that could
"reawaken" nerve impulses that were "dormant" even when "the best standard method
had failed."[38] As she explained to reporters, she sought medical advice about the scientific
basis of her work and the appropriate moments for its application, not about its efficacy.
"I do not want medical men to discuss whether or not my work is valuable, because I know
what it will do" she said defiantly. "I want them to tell me how best this new knowledge
of rapidly restoring paralysed people to health and strength can be applied where it is
needed."[39] Kenny also began to believe there was a medical conspiracy against her, telling
the *Women's Weekly* magazine that the "treatise" that she and Guinane had written was

"the only copy in the world" and therefore "great care had to be taken to safeguard it falling into unscrupulous hands."[40] Later she claimed that "a doctor had burnt a chart which had shown improvement in a patient at her clinic."[41] She also became more careful of her own moral reputation. She told an old friend that she was going to discharge one of her nurses who was keeping company with "a very reputable chap" because Kenny had heard that the friendship was a little too intimate and her enemies would try to ruin her with any rumors of indiscreet conduct.[42]

Parents and family members publicized her dramatic results, praising their efficacy and her moral character. In the *North Queensland Register* one father described his son whom "medical men [had] pronounced a permanent cripple." Kenny had taken photographs of the boy's withered limb and had the leg measured by a physician supervising her work. When Cilento examined the child after 4 months of Kenny treatment, he admitted to the father that the boy's progress was remarkable.[43] This public support gave her work political momentum. With the approval of the state government Kenny opened an outpatient clinic on George Street, Brisbane, in June 1935.[44] A few months later, perhaps pressured by medical critics, the government set up a Royal Commission to study her work. Initially Kenny said she was delighted by this action. The commission's members were all well-known physicians, including Anneas McDonnell, Kenny's mentor from Toowoomba, and it was chaired by orthopedist Charles Thelander, a cousin of hers.[45]

The Queensland Commission's 1938 report took up 37 pages in the *Medical Journal of Australia* and was summarized in the *British Medical Journal* and *JAMA*.[46] Like most Australian physicians the commission members did not approve of Kenny's methods or her ideas. They drew on a critical review of Kenny and Guinane's 1937 textbook by Sydney surgeon Lennox Teece who warned about the dangers of overstretching and deformity if immobilization were rejected and doubted that any paralyzed muscles had been "reactivated" by her methods.[47] The Queensland commission declared that immobilization was *"essential"* in polio care and any abandonment was a *"grievous error* and fraught with great danger."[48] Like Teece the commission also dismissed Kenny's work with children with cerebral palsy. Given special facilities and time, the commission argued, most "spastic" children did "improve with age apart from any treatment whatever."[49] Admirers of her work, the commission explained, had been blinded by Kenny's "strong personality" and "her own conviction of technical competence" rather than the actual efficacy of her methods.[50] "Doctors' Sharp 'No:' Find Kenny System A Failure" announced the *Sydney Sun*. The article concluded that a properly trained physical therapist could have obtained similar results given the same opportunity for concentrated attention.[51] More harshly the *Australasian* pointed out that many "cripples" had "wasted their time and public money on a repetition of treatment—modified in some cases for the worse."[52]

By the time the Queensland commission was finishing its report, however, Kenny had already left Australia. In 1937 she traveled to London where she convinced health officials to allow her to introduce her methods in the Queen Mary's Hospital in Carshalton, Surrey, a children's convalescent hospital run by the London County Council. She was in charge of 3 wards, caring for around 20 patients with polio and 8 with cerebral palsy, and her work was supervised by a group of orthopedic specialists. Later she commented on the specialists' disdain, but in this period she felt hopeful that the surgeons, perhaps inspired by the hospital's enthusiastic nurses and physical therapists, were taking her work seriously.[53] In late 1937 she returned from England to care for her ailing mother and was engulfed by more polio outbreaks. She trained nurses and worked at a children's rehabilitation hospital in Hampton, a Melbourne suburb.[54] Increasingly confident, Kenny responded to reporters' queries mischievously, reminding them about the patients being treated at Queen Mary's in England where "her ideas" were having "scientific and public investigation." She denied that she had ever promised a "100 percent cure" or that her patients were improved as a result of her "personality," retorting "I thought that with intelligent men, the age of witchcraft and 'hooey' had gone. Loyalty to me is inspired by [the] improved condition of my patients."[55] In a technique she would later use many times she showed before-and-after photographs of her patients to counter the commission's claims that some had shown "no appreciable recovery."[56] A few of Kenny's adult patients wrote to local newspapers praising her "invaluable work" and the Queensland government that had given them access to it.[57] In the *Brisbane Courier-Mail* one former patient made much of Kenny's ethical veracity: "if she knows she cannot help the patient she immediately says so." This former patient also questioned the commission's qualifications, suggesting "instead of a commission of medical men, why not a commission of patients or their parents?"[58] But in a statement repeated by critics for the rest of Kenny's life, Sydney orthopedist Max Hertz proclaimed that "the treatment has features that are new and features that are good, but where they are good they are not new and where they are new they are not good."[59]

Kenny had made much of the fact that her work at Queen Mary's Hospital was being investigated scientifically. She was thus very disappointed when a few months later the London specialists published an unenthusiastic report in the *British Medical Journal*. They admitted that none of her patients treated without splinting had developed "contractures" but nonetheless did not approve of Kenny's refusal to use splints or her claim that splinting would cause muscular impulses to "wither... [and] die beyond the hope of resuscitation." Despite her promises she had not achieved any "permanent cure[s]" and her use of early muscle exercises though "harmless" was "of unproved value."[60] It was a sign that Kenny's work had reached a national medical audience that the *Medical Journal of Australia* then published a letter from Kenny protesting this report by noting that physicians at the Hampton hospital had recently "drawn attention to the evils of improper splinting," praised her identification of the condition of muscle spasm as "a definite contribution to the treatment of poliomyelitis," and urged "further research... both clinically and academically, into this disease."[61] Her attention to the clinical sign of muscle spasm was new. She had not mentioned it in her 1937 text, but later claimed that she had discussed it in London and the specialists had told her it was new to them.[62]

Prominent physicians continued to dislike Kenny and her attacks on standard polio care, and sought to defend themselves against her accusations that they neglected their patients. Thus, the *Medical Journal of Australia* paired Kenny's response with an article by Melbourne polio expert Jean Macnamara. Without denying her own advocacy of splinting, Macnamara nonetheless protested strongly against any suggestion that she did not use physical therapies or kept patients confined for a long period of time.[63] Most experts agreed with Macnamara but a few remained intrigued by the idea that immobilization might be harmful. The journal's next issue contained a letter that praised Kenny for helping "to break down the pernicious form of treatment" of "overlong reliance" on rest and splints.[64]

Perhaps as a result of such confusion among experts or the power of public support Kenny's influence expanded. With the support of Billy Hughes, the federal minister of health, and a wealthy philanthropist, she had set up a clinic attached to the Royal North Shore Hospital in Sydney that was in Hughes' constituency.[65] Now the New South Wales minister for health, citing evidence that North Shore patients had shown "improvement," opened the state's second Kenny clinic at Newcastle Hospital.[66] Most importantly, the Queensland government offered Kenny control of Ward 7 at the Brisbane General Hospital. It was highly unusual to have a nonphysician in charge of inpatients at a large city hospital. As one Brisbane physician later recalled, she "wasn't under anybody" and she reported directly to the minister of health.[67]

Kenny's success in Brisbane was partly the result of alliances with influential administrators. Abraham Fryberg, for example, who had directed Kenny's George Street clinic in 1936, continued to support her after he joined the Queensland health department.[68] An even more powerful ally was Aubrey Pye, a prominent surgeon who directed the entire Brisbane Hospital complex. During the late 1930s Pye became the gatekeeper for every clinical demonstration she sought to make.[69] Pediatric surgeon Felix Arden, the director of the Children's Hospital in the Brisbane Hospital complex, whose own father was in a wheelchair, was sympathetic to the difficulties faced by physically disabled people. Arden asked parents whose children were sent to the Children's Hospital if they wanted Kenny or orthodox methods of treatment. If they expressed no preference he alternated the patients fifty/fifty.[70] Elsewhere Kenny's clinics received far less administrative support. At the North Shore hospital her outpatient clinic, housed in the basement of one of hospital buildings, was visited by neither the hospital's medical director nor the hospital residents. Other clinics suffered similar neglect. But this disregard afforded Kenny and her staff complete clinical control.[71]

In a series of lectures and clinical demonstrations at the Brisbane hospital a more confident Kenny began to articulate bolder claims. Not only did splints worsen muscle spasm, she argued, but the use of iron lungs could harm patients, even those with serious respiratory paralysis. She shocked hospital physicians by taking one child out of an iron lung and treating him with hot packs. The child did not die and learned to breathe on his own.[72] Her efforts to explain how her methods worked were less successful. She argued that the conditions created by immobilization—lessened circulation, poor nutrition of the skin, increased joint stiffness—led to diminished nerve impulses. Immobilization also interfered with "the normal function of the subconscious mind" and gave patients "an adverse psychological outlook." The principles of the "orthodox system" were, she said, the opposite of the principles of her system of treatment. If muscle spasm was unrecognized and untreated the consequences were dire. She spoke awkwardly of maintaining "maximum vitality and volitional control" through an "efficient" circulatory system that allowed a patient to maintain an uninterrupted stream of "neural impulses." To explain why some patients found it difficult to move muscles that were no longer in pain or spasm she began to use the term "alienated" or speak of "a state of diminished awareness of the affected parts." Convinced that he no longer had any control over paralyzed muscles, the patient lay in bed "frightened to move or [to] permit anyone to move him."[73] Other than neuroanatomist Herbert Wilkinson whose foreword in her 1937 textbook had speculated on the functioning of motor neurons and muscle fibers, Kenny found that none of her Australian allies could explain why her methods worked.[74] She was sure that somewhere experts would know how to explain them.

Kenny was convinced that polio care must be practiced her way. Changing the way polio care was practiced, she recognized, involved a vast array of cultural and social resources, not just a few clinics and a handful of medical allies. It also required changing how clinicians understood the pathophysiology of polio. Despite her use of unorthodox methods, Kenny's broader view of clinical change was based on a strong faith in scientific explanations to gird her clinical work and lead physicians to adopt it. Investigations by "men of science," she hoped, would lead physicians to take seriously "the signs and symptoms…previously left unnoticed and unattended."[75] Aware that some nurses she had trained were returning to institutions full of antagonistic colleagues, she urged hospital officials to recognize them as specialists in the "Kenny system of treatment," perhaps with a special certificate to help them gain appropriate status in their hospitals.[76]

In September 1939 Britain and Australia declared war on Germany and government officials paid more attention to readying troops than to domestic disease. Laudatory statements by physicians, Kenny discovered, were now "buried by war news."[77] After reading an admission in *JAMA* by a polio specialist that polio had no effective therapy, Kenny was sure that the United States, a country not immersed in the European conflict, needed her help.[78] This idea was strengthened when Alan Lee, a sympathetic Brisbane surgeon, returned from a trip there and told her about the founding of the NFIP. Lee, who had spoken to Mayo Clinic orthopedist Melvin Henderson about his work with the foundation, urged Kenny to visit the Mayo Clinic.[79] Pye, Fryberg, Wilkinson, and her other Brisbane allies helped organize her trip to America including Hanlon's approval of £300 to cover the round-trip fare and a letter of introduction to the head of the NFIP from the Premier of Queensland.[80] Without a clear idea about how American medicine worked, Kenny left for the United States, believing that American physicians would be more open than their Australian and British counterparts.

A MEDICAL FRONTIER

Kenny knew she needed to find an arresting way to sell her ideas without sounding like a quack. Attacks on patent medicine promoters and unorthodox practitioners were part of a widely publicized policy of the American Medical Association (AMA). Inspired by the German model of medical education and reinforced by education reformer Abraham Flexner's 1910 *Report*, America's physicians claimed to be social experts free of creed or partisanship. In theory, doctors in white coats were aloof from the commercialized world, although a number continued to appear in advertisements for cigarettes, patent medicines, detergents, and other products. The Great Depression had buffeted the stability of this medical culture. Many physicians who had seen themselves as independent businessmen were forced to consider other forms of work, including group practice, contract practice for a school system or a factory, or government health positions. Private practitioners retreated into their local medical societies and civic clubs, resentful of the privileges claimed by elite specialists at medical schools and teaching hospitals. Seeking a politics that would bind these groups across class and regional lines, the AMA held tightly to certain ethical guidelines defining professional legitimacy. One principle was the restriction on selling: no respectable physician should directly advertise his services to the public or claim any special abilities or techniques that would "cure" disease. How then could an unknown nurse promote a method that contradicted mainstream practice to a professional community in which selling had such base, shoddy implications?

Kenny intended to demonstrate her professional respectability through her dignified appearance, her unusual accent, and written testimonials from Australian doctors and politicians. Her letters of introduction stated that she had made a distinctive "contribution" to polio care and that she had "given her services entirely voluntarily" and did not "seek personal gain."[81] They were mostly, however, written by unknown physicians, including government health officials who in both Australia and America were seen as partisan appointees. Kenny wanted a chance to demonstrate her method on paralyzed patients in order to convince American experts to try them, recognize their value, and call for the transformation of polio care everywhere. In seeking out NFIP officials and Mayo Clinic physicians Kenny sought formal, official approval of her work, something she assumed she would never get from leaders of the organized American profession if they were anything like the elite physicians she had encountered in Australia. She hoped that a polio philanthropy would be less beholden to the medical establishment and that her Brisbane allies' personal connections to Mayo specialists would give her an opportunity to show her methods in a more welcoming atmosphere than Australian specialists had provided.

Kenny's appeal also drew on a popular notion of the open-minded American. Just as science popularizer Paul De Kruif imagined scientists *hunting* microbes and *fighting* hunger and death, so Kenny saw the American physician as a kind of frontiersman.[82] This stereotype drew on the antielitist heroes she had seen in Hollywood movies at the Brisbane cinema, where she had often escaped from professional tensions during the 1930s. Cinematic heroes were courteous to ladies, strangers, and even friendly Indians; they were receptive to challenge and quick to adapt unusual technological means to achieve their mastery of nature and fight against evil. They laughed at orthodox conservatism, and achieved love and riches by ignoring or conquering it. Doctors in this distinctive culture, Kenny believed, had that "quality which has put the United States in the forefront in almost every department of science—that is, an eagerness to know what it is really all about, in order that he may not be the one left behind if there is something to it."[83] Kenny was an innovator; this new audience valued—perhaps even preferred—the new and improved.

Kenny had been certain that in the United States, as in Australia and Britain, there was a polio orthodoxy she would need to identify and challenge. Before O'Connor returned to New York, she was invited to the NFIP headquarters at 120 Broadway to meet Peter Cusack, the NFIP's executive secretary. Greeting her "with the utmost courtesy" Cusack "showed interest" in the material Kenny gave him and in return gave her *Bulletin No. 242*, a Public Health Service pamphlet on polio care written by physical therapists Henry Kendall and Florence Kendall. This pamphlet, which Kenny studied "carefully," had, as she saw it, the combined formal approval both of the nation's medical establishment and its federal government. The Kendalls argued that weak muscles must be protected from fatigue, shortening, and overstretching by the use of splinting and rest to maintain joints in a neutral position.[84]

In approaching American physicians, Kenny faced a fundamental strategic decision. Should she present her work simply as an improvement to rehabilitative therapy, or should she claim that orthodox polio care was based on a flawed understanding of the disease? In 1940 Kenny did not really have a well-developed *theory* of polio. She spoke of distinctive clinical signs that only she had recognized, and warned that if they were not treated patients would be left deformed. She knew her method was distinctive, indeed opposed to elements of standard care.[85] Recalling conservative Australian physicians who saw her as an ignorant upstart she came to believe that only the boldest approach would allow her to open eyes and change minds.

Kenny's sense that there was a single, approved method of polio care in the United States was intensified at another meeting with physicians at the Ruptured and Crippled. As she read a paper on her work, "the look of something like boredom" spread over their faces. Some of the men, she recalled later, took naps as she talked, and "one member of the group with a cartoonist kink amused himself by drawing an outline of my features on his cuff."[86] This kind of disdain and ridicule was familiar to her; it had occurred during her demonstration at the Brisbane General Hospital in 1933. Her suspicion that minor NFIP officials were trying to get rid of her before O'Connor returned was reinforced when Cusack urged her to leave New York and go to Chicago to speak to the head of the AMA's Council on Physical Therapy. Reflecting on her many antagonistic experiences with Australian physicians, Kenny had planned to avoid the headquarters of the AMA and turned down Cusack's proposal.[87] She was, however, willing to test the openness of New York's scientific establishment, and using a letter of introduction she began explaining her ideas on the phone to a prominent research worker. She had not gone far when this man (probably Thomas Rivers, a prominent virologist at the Rockefeller Institute who was the head of the NFIP's advisory committee on scientific research) advised her to follow Cusack's advice, adding, "I do not think I wish to meet you." Unable to curb her "nerves and temper" Kenny retorted "I do not only *think* I have no wish to meet *you*. I am sure of it." So, she reflected later, "ended my first effort to make contact with a research institution in the United States."[88]

POLIO PHILANTHROPY

Kenny now had an introduction from the NFIP to a Chicago specialist in physical medicine as well as introductory letters from Australia to physicians at the Mayo Clinic. In New York she had faced disdain, condescension, and dismissal. But nonetheless she stayed there instead of traveling west. What was she waiting for?

The NFIP, as Kenny shrewdly recognized, was becoming a crucial institution in funding polio care. Formally incorporated only 2 years earlier, it was in the midst of reshaping itself into what became a model for all voluntary health agencies: a sophisticated disease philanthropy committed to funding research, professional training, and patient care on a national scale. Yet it had already had to weather accusations of corruption and dangerous experimentation. Roosevelt had bought the Warm Springs resort in 1926 and established the Georgia Warm Springs Foundation (GWSF), a nonprofit corporation to help him raise funds for it. Both the GWSF and the resort had been accused of corruption and racism, and had been tied too closely to Roosevelt's own political fortunes. The GWSF, further, had become a forum for activist polio survivors who, inspired by their community at Warm Springs, attacked the widespread neglect of patients with polio and other disabled Americans. Calling themselves the Polio Crusaders, the group had called for expanding the rights of the disabled. By 1933, however, Roosevelt's presidential advisors realized that disabled children were more appealing and far less dangerous than vocal adult subjects. A new fundraising organization based around the president's birthday subsumed the GWSF and removed disability rights from its national agenda. Despite efforts by the newly established Birthday Ball Committee to encourage local communities to expand their own centers, Warm Springs continued to be considered a national center for polio rehabilitation.

An even more dramatic setback occurred in 1935 when a polio vaccine supported by the Birthday Ball Committee led to the paralysis and death of 11 children. The vaccine disaster followed by disappointing trials of a zinc sulfate nasal spray convinced O'Connor that the NFIP must stop funding what a science writer later called "trial-and-error 'miracle cures.'"[89] By 1940 a reorganized NFIP had developed a new strategy of providing grants for mostly basic science research approved by elite "known" scientists and clinicians. The NFIP's major aim was paying for medical care for patients with polio who could not afford it and it was structured around a sophisticated fundraising program based on the efforts of local and regional chapters run by volunteers but including influential physicians and welfare officials. An invigorated professionally trained public relations staff continued to market hope along with fear, stressing the likelihood that anyone's child could be a victim, the pathetic disabled polio survivor, and the civic virtue of giving.

Although the NFIP claimed it was not in the business of judging polio therapies, that was not quite true. It had to define best polio care when it funded training in the latest methods of diagnosis, treatment, and prevention. The pamphlets it distributed similarly laid out therapies reflecting a particular vision of polio's pathology. Thus, *The Nursing Care of Patients with Infantile Paralysis* emphasized the need for rest during polio's early stage and the usefulness of "orthopedic appliances" such as frames and splints to protect muscles from overstretching.[90] The NFIP also sponsored polio exhibits at national conferences such as the National Congress of Physiotherapy and the American Academy of Orthopedic Surgeons.[91] While the NFIP never resolved how to define best practice, by the early 1940s it followed the least partisan policy possible, agreeing to pay for any form of therapy recommended by a physician who was legally recognized by a state's licensing laws. The NFIP's research policies, however, became far stricter and more centralized: local and state chapters were forbidden to use any of their funds for research and grants were offered only to individuals or groups based at an institution that the NFIP recognized as equipped to pursue scientific work.

NFIP officials expected Kenny to be another kook but were hesitant to dismiss someone recommended by physicians, however unknown. Kenny's reiteration of the many letters after their names—M.S., F.R.C.S., F.R.A.C.P.—was powerful in a country without Royal Colleges and with diverse medical standards. Her claim to be a "representative" of the Australian government was even more impressive. NFIP officials contacted officials in Washington to verify this claim. Unknown to Kenny as she waited in New York, Richard Casey at the Australian embassy (then known as the Legation) sent a telegram to Canberra to ask whether Kenny was in fact "sponsored by the Australian Government."[92] An Australian federal health official based in Brisbane had a "long talk" with Raphael

Cilento, now both Queensland's health director-general and head of the state's medical society. Cilento, no friend of Kenny's, claimed that "Sister Kenny had herself decided to go to America" and showed the official a copy of Forgan Smith's letter to the NFIP, pointing out its "non-committal" tone.[93] In a less antagonistic manner, the Canberra office informed Casey that although the Australian government had not sponsored Kenny, the Queensland government had given her £300 and a letter of introduction to the NFIP.[94] NFIP officials did not confront Kenny with this information, but it may well have influenced their cautious dealings with her and their care to have her assessed by eminent American physicians.

KENNY MEETS THE NFIP

Officials at the NFIP had long experience with people who demanded money for their polio "cure." Even more than tuberculosis or cancer, polio had gained public prominence. Roosevelt's experience suggested that anyone could potentially become a victim of polio paralysis, and the frequency and unpredictability of polio epidemics further frightened the public. Before the late 1940s the federal government played only a limited role in funding medical research, so disease-oriented charities along with major foundations such as Rockefeller, Carnegie, Russell Sage, and Kellogg as well as some municipal and state health departments were the major sources of research funds.

Roosevelt was frequently sent letters with ideas about preventing and curing polio, and these were now forwarded to the NFIP. In February 1940, a few months before Kenny appeared, O'Connor had been sent 2 letters addressed to the President. One was from a nurse with a "cure" for polio called "Via Pak" who wanted an opportunity to "demonstrate its effectiveness."[95] The second was from a wealthy woman who, impressed by the work of a Dr. John van Paing of Washington D.C., offered to give the government 30 acres including 2 large warm water pools in order to set up a polio institution like Warm Springs where medical experts from the NFIP could investigate van Paing's treatment.[96]

The man in charge of the NFIP was a tough-minded Irish Catholic in an era when Catholics faced widespread social discrimination. Basil O'Connor had grown up in a working-class family in Taunton, Massachusetts. He had studied at Dartmouth College, playing violin in a dance band to support himself, and found a sponsor to help him attend Harvard Law School, one of the few ways the rare Catholic or Jewish graduate could then gain a position in a prominent law firm. O'Connor moved to New York City in 1919 where he worked as a lawyer for oil companies and became a wealthy Wall Street lawyer as well as a donor to Catholic charities. Irish Catholics were a crucial part of the Democratic Party's organization. Not only was Basil's brother John a New York City Congressman but in the early 1920s Basil O'Connor chose Franklin Roosevelt as his legal partner. Roosevelt, despite his paralysis, was determined to return to political life and O'Connor could see how useful Roosevelt's name and connections would be for their law firm. O'Connor became one of Roosevelt's confidants and was one of the few people invited to Warm Springs where Roosevelt could relax in an openly disabled world.[97]

Delighted to have a chance to speak to O'Connor, Kenny spent "almost two hours" talking and explaining. Years later she would tell audiences eager to hear the worst that O'Connor had treated her coldly, but in the early 1940s while her relationship with the

NFIP prospered, she reported that she had enjoyed meeting him. O'Connor carefully explained to her the NFIP policy of awarding grants only to individuals based at an institution that had requested funding from the NFIP and then only if the project "met the approval of the [NFIP's] medical advisory board." Kenny was convinced by "the sincerity of purpose" behind this policy and "the soundness of its argument." It was, she concluded, "only natural that a lawyer would hesitate to dictate a policy to men who were specialists in the field of medicine."[98] O'Connor later recalled that after that first meeting he said to Don Gudakunst, the NFIP's medical director, "I think she's a crackpot, but I'm not so sure she may not have something."[99]

Kenny decided she would go to Chicago to visit the AMA's Council on Physical Therapy as Cusack had suggested and then fulfill her obligation to visit the Mayo Clinic, which her Brisbane allies expected her to do.[100] Kenny suspected that representatives of America's organized profession would be no more open to her than their British and Australian counterparts. She was right. In Chicago, Howard Carter, the secretary of the AMA's Council on Physical Therapy, greeted her with the unfriendly remark: "I don't understand just what it is you want. I was under the impression that you belonged to some religious order and had something to sell." Ignoring the confusion over her title Kenny focused on the accusation that she was just a greedy charlatan. On the contrary, she replied tartly, she had "something to give to America if America were willing to accept it." Skeptical, Carter made an appointment for her with John Coulter, head of the Department of Physical Therapy at Northwestern University's medical school.[101] A respected specialist in physical medicine, Coulter appeared genuinely interested. He asked Kenny to autograph his own copy of her 1937 textbook and invited her to meet the 2 women physical therapists with whom he worked. Kenny had always sought out the most senior male experts involved in polio care—usually orthopedic surgeons—and she recognized that she was being put in her gendered place as a female technician. Coulter's therapists told Kenny that for her method to make sense the disease in Australia "must differ radically from that found in any other part of the world."[102] Prepared for this argument, Kenny replied that she believed she could prove "the disease was the same everywhere" but that she "was the only one who had recognized its true symptoms." One of the therapists retorted scornfully, "do you mean to tell me that I have been massaging monkeys for two years for symptoms of a disease that does not exist?" In words that may have been softened in her later recollections, Kenny replied that such therapy was "certainly doing damage."[103]

Disheartened by her experiences in Chicago, Kenny traveled on to Rochester seeing "nothing ahead but to return to Australia."[104] She contacted Mayo Clinic orthopedist Melvin Henderson, using her letter of introduction to him from Herbert Wilkinson, the Queensland neuroanatomist who had written the preface to her 1937 textbook.[105] Henderson was courteous but wary. He had already been president of the American Orthopedic Association and the American Board of Orthopaedic Surgeons, and was the director of Mayo's nursing school at Colonial Hospital, one of Mayo's affiliated hospitals where he was chief of staff. He privately assured Wilkinson that he would be glad to see Kenny but warned that all his Mayo patients were private and would therefore not be suitable for "demonstration purposes."[106]

Henderson introduced Kenny to his colleague Frank Krusen, one of the founders of a group of physicians practicing physical medicine (later the American Academy of Physical Medicine and Rehabilitation). At the Mayo Clinic Krusen directed the nation's first

3-year physical medicine residency program. He had written physical therapy textbooks for physicians and nurses and also directed the Mayo Clinic's physical therapy training program, which had graduated its first class only a year earlier.[107] Krusen talked to Kenny "at intervals" for 2 days and was, he admitted a few years later, "taken aback by her belligerent attitude." However, learning that the Queensland government had sponsored some of her clinics and that a few Australian physicians were enthusiastic about her treatment, he and Henderson decided that some physicians should "observe her work more closely." Sensing, however, that Kenny might not be easy to work with, they urged her to go to Minneapolis where there was a large public hospital as well as a state orthopedic hospital.[108]

In the Twin Cities Kenny was, for the first time, able to treat American patients, although only the "hopeless" ones. Her clinical results, more than her written testimonials, intrigued a few, well-connected local surgeons, including Wallace Cole, head of the University of Minnesota's orthopedic department.[109] At the Gillette State Hospital, renowned as one of the few state-funded orthopedic hospitals in the country, Kenny saw familiar conditions: "little patients lying in their beds, the old look of resignation on their faces, their frail bodies strapped into frames or laden with splints and casts" and "the pelvic tilts, the apparent leg shortening, the dropped feet, the stiff and distorted spines, and the useless abdominals." At the Shriners Hospital she removed the splints and braces of a boy with a deformed spine who had made no improvement in 5 months and pointed out the "muscle condition" that "must be treated." At the Children's Hospital in St. Paul she examined another boy left with deformed feet "despite the best efforts of the supervising surgeon" and after treating him for just a few days was able to demonstrate clinical improvements that impressed the hospital's medical staff.[110]

It was against this background of desperate parents and intrigued surgeons that Kenny gave a lecture to physicians at the University of Minnesota in which she spoke of the treatment she had "evolved" for "symptoms which were the opposite of those generally accepted." These symptoms, she argued, had not just been overlooked but contradicted the accepted picture of polio paralysis. "I can clearly see the difficulty you are experiencing in attempting to follow the lectures I am giving," she told the physicians in her audience, but "if you wish to be successful [you have to]...disregard all measures...you have been taught."[111]

Unlike the many times when her conclusions had failed to convince her listeners on this occasion Kenny began to feel encouraged.[112] Miland Knapp, head of the university's physical therapy department, admitted later that he and his colleagues "did not have the slightest idea of what she was talking about when she started." But Knapp, a patient man, tried to understand what Kenny was saying.[113] He invited her to St. Barnabas Hospital to see one of his patients, a boy with a paralyzed arm in splints where "after several months of ineffectual treatment, doctor, patient and parents were on the ragged edge." Kenny took off the boy's splint and demonstrated several clinical signs that Knapp "had not previously recognized." Under her care the boy began to improve and a few months later was able to shovel snow for his family. Knapp was shocked by the patient's initial improvements for he had been taught that if an arm in an airplane splint was brought down "even once" it would lose the positive effects of several months care. He and his wife invited Kenny and Mary to stay at their house for about 2 weeks. They enjoyed Kenny's "wonderful sense of humor," but disliked the casually domineering way she treated her ward, demanding, for example, that Mary go to bed at 8 pm.[114]

Physicians like Knapp and Cole were members of a local and regional elite, with prestigious university and hospital positions, and Henderson and Krusen were prominent national figures. While doctors who specialized in physical medicine struggled for professional respect, orthopedic surgeons were known for being conservative and insular. The responsiveness that Kenny experienced in Minnesota was surprising.[115]

Certainly, as Kenny spoke of "deformities" and their prevention, she was careful to remain respectful of surgery itself, telling her audience that her methods would not provide a substitution for the orthopedic operations typically performed on patients with polio once their disabilities were clearly not going to improve. Further, it was clear to many of her listeners that whatever their other benefits, her methods would dramatically alter an aspect of polio care that made the bad situation of paralysis worse. Instead of stiff patients lying in pain in splints or a frame, her patients lay comfortably in their hospital beds.

CLINICAL AND POLITICAL ACUITY

Kenny had met the right people—Basil O'Connor, Kristian Hansson, and John Coulter—and she did not act like a quack. But neither was she a deferential nurse. She spoke confidently about the physicians who had attacked her work and the medical traditions she was challenging. Most of all, her hands and her way of working were transformative. She became, many people commented, a different person when she worked with patients, speaking gently and with great patience. And her words of hope were so different from the pessimistic tone that most doctors used in offering their prognosis to patients and families.

Kenny's challenge to polio care aptly pointed to a vacuum in medical research and clinical practice. Her methods seemed initially an innocuous and promising way to redirect polio therapy. But Kenny was not willing to have her work adapted; she wished to transform understanding of the disease and its treatment, and she made her claims to therapeutic change explicit and assertive. Taking off casts and splints was dramatic and provocative. What she was offering, she reiterated, was not a simple progression of improved practice. To understand why she received the impressive results she did her medical audiences needed to see polio and the paralyzed body *her* way. Claiming innovation has always been a powerful step in the history of medicine. Kenny wanted to be recognized as an important innovator. In her later stories she portrayed herself as the ridiculed discoverer whose work could be valued only by the open-minded scientific observer, a familiar figure to anyone who had seen the movies *The Story of Louis Pasteur* or *Dr. Ehrlich's Magic Bullet*. But in 1940 she tended to emphasize less the process of discovery than the process of acceptance, telling one audience she was "most grateful to have been so happily placed in a hospital where I receive the whole hearted cooperation of the Medical and Nursing staff" for "the world looks to America for many things, more especially for reformation in the treatment of the disease anterior Poliomyelitis."[116] But increasingly such gratitude was not enough.

A turning point came when orthopedic surgeon John Florian Pohl invited Kenny to examine one of his private patients, Henry Haverstock Jr., who had returned from 4 months at Warm Springs still unable to walk or even sit up. Born in 1903, Pohl had worked as a school teacher before studying medicine at Minnesota's medical school, and then continued his studies with orthopedist Arthur Legg at Harvard. He now had a successful private practice and directed the city hospital's polio wards but had no formal teaching position at the medical school and was little known outside the state.[117]

Pohl's patient was 17 years old, the "charming and brilliant son" of a local lawyer, facing a future without a college education or professional career. He had come home from Warm Springs wearing locked braces on both legs extending to his hips, a metal stomach corset, and braces on both feet and his left hand. After removing all the apparatus and examining him, Kenny told his parents that he was "suffering painfully because the true symptoms of the disease had never been treated."[118]

Kenny then initiated a policy that put her in good standing not only with Pohl but also with other local physicians with wealthy private patients. Instead of saying that she would treat the boy in his home, she demanded that he be admitted to a hospital where she would treat him, thus setting herself up not as a financial competitor of the boy's doctor but as a professional ally. At the hospital where Pohl sent Haverstock, however, Kenny later reported, "two very prominent orthopedic men" complained to the hospital's director that "if he didn't get rid of that 'quack'—meaning me, of course—the hospital would be ruined." Fortunately, Kenny reflected, the director overruled them.[119] Within a few months Haverstock could raise himself with his hands to a sitting position, get off the treatment table, and walk with the aid of 2 half-crutches.[120]

Kenny's work with Haverstock was also a turning point in her relationship with the city's business establishment. Haverstock's father became a powerful supporter and introduced her to local businessmen and their wives. The son later graduated from the University of Minnesota and became a lawyer; his physical and professional achievements provided dramatic evidence of the veracity of Kenny's claims.

Impressed by the enthusiasm of Pohl and Knapp, Cole, the university's senior orthopedist, asked the NFIP to pay for a study of Kenny's method at the University of Minnesota. In this era of informal research funding, there were few forms to fill out. O'Connor agreed to finance Kenny's living expenses for 6 months as long as the NFIP was "kept informed of Miss Kenny's work."[121] Her sponsors also had to gain the support of city officials, for Kenny claimed that her methods were most effective with patients in the acute stage of the disease. As such patients were considered contagious, only the city hospital, unlike the University of Minnesota's hospital and most other voluntary hospitals, accepted them. Pohl introduced Kenny to the city's Board of Public Welfare where in a "deep, matter-of-fact monotone" she read "letter after long letter" by Australian doctors, patients, and parents. "Her braggadocio struck us as a breach of professional decorum," one official recalled, yet as "our best local medical men thought she had something valuable to offer," he and the rest of the board agreed to allow her to treat patients in the city hospital.[122] Knapp also arranged for her to give a series of lectures, which were attended, according to Kenny, by "eager, intelligent young doctors and physiotherapists who were always ready with questions the moment I had ceased speaking."[123] Back in Brisbane, Chuter, delighted to hear of her success, teased her by asking if she had yet met President Roosevelt, and remarked that it was "humorous" to think that not so long ago she was dismissed as an unlicensed "masseuse."[124]

By November 1940 Kenny began to give talks to women's clubs and developed a group of influential allies whose allegiance became increasingly clear to NFIP officials in New York City. One local woman supporter, responding to Kenny's complaints about the tardiness of NFIP funding, noted that many local people had offered to provide funds, but Kenny refused to accept "aid from anyone outside the Foundation...as her country wrote you and she presented her introduction to you." In a criticism that would be repeated many times in subsequent years, the supporter complained that "millions of dollars" had been contributed by the American public "for the express purpose" of alleviating polio, yet the NFIP had ignored "countless testimonials to be had from patients, parents, doctors, general hospitals, and scores of other people to bear witness to the positively miraculous results she has obtained."[125] This letter sounded themes that would become very familiar to O'Connor: the sense of the NFIP as a national civic organization, Kenny as the unwitting victim of unpleasant policies that left her without proper funding to continue her work, and the worth of the work itself proven by "testimonials"—all ideas that gained greater political force by the mid-1940s.

Kenny's work at Station K, her ward at the Minneapolis General Hospital, was not easy. During her first 6 months she and Mary struggled to overcome the resistance of members of the hospital staff who saw her methods as dangerous and irrational. Kenny argued that traditional ways of testing muscles exacerbated muscle spasm, but physical therapists ignored this argument and during the night while she was away from the hospital would test the muscles of her patients.[126] In other instances individual physicians paid no attention to Kenny's claim to clinical authority. One of her patients recalled that his physician prescribed arm and leg splints saying "you're my patient, so I'm going to do what I think is right." When Kenny came back she cut off the splints and threw them on the floor. To horrified patients and nurses she said reassuringly "he's just a young doctor; I'll have a talk with him."[127] In a single ward she could hope to counteract such actions, but how would her work manage to transform institutional practice and professional resistance across the country?

MONEY AND POLIO

Money was always central in Kenny's American career, partly because she made much of presenting her work as a "gift." In Australia she had been paid as a private duty nurse, supplemented by her Army war pension and royalties from the Sylvia stretcher she had designed and patented.[128] She had expected to be able to draw on some of her Australian savings in America, but during the war Australia had followed Britain's lead by restricting the amount of currency that could leave the country.[129] Increasingly anxious that the NFIP was not fulfilling its promise to pay her expenses Kenny wrote a number of times to O'Connor reminding him that the NFIP had agreed to "be responsible for my expenses during this demonstration." She was also becoming annoyed with the NFIP's funding arrangement, whereby she had to request money from Cole who then contacted the NFIP's head office in New York before giving her a check.[130]

It is at this point that Mary became a more central figure. After Kenny's mother had died in 1937 Mary continued her training as a Kenny technician by moving to Brisbane to work at the outpatient clinic.[131] By the time she and Kenny arrived in America, Mary was crucial in Kenny's life, providing emotional ballast and balancing Kenny's pride and temper with a softer, more pragmatic approach. Kenny had brought her to America partly as a companion and clinical assistant and partly as a servant. In Kenny's 1943 autobiography Mary appears as a wide-eyed child, amazed at America's scenic beauty and technological marvels like automats, but it is clear that Mary's less combative attitude helped Kenny to achieve her goals. Thus, when their funds were dwindling after 3 months in the United States, Kenny phoned Henry Haverstock's parents and told them that she had to return to Australia. Haverstock's father immediately contacted Kenny at home and offered her money, which Kenny refused to accept. It was Mary to whom the father then addressed an envelope containing $40 that he left in their mail box. And, according to Kenny, it was Mary who "pleaded with me to stay."[132] Kenny does not mention whether she allowed Mary to keep this money, but she certainly encouraged the Haverstock family to pressure physicians at the medical school and Minnesota's Republican Senator Henrik Shipstead, a member of the Senate Committee on Foreign Relations, to contact the Australian ambassador.[133] Not long after this encounter Cole phoned Kenny to say that the NFIP had sent $400 for her expenses.[134]

Minnesota's local NFIP officials had been initially skeptical of the New York office's decision to fund Kenny's work. In September 1940 Arthur Reynolds, a prominent Democrat and the chairman of the state chapter, warned the NFIP's New York office about divisions among local physicians "as to her worth and her proper place." To Reynolds Kenny seemed "more or less of a publicity hound" and he wondered whether O'Connor wanted local officials "to treat her nice and send her on her way as quickly as possible?"[135] O'Connor explained that in 6 months, after a full report from Minneapolis physicians at the medical school, the NFIP would be able "to appraise the value of Miss Elizabeth Kenny's methods of treatment."[136] A few months later Reynolds' attitude had softened and he told O'Connor that among most "medical people" the "consensus of opinion is favorable" about the value of Kenny's work. The state chapter began to pay for 16 patients under her care at the city hospital. The money question continued to fester, however, and Reynolds was outraged to hear that Kenny had said during a talk at a women's club in Minneapolis that she *was paying her own personal expenses.*"[137] The question of who deserved credit for funding Kenny's work later became a publicized and politicized issue.

Nor did Kenny consider that her needs should be in any way secondary, even to the concerns of the nation's President. In September 1940 she wrote to Roosevelt, explaining that she was an "official visitor" with an "official visa" who for the past 3 months had "given lectures and demonstration to a class of medical men and physiotherapists and nurses." Despite assurances to "defray her personal expenses" the NFIP had not yet done so, and "owing to war conditions, it is impossible for me to receive sufficient money from my own Country."[138] After Cole paid her with NFIP funds, Kenny wrote to Roosevelt again, reminding him that almost a third of the cases of crippling in the United States were caused by polio. Since "this enemy knows no frontiers," she wrote, "I consider the question is of national importance to your country." Without explicitly asking for money, she complained that the NFIP funds did not cover her expenses, which she estimated at

$180 a month to cover rent, telephone, gas, electric light, food, and transportation to and from the hospitals she visited.[139]

All letters from the public about the NFIP and polio, whether directed to Roosevelt, his wife, or other prominent figures, were forwarded to O'Connor and his staff. Annoyed at Kenny's audacity at approaching Roosevelt directly, O'Connor contacted Cole, whom he saw as her formal supervisor. Her second long letter, O'Connor reported, which described "somewhat in detail the remarkable cures she has been effecting [sic] in your area" without NFIP funding was incorrect, for the NFIP had already sent her funds. Thus, "one could hardly say that Sister Kenny's statement to President Roosevelt was playing cricket."[140] Cole apologized to Kenny, explaining that he had been away for a month before all the necessary forms were filled in and argued that the NFIP was not "in any way… to blame in this matter and if there has been any delay it should be placed only at my door."[141] Later Kenny praised "the great, humane and unbiased attitude of men" like Cole, Knapp, and Pohl, but in day-to-day affairs she clearly saw such delays as slights.[142] Going to the top and using local and national political connections were techniques she had developed during her years in Australia when she sought to gain government support for clinics despite opposition from Brisbane specialists.

Kenny then sent what she called a "brief report" to Cole and O'Connor "to place before you the evidence I have produced during the past three months." In 9 typed pages she compared the Minneapolis physicians to the Queensland Royal Commission and the London County Council, arguing that their "unbiased attitude" had led them to provide "the material I so much desired to demonstrate and prove my ideas to be correct, although so much opposed to orthodoxy." She also praised "the open mindedness of the members of the American medical profession who have listened and granted me the privilege of demonstrating my ideas under their personal observation" and the NFIP for its "financial assistance."[143] In a letter to Chuter she boasted of her successes at a university that was "the largest in the U.S.A. in one campus" and described with delight a formal dinner at the University Club during the Northwestern Pediatric Conference where she had been seated between the president of the pediatric society and the chief orthopedic surgeon of the General Hospital.[144]

1940 was not an epidemic year for polio in Minnesota, and between June and December Kenny treated only 24 acute patients. The Minneapolis physicians knew that this number of cases was not sufficient for a convincing conclusion about her work, as improvement might also have resulted from spontaneous recovery. Kenny had initially been asked to stay only for 6 months, but Cole and Knapp wanted to retain her as both teacher and clinician. They therefore asked the NFIP to allow her to stay during another polio season so that doctors, nurses, and physical therapists could become better acquainted with her methods.[145]

Most crucially, these physicians began to publish clinical reports that linked their careers with Kenny and her work. Cole and Knapp wrote a preliminary study of her first patients that was presented at a NFIP meeting in New York that December. Their report, cautious but positive, convinced O'Connor and the NFIP's advisory committee to continue funding Kenny at the University of Minnesota, and when she announced that she would have to return to Australia for a few months, the NFIP agreed to pay her travel expenses.[146] Kenny was going to Australia ostensibly to help her Brisbane staff deal with a polio outbreak but she intended to return to Minnesota with 2 Australian technicians.

The NFIP agreed to pay their expenses as well. Kenny later recalled that she had suggested to Mary that she also return to Australia but that Mary wanted to stay with the Minneapolis patients and continue training local physical therapists and therefore "begged to remain and for me to return." Mary stayed behind not only to supervise the work in Minneapolis but also as a quiet symbol of the power of the work without its most vocal and at times refractory proponent.[147]

By the time Kenny returned the dynamics of the relationship among the Australian nurse, NFIP officials, and University of Minnesota physicians had become established. It was an uneasy relationship in which Kenny refused to be easily slotted into the role of subservient nurse. She appeared neither grateful nor amenable; she was difficult, ambitious, easily irritated, and defensive. Yet she was also good company, telling stories of her war experiences and her bush nursing in an era when social graces of participants before and after professional meetings were crucial parts of a medical professional's reputation. NFIP officials and Kenny's medical supervisors hoped that they could extract what was good about her methods and then send her back to Australia. They would be disappointed.

NOTES

1. Elizabeth Kenny with Martha Ostenso *And They Shall Walk: The Life Story of Sister Elizabeth Kenny* (New York: Dodd, Mead, 1943), 201, 206; "For Poliomyelitis Test: Australian Nurse Leaves Coast to Discuss New Treatment Here" *New York Times* April 18 1940; William Forgan Smith to Dear Sir [Basil O'Connor], March 11 1940, Series A981/1, United States 148, Australian Archives, ACT Regional Office, Canberra, ACT, Australia (hereafter AA-ACT).

2. Kenny with Ostenso *And They Shall Walk*, 206.

3. Kristian Gosta Hansson "After-Treatment of Poliomyelitis" *JAMA* (July 1939) 113: 32–35. For a reference to this article "where it admitted, that nowhere in the world is there a treatment for this disease in the acute stage," see Kenny to Sir [Charles Chuter], January 19 1940, Home Secretary's Office, Special Batches, Kenny Clinics, 1941–1949, A/31753, Queensland State Archives, Brisbane (hereafter QSA).

4. Kenny with Ostenso *And They Shall Walk*, 207.

5. Richard Casey to John McEwen, June 5 1940, cited in W. J. Hudson *Casey* (Melbourne: Melbourne University Press, 1986), 116–117.

6. Marvin L. Kline "The Most Unforgettable Character I've Met" *Reader's Digest* (August 1959), 75: 204.

7. Kenny with Ostenso *And They Shall Walk*, 17.

8. Kenny with Ostenso *And They Shall Walk*, 12–13, 62; Wade Alexander *Sister Elizabeth Kenny: Maverick Heroine of the Polio Treatment Controversy* (Rockhampton: Central Queensland University Press, 2002), 17–30. For examples of efforts to assess how much nursing training Kenny had, see Alexander *Maverick*, 23–24; Victor Cohn *Sister Kenny: The Woman Who Challenged the Doctors* (Minneapolis: University of Minnesota Press, 1975), 37. McDonnell (1864–1939), the son of Irish immigrants and a graduate of Sydney's medical school, became a general surgeon after traveling to Japan, England, and the United States, and set up practice in Toowoomba in the 1890s; by the 1930s he was a member of the state medical society, the Australian Trained Nurses Association Council, and a medical examiner for Toowoomba's Nurses Board; see Alexander *Maverick*, 20–21; Cohn *Sister Kenny*, 27–29, 43–45.

9. Kenny with Ostenso *And They Shall Walk*, 23–24.

10. Kenny with Ostenso *And They Shall Walk*, ix, 32, 38–40; see Alexander *Maverick*, 29–39. Wilson states that she was discharged from the Nursing Service in 1919; John R. Wilson *Through Kenny's Eyes: An Exploration of Sister Elizabeth Kenny's Views about Nursing* (Townsville: Royal College of Nursing Australia, 1995), 37.

11. Alexander *Maverick*, 46–47; [Cohn interview with] Mary and Stuart McCracken, April 14 1953, Victor Cohn Papers in Elizabeth Kenny Papers, Minnesota Historical Society, St Paul (hereafter MHS-K); Cohn *Sister Kenny*, 69–70. Lucy Lily Stewart was born on October 31 1916, and was officially adopted May 4 1926.

12. Kenny *And They Shall Walk*, 76–77, 119; Alexander *Maverick*, 45–50.

13. George Draper "Infantile Paralysis" *Harper's Monthly Magazine* (February 1930) 160: 368.

14. John R. Paul *A History of Poliomyelitis* (New Haven: Yale University Press, 1971), 190–199.

15. [Editorial] "Poliomyelitis and Its Early Treatment" *Medical Journal of Australia* (September 21 1935) 2: 385–386; J. Steigrad "The Early Treatment of Poliomyelitis" *Medical Journal of Australia* (May 7 1938) 1: 801–804.

16. "Queensland Nurse's Generous Action! Sister Kenny's Treatment for Paralysis a Gift for the Sick Poor" *Australian Women's Weekly* February 23 1935, 4.

17. See Cohn *Sister Kenny*, 97; "Sister Kenny" *[Sydney] People Magazine* June 20 1951, 3.

18. See Wendy Selby "Motherhood and the Golden Casket: An Odd Couple" *Journal of the Royal History Society of Queensland* (1992) 24: 406–413. Queensland was the first Australian state to own and operate a lottery. It was established during the Great War to raise money for veterans and war widows, and in 1919 was used to raise money for Children's Hospital repairs, and in 1920 its revenue was part of a special fund for maternal and infant welfare and then to finance public hospitals, possibly as a result of the actions of Charles Chuter who was then managing the finances of the Brisbane Hospital and by 1924 was president of the Golden Casket Committee; this lottery was not formalized legally until 1931.

19. See John H. Tyrer *History of the Brisbane Hospital and Its Affiliates: A Pilgrim's Progress* (Brisbane: Boolarong Publication, 1993); Anne Crichton *Slowly Taking Control: Australian Government and Health Care Provision 1788–1988* (Sydney: Allen & Unwin, 1990).

20. On Chuter see Alexander *Maverick*, 52; Aubrey Pye, interview by Douglas Gordon and Ralph Doherty, November 8 1980 [transcript of sound recording], Fryer Library and Special Collections, University of Queensland, St. Lucia (hereafter Fryer Library); see also James A. Gillespie *The Price of Health: Australian Governments and Medical Politics 1910–1960* (Sydney: New South Wales University Press, 1988); Ross Patrick *A History of Health and Medicine in Queensland* (St. Lucia: University of Queensland Press, 1987).

21. See Alexander *Maverick*, 57–58; and see "Appendix A: Report by Dr. Harold Crawford, Brisbane (President, Queensland Branch, A.M.A.) on a Demonstration on 5th September, 1933, by Sister E. Kenny" in R. W. Cilento "Report on Sister E. Kenny's After-Treatment of Cases of Paralysis Following Poliomyelitis," Ms. 44/109, Fryer Library, [18].

22. Cohn *Sister Kenny*, 85–86; Kenny with Ostenso *And They Shall Walk*, 94. See also "Appendix A: Report by Dr. Harold Crawford" in Cilento "Report on Sister E. Kenny's After-Treatment," [18]; S. F. McDonald to Dear Mr. Dickson, March 30 1946 [enclosed in] C. H. Dickson to Dear Professor Myers, May 3 1946, Box 19, Sister Kenny Institute, 1938–1946, Jay Arthur Myers Papers, University of Minnesota Archives and Special Collections, Minneapolis (hereafter UMN-ASC).

23. "Appendix A: Report by Dr. Harold Crawford" in Cilento "Report on Sister E. Kenny's After-Treatments," [19]; see also Pye, interview 1980, Fryer Library.

24. Philippa Martyr "'A Small Price to Pay for Peace': The Elizabeth Kenny Controversy Reexamined" *Australian Historical Studies* (1997) 27: 47–65; "Sister Kenny Visits Bendigo Hospital and Tells Her Experiences" *Bendigo Advertiser* January 10 1938.

25. For the claim that Kenny's mother had contacted Sir Littleton Groome, their local representative, to pressure Hanlon, see Cohn *Sister Kenny*, 86–87.

26. Elizabeth Kenny, *Infantile Paralysis and Cerebral Diplegia: Methods Used for the Restoration of Function* (Sydney: Angus and Robertson, 1937), 4.

27. See Alexander *Maverick*, 55–61; Kenny to Dear Mr. Nichols, September 18 1944, Cohn Papers, MHS-K; Cohn *Sister Kenny*, 82–92.

28. [Cohn interview with] James Guinane, November 23 1955, Cohn Papers, MHS-K; see also Cohn *Sister Kenny*, 82–92; [Cohn second interview with] Dr. Philip L. K. Addison, October 25 1955, Cohn Papers, MHS-K.

29. Kenny, *Infantile Paralysis and Cerebral Diplegia*, 19, 11, 64; see also "Reviews: Muscle Reeducation" *Medical Journal of Australia* (May 8 1937) 1: 713–714; J. V. Guinane "Introductory Notes" Kenny, *Infantile Paralysis and Cerebral Diplegia*, xvii–xxxiii.

30. See Alexander *Maverick*, 58–59, 63–65.

31. R. W. Cilento "Report on The Muscle Re-Education Clinic, Townsville (Sister E. Kenny), and its Work" [August 9 1934] Box 13, Elizabeth Kenny Collection, Fryer Library, 4–5.

32. On Cilento see Fedora Gould Fisher *Raphael Cilento: A Biography* (St. Lucia: University of Queensland Press, 1994); Milton J. Lewis *The People's Health: Public Health in Australia, 1788–1950* (London: Praeger Publishers, 2003); Warwick Anderson *The Cultivation of Whiteness: Science, Health and Racial Destiny in Australia* (Melbourne: Melbourne University Press, 2002); Douglas Gordon "Sir Raphael West Cilento" *Medical Journal of Australia* (September 16 1985) 143: 259–260; Alexander *Maverick*, 62–66.

33. Cilento "Report on Sister E. Kenny's After-Treatment," 8–9, 12–14, 15–16; Cilento "Report on The Muscle Re-Education Clinic, Townsville," 4–5.

34. "Infantile Paralysis: Clinic for Brisbane" *Townsville Daily Bulletin* May 15 1935; "Sister Kenny: Brisbane Bombshell" *Townsville Daily Bulletin* May 14 1935; [Cohn interview with] Sir Raphael Cilento, November 16 1955, Cohn Papers, MHS-K. On Wilhelmina G. Wright see Alexander *Maverick*, 79–80. Wright's 1912 article "Muscle Training in the Treatment of Infantile Paralysis" from the *Boston Medical and Surgical Journal* was republished by the U.S. Public Health Service.

35. "Sister Kenny: Brisbane Bombshell" *Townsville Daily Bulletin* May 14 1935; "Infantile Paralysis: Clinic for Brisbane" *Townsville Daily Bulletin* May 15 1935.

36. Cilento "Report on Sister E. Kenny's After-Treatment," 8–9. This fight even reached the *Lancet*; see "Australia: The Treatment of Infantile Paralysis" *Lancet* (June 15 1935) 1: 1408–1409.

37. "'I Am Nobody's Servant': Status of Sister Kenny's Clinic" *Brisbane Courier Mail* March 2 1935; [Cohn interview with] Sir Raphael Cilento, November 16 1955, Cohn Papers, MHS-K; "'My Work Will Go On In Spite Of Criticism': Sister Kenny's Declaration: 'Too Important to Permit of Controversy'" *Brisbane Telegraph* March 27 1935.

38. Kenny, *Infantile Paralysis and Cerebral Diplegia*, xxiv.

39. "Queensland Nurse's Generous Action!," 4.

40. Ibid.

41. "Sister Kenny's Paralysis Method: The Statements For and Against" *Australasian* January 15 1938; see also Cohn *Sister Kenny*, 100.

42. Tom Aikens to Dear Pal [Cohn] [December 1955], Cohn Papers, MHS-K. For additional tales of conspiracy see Kenny with Ostenso *And They Shall Walk*, 117–121.

43. G. W. Rainnie, letter to editor, *North Queensland Register*, April 20 1935.

44. "Sister Kenny: Brisbane Bombshell" *Townsville Daily Bulletin* May 14 1935; "Sister Kenny: City Council Motion" *Townsville Daily Bulletin* May 17 1935; see also Alexander *Maverick*, 68–69; Cohn *Sister Kenny*, 96–97, 106.

45. See Alexander *Maverick*, 81; "Sister Kenny Was Political Pawn in Queensland" *[Sydney] Smith's Weekly* January 15 1938; On Thelander see Betty Newell and Rodney Thelander *Footprints: Life and Times of Charles Thelander, 1883–1959* ([Brisbane] Queensland: Figtree Pocket, 1995).

46. "Report of the Queensland Royal Commission on Modern Methods for the Treatment of Infantile Paralysis" *Medical Journal of Australia* (January 29 1938) 1: 187–224; "Treatment of Infantile Paralysis By Sister Kenny's Method: Report of Queensland Commission" *British Medical Journal* (February 12 1938) 1: 350; "Australia (From Our Regular Correspondent): A New (?) [sic] System of Orthopedics" *JAMA* (March 19 1938) 110: 910–911. The commissioners were Charles August Thelander (chair), Aeneas John McDonnell, Leslie John Jarvis Nye, John Bostock, J. Rudolph Sergius Lahz, Alexander Edgar Paterson, James Vincent Joseph Duhig, and Leslie Wylie Norman Gibson.

47. "Report of the Queensland Royal Commission," 191, 205; "Appendix B: Review of Miss Kenny's Text-Book by Dr. Lennox Teece, October 1 1937" in "Report of the Queensland Royal Commission," 220, 222; see "Muscle Reeducation" [review of Kenny *Infantile Paralysis and Cerebral Diplegia: Methods Used for the Restoration of Function]* *Medical Journal of Australia* (May 8 1937) 1: 713–714. As part of the Commission's investigation Kenny had identified about a dozen disabled patients and provided a prognosis for each one, based on her assessment of how much they would improve after about a year of her treatment.

48. "Report of the Queensland Royal Commission," 201–203, 190.

49. "Report of the Queensland Royal Commission," 204, 222–223. The commission especially disliked the defense of Kenny's cerebral palsy work by F. H. Mills, a young Sydney physician in the *British Medical Journal* a year earlier. Mills had also attacked certain orthopedic operations as likely to "increase spasticity," a claim the commission considered "so ridiculous as to need no further comment"; F. H. Mills "Treatment of Spastic Paralysis" *British Medical Journal* (August 25 1937) 2: 414–417; see also F. H. Mills "Treatment of Acute Poliomyelitis: An Analysis of Sister Kenny's Methods" *British Medical Journal* (January 22 1938) 1: 168–170. On a letter that Mills wrote to the Victorian minister of health in 1938 praising Kenny's work see Alexander *Maverick*, 101.

50. "Report of the Queensland Royal Commission," 213–214, 219; Cilento [Report, August 1934] quoted in "Report of the Queensland Royal Commission," 189; see Alexander *Maverick*, 81, 92–98.

51. "Doctors' Sharp 'No:' Find Kenny System A Failure" *Sydney Sun* January 5 1938; "Sister Kenny Explains Her Treatment of Paralysis" *Sunday Sun and Guardian* January 16 1938.

52. "Sister Kenny's Paralysis Method: The Statements For and Against" *Australasian* January 15 1938.

53. On Kenny in London see Alexander *Maverick*, 87–92.

54. Anne Killalea *The Great Scourge: The Tasmanian Infantile Paralysis Epidemic 1937–1938* (Hobart: Tasmanian Historical Research Association, 1995), 23. On the founding of the Kenny Clinic in Hobart see Killalea *The Great Scourge*, 11, 24; "Sister Kenny's Paralysis Method: The Statements For and Against" *Australasian* January 15 1938; "Sister Kenny's Camera Clouts For Her Critics" *Melbourne Truth* February 5 1938; Jean Macnamara "Elizabeth Kenny" *Medical Journal of Australia* (February 17 1953) 1: 85.

55. "Doctors' Sharp 'No:' Find Kenny System A Failure" *Sydney Sun* January 5 1938; "Sister Kenny's Trenchant Reply to Commission: Says Her Method Was Never Viewed" *Melbourne Truth* January 9 1938; "'Would Be Humorous If It Were Not Ludicrous:' Sister Kenny Replies to Sir Cilento" *Brisbane Telegraph* January 1938, Home Secretary's Office, Special Batches, A/31752, 1938–1940, QSA; "'So Weary of Untruths' Sister Kenny's Denials" *Melbourne Argus* January 12 1938; see also Alexander *Maverick*, 99–102.

56. "Sister Kenny's Camera Clouts For Her Critics" *Melbourne Truth* February 5 1938.

57. See Miss Ethel Dunne, letter to editor, *Brisbane Telegraph* January 17 1938. A sympathetic report on Kenny's patients in the *Brisbane Telegraph* highlighted those who were now independent including a South African man who had moved from a wheelchair to crutches and a "spastic" girl who could now recite nursery rhymes; "Patients of Sister Kenny Tell of Their Recovery" *Brisbane Telegraph* January 7 1938.

58. N. Thompson "Paralysis Patient's Story" *Brisbane Courier-Mail* January 16 1938.

59. "Sister Kenny Was Political Pawn in Queensland" *[Sydney] Smith's Weekly* January 15 1938; see also John G. Kuhns et al. "Sixty-Seventh Report of Progress in Orthopedic Surgery" *Archives of Surgery* (1938) 37: 1035; "Australia (From Our Regular Correspondent)," 910–911.

60. H. A. T. Fairbanks, Macdonald Critchley, E. I. Lloyd, C. Lambrinudi, R. C. Elmslie, George M. Gray, and Henry O. West "Infantile Paralysis and Cerebral Diplegia Clinic at Carshalton" *British Medical Journal* (October 22 1938) 1: 852–854; "Medical Practice: Report of the Committee Appointed to Observe the Kenny Method of Treatment for Paralysis at London" *Medical Journal of Australia* (December 31 1938) 2: 1133–1137. See also Kenny with Ostenso *And They Shall Walk*, 141–142; Alexander *Maverick*, 101–102.

61. E. Kenny, letter to editor, *Medical Journal of Australia* (March 4 1939) 1: 368–369; Kenny with Ostenso *And They Shall Walk*, 141–142; W. R. Forster and E. E. Price "Medical Practice: Report on an Investigation of Twenty-Three Cases of Poliomyelitis in Which the 'Kenny System' of Treatment Was Used" *Medical Journal of Australia* (February 25 1939) 1: 321–325; see also Alexander *Maverick*, 103–104. She reiterated these comments in a letter to Australia's prime minister, emphasizing that "two medical men of high degree should not be passed over"; Kenny to Dear Mr. [Arthur] Fadden, May 15 1939, Series A-1928, 802/17/ Section, 3, AA-ACT.

62. Elizabeth Kenny *Treatment of Infantile Paralysis in the Acute Stage* (Minneapolis: Bruce Publishing Company, 1941), 26, 119. She also claimed that she had told the Brisbane Hospital audience in 1933 that the exaggerated groove in the patient's neck was the result of spasm; Kenny *Treatment of Infantile Paralysis*, 146.

63. Jean Macnamara "The Treatment of Infantile Paralysis" *Medical Journal of Australia* (March 8 1939) 1: 562–563. Macnamara (1899–1968) was a respected orthopedist with a private practice that emphasized polio care, and was a consultant at the physical medicine department of Melbourne's Royal Children's Hospital. She had been an advisor to Victoria's polio committee in the late 1920s and then to other state official bodies. She had spent over a year in Britain and the United States on a Rockefeller Foundation traveling scholarship (1931–1933) where she had met Agnes Hunt at the Shropshire Orthopaedic Hospital and

developed new ideas for splinting and rehabilitation. Her renown as an orthopedist had led to the honor Dame of the British Empire in 1935; Ann G. Smith "Macnamara, Dame Annie Jean (1899–1968)" *Australian Dictionary of Biography*, Volume 10 (Melbourne: Melbourne University Press, 1986), 345–347; see also Desmond Zwar *The Dame: The Life and Times Of Dame Jean Macnamara Medical Pioneer* (Melbourne: Macmillan & Co Limited, 1984). Kenny had met Macnamara at a 1936 conference on "the crippled child" in Canberra, and been rebuked by Lady Ella Latham, a wealthy philanthropist who was the head trustee of Melbourne's Royal Children's Hospital, a reminder for Kenny that many elite Australians shared Brisbane specialists' disdain for her; see Kenny with Ostenso *And They Shall Walk*, 127–129; Alexander *Maverick*, 82. On Latham see Howard E. Williams *From Charity to Teaching Hospital: Ella Latham's Presidency 1933–1945, the Royal Children's Hospital, Melbourne* (Glenroy, Vic: Book Generation, 1989).

64. W. Kent Hughes, letter to editor, *Medical Journal of Australia* (March 18 1939) 1: 448.

65. Cohn *Sister Kenny*, 93; Alexander *Maverick*, 83, 94, 99.

66. "Sister Kenny Explains Her Treatment of Paralysis" *Sunday Sun and Guardian* January 16 1938; "Sister Kenny's Paralysis Method: The Statements For and Against" *Australasian* January 15 1938; see also "The Treatment of Paralysis at the Elizabeth Kenny Clinic Royal North Shore Hospital of Sydney" *Medical Journal of Australia* (November 13 1937) 2: 888–894.

67. Felix Arden, interview with Naomi Rogers, September 29 1992, Brisbane, Queensland; Alexander *Maverick*, 105–106. She told the hospital administrator that she wanted this ward painted blue in the same shade as her treatment room in the Townsville clinic; Kenny to Dear Dr. Pye, April 26 1939, Home Secretary's Office, Special Batches, A/31752, 1938–1940, QSA.

68. [Cohn interview with] Abe Fryberg, [1953], Cohn Papers, MHS-K; see also Arden, interview with Rogers, 1992; and Abraham Fryberg "Experiences of a Medical Administrator: Address to College of Medical Administrators, Melbourne, 29th May 1968" *The Quarterly* ([first published in Royal Australasian College of Medical Administrators First Annual Report, May 1968] reprinted December 2007) http://racma.edu.au/index.php?option=com_content &view=article&id=104:experiences-of-a-medical-administrator&catid=8:the-quarterly-vol4 0-no4-december-2007&Itemid=182. Fryberg (1901–1993) had stopped his clinical practice and become a health administrator after losing his arm in a car accident in the early 1930s. He received his Graduate Diploma in Public Health from the University of Sydney in 1936, and was appointed Queensland Director-General in 1947; he retired in 1967.

69. Arden, interview with Rogers, 1992; see also Pye, interview 1980, Fryer Library; and Cohn *Sister Kenny*, 118. Aubrey David Dick Pye (1901–1994) was a Fellow of the Royal College of Surgeons of Edinburgh and the Royal Australian College of Surgeons, and was the Brisbane Hospital director from 1932 to 1967; in the first decade he was the only physician member of the Brisbane and South Coast Hospitals Board.

70. Arden, interview with Rogers, 1992; Anthony Arden "Felix Wilfrid Arden," Volume XI, page 25, RCP Munks Roll; http://munksroll.rcplondon.ac.uk/Biography/Details/5130. Felix Arden (1910–2002) was the medical superintendent of the Children's Hospital [Hospital for Sick Children in Brisbane, renamed The Royal Children's Hospital in 1968] from 1938 to 1946 and then entered private practice.

71. J. D. Radcliff to Dear Sir [General Superintendent, Brisbane Hospital] May 15 1939, Kenny Collection, Fryer Library; Kenneth W. Starr *A Report to the Minister for Health, N.S.W. on Sister Kenny's Method of the Treatment of Infantile Paralysis* (Newcastle: N. Morriss, May 1939); on Starr's report see Alexander *Maverick*, 104–108.

72. Kenny to Sir [Mr. Watson, Under Secretary, Chief Secretary's Department], February 14 1940, Home Secretary's Office, Special Batches, Kenny Clinics, 1941–1949, A/31753, QSA; Kenny "Complications Due to Immobilisation in Cases of Anterior Poliomyelitis," [1939], [enclosed in] Kenny to Dear Dr. Pye, August 18 1939, Home Secretary's Office, Special Batches, Kenny Clinics, 1938–1940, A/31752, QSA; [Cohn interview with] H. J. Wilkinson, April 24 1953, Cohn Papers, MHS-K.

73. Kenny "Complications Due to Immobilisation in Cases of Anterior Poliomyelitis" [1939], [enclosed in] Kenny to Dear Dr. Pye, August 18 1939, Home Secretary's Office, Special Batches, Kenny Clinics, 1938–1940, A/31752, QSA; Kenny *Treatment of Infantile Paralysis*, 20–26, 47–49; Kenny to Dear Dr. Pye, August 18 1939, Home Secretary's Office, Special Batches, Kenny Clinics, 1938–1940, A/31752, QSA; and see Kenny to Dear Sir [Manager of Brisbane and South Coast Hospitals Board], September 19 1939, Kenny Collection, Fryer Library.

74. Herbert J. Wilkinson "Foreword" Kenny, *Infantile Paralysis and Cerebral Diplegia*, i–xvii.

75. Kenny to Dear Sir, November 25 1938, John R. Wilson Collection, Quoiba, Tasmania (hereafter Wilson Collection).

76. Kenny to Dear Sir [Manager of Brisbane and South Coast Hospitals Board], September 19 1939, Kenny Collection, Fryer Library.

77. Cohn *Sister Kenny*, 119. See, for example, Sydney orthopedist Allen Fletcher who came with 2 colleagues to see her work at the Brisbane outpatient clinic and in Ward 7 and told the *Brisbane Telegraph* that they agreed that "of all treatment we have seen of the early stages of anterior poliomyelitis the method evolved by Sister Kenny offers greater hopes than any other"; Alan Fletcher to Dear Sister Kenny, December 18 1939, Australia 1939–1952, MHS-K; see Alexander *Maverick*, 110–111. Fletcher also sent a statement to the federal minister of health saying that they "were much impressed by the condition of the patients" and "that it would be nothing short of a crime if her methods are not made available to every sufferer from infantile paralysis"; Alan Fletcher to Minister for Health, December 18 1939; Series A981/1, United States 148, AA-ACT.

78. K.G. Hansson "After-Treatment of Poliomyelitis" *JAMA* (July 1939) 113: 32–35; Kenny to Dear Sir [Manager of Brisbane and South Coast Hospitals Board], September 19 1939, Kenny, Fryer Library; see also Alexander *Maverick*, 110.

79. Kenny to Sir [E. M. Hanlon], February 19 1940, Home Secretary's Office, Special Batches, Kenny Clinics, 1941–1949, A/31753, QSA.

80. [Cohn interview with] Jarvis Nye, April 23 1953, Cohn Papers, MHS-K; see also Alexander *Maverick*, 112; E. M. Hanlon to Dear Miss Kenny, February 21 1940, Home Secretary's Office, Special Batches, Kenny Clinics, 1941–1949, A/31753, QSA. Note that she had sent letters to federal and state officials pointing out both "the humane value of the work" and its potential "financial gain" for the federal and state governments; see, for example, Kenny to Sir [Mr. Watson, Under Secretary, Chief Secretary's Department], February 14 1940, Home Secretary's Office, Special Batches, Kenny Clinics, 1941–1949, A/31753, QSA.

81. Lee, Nye, Pye, Arden, and Fryberg To Whom It May Concern March 12, 1940; Series A981/1, United States 148, AA-ACT; Forgan Smith to Dear Sir [Basil O'Connor], March 11 1940, Series A981/1, United States 148, AA-ACT; Alan Fletcher to Minister for Health, December 18 1939; Series A981/1, United States 148, AA-ACT.

82. See, for example, Paul de Kruif *Microbe Hunters* (New York: Harcourt, Brace Jovanovich, 1926); de Kruif *Men Against Death* (New York: Harcourt, Brace & Co., 1932); de Kruif *The Fight for Life* (New York: Harcourt Brace, 1938).

83. Kenny with Ostenso *And They Shall Walk*, 207. See also Kenny to Mrs. M. G. McCrae, January 16 1942, in Box 3, Folder 12, OM 65-17, Charles Chuter Papers, John Oxley Library, State Library of Queensland, Brisbane (hereafter Oxley-SLQ).

84. Kenny with Ostenso *And They Shall Walk*, 209; Henry Otis Kendall and Florence P. Kendall *Care During the Recovery Period in Paralytic Poliomyelitis* (Washington, DC: Government Printing Office, 1938, revised 1939, Public Health Service Bulletin No. 242). This Bulletin was cited consistently in Kenny's 1941 textbook; Kenny *Treatment of Infantile Paralysis*. In 1944 Kenny claimed that Cusack had given her the pamphlet saying that "this was the accepted work of the United States of America and no institution was interested in investigating my presentation"; Kenny "My Message to the People of the United States of America," [1944] Evidence-Reports, Box 1, MHS-K.

85. "My method introduces an entirely original conception in the treatment of poliomyelitis" that was "exactly the opposite to methods now employed"; "Australia Brings American Medicine New Method of Treating Infantile Paralysis" *Los Angeles Times* April 16 1940; see Cohn *Sister Kenny*, 126.

86. Kenny with Ostenso *And They Shall Walk*, 209.

87. Kenny with Ostenso *And They Shall Walk*, 210.

88. Kenny with Ostenso *And They Shall Walk*, 210–211; see also Paul *A History*, 313. Rivers' later version of refusing to meet Kenny is only slightly different; see Saul Benison *Tom Rivers: Reflections on a Life in Medicine and Science* (Cambridge: MIT Press, 1967), 282–284; see also Tony Gould *A Summer Plague: Polio and Its Survivors* (New Haven: Yale University Press, 1995), 96.

89. Richard Carter *The Gentle Legions* (Garden City, NY: Doubleday, 1961), 116–121.

90. Jessie L. Stevenson *The Nursing Care of Patients with Infantile Paralysis* (New York: National Foundation for Infantile Paralysis, 1940).

91. Roy L. Chambliss, Jr. "A Social History of the National Foundation of Infantile Paralysis, Inc, 1938–1948," Master of Science in Social Service dissertation, Fordham University School of Social Service, New York, 1950, Public Relations, History, March of Dimes Archives, White Plains, New York (hereafter MOD), 83.

92. Telegram from Australian Legation to Department of External Affairs, Canberra, April 18 1940, Series A981/1, United States 148, AA-ACT. On Casey see Hudson *Casey*.

93. Chief Quarantine Officer [Brisbane] to J. H. L. Cumpston, April 22 1940, Series A981/1, United States 148, AA-ACT.

94. Director-General of Health to Secretary, Department of External Affairs, Memorandum, April 23 1940, Series A981/1, United States 148, AA-ACT; External Affairs to Australian Legation, April 24 1940, telegram, Series A981/1, United States 148, AA-ACT; External Affairs to Australian Legation, May 7 1940, Series A981/1, United States 148, AA-ACT.

95. Mrs. Salena Thomas, R.N. to Roosevelt, February 28 1940 [abstract] FDR-OF-1930, Infantile Paralysis 1934–1942, Box 1, Franklin Delano Roosevelt Presidential Library and Museum Archives, Hyde Park (hereafter FDR Papers).

96. C. H. Scott to M. A. LeHand [forwarded to Basil O'Connor], February 2 1940 [abstract] FDR-PPF-4885 (Comm. Celeb. President's Birthday Cross-Refs 1939–1940), FDR Papers; also C. H Scott to Wilson Comptons [abstract], [January] 1940, FDR-OF-1930, Infantile Paralysis 1934–1942, Box 1, FDR Papers; these inquiries were also sent to Eleanor Roosevelt.

97. O'Connor graduated from Dartmouth in 1912 and from Harvard Law School in 1915. While his dapper clothes and luxurious lifestyle were at times attacked as signs of "excessive fund raising and egregious razzle-dazzle," O'Connor boasted that he received no salary from

the NFIP and that his insistence "on traveling de luxe" was a deliberate tactic designed to show everyone that the NFIP was "something special"; Paul *A History*, 308–309; Alden Whitman "Basil O'Connor, Polio Crusader, Died" *New York Times* March 10 1972; Carter *The Gentle Legions*, 100–106; Timothy Takaro "The Man in the Middle" *Dartmouth Medicine* (Fall 2004) 29: 52–57.

98. Kenny with Ostenso *And They Shall Walk*, 211; see also O'Connor's recollection that he and Gudakunst had listened to her for 3 hours, [Cohn interview with] Basil O'Connor, June 20 1955, Cohn Papers, MHS-K.

99. [Cohn interview with] Basil O'Connor, June 20 1955, Cohn Papers, MHS-K.

100. Kenny with Ostenso *And They Shall Walk*, 212, 213.

101. Kenny with Ostenso *And They Shall Walk*, 212. For a slightly different version of the Chicago visit in which Fishbein suggested that O'Connor send Kenny to Chicago so that Harry Mock, head of the AMA's Council on Physical Therapy, could interview her see Morris Fishbein *Morris Fishbein, M.D. An Autobiography* (Garden City, NY: Doubleday & Co., 1969), 230–231. According to Kenny she had "personally interviewed" Mr. Carter and Dr. Coulter "both of whom informed me no material was available in Chicago;" Kenny to Dear Dr. Gudakunst, June 10 1940, Public Relations, Kenny Files, March of Dimes (hereafter MOD-K); see also Kenny to Dear Mr. Chuter, May 28 1940, Home Secretary's Office, Special Batches, Kenny Clinics, 1941–1949, A/31753, QSA.

102. Kenny with Ostenso *And They Shall Walk*, 212–213; Paul *A History*, 225–231; The same argument was used to dismiss work by Australian virologists Francis Macfarlane Burnet and Jean Macnamara, who had published crucial but largely ignored research in 1931 showing more than one type of polio virus; Paul *A History*, 239.

103. Kenny with Ostenso *And They Shall Walk*, 213. The therapists were probably Gertrude Beard and her assistant Elizabeth Wood.

104. Kenny with Ostenso *And They Shall Walk*, 213–214, 218.

105. H. J. Wilkinson to M. Henderson, March 8 1940, Inv. Physicians Letter, 1939–1940, MHS-K; see also Geoffrey Kenny "Wilkinson, Herbert John (1891–1963)" in *Australian Dictionary of Biography* (Melbourne: Melbourne University Press, 2002), 16: 547–548; Wilkinson "Foreword" Kenny *Infantile Paralysis and Cerebral Diplegia*, i–xvii. He had visited Europe and the United States as a Rockefeller Fellow a decade earlier.

106. Melvin S. Henderson to Dear Dr. Wilkinson, April 9 1940, Home Secretary's Office, Special Batches, Kenny Clinics, 1941–1949, A/31753, QSA. Henderson told Wilkinson he had spoken to Cole who was in charge of Gillette Hospital for Crippled Children, which was used by the University for teaching purposes and that "Dr. Cole would like very much to have Sister Kenny visit Gillette Hospital."

107. Frank H. Krusen *Physical Medicine: The Employment of Physical Agents for Diagnosis and Therapy* (Philadelphia, PA: W. B. Saunders Company, 1941); Krusen and John Kolmer *Light Therapy* (New York: Paul B. Hoeber, 1933); Krusen *Physical Therapy in Arthritis* (New York: Paul B. Hoeber, 1937). See also Kenny to Dear Mr. Chuter, May 28 1940, Home Secretary's Office, Special Batches, Kenny Clinics, 1941–1949, A/31753, QSA. A tuberculosis survivor, Frank Hammond Krusen (1898–1973) (Jefferson MD) had set up the first physical therapy training program for physicians at Temple University Hospital in 1929. At the Mayo Clinic he directed the nation's first 3-year physical medicine residency program. He had written physical therapy textbooks for physicians and nurses and also directed the Mayo Clinic's physical therapy training program, which had graduated its first class only a year earlier; "Dr. Frank Krusen of Mayo Clinic, 75" *New York Times* September 18 1973; Glenn Gritzer and Arnold Arluke *The Making of*

Rehabilitation: The Political Economy of Medical Specialization, 1890–1980 (Berkeley: University of California Press, 1985), 87–88. Krusen had coined the term "Physiatrist" as a way of distinguishing physician specialists from physical therapists; G. Keith Stillwell "In Memoriam: Frank H. Krusen, M.D. 1898–1973" *Archives of Physical Medicine and Rehabilitation* (November 1973) 54: 493–495.

108. Krusen, "Observations on the Kenny Treatment of Poliomyelitis" *Proceedings of the Staff Meetings of the Mayo Clinic* (August 12 1942) 17: 450; [Cohn interview with] Frank Krusen, March 24 1953, Cohn Papers, MHS-K.

109. Henderson had given Kenny an introduction to Wallace Cole, head of orthopedic surgery at the University of Minnesota; Melvin S. Henderson to Dear Dr. Wilkinson, April 9 1940, Home Secretary's Office, Special Batches, Kenny Clinics, 1941–1949, A/31753, QSA.

110. Kenny with Ostenso *And They Shall Walk*, 217–220; see also Kenny to Dear Mr. President, September 2 1940, Public Relations, MOD-K.

111. Kenny with Ostenso *And They Shall Walk*, 220–221; Kenny "Paper Read at the Northwestern Pediatric Conference, Nov. 14, 1940, Saint Paul University Club, "Kendall Collection"; "Lecture given at Minneapolis General Hospital, August 12 1940" in Kenny *Treatment of Infantile Paralysis*, 116.

112. Kenny with Ostenso *And They Shall Walk*, 220–221.

113. Krusen "Observations," 450. See also Krusen on Knapp as "the most patient soul that ever lived"; [Cohn interview with] Frank Krusen, March 24 1953, Cohn Papers, MHS-K. Miland Knapp had received his MD from the University of Minnesota in 1929 and became interested in physical medicine but had struggled unsuccessfully to set up a specialty practice limited to physical therapy in Chicago, despite support from John Coulter, until he had returned to Minneapolis where he was appointed as the head of a physical therapy department at the Minnesota General Hospital; [Cohn third interview with] Miland Knapp, August 24 1963, Cohn Papers, MHS-K; see also Russell J. N. Dean *Rehabilitation for America's Disabled* (New York: Hastings House, 1972), 56–58.

114. Kenny with Ostenso *And They Shall Walk*, 221; Alexander *Maverick*, 118–119; Krusen "Observations," 451; [Cohn third interview with] Miland Knapp, August 24 1963, Cohn Papers, MHS-K.

115. For a suggestion about Midwestern openness see Alexander *Maverick*, 128–129.

116. Kenny "Paper Read at the Northwestern Pediatric Conference, Nov. 14, 1940, Saint Paul University Club."

117. Mary Pohl, interview with Naomi Rogers, August 21 2003, Tallahassee, Florida; "John F. Pohl" [Biographical Information] in Supplementary Data, Committee to Review Request of Elizabeth Kenny Institute to National Foundation for Infantile Paralysis: General, Medical Sciences, 1944, National Academy of Sciences, Washington, D.C. He also visited the Manchester Royal Infirmary and then spent a year as a resident in neurosurgery at the Boston Children's Hospital.

118. Kenny with Ostenso *And They Shall Walk*, 225–227; Henry M. Haverstock To Whom It May Concern, September 4 1940, Public Relations, MOD-K. Haverstock later remembered his parents asking her to stop reading her testimonials and begin her examination; Gould *Summer Plague*, 96–98; Alexander *Maverick*, 118–119.

119. Kenny with Ostenso *And They Shall Walk*, 225–227.

120. Kenny *Treatment of Infantile Paralysis*, 270.

121. O'Connor to Cole, September 10 1940, FDR-OF-1930, Infantile Paralysis 1934–1942 Box 1, FDR Papers.

122. Kline "The Most Unforgettable Character I've Met," 203–208; see also Harold S. Diehl "Summary of the Relationship of the Medical School of the University of Minnesota to the work of Sister Elizabeth Kenny" May 1944, Public Relations, MOD-K.

123. Kenny with Ostenso *And They Shall Walk*, 223.

124. Chuter to Dear Sister Kenny, July 15 1940, Wilson Collection.

125. Evelyn P. Holmberg to Dear Sir [O'Connor], November 13 1940, Public Relations, MOD--K.

126. Kenny "Report of Activities: June, 1940–1943," FDR-OF-5188, Sister Elizabeth Kenny Institute, 1940–1944, FDR Papers.

127. Robert Gurney in Edmund J. Sass with George Gottfried and Anthony Sorem eds. *Polio's Legacy: An Oral History* (Lanham, MD: University Press of America, 1996), 25.

128. See Alexander *Maverick*, 45–50.

129. Kenny to Dear Dr. Diehl, June 21 1943, Dr. Harold S. Diehl, 1941–1944, MHS-K.

130. Kenny to Dear Sir [O'Connor], June 24 1940, Public Relations, MOD-K; on the delay between May and September see Diehl "Summary."

131. Alexander *Maverick*, 85–87, 92; [Cohn interview with] Mary and Stuart McCracken, April 14 1953, Cohn Papers, MHS-K; Cohn *Sister Kenny*, 69–70. Mary Moore Kenny died on December 20 1937 when she was 93; [Chris Sharpe] Interview with Mary Stewart Kenny McCracken and Stuart McCracken, July 3–4 1998, Chris Sharpe Collection, in author's possession.

132. Kenny to Dear Dr. Diehl, June 21 1943, Dr. Harold S. Diehl, 1941–1944, MHS-K. See also Abe Altrowitz "Under Your Hat" *Minneapolis Tribune* November 1943, Box 19, Sister Kenny Institute 1938–1948, Myers Papers, UMN-ASC.

133. Henry W. Haverstock to Senator Henrik Shipstead, July 3 1940, Series A981/1, United States 148, AA-ACT. Shipstead (1881–1960), a dentist, was elected first to the Senate as a member of the Farmer-Labor Party in 1922, and later in 1940 as a Republican. Kenny also wrote directly to Richard Casey at the Australian legation, suggesting the Australian government provide $150 a month to "assist and promote a friendly feeling so much to be desired in the present troublesome times" and "earn the gratitude of the people of the United States of America forever"; Kenny to Australian Legation, July 6 1940, Series A981/1, United States 148, AA-ACT; see also Henrik Shipstead to Australian Legation, July 6 1940, Series A981/1, United States 148, AA-ACT. With the knowledge he had gained from earlier inquiries, Casey was not sympathetic. He reminded Kenny and Shipstead that Kenny's visit "was not sponsored in any way" by the Australian government. He further pointed out that during the European war "the need at the present time [was] to conserve as many dollars as possible in this country"; R. G. Casey to Kenny, July 12 1940, Series A981/1, United States 148, AA-ACT; R. G. Casey to Shipstead, July 12 1940, Series A981/1, United States 148, AA-ACT.

134. Kenny to Dear Dr. Diehl, June 21 1943, Dr. Harold S. Diehl, 1941–1944, MHS-K; Kenny to Gentleman, July 3 1940, Series A981/1, United States 148, AA-ACT.

135. Arthur D. Reynolds to Keith Morgan, September 5 1940, Public Relations, MOD-K.

136. O'Connor to Reynolds, September 17 1940, Public Relations, MOD-K.

137. Reynolds to O'Connor, November 29 1940, Public Relations, MOD-K. Note that she told reporters in 1940 that her 20 years of effort had been "entirely gratuitous"; "Australia Brings American Medicine New Method of Treatment Infantile Paralysis" *Los Angeles Times* April 16 1940; see also "She reports that she is doing this work free of charge in the interest of science"; Henry M. Haverstock To Whom It May Concern, September 4 1940, Public Relations, MOD-K.

138. Kenny to Dear Mr. President, September 2 1940, Public Relations, MOD-K; Kenny to Roosevelt, September 2 1940 [abstract] FDR-OF-5188, Sister Elizabeth Kenny Institute 1940–1944, FDR Papers; see also Henry M. Haverstock To Whom It May Concern, September 4 1940, Public Relations, MOD-K.

139. Kenny to Dear Mr. President, September 6 1940, Public Relations, MOD-K; Kenny to Roosevelt, September 6 1940 [abstract], FDR-OF-5188, Sister Elizabeth Kenny Institute 1940–1944, FDR Papers.

140. O'Connor to Cole, September 10 1940, FDR-OF-1930, Infantile Paralysis 1934–1942, Box 1, FDR Papers.

141. Cole to Kenny, September 9 1940, Cole, Dr. Wallace H. 1940–1947, MHS-K. Between August and November 1940 Kenny received $180 a month; Diehl to My Dear Sister Kenny, April 13 1944, Dr. Harold S. Diehl, 1941–1944, MHS-K.

142. Kenny *And They Shall Walk*, 254.

143. Kenny to Dear Dr. Cole, September 12 1940, Public Relations, MOD-K.

144. Kenny to Dear Mr. Chuter, May 28 1940, Home Secretary's Office, Special Batches, Kenny Clinics, 1941–1949, A/31753, QSA; see also Kenny to Dear Mr. Chuter, November 15 1940, Home Secretary's Office, Special Batches, Kenny Clinics, 1941–1949, A/31753, QSA.

145. Diehl, "Summary."

146. Miland E. Knapp to Dear Doctor Diehl, March 10 1944, [accessed in 1992 before recent re-cataloging] Am 15.8, Folder 1, UMN-ASC; Wallace H. Cole and Miland E. Knapp "The Kenny Treatment of Infantile Paralysis: A Preliminary Report" *Journal of the American Medical Association* (June 7 1941) 116: 2577–2580; and see Wallace H. Cole, John F. Pohl, and Miland E. Knapp "The Kenny Method of Treatment for Infantile Paralysis" *Archives of Physical Therapy* (1942) 23: 399–418, also published as a separate pamphlet by the National Foundation for Infantile Paralysis (Publication No. 40, 1942); see also Diehl "Summary."

147. Kenny to Dear Dr. Diehl, June 21 1943, Dr. Harold S. Diehl, 1941–1944, MHS-K.

FURTHER READING

On polio in Australia see Kerry Highley "Mending Bodies: Polio in Australia," Ph.D. thesis in History of Medicine, 2009, Australian National University, ACT; Anne Killalea *The Great Scourge: The Tasmanian Infantile Paralysis Epidemic 1937–1938* (Hobart: Tasmanian Historical Research Association, 1995); Milton J. Lewis *The People's Health: Public Health in Australia, 1950 to the Present* (Westport: Praeger Publishers, 2003), 37–42; Barry Smith "The Victorian Poliomyelitis Epidemic 1937–1938" in John C. Calwell et al. ed. *What We Know About [the] Health Transition: The Cultural, Social and Behavioural Determinates of Health: The Proceedings of an International Workshop, Canberra, May 1989* (ANU Printing Service, Canberra, [1990], vol. 2), 866–881; John Smith "The Polio Epidemics in Australia 1895–1962 With Specific Reference to Western Australia," Ph.D. thesis in History, 1997, Edith Cowan University, Perth.

On polio in North America see Tony Gould *A Summer Plague: Polio and Its Survivors* (New Haven: Yale University Press, 1995); David M. Oshinsky *Polio: An American Story* (New York: Oxford University Press, 2005); John R. Paul, *A History of Poliomyelitis* (New Haven: Yale University Press, 1971); Naomi Rogers *Dirt and Disease: Polio before FDR* (New Brunswick, NJ: Rutgers University Press, 1992); Christopher Rutty "Do Something! Do Anything! Poliomyelitis in Canada, 1927–1962," Ph.D. Thesis, 1995,

University of Toronto; Rutty "The Middle-Class Plague: Epidemic Polio and the Canadian State, 1936–1937" *Canadian Bulletin of Medical History* (1996) 13: 277–314; Jane S. Smith *Patenting the Sun: Polio and the Salk Vaccine* (New York: William Morrow, 1990); Daniel J. Wilson *Living with Polio: The Epidemic and its Survivors* (Chicago: University of Chicago Press, 2005).

On nursing in Australia see Elizabeth Burchill *Australian Nurses since Nightingale 1860–1990* (Richmond: Spectrum Publications, 1992); Angela Cushing *A Contextual Perspective to Female Nursing in Victoria, 1850–1914* (Geelong: Deakin University Press, 1993); Mary Dickenson *An Unsentimental Union: The NSW Nurses Association 1931–1992* (Sydney: Hale and Ironmonger, 1993); Judith Godden and Carol Helmstadter "Woman's Mission and Professional Knowledge: Nightingale Nursing in Colonial Australia and Canada" *Social History of Medicine* (2004) 17: 157–174; Rupert Goodman ed. *Queensland Nurses: Boer War to Vietnam* (Bowen Hills: Boolarong Publications, 1985); Helen Gregory *A Tradition of Care: A History of Nursing at the Royal Brisbane Hospital* (Brisbane: Boolarong Publication, 1988); Ruth Lynette Russell *From Nightingale to Now: Nurse Education in Australia* (Sydney: Harcourt, Brace Jovanovich, 1990); Bartz Schultz *A Tapestry of Service: The Evolution of Nursing in Australia* (Melbourne: Churchill Livingstone, 1991); Glenda Strachan *Labour of Love: The History of the Nurses Association in Queensland 1860–1950* (St. Leonards, NSW: Allen & Unwin, 1996).

On nursing in North America see Patricia D'Antonio *American Nursing: A History of Knowledge, Authority, and the Meaning of Work* (Baltimore: Johns Hopkins University Press, 2010); Kathryn McPherson *Bedside Matters: The Transformation of Canadian Nursing, 1900–1990* (Toronto: Oxford University Press, 1996); Barbara Melosh *The Physician's Hand: Work Culture and Conflict in American Nursing* (Philadelphia: Temple University Press, 1982); Susan M. Reverby *Ordered to Care: The Dilemma of American Nursing, 1850–1945* (Cambridge: Cambridge University Press, 1987).

There is no complete history of the National Foundation but see Angela N. H. Creager *The Life of a Virus: Tobacco Mosaic Virus as an Experimental Model, 1930–1965* (Chicago: University of Chicago, 2001); Scott Cutlip *Fund Raising in the United States* (New Brunswick: Rutgers University Press, 1965); Tony Gould *A Summer Plague: Polio and Its Survivors* (New Haven: Yale University Press, 1995); Sydney A. Halpern *Lesser Harms: The Morality of Risk in Medical Research* (Chicago: University of Chicago Press, 2004); Lawrence Friedman and Mark McGarvie eds. *Charity, Philanthropy, and Civility in American History* (New York: Cambridge University Press, 2002); Stephen E. Mawdsley "'Dancing on Eggs': Charles H. Bynum, Racial Politics, and the National Foundation for Infantile Paralysis, 1938–1943" *Bulletin of the History of Medicine* (2010) 84: 217–247; David M. Oshinsky *Polio: An American Story* (New York: Oxford University Press, 2005); John R. Paul *A History of Poliomyelitis* (New Haven: Yale University Press, 1971); David W. Rose *March of Dimes: Images of America* (Charleston: Arcadia, 2003); Jane S. Smith *Patenting the Sun: Polio and the Salk Vaccine* (New York: William Morrow, 1990); Olivier Zunz *Philanthropy in America: A History* (Princeton: Princeton University Press, 2012).

On Kenny see Wade Alexander *Sister Elizabeth Kenny: Maverick Heroine of the Polio Treatment Controversy* (Rockhampton: Central Queensland University Press, 2002); Victor Cohn *Sister Kenny: The Woman Who Challenged the Doctors* (Minneapolis: University of Minnesota Press, 1975); Philippa Martyr *Paradise of Quacks: An Alternative History of Medicine in Australia* (Paddington N.S.W.: Macleay Press, 2002); Philippa Martyr "'A Small Price to Pay for Peace': The Elizabeth Kenny Controversy Reexamined" *Australian Historical Studies* (1997)

27: 47–65; Evan Willis "Sister Elizabeth Kenny and the Evolution of the Occupational Division of Labour in Health Care" *Australian and New Zealand Journal of Sociology* (1979) 15: 30–38; John R. Wilson "Sister Elizabeth Kenny's Trial by Royal Commission" *History of Nursing Journal* (1992–1993) 4: 91–99; John R. Wilson "The Sister Kenny Clinics: What Endures?" *Australian Journal of Advanced Nursing* (1986) 3: 13–21; John R. Wilson *Through Kenny's Eyes: An Exploration of Sister Elizabeth Kenny's Views about Nursing* (Townsville: Royal College of Nursing Australia, 1995).

On American medicine and consumerism in the early to mid-twentieth century see Deborah Stone "The Doctor as Businessman: The Changing Politics of a Cultural Icon" *Journal of Health Politics, Policy and Law* (1997) 22: 533–556; Nancy Tomes "The Great American Medicine Show Revisited" *Bulletin of the History of Medicine* (2005) 79: 627–663; Nancy Tomes "Merchants of Health: Medicine and Consumer Culture in the United States, 1900–1940" *Journal of American History* (2001) 88: 519–547; James Harvey Young *The Medical Messiahs: A Social History of Health Quackery in Twentieth-Century America* (Princeton: Princeton University Press, 1967).

On homogenization of the American medical profession see Robert B. Baker, Arthur L. Caplan, Linda L. Emanuel, and Stephen R. Latham eds. *The American Medical Ethics Revolution: How the AMA's Code of Ethics Has Transformed Physicians' Relationships to Patients, Professionals, and Society* (Baltimore: Johns Hopkins University Press, 1999); Barbara Barzansky and Norman Gevitz eds. *Beyond Flexner: Medical Education in the Twentieth Century* (Westport: Greenwood Press, 1992); Gert H. Brieger "Getting Into Medical School in the Good Old Days: Good for Whom?" *Annals of Internal Medicine* (1993) 119: 1138–1143; James G. Burrow *AMA: Voice of American Medicine* (Baltimore: Johns Hopkins University Press, 1963); Jonathan Engel *Doctors and Reformers: Discussion and Debate over Health Policy 1925–1950* (Charleston: University of South Carolina Press, 2002); Michael R. Grey *New Deal Medicine: The Rural Health Programs of the Farm Security Administration* (Baltimore: Johns Hopkins University Press, 1999); Susan E. Lederer *Subjected to Science: Human Experimentation in American before the Second World War* (Baltimore: Johns Hopkins University Press, 1995); Kenneth M. Ludmerer *Time to Heal: American Medicine from the Turn of the Century to the Era of Managed Care* (New York: Oxford University Press, 1999); Dan A. Oren *Joining the Club: A History of Jews and Yale* (New Haven: Yale University Press, 1985); Elton Rayak *Professional Power and American Medicine: The Economics of the American Medical Association* (Cleveland: World Publishing Company, 1967); Janet Tighe "Never Knowing One's Place: Temple University School of Medicine and the American Medical Education Hierarchy" *Transactions and Studies of the College of Physicians of Philadelphia* (1990) 12: 311–334.

On the history of Warm Springs and disability politics in this period see Daniel Holland "Franklin D. Roosevelt's Shangri-La: Foreshadowing the Independent Living Movement in Warm Springs, Georgia, 1926–1945" *Disability & Society* (2006) 21: 513–535; Paul K. Longmore and David Goldberger "The League of the Physically Handicapped and the Great Depression: A Case Study in the New Disability History" *Journal of American History* (2000) 87: 888–922; Naomi Rogers "Polio Chronicles: Warm Springs and Disability Politics in the 1930s" *Asclepio: Revista de Historia de la Medicine y de la Ciencia* (2009) 61: 143–174; Naomi Rogers "Race and the Politics of Polio: Warm Springs, Tuskegee and the March of Dimes" *American Journal of Public Health* (2007) 97: 2–13.

2

The Battle Begins

WORKING UNDER THE auspices of the University of Minnesota and funded by the National Foundation for Infantile Paralysis (NFIP) Kenny made the Twin Cities her base. Along with her Australian assistants she treated patients in local hospitals, taught local nurses and physical therapists, and lectured to physicians. The Minneapolis health department received floods of letters from people who had read that Kenny had "demonstrated cures in 17 out of 36 cases" and came with their children hoping for a similar result. The University of Minnesota's hospital opened a special polio clinic for patients from outside the state, while the city hospital continued to treat local patients.[1] In June 1941 *JAMA* published the first serious study of Kenny's patients by physicians from the university's medical school praising her methods and defending her new symptoms. After this publication in the nation's most prominent medical journal augmented by stories in the popular press Kenny's work in Minneapolis began to attract wider attention. Kenny began to travel to medical societies and hospitals lecturing and demonstrating her methods.

Not willing to base its assessment of her credibility solely on the authority of sympathetic local physicians, the NFIP sent a group of skeptical physical therapists to Minneapolis, a meeting destined to end disastrously. The visiting therapists were intrigued and yet also irritated by this usurper. They debated not only her practices and theories but also her personality, especially her shocking lack of deference. The meeting left 2 Baltimore therapists convinced that both Kenny and her work were irrational and probably harmful while the other 3 remained willing to be impressed. Even though the 2 critical therapists sent the NFIP a report rejecting Kenny's methods and her attacks on standard polio therapy, the NFIP nonetheless continued to support her work and began to urge its local and state chapters to send doctors, nurses, and physical therapists to learn this new method. Simultaneously the NFIP assured skeptics that its medical advisors were still evaluating its value. Basil O'Connor sent his medical director and a few other physicians to Minneapolis to get additional reports and kept in close touch with Morris Fishbein, the American Medical Association's (AMA's) powerful general secretary. Behind the scenes Fishbein not only shaped the first formal publications by Minnesota physicians but also edited and censored journalists' stories of Kenny and her work to make sure they did not exaggerate her achievements. In her own effort to gain national attention and public sympathy, using skills well honed in Australia, Kenny cooperated with the *Reader's Digest* for an article that made her into a heroic figure and also compiled her lectures into a textbook that was published by a local publisher. Efforts by the NFIP and Fishbein to try to rein her in were in vain.

NFIP CAUTION

Although NFIP officials hoped Kenny's work would be a major step toward achieving victory over polio, they hesitated. Like many other American disease philanthropies, the NFIP had been established by people outside the medical profession, and its local and state chapters were still mostly directed by members of the public. All research funding, however, was supervised by nationally recognized physicians who met once or twice a year to assess worthy applications. Led by the conservative virologist Thomas Rivers, the NFIP's advisory committee on scientific research funded mostly laboratory investigations of the characteristics of the polio virus.[2]

The funding of polio therapies or other clinical research was overseen by the NFIP's Aftereffects Committee, chaired by orthopedic surgeon Philip Lewin. Its members were orthopedists known for their skepticism. Any unusual innovator, especially someone who was not a specialist or who worked outside an elite medical school, was not taken seriously. Indeed the NFIP prided itself on its unwelcoming attitude to aspiring clinical discoverers, especially men or women who had discovered a polio "cure" and therapists who ran alternative healing centers. At his first meeting with Kenny in 1940, O'Connor had made it clear that the NFIP would consider sponsoring her work only if it were supervised by physicians at a recognized medical institution.[3] These cautious policies were all efforts to appease the wider culture of American medicine in which skepticism was the sine qua non of the professional, the opposite of the public's interest in every amazing healer. Yet the NFIP was now funding a nurse, who, local papers claimed, was remarkable, perhaps even a kind of miracle worker. Physicians at the Mayo Clinic like physical medicine specialist Frank Krusen had so far kept their distance, a clear difference from city officials and local physicians who had allowed Kenny and her assistants to practice in the city hospital and instruct its nursing staff.

Most of the research funded by the NFIP in the late 1930s and early 1940s had little to do with polio's clinical symptoms. Conferences on polio usually did not include clinicians or physiologists, reflecting both the dearth of physiological polio research and the sense that there were few new facts to be learned. The failure of trials of a chemical nasal spray in the 1930s had led many investigators to question the validity of the concept of the nose and mouth as the virus's natural portal of entry.[4] The idea of alternate routes through the body was slowly moving polio away from its fixed neurological categorization. Although Yale epidemiologist John Paul admitted he could offer "no good explanation to account for the presence of the virus in the intestinal tract," he and his Yale colleagues were confident that they had found the virus in the sewers of New Haven and New York. This unusual evidence suggested that polio might not solely be a neurological infection and that levels of the virus might be endemic among communities without causing dramatic paralytic symptoms.[5] No one was certain exactly how the polio virus spread through the body or from one person to another or what predicted an individual's resistance to developing paralysis. Reflecting this confusion, the NFIP funded studies on the influence of dietary deficiencies (University of Wisconsin); metabolic factors influencing damage to nerve cells (New York University); the effect of chemicals on the virus (Michigan Department of Health); the role of the virus in dust, nervous tissue, and stools (Stanford University); vitamins, calories, and nutrition (University of Pennsylvania and Wayne University); hormones and diet (University of Utah); and epidemiological factors including domestic animals as a reservoir (University of Chicago).[6]

Kenny's challenge to polio care pointed to a vacuum in medical research and in clinical practice. In every medical textbook the polio virus was believed to damage or destroy nerve cells, leading to paralysis through the disruption or severing of connections between nerves and muscles. But in Kenny's view the polio virus affected not only the nervous system, but also the rest of the body, especially the muscles, tissue, and skin. To explain why some patients improved and others did not she blamed the pessimistic attitude of many professionals, as well as their ignorance of what was causing the patient's symptoms, particularly pain and spasm, which she felt clinicians did not recognize or take seriously. For many patients, she believed, the virus did not destroy the connection between nerve and muscle but left some muscles in spasm, the result of disordered corresponding nerve cells. Connections between nerves and muscles could therefore be repaired through directed muscle therapy. Kenny believed that her knowledge of paralyzed muscles and their function enabled her to see a different disease when she looked at polio patients. Thus, she argued that the whole orthodox concept of polio was incorrect: doctors did not understand the "true symptoms" of the disease and therefore treated the wrong disease.

Still, Kenny's work was easily categorized as continuing elements of already existing polio care rather than as an innovation. Techniques for the management of pain and for muscle training were the province of orthopedic nurses and physical therapists supervised by orthopedists and the small group of doctors who specialized in physical medicine. To defuse any suspicions that local physicians had somehow been swayed by Kenny's personality and by the enthusiasm of the public and lost their ability to judge her work with scientific objectivity, the NFIP needed to organize some form of outside assessment. As a way of identifying this work as a potential contribution to physical therapy rather to the more prestigious fields of polio science or clinical diagnosis, the NFIP decided to send Kenny's supposed peers to assess this work: nationally recognized physical therapists. This was an effort to pigeonhole Kenny as a nurse with a useful technical innovation.

This was a meeting destined to ignite tensions. The therapists came, uneasy about the extravagant claims they had heard but recognizing that local therapists and their medical supervisors were taking this unusual nurse seriously. For her part, Kenny greeted the visitors suspiciously. She had little experience with sympathetic physical therapists. In the 1930s therapists at the Brisbane General Hospital had laughed at her during a clinical demonstration, and the Queensland branch of the Australian Massage Association had rejected her trained nurses from hospital positions as they lacked proper training in physical therapy.

Still, her initial experience in Minneapolis pleasantly surprised her. She had begun teaching a small group of local physical therapists and nurses, and, with the support of senior hospital clinicians, found it possible to challenge their previous ideas and practices. Many of the local therapists had expressed great enthusiasm about Kenny's work. The local branch of the American Physical Therapy Association (APTA), "a very earnest group of women" she recalled in her autobiography, had invited her to dinner to talk about her work. These women, Kenny noted, became "devoted exponents of my conception of infantile paralysis" and later were among the first to get certificates from her training course at the university.[7] By January 1941 around 20 physical therapists from the Twin Cities were spending "practically all of their free time" with Kenny, giving up their Saturdays and Sundays.[8] Nonetheless, she feared that outside therapists would be likely to judge any innovative clinical practice that looked odd as wrong and harmful.

Kenny's keen sense of the workings of gender and medical authority had left her convinced that changing polio's clinical care could not be achieved solely by convincing nurses and physical therapists. She saw physical therapists and nurses as simply foot soldiers in the war against polio. To have clinical change properly and scientifically achieved, the crucial task, as she saw it, was to convince America's prominent physicians, who could then issue definite statements that would assure their skeptical peers of the worth of her work and the importance of rejecting old ways and embracing the new. These visitors were technicians without sufficient medical training or status to assess her new understanding of the symptoms of polio. This view, indeed, was shared by many orthopedic surgeons who also saw physical therapists as "hands" who carried out doctors' orders, not as specialists with a distinctive understanding of medical practices based on scientific knowledge.

Kenny herself acted not like any ordinary nurse but as a cross between an inventor and a scientific discoverer. She spoke to doctors assertively, sometimes arrogantly. In Australia she had become used to how the worth of her work was linked to her character. In 1937 a Sydney orthopedist had denigrated her with faint praise as "a woman of enthusiasm, energy and organizing ability," and her Queensland antagonist Raphael Cilento saw her as

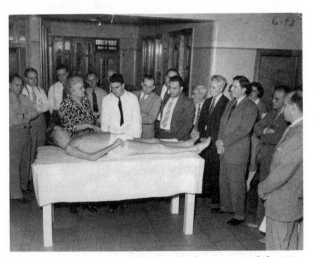

FIGURE 2.1 Kenny explaining her method to a group of physicians in a corridor of the Minneapolis General Hospital [1942]. Box 9, Elizabeth Kenny Papers, Minnesota Historical Society, St Paul.

"a most difficult woman to work with" and "somewhat intolerant of other people's views."[9] Certainly, one of the ways she was "difficult" was the fact that as a nurse—and therefore a woman and a professional inferior—she dared to tell physicians that they were wrong.

To inculcate clinical change required recognition of the politics of medicine, and its sources of cultural and institutional power. Gender—especially as it was expressed in the hierarchy of medical schools and hospitals—was a crucial ingredient in this equation. Kenny had enjoyed an unusual amount of clinical and professional autonomy as the result of her work as a bush nurse, a private duty nurse, and director of her own clinics and wards. This work provided her with clinical, pedagogical, and administrative experience. She saw the way hospital nurses were supposed to keep their eyes to the floor and their hands behind their backs when they talked to physicians. She taught many physical therapists and nurses who became her friends, but she rarely joined their typical socializing. The close connections she most desired were with physicians; and this goal structured her work in Minneapolis as she prevailed on medical experts to visit her, watch her work, and listen to her lecture.

THE THERAPISTS

In the wintry January of 1941 the 5 physical therapists sent by the NFIP arrived eager to see Kenny's work for themselves. There was Alice Plastridge, head therapist at Warm Springs; Gertrude Beard, senior therapist at Northwestern's medical school; Mildred Elson, editor of the APTA's *Physiotherapy Review*; and Florence and Henry Kendall, a husband and wife team who directed the physical therapy department of the Baltimore Children's Hospital-School. The Kendall's 1938 pamphlet *Care During the Recovery Period in Paralytic Poliomyelitis*, which was distributed by the Public Health Service, was one of the defining texts on polio therapy, and Kenny had been given it by the NFIP's executive secretary when she was still in New York.[10]

These 4 women and one man brought with them the skepticism of science and the pride of professionalism. More than anyone in America they knew the "orthodoxy" of polio treatment and what it had and had not achieved. Kenny's work had already been creating a lot of controversy in physical therapy circles. Everyone was anxious to hear if Kenny was a crazy quack or if she really had a scientifically sound solution to the difficult problems of polio care, including, as one nurse described it, the agony of listening to "frequent fits of crying bordering on hysteria" coming from children's polio wards at night.[11]

The professional field of physical therapy had moved away from its origins in military reconstruction during and after World War I, and was now practiced by an unusual mixture of disabled male veterans and athletic young women. By the 1920s many therapists worked in the expanding network of veterans' hospitals run by the new Veterans Administration. Outside these facilities, physical therapy was considered a luxury. Most hospital trustees were not convinced that paying for a heated pool, ultraviolet lamps, or exercise tables was necessary, and the physical therapy department in many hospitals consisted of a single therapist working in a basement or a back room. The few physicians who prescribed such therapies and were enthusiastic about rehabilitative medicine were treated with "frank hostility" by their colleagues.[12]

As growing numbers of polio epidemics made child patients rather than wounded soldiers the defining focus of physical therapy work, the site of practice shifted from veterans' hospitals to children's hospitals and children's rehabilitative centers (known as "crippled children's homes"). Boosted by federal funding through the 1935 Social Security Act, state services for children with physical disabilities expanded along with continuing support by service groups such as the Shriners.

Polio provided a major impetus to the development of the American physical therapy profession. By the early 1940s polio had become the nation's most prominent disabling disease, although it was not as statistically significant as tuberculosis, birth injuries, or rheumatic heart disease. With funds from the NFIP and from state Crippled Children's Bureaus to pay for care and for orthopedic equipment such as braces and crutches, rehabilitation came to be recognized as a crucial element in recovery from polio paralysis. Nonetheless, the physical therapy profession grew slowly. In 1941 there were only 16 approved schools for physical therapy training, and when war was declared at the end of the year there were fewer than 1,200 qualified physical therapists in the United States.[13]

Alice Lou Plastridge (1889–1993) was a prominent clinician whose career reflected the best polio training of her generation. After graduating from Mount Holyoke in 1911 she worked first as a physical education teacher and then in 1916 was trained in physical therapy by Boston orthopedist Robert Lovett and his physical therapist Wilhemine Wright during the worst polio epidemic that had hit the nation to date. Plastridge moved to Chicago where she worked as a private practitioner, and in the mid-1920s accompanied one of her patients, the daughter of a wealthy manufacturer, to Warm Springs. In 1926 Plastridge traveled to Hyde Park to work with Roosevelt who, the therapist later recalled, "was sort of at a stalemate in his therapy." She recognized that his legs were unlikely to improve, but she was able to teach him to use crutches more efficiently. By 1930 she had been appointed senior physical therapist at Warm Springs and later helped organize a physical therapy training program there.[14] Plastridge's work at Warm Springs gave her a sense both of the strength and physical limitations of bodies disabled by polio, and she trained her therapists to help patients create lives that accepted these limitations.

Gertrude Beard (1887–1971) and Mildred Elson (1900–1987), like Plastridge, were of Kenny's generation and had seen the flowering of physical therapy during the 1910s and the rise and fall of many overly optimistic therapeutic systems. They were concerned that Kenny's method—naturally grasped by desperate parents with disabled children— should not detract from the respectability of American physical therapy. Elson was a founding member of the APTA, the editor of its professional journal, and later its first salaried executive director. A professional organizer, she sought to improve her profession's educational standards and its relations with physicians and hospital administrators.[15] Beard, a Chicago physical therapist, had trained first as a nurse, and like Kenny, had worked as an army nurse during the Great War. She had developed physical therapy at Chicago's Wesley Hospital and at Northwestern University and, unusual among her peers, she had published research articles on muscle physiology.[16]

Florence and Henry Kendall were a decade or so younger than Kenny and the other therapists and were the standard bearers of orthodox polio care, much of which they had developed. Working with Johns Hopkins orthopedic surgeons they had transformed the Children's Hospital-School in Baltimore from a forlorn crippled children's home into a leading rehabilitative facility that attracted even Warm Springs patients dissatisfied with their progress.[17] Hospital-schools were popular institutions founded during the 1910s and 1920s to rehabilitate physically disabled children somatically and morally.[18]

The Baltimore facility had been founded in 1905 by the local Crippled Children Society and, like other hospital-schools around the country, was shifting its therapeutic focus in response to increasing numbers of patients with polio.[19] Although some orthopedic interns and residents from Johns Hopkins worked at the Hospital-School supervised by its senior orthopedist George Bennett, in most respects the Hospital-School was isolated from the major medical activities of the city, reflecting the poor reputation of rehabilitative medicine, a field that dealt with the slow and sometimes hopeless task of trying to heal the disabled. When in 1935 Florence Peterson, who had been trained to care for both military and polio patients, married blind veteran and rehabilitative expert Henry Kendall, the couple was able to combine rehabilitative therapy and the model of an autonomous disabled professional in a creative and long-lasting partnership. The Kendalls, who had 3 daughters together, became a respected and admired clinical team.

Henry Otis Kendall (1898–1979) was typical of the men who practiced physical therapy in this era: a disabled veteran who had gained professional training as part of his own rehabilitative therapy. The youngest of 13 children from a poor mountain family in Smithsberg, Maryland, Kendall had joined the Army in 1917 and become a sapper in the 41st Engineers. After a shell hit his face, destroying one eye and injuring the other, he was sent to the Evergreen School for the Blind in Baltimore where he learned physical therapy.[20] He began working at the Hospital-School in 1920 and became director of its physical therapy department, which also functioned as a facility for professional expansion. Its training program was affiliated first with Johns Hopkins and later with the University of Maryland. In the 1930s the Kendalls founded Maryland's first APTA chapter.[21] Kendall's colleagues were able to integrate or at least ignore his disability in a field in which disabled men with a military background were considered appropriate directors of the care of disabled patients.

Florence May Peterson (1910–2006) had graduated from the University of Minnesota in 1930 with a major in physical education and then studied physical therapy at the Walter Reed Army Hospital in Washington, D.C. During her student years, most of her patients were veterans suffering nerve and muscle injuries. But in a shift that reflected the growing significance of polio care for physical therapists, she spent 9 months during her second year caring for a polio patient in the Baltimore Children's Hospital-School under the direction of Henry Kendall. She then joined the Hospital-School's physical therapy department where she worked for the next 50 years.[22]

As polio experts the Kendalls saw themselves in a lineage beginning with Boston orthopedists Robert Lovett and Arthur Legg, and expanded through a network of physical therapists across the country including Janet Merrill in Boston, Alice Plastridge in Warm Springs, Gertrude Beard in Chicago, and Catherine Worthingham at Stanford. Polio care at the Hospital-School was conservative, based on the principles of rest and muscle protection, and structured around the fear, articulated in the Kendalls' *PHS Bulletin*, that inappropriately stretched muscles would further deform a patient struggling to regain muscle function.[23] The Kendalls criticized the widespread enthusiasm for water therapy and popularized their methods with a one-hour, 5-reel film shown at the 1937 annual meeting of the AMA and the 1938 annual meeting of the APTA.[24] But although widely known and emulated, the Kendall method did not provide the results that many polio survivors hoped for. It tended to produce stiff joints, weak muscles, and shortened limbs, and patients treated using this method often required a series of orthopedic operations.[25]

Feeling embattled, the Kendalls arrived in Minneapolis already prepared to see Kenny as yet another critic attacking the standard polio therapy they had developed. At the same time as they had learned of the NFIP's support of Kenny's work, the Kendalls had been given a draft of an article by St. Louis orthopedists H. Relton McCarroll and Craig Crego, later published in the *Journal of Bone and Joint Surgery*. In this study of 160 polio patients at the Shriners' Hospital for Crippled Children between 1935 and 1940, McCarroll and Crego found that no matter which method of polio therapy they used, including the Kendalls', there was no improvement in their patients. They had first treated patients with familiar immobilizing methods of solid plaster for 3 to 4 months, followed by plaster splints or bivalved plaster casts alternating with exercises in a heated pool or massage on a table, and had "very disappointing" results. In 1936 the orthopedists altered this therapy by hiring a physical therapist "trained by Mr. Kendall [and]...thoroughly familiar with his ideas and the details of his method of treatment." They gave her a ward of patients to treat, which they argued was a way of ensuring an "impartial trial" of the Kendall method. The therapist used 1 to 3 months of immobilization and rest followed by physical therapy for 3 to 6 months, but in McCarroll and Crego's estimation, "the results in that year were no better." In 1938 the surgeons read a description of Kenny's work in the *British Medical Journal*, which they characterized as "intensive physiotherapy." Although they did not use the Kenny method themselves, they did try to develop a therapy "between these two extremes," and for a period of 2 years treated patients with limited immobilization and various forms of exercise "without preconceived ideas as to the relative value of any particular form of therapy." The results for this group were also no better. Most striking in their study was a group of 14 polio patients who received what the surgeons called "no treatment." Reflecting the role of geography and also perhaps parental suspicion of surgeons and hospitals, these children were not seen by a physician until several months after the onset of paralysis. The parents refused to follow advice about rest or splinting and told the hospital staff that they believed "the paralysis would progress unless the child was forced to use the involved extremities and exercise them as much as possible." The surgeons concluded that the length of time since the initial infection suggested that no therapy would now aid these patients. To the surgeons' consternation, this "no treatment" group had the "highest percentage of satisfactory brace-free extremities" (19 percent), yet they had been the furthest from the best professional care. Despite these results, however, McCarroll and Crego concluded that careful immobilization was essential to prevent deformities from muscle imbalance. Rather than suggesting that paralyzed children living far from an orthopedic hospital might have benefited from the avoidance of standard therapies, McCarroll and Crego stressed the "underlying pathological process" of the polio virus. With the destructive power of the virus during the acute illness, they declared, "the die for the final picture is cast."[26] In their view combating residual paralysis was essentially out of the control of any physical therapist, much less a parent, and only an orthopedic surgeon could address the physical abnormalities that resulted from paralysis through surgery.

Kenny, the Kendalls, and most other American physical therapists rejected a clinical conclusion that made rehabilitative therapy irrelevant. The Kendalls were especially appalled at McCarroll and Crego's characterization of their own work. The surgeons had boasted that they had relied on a Kendall-trained physical therapist and that Henry Kendall had come to St. Louis to oversee the work of this therapist. In fact, both Kendalls had visited the Shriners Hospital in 1937 and as Florence later recalled, "indelibly imprinted in my memory is the moment of shock and incredulity we experienced walking into the [therapist's] ward and finding all of the patients with involved extremities encased in solid plaster! Our first reaction was, 'You must get the patients out of the plaster!'"[27] Nonetheless, the St. Louis study and later Kenny's frequent references to it reinforced many American professionals' sense that the Kendall method was the "immobilization" method and the epitome of orthodox polio care.

THE MEETING IN JANUARY

The therapists had not intended to converge on Minneapolis at the same time, but shortly before Christmas, Kenny slipped on the ice and broke her wrist. Early in January, John Pohl wrote to all of them, asking them to visit together so "that she will not be faced with repeating her demonstrations," for she "feels that her strength will only allow her about three days of work and talking at any one stretch."[28] Reading between the lines, Pohl's message suggests that Kenny was aware of how much emotional and physical strength it would take to confront this onslaught of visiting experts and was perhaps hoping to gain some sympathy for her injury, which was in a plaster cast and "debarred me from demonstrating any treatment satisfactorily."[29] Her fall had only deepened the frustration she had been feeling about the progress of her work both in Australia and in the United States. There was now a small polio epidemic in Queensland, and she feared the nurses she had trained at the Brisbane General Hospital would not be able to cope with so many acute patients.[30] She was also beginning to sense that her Minneapolis audiences were watching rather than listening, and that she and Mary were being used as demonstrators rather than as teachers: "it appeared as if I was expected to go on demonstrating indefinitely, when my one hope was that I might teach others and make them proficient in my methods."[31] Her demonstrations were being seen as a kind of show rather than as an integral part of a training program.

The January visit did not go well. The visitors were conversant with polio's physiology and neurology, and were confident that they could understand and critique Kenny's theories, especially her claim that she had identified symptoms that required a new kind of therapy and whose success indicated a previously unrecognized physiological process. Kenny had expected to find the experts skeptical and defensive, and her expectations were fulfilled. "I regret to say," Kenny later reported to Baltimore orthopedist George Bennett, that "it was impossible for me to demonstrate my work to these visitors, owing principally to the fact that they were absolutely non-receptive."[32]

On the first day Kenny invited the group to the city hospital's auditorium to hear her lecture. The lecture was based on evidence from Australian and local patients, interspersed with many references to doctors' responses to her work. Her method, she claimed, "evolved by myself...presents the disease in a different light from that accepted by orthodoxy throughout the world." She listed the authorities she disagreed with, beginning with the Queensland Royal Commission, British orthopedic specialist Sir Robert Jones, Australian polio expert Jean Macnamara, New York's Kristian Hansson, the Kendalls, George Bennett and Robert Johnson of Baltimore, and Robert Lovett, Arthur Legg, and Janet Merrill of Boston. These authorities believed that splinting prevented deformities but nonetheless deformities occurred in their patients. "Deformities do not occur with our system," Kenny announced boldly, even among patients "who have received the best orthodox treatment in Australia and America, including Georgia Warm Springs." "I do not claim," she said, careful to distinguish herself from the exaggerated press, "that a complete cure for the disease anterior poliomyelitis has been established." But disabilities could be significantly reduced "by putting into practice the original conceptions which I have presented to medical men and which have been acknowledged by them to be of great benefit to mankind."[33] Here was caution matched with breathtaking confidence.

This lecture, which consisted "mainly of her life history and the story of her success against great odds," the Kendalls said later, "gave us the impression that Sister Kenny would have us accept her work on the basis that she had proved it to a great many Australian and English Doctors."[34] They disliked the way Kenny dismissed their own work and that of other polio authorities and saw her references to physicians who acknowledged the benefit of Kenny's methods as puffery. Kenny was later outraged to read their assessment, which trivialized her detailed discussion of how she had developed her method and defended it against skeptics. In fact, she protested to O'Connor a few months later, "the history of my work and research which formed the basis of this lecture is supposed to be of great interest to all listeners."[35]

After the lecture Kenny presented some of her polio patients with before-and-after slides, each showing prominent clinical problems solved by Kenny therapies. One boy at the city hospital had difficulty swallowing. Within 10 hours after she had identified the spasm in his posterior neck muscles to the medical supervisor and explained how to treat it, the patient was able to sit up and eat a hearty meal, and in 6 weeks he made a complete recovery. Another boy at the university hospital was in an iron lung. Kenny had "advised immediate removal from the respirator," and, after treatment for the spasm in his neck and shoulders and the mental alienation in his anterior muscles, he was able to breathe freely, eat well, and had "all muscles functioning." A "prominent pediatrician" in Minneapolis had urged her to use splints to aid a girl receiving the Kenny treatment for bilateral foot drop. Kenny refused, arguing that the patient's posterior muscles were in painful spasm and were unable to relax to allow the opposing muscles to return to their normal resting place. After treatment for spasm and mental alienation and without the use of any supports, the girl recovered.[36] In Australia, as late as 1940, she had argued that she made "no claims of perfection in my methods [for]...no technique is perfect and that there is always the possibility of improvements as knowledge advances."[37] But in Minnesota this conciliatory tone had disappeared.

Kenny tried to have her visitors recognize that the symptoms she was describing were "exactly opposite to those recognized by Orthodoxy," urging them "to understand that if I had to make any harsh remarks about the Orthodox method, it was only meant for our mutual benefit. As I understood, we were all out for the benefit of the afflicted." After seeing Kenny's slides of twisted and stiff posterior neck muscles compared to patients who had received the Kenny treatment and were now normal, Florence immediately remarked that "all of these cases recover anyhow," adding that this kind of spasm "recovers very quickly." Hearing this allusion "to a condition that she and her husband deny existed in their book," Kenny pointed out that Florence "was admitting the source of a symptom that was not supposed to exist."[38] The Kendalls retorted that "there was a confusion of terms," for the term "spastic" was not the same as "spasm or contracture" and that in any case orthodoxy did recognize the condition of muscle spasm in acute polio. When Kenny protested that their *PHS Bulletin* had not mentioned the term, they replied that "the Bulletin does not deal with acute but with convalescent poliomyelitis."[39]

After this tense encounter, Kenny invited the visitors to be her guests at a luncheon but the Kendalls had already made plans to have lunch with John Pohl. Annoyed at this rebuff, Kenny gave the other 3 therapists who did accept her lunch invitation a "private showing" later that afternoon where she demonstrated the details of her work and put some of her patients in the city hospital "through a severe test to show what she considered normal."[40] Not only did she relax in these less combative environments she also joked and showed a side of herself that the Kendalls never saw.[41]

On the following day the Kendalls hoped to be shown the concrete details of Kenny's techniques. Instead Kenny began by discussing "certain inaccuracies in accepted theories" including "muscle testing and its dire results." She then presented some of her recovered patients. "The audience was interested," she reflected later, "but the task was irksome," for the observers were looking at results from a treatment for symptoms "they did not recognize."[42]

When Kenny finally presented her patients she was challenged by the Kendalls over her diagnoses. In the Kendalls' notes from that day Kenny insisted that a paralyzed foot was now normal, although they felt that it "showed marked proration & flatness of long arch." When explaining the cause of an arm's paralysis, Kenny claimed it was the result of a spasm in the pectoral major muscle but Henry "raised arm thru range of motion & showed *that* range was entirely N[ormal]."[43] Kenny then asked Henry to describe the deformities he saw in certain patients and to explain their cause "according to Orthodoxy." When he finished she pointed out how his explanations differed from her own views.[44] Kenny then shocked her audience by declaring that she rejected any use of muscle testing in polio for "the extreme effort necessary on the part of the patient would only exaggerate the inco[-]ordination" and also cause "further spasm and contractures."[45] This was a direct attack on the physical therapists' standard tool of assessment.

On the third day the physical therapists met Kenny at Station K, her city hospital ward. The Kendalls were eager to see Kenny's techniques in action, but were not surprised when Kenny announced that she first "wished to discuss principles regarding treatment." Speaking as an expert with a touch of arrogance, Florence told Kenny that "we thought she had a contribution to make in her treatment" and that "by being open-minded and discussing the problem . . . we probably would find there were not as many points of difference as appear on the surface."[46] The Kendalls saw themselves as trying to be agreeable but Kenny "became very much annoyed" and replied "you say there is no difference between my treatment and yours, and I maintain they are entirely opposite," adding that she had already proved her work in Australia. After further discussion the Kendalls concluded that "it was obvious that to disagree with Sister Kenny or question her was as great a mistake as agreeing with her." They said they wanted to discontinue any discussion until the doctors arrived, reminding Kenny that "Dr. Pohl had invited us to observe treatment." Kenny replied dismissively that "she didn't care what Dr. Pohl had invited us to do, she did not intend to show us any treatment." With rising ire she also criticized the NFIP "for sending us out" and "permitting us to write a report on the basis of a three-day visit." The NFIP had told them to stay as long as they needed to, the Kendalls countered, and it was Pohl who had suggested 3 days "otherwise we would have planned to stay longer."

Unless they were permitted to see treatment, they warned, "we would have to state in our report that we were refused the opportunity," and Henry angrily added "we're going to stay just long enough to expose you."[47] The meeting broke up when the Kendalls left to talk to Pohl. According to Kenny, she waited for an hour for them to return, but the Kendalls recalled instead that she left the hospital "in a huff" threatening to leave for Australia.[48]

Alice Plastridge stood somewhat apart from the heated exchanges between Kenny and the Kendalls. Her work at Warm Springs based around its thermal spring pools with patients in the convalescent rather than the acute stage had shown her the potential of muscle exercises and heat. Warm Springs also emphasized functionality over straightening twisted bodies, which may have led Plastridge to be less concerned by Kenny's rejection of testing muscles to assess the exact extent of their weakness. Indeed, orthopedist Charles Irwin, Plastridge's Warm Springs supervisor, had argued in *JAMA* that "no immediate effort should be made to make a complete muscle analysis" in polio for "it causes the patient too much discomfort" and until tenderness subsides "it can't possibly be correct."[49]

Plastridge had come to Minnesota with an open mind. She arrived 2 days before her meeting with Kenny in order to talk to local therapists who were being trained by Kenny. These therapists explained some of "the underlying principles of this treatment" to her and tried to clarify Kenny's "seemingly contradictory theories." With the comment "forewarned is forearmed," they warned Plastridge about Kenny's tendency to hear every question as a criticism, which was the result, they explained, of her effort "for so many years to get her ideas across and prove the worth of her work" with "ridicule…heaped upon her for so long." Thus, the "only way of learning her theories" was "to let her do *all* the talking." Plastridge should therefore not ask questions or raise objections for she might be "singled out for derision and unanswerable questions." The lessons she learned from these therapists, Plastridge reflected, "made me a little more tolerant of Sister Kenny's peculiarities."[50]

Plastridge was especially interested in Kenny's claim to have healed Henry Haverstock, a former Warm Springs patient whose case had professional significance for her. Haverstock's case had been featured by local newspapers with, Plastridge noted, "remarkable claims made about his progress." She went to examine him herself and sent a separate report to her supervisor in Georgia. Before Haverstock had come to Warm Springs, Plastridge noted, he had been extremely active at home, "even trying to walk." As a result, his muscles were "so fatigued and so weak" that the Warm Springs staff had advised "complete rest, in plaster" for the first 2 months before he was allowed to exercise in the pools. He was finally taught to walk with the aid of leg splints, a canvas stomach corset, and crutches, and after 4 months was sent home.[51] All this equipment had been removed by Kenny who claimed that her method was treating his "true symptoms."[52] In Plastridge's assessment after some months of Kenny's treatment he "showed a very pendulous abdomen and hyperextension of the right knee" as well as a "Trendelenberg limp [the result of a weak gluteus medius muscle]." Haverstock tried to show Plastridge how he could walk but could only manage 3 steps; she felt that the stability that might be gained from using a brace on his right leg and a pair of crutches would have given him more self-confidence and "increased rather than decreased his independence."[53] A year later, Haverstock was featured in national magazines as a college student who could climb 3 flights of stairs daily to different classrooms and in *JAMA* John Pohl used his case as a prominent example of the worth of Kenny's work.[54] But in 1941 Haverstock's limited recovery did not provide evidence to convince visitors that Kenny's methods enabled convalescent patients to improve their strength and functionality. Thus Plastridge did not consider Kenny's results with Haverstock and other patients with long-standing paralysis "very different from those obtained by any conscientious physical therapist."[55]

Kenny's results, though, convinced all the visiting therapists that her methods were of great psychological benefit to patients.[56] Plastridge, Elson, and Beard had observed her methods in the afternoon session that the Kendalls had not attended. Plastridge was especially impressed with the way Kenny worked with patients whereby every movement was "done with the most meticulous care." This new method, Plastridge agreed, "aids circulation, muscle tone and (what is most important to Sister Kenny) it aids in keeping up the patients' 'mental awareness'" so that "the patient never forgets how to make the effort to move the different parts of his body."[57] Plastridge's positive assessment reflected her more nuanced view of Kenny herself, gained through observing her not only as a didactic lecturer, but as a genial host and as a clinician at the bedside. Unfortunately Elson and Beard left no record of their experiences.

Kenny's belligerent attitude frustrated all of her visitors, but Plastridge tried to separate the woman from the work. Kenny was the kind of person, she admitted, who "raises your ire to the boiling point with her aggressiveness and unreasonableness." She considered her too "intolerant and impatient" to allow opportunities "for free discussion" and therefore not "a good lecturer or teacher—neither scientific nor logical in her explanations, although she does know her anatomy and probably her neurology." But Plastridge admired her "imposing, almost majestic bearing [and her] ... fine sense of humor," as well as "her fund of stories and anecdotes from her own nursing experiences and extensive travels." Impressed by Kenny's "unusually good results," Plastridge, like many observers, could not believe it was "possible they could all be a matter of chance." Unlike the Kendalls she was willing to speculate about the validity of Kenny's ideas, concluding that "whether her theories are scientifically sound or not only time and further investigation will prove." She also anticipated that Kenny's controversial theories would give "a tremendous stimulation to further research in this field" for Kenny's claims had already "made many of us take serious stock of ourselves, and the type of physical therapy we are doing."[58]

The Kendalls were given a copy of Plastridge's comments, but they remained unconvinced. They completed their own 13-page report to the NFIP a few months after the visit in which they defended their criticisms of Kenny's work, trying not to discuss their dislike of her character. They had, they said, sought to "distinguish between the real and apparent" value of this new method. "The Orthodox conception," they emphasized, did recognize "early spasm (which accompanies meningeal irritation), *followed by* flaccidity in muscles (which accompanies onset of paralysis)." Yet Kenny "fails to recognize this transition from the symptoms of spasm to the symptoms of flaccidity." Her outrageous claim that muscle tests were harmful was part of a pattern of what they saw as a lack of rigor: deficient clinical records and an inappropriate reliance on qualitative evidence.[59] Comparing her to the standards of their own well-respected institution, they remarked in their private notes, "SK's notes and charts are kept at home—not at the hosp!"[60] The credit Kenny claimed for all recoveries ignored the likelihood that many of her patients had made a spontaneous recovery and therefore made accurate comparisons impossible. Her claims required a thorough statistical study including complete case histories and muscle examinations for all patients at the end of 6 weeks, but "unfortunately Sister Kenny advocates that it [testing] tends to produce 'mental alienation.' "[61]

The Kendalls openly disagreed with Kenny's assessment of some of her patients, doubted her theories, remained convinced that muscles without proper support would be damaged, and were appalled to hear Kenny reject the muscle test, the major tool of their own clinical and research program. They also disliked her confusing terminology. In their view, "she used terms freely and interchangeably, without regard for clear cut meanings of those terms" and her "knowledge of muscle function was not only very incomplete [but]...quite inaccurate."[62] They had been ready to accept that her unusual terms were the result of language differences, an argument proffered by Knapp who had warned the visitors "how easy it was to misunderstand Sister Kenny because of the differences in the meanings of words—even in English-speaking countries like Australia."[63] But Kenny made clear that she was not just giving new names to familiar symptoms in an exotic accent. Hers was a new language for new ideas. What was new, she tried to explain, were the distinctive symptoms she had identified that made polio—at least in its acute stage—a new disease, rendering any debate based on the orthodox conception of polio irrelevant. The Kendalls interpreted this as sloppy thinking; they did not see clinical signs such as spasm as crucial in the construction of polio itself. Thus, during a discussion of a shoulder whose muscle Kenny claimed was in spasm, the Kendalls found "no contraction." Their notes read: "When facts pointed out she became confused & made statement— 'We are talking about a diff. disease.' H.O.K. said 'Oh no—I'm talking about muscles & deformities, not the disease.' "[64] But to Kenny "muscles & deformities" were a critical, neglected element of polio care that proved both ineffective treatment and damaging physiological disruption. Kenny's distinction between "affected" muscles and "alienated" muscles frustrated all the therapists, and the Kendalls concluded that her classification of "spasm" was neither a new symptom nor one that required distinctive treatment. She also seemed not particularly interested in a scientific explanation for the cause of these new symptoms. Her vague comment that muscle spasm was "caused by irritation in the spinal cord" was unconvincing. Of course Kenny also said that she had come to America to find scientific researchers who could explain the complex mechanism underlying the distinctive symptoms she had identified.[65]

In any case, the Kendalls argued, most of her ideas and techniques were "not so radically different from our own, even though differently applied." As early as the 1916 polio epidemic, hospitalized patients in the acute stage after leaving the contagious disease hospital were placed in tubs of hot water while pain was severe; thus, "heat, in one form or another, is not new." The maintenance of a normal mental attitude "has long been taken for granted as one of the most important phases of the recovery period." As for exercises to regain muscle function, "a great deal depends upon the experience, conscientiousness and patience of the physical therapist" and, whether called muscle consciousness or mental alienation, "that is definitely one of the things we have worked for the hardest." Many of her techniques were part of standard polio care: hot packs to stabilize body parts and a foot board and a wooden plank under the mattress as methods of immobilization. Such techniques, however, they feared, would not adequately protect weak or paralyzed muscles. Kenny's early introduction of muscle training, allowing a patient complete free-dom of joint movement, was even more harmful. Her claim about the danger of rest made no sense to the Kendalls, for the idea that rest could aid "the inflamed or potentially paralyzed part" had scientific confirmation from studies of polio for almost 100 years. Although these studies, they admitted, were almost all based on clinical evidence rather than laboratory evidence, they were nonetheless so extensive that there should be no debate over "the necessity of protecting weak muscles in cases of nerve injury."[66] She should not, they concluded, be given responsibility in the treatment of patients in the acute stage or "be entrusted with teaching the principles of muscle actions."[67] In their harshest assessment, they felt her idea that "brain power" could be reinvigorated by phys-ical therapy contradicted "the results of scientific studies by the most competent minds in medicine, and accordingly must be relegated to 'cultism' until further evidence is forth-coming."[68] The Kendalls sent their report to the NFIP and to *JAMA*, but Morris Fishbein decided not to publish it, seeing it as a bitter attack on Kenny's method.[69]

The Kendalls began circulating their report to fellow professionals but were disap-pointed to find that the politics of polio had shifted away from their views. When Florence Kendall asked Catherine Worthingham, president of the APTA, for her reactions to the report, she was surprised to find that Worthingham reduced their many objections to the issue of terminology. Although Worthingham agreed that Kenny's choice of terms was unfortunate, Worthingham and the APTA's Governing Board believed "it would be very unwise to bring it up now," and she reminded Florence there were "so many things that are important to us in our relationship to other organizations that it would be unfortu-nate to cloud the issues with the discussion of terminology."[70] Thus, as Worthingham was noting obliquely, Kenny's work had drawn attention to the significance of physical therapy in polio care and thereby reinforced the relationship between the APTA and the NFIP, so the APTA would not want to take a public stance against the NFIP-sponsored nurse by making what might seem picky complaints about her terms. During the 1940s NFIP-funded physical therapists' specialized training and professional development con-tributed to the expansion of the profession in both numbers and respectability.

Following this strategy of cooperation and appeasement, Worthingham asked Kenny to participate in an NFIP-funded study of "Physical Therapy Treatment in Poliomyelitis" a few months after the therapists' visit to Minneapolis. The APTA, Worthingham explained, was sending questionnaires to hospitals, crippled children's schools, private practitioners, charity and governmental agencies, and physical therapy training schools in preparation for a conference to evaluate the collected material and to make "recom-mendations as to methods of approach."[71] Kenny replied predictably. Such a survey, she said, would be of "no value" for "all observers [had admitted] . . . that I have evolved a satisfactory and commendable treatment . . . which holds out more hope for recovery than any other method produced anywhere." She was "pained and surprised" that money would be spent funding yet another study considering that "for twenty-five years results have been tabled and compared and no advance has been made."[72] This query promoted Kenny to remind O'Connor that the funds of his "very splendid organization" should "be better employed" if they were "used to teach technicians the method while I am still available, rather than go over old ground." She reiterated her provocative claim that the twisted bodies of disabled children were largely the result of inappropriate and ineffec-tive therapy—"the after-effects of orthodox treatment"—rather than the disease itself.[73]

Kenny's method rapidly became seen as a legitimate polio therapy. As early as November 1941 Emil Rosner, a physical therapist at the New York Hospital for Joint Diseases, boasted to the Kendalls that he was "familiar with the Sister Kenny Method, the Mayo Clinic Method, the Janet Merrill Method, and the Hansson Method—and your splendid work."[74] Rosner had not recognized that the Kendalls did not consider Kenny's work in the same pantheon as other respected polio authorities.

CRAFT AND CONTROL

Kenny did not see the Kendalls' report for some time. Not long after the therapists' visit, she left for Australia, ostensibly to supervise her Brisbane clinic staff during a local polio epidemic. NFIP officials assured her that they would continue to pay the living expenses of herself and Mary, who remained behind to continue the work. The NFIP also agreed to pay for both travel and living expenses of the 2 Australian therapists (Kenny's nephew Stanley Willis (Bill) Bell and Brisbane nurse Valerie Harvey) she would bring back to Minnesota.[75]

Both Kenny and the medical school needed to prove that Kenny's results were not the result of suggestibility either to her patients or to local physicians. Her trip to Australia helped "spike...a romantic theory in which many had indulged," a reporter noted later, the theory that Kenny's method worked "by dominating the patient's mind" and that "perhaps she was a faith healer with some of the talents of a hypnotist."[76] Thus, Kenny's absence helped solidify the scientific nature of her work as, under Mary's calm supervision, treatment and clinical improvements went on without her.[77]

Kenny spent 3 months in Australia. Her medical supporters in Brisbane, in a gesture they considered open-minded, were allowing parents to choose whether to have their paralyzed children cared for by Kenny-trained technicians at the Brisbane General Hospital or in the wards where medical orthodoxy reigned. According to Kenny's recollections "almost eighty percent chose the Kenny treatment." Nonetheless, she felt such a situation was "not in keeping with the dignity of the medical profession," and the choice "was not between a better and a worse method...[but] really a choice between the right and the wrong, the correct and the incorrect." She was further distressed to learn from Abraham Fryberg, the hospital's superintendent, that in the orthodox wards polio treatment was "compounded from as much of the Kenny method as they [the staff] could remember" from her earlier lectures. Not only did such practice suggest a bastardized version of her work, but most of those techniques, she protested, had been designed for convalescent rather than acute care. Unable to alter the hospital's polio admissions policy or its practice in the orthodox wards, Kenny concluded that "I was still a bush nurse who was supposed to know nothing except what lay within the narrow limits of her own sphere."[78] She was, however, delighted to be sent a draft copy of a positive report on her work by Cole and Knapp. She showed the report to Australian government officials, drawing attention to their statement that "we personally firmly believe that this method will be the basis of the future treatment of infantile paralysis."[79]

By the time she returned to the Twin Cities, local officials and physicians at the university had decided that her work was worth learning. She was now in charge of wards in both the city hospital (Station K) and in the university hospital (Station 43), and was growing confident that her base in Minneapolis would enable her to alter the minds of doctors, nurses, and physical therapists across America. "I have a very nice set up at the University," she wrote to a Brisbane ally, "and am in the proud position of being consultant in all the hospitals of the Twin Cities for all polio cases."[80] Local boosters in Minnesota had already begun to retell Kenny's story as one of civic acumen. "Minneapolis was the only city in America to give her a friendly hearing," the *Minneapolis Star-Journal* claimed, "previously she had offered her services to New York, Chicago, Denver and San Francisco."[81] The *Star-Journal* featured patients like Bob Gurney, an 18-year-old patient from St. Paul who had been paralyzed by polio "so bad[ly] [that] I could only wink my eyes," but was now leaving the hospital and planning to return to high school.[82]

By the time America's 1941 polio season arrived the Kendalls' doubts were subsumed by a wave of professional and public interest provoked by Cole and Knapp's enthusiastic article on "The Kenny Treatment of Infantile Paralysis" published in *JAMA* that June.[83] But in print the article looked quite different from the draft Kenny had read. The careful crafting of this report for publication showed the hand of Morris Fishbein who was trying to dampen what the *New York Times* later called the "silent controversy raging behind closed doors in medical circles ever since Miss Kenny introduced her method of treatment in this country."[84] *JAMA* was the most important medical journal in North America and as its editor Fishbein was one of the most influential American physicians. Throughout the 1940s *JAMA*'s high circulation numbers matched the circulation of the next 6 largest medical journals combined.[85] Fishbein wanted to be very careful in approving this first *JAMA* article on Kenny's work. In his role as chair of the NFIP Committee on Information he had "returned it to be dissected by a special committee" and had "finally accepted [it] with some misgivings and published [it] with many deletions."[86] Fishbein asked Frank Krusen, the Mayo specialist in physical medicine, to head this "special committee." Some of the behind-the-scenes machinations can be guessed at from a private note Knapp sent to Krusen apologizing for asking him "to sign a statement explaining an article you have not seen about work you have not observed." Knapp added that he had been told this should be done in order to "prevent 'the report from being misunderstood.'"[87] In another glaring change, the published article did not use John Pohl's name even though he had done much of the work, but Fishbein did publish a separate article by Pohl 10 months later.[88]

The preface to Cole and Knapp's published report was full of caveats warning that the report was only preliminary, that "several years must elapse before a definite evaluation of the method" could be made, and that "it is, of course, recognized that spontaneous recovery may occur." The preface authors did acknowledge that "the currently accepted methods of treatment of the disease are far from satisfactory" and they urged that Kenny's method "should be given a fair trial and should be studied with open minds." In examples that contradicted this, however, the preface included lengthy quotations from earlier critical reports on Kenny's work by British and Australian physicians.[89]

In the rest of the article, written in a distinctly different tone, Cole and Knapp not only praised Kenny's "highly refined and detailed method of muscle reeducation" but also her rejection of splinting, a technique that they pointed out did not prevent deformities. With confidence they explained that "obviously in this treatment there is no place for 'muscle testing' as usually performed…for this testing can definitely cause 'incoordination' and may slow down the patient's recovery." The 26 acute patients they had observed treated with Kenny's methods and without splinting were "much more comfortable and cheerful," and, to date, not one had developed "contractures or deformities following this treatment." Most strikingly, they defended Kenny's ideas of incoordination and alienation, explaining that muscle training could "maintain normal nerve pathways and restore those which are damaged." While they agreed that these ideas were new they made much of the evidence of efficacy. And how had Kenny been able to identify something unrecognized by generations of polio experts? In the Australian bush her "keen, analytical mind [was] unprejudiced by previous contact with theory or training in the prevalent conception of treatment of this disease... [and] without knowledge of postmortem pathologic appearances."[90] Insight through ignorance was a strange defense made by physicians about a clinician. But Cole and Knapp recognized how many of their peers were dissatisfied with not only current therapeutic options but also polio scientists' seemingly endless attention to pathological lesions in monkeys rather than pain and disability in living patients.

The *JAMA* article became the basis of numerous stories in the popular press. Accompanied by a picture of Kenny in a wide-brimmed black hat, a *Time* article described the "new and apparently successful treatment for infantile paralysis—reversing all accepted methods of treating the disease." "No doctor invented this method," the magazine noted, "but a nurse in the Australian bush." Still, in an effort to mend the disturbed gender relations and to make this medical discovery less transgressive, *Time* explained that Cole and Knapp had invited "strapping, soft-spoken Sister Kenny" to work in local hospitals. [91] Thus, Kenny was presented as a nurse with stereotypically deferential characteristics whose work had been recognized by insightful medical men.

Kenny immediately saw that this article was not the same as the version she had read in Australia. She identified Fishbein's editorial hand even before O'Connor told her that Fishbein had required the article "be edited and prefaced."[92] Cole and Knapp, Kenny believed, had provided a ringing endorsement of her work. Yet sentences in the draft such as "we have been favorably impressed with this work both as to rationale of therapy and as to results so far observed" were replaced by the more tepid claim that results were better than "previous generally accepted therapeutic procedures." The sentence "we personally firmly believe that this method will be the basis of the future treatment in infantile paralysis" was missing.[93]

The most serious alteration in Kenny's view was Cole and Knapp's original statement that "muscle spasm is a constant accompaniment of the muscle pain of acute anterior poliomyelitis, and it may be the real and sole cause of the pain," which now read "she believes that muscle spasm is a constant accompaniment of the muscular pain of acute poliomyelitis." Kenny could see the epistemological shift in this phrasing. "The statement was made by the observers, not by me," she pointed out to O'Connor, but the *JAMA* version "would lead your readers to believe this announcement was made by me. I am not qualified to suggest or make the statement that spasm may be the real or sole cause of the pain. I consider the medical supervisors are qualified to do so."[94] This effort to distant the authorship of medical claims about her work was part of a process she had honed during the 1930s in response to critical reports on her work. Public approval by physicians was crucial for the status of her clinical and teaching work. These alterations, she warned, had "completely cut the ground from beneath my feet as far as teaching my method is concerned." The NFIP had paid for her to return with 2 technicians in order to teach this method, but "in order to teach, the students must first understand there is something of value to learn, otherwise I would only be wasting valuable time."[95]

In June 1941 Kenny and Pohl appeared again before the city's Board of Public Welfare. Aware that he was becoming one of Kenny's most prominent medical supporters, Pohl declared, "I think it would be criminal to treat any child afflicted with acute infantile paralysis by the methods we formerly employed," praise echoed by the director of the city hospital and by the city's health commissioner. The board voted to fund 2 graduate nurses who would work with Kenny for a year and then be able to "carry on the work." The board also seconded the university's request to the NFIP for a $10,000 grant to set up a 25-bed polio clinic at the university hospital.[96] When the NFIP agreed to fund the new clinic and the training of technicians as well as cover the expenses of Kenny, Bell, Harvey, and Mary Kenny for another 8 months, officials at the NFIP and the medical school believed that these decisions had been made among themselves. NFIP officials, with Fishbein's assistance, hoped to keep Kenny in line and ensure that her clinical and teaching work remained under the supervision of medical school faculty.

But even in this early period, Kenny was able to reach over the heads of NFIP officers and senior AMA members and claim the independence she wanted. She began to complain to local reporters and NFIP officials that the NFIP had not praised the worth of her work publicly. Without a "definite statement" by the NFIP or *JAMA*, Kenny declared, she and her Australian staff would only "carry on for a short time," and, she told O'Connor, "I am sure my country will arrange for the reimbursement of all funds spent and for my return to Australia." "Other countries desire my presence," she reminded readers of the *Minneapolis Star-Journal*, but if her work was publicly acknowledged "I am prepared to stay and teach."[97]

At the same time as she was threatening to leave Kenny urged O'Connor and his medical director Don Gudakunst to visit Minneapolis so that she could demonstrate her work and provide them with defining evidence that could be followed up by a formal statement from the NFIP.[98] O'Connor tried to explain to Kenny why any visit by him or Gudakunst to Minneapolis would not confirm her work's value, explaining that the NFIP was cooperating with "its grantee, the Medical School of the University of Minnesota" and it would be unwise for the NFIP "to attempt to make any separate evaluation of that method." He refused to bow to Kenny's threat to leave along with her staff, reminding her that the final evaluation of the work lay with physicians at Minnesota's medical school, which would be done with or without "your continued presence."[99] But his effort to have Kenny recognize the difference between the director of an organization and its expert advisors failed. O'Connor was the head of NFIP; he had agreed to fund her work; he should put the weight of his organization behind it. It made no sense for the NFIP to encourage polio professionals to use her work at the same time the work was continuing to be evaluated. Kenny had come back from Australia determined to have her work formally approved and then spread across the country. She did not see herself as dependent on the medical school or the NFIP, points she reiterated in longer and longer letters to O'Connor.

FISHBEIN AND KENNY

As the AMA's cultural censor behind the scenes and as a professional editor aware of the lasting power of the written word, Fishbein tended not to put much on paper. He usually responded by phone and thus we do not know how he answered O'Connor who sent him a copy of an especially long letter from Kenny with the query "How should I answer this?." Fishbein did send O'Connor a comic note a few months later wishing him "profound sympathy in this affliction."[100] Increasingly Fishbein recognized the potentially unsettling power of Kenny and her work, especially as reporters began to tell the story of a nurse who trumps the doctors and challenges medical orthodoxy. Indeed he was one of the first American physicians to understand the threat Kenny posed in gender relations, medical authority, and professional orthodoxy. But initially he saw her as just another quack, the designation he applied to most of his antagonists. His best-selling 1925 expose *The Medical Follies; an Analysis of the Foibles of Some Healing Cults, Including Osteopathy, Homeopathy, Chiropractic, and The Electronic Reactions of Abrams, with Essays on the Antivivisectionists, Health Legislation, Physical Culture, Birth Control, and Rejuvenation* revised in 1927 to include *the Cult of Beauty, the Craze for Reduction, Rejuvenation, Eclecticism, Bread and Dietary Fads, [and] Physical Therapy* had sought to convince the American public that all these groups should be considered harmful to the progress of medical science.[101] During the 1920s and 1930s he had led fierce attacks on alternative practitioners and proponents of government health insurance, and defended medical societies that were resisting group practice. In the late 1930s, after members of Washington, D.C.'s medical society sought to censor local physicians who had formed a group practice, New Deal officials, frustrated with AMA leaders' intransigence over federal efforts to expand health and welfare services, named Fishbein along with members of the local society in an antitrust case brought by the Justice Department. Fishbein was confident that his own power as well as the rising status of American physicians and the AMA would continue, irrespective of the outcome of this case.

Monitoring the Kenny story seemed to Fishbein to be a question of cultural rather than scientific politics. Not only did he control what was published in *JAMA* but as chair of the NFIP's Committee on Information, Fishbein had dictatorial power over the popular press as well. After the publication of Cole and Knapp's *JAMA* article, Fishbein received drafts of numerous articles on Kenny. He approved an article for the *Saturday Evening Post* by Robert Yoder, a *Chicago Daily News* journalist.[102] However, Fishbein rejected the overly effusive "Infantile Paralysis Loses the First Round" when its author, freelance writer Walter Quigley, seemed unwilling to be deferential enough.[103] Reminding Quigley that he was one of NFIP's medical advisors, Fishbein explained that "for me to undertake to pass on your manuscript" Quigley would need to correct the identified mistakes and his "several unwarranted inferences." If he did this, "we will be glad to have you indicate to the prospective publisher that the manuscript has been passed on by the [NFIP] Committee on Information."[104] "There are indications that he is trying to be very much of a smart aleck in this affair," Fishbein concluded in a separate note to O'Connor, and "it is obvious from his manuscript that he knows nothing whatever about the subject."[105] Recognizing the threat behind Fishbein's words, Quigley apologized abjectly, saying he was "anxious to get this accurate" and would "rewrite the MSS to make it correct."[106] But his backtracking was too late, and without Fishbein's approval no magazine agreed to publish Quigley's piece.

Robert Potter, the science editor of the Hearst newspapers' Sunday magazine *American Weekly*, fared better. Potter agreed to "cooperate fully with the Foundation to see that every word of the article and every fact is in accordance with the present medical knowledge." "There will be no need to try to sensationalize such an article," he assured Gudakunst, as "the human interest facts of a nurse in the Australian bush making a contribution to the aftercare of infantile paralysis are so good, in themselves, that the article can stand on its own feet."[107] Fishbein found Potter, unlike Quigley, "was glad to accept advice and suggestions and was most appreciative of what was done for him."[108] Nonetheless, he warned Potter that, like many other writers, he had "approached the subject with a view to sensationalism." Fishbein proposed the substitution of "remarkable" for "amazing," "distressing pain" for "terrific pain," and "the preferable way" for "the only correct way." Do not say "the Kenny treatment is the answer," Fishbein advised him, "when the scientific statement would be 'may be the answer,'" or "'the medical profession has been fooled too often'... when the correct statement would be that 'the medical profession has been fooled on occasion.'" Potter should also delete the paragraph that quoted Pohl "saying that it would be criminal to treat a child with any method except the Kenny treatment." It would indeed, Fishbein argued, be criminal not to give a child diphtheria antitoxin "because that technic [sic] is well established," but there was "not as yet any convincing evidence that the Kenny treatment alone is better than other methods of orthopedic care." These suggestions, Fishbein assured Potter, were offered "simply to make your article scientifically safe."[109] Potter not only found Fishbein difficult to please but when he traveled to Minneapolis, despite the NFIP's assurance that he would have full cooperation, he found a "gun-shy" Knapp who refused to comment further "without specific authorization from Mr. O'Connor" and Kenny "bottled up like [a] stuffed herring by [the] Docs." "My private belief," Potter complained to the NFIP's New York office, "is that I'm getting [a] royal runaround and the brush off reserved for local reporters." If he could "get nothing better," he threatened, he could "make a swell yarn out of the run around which would be swell exposure of medical high handedness and stupidity."[110] Potter's article appeared in August 1941, presenting Kenny as a woman with an exotic, rural background and gentle hands.[111] And Fishbein began to keep "careful records" on Kenny.[112]

THE POWER OF SEEING

Convinced that the Kenny method described in Cole and Knapp's *JAMA* article was an important step toward improving polio therapy, a number of physicians, nurses, and physical therapists wanted to see the nurse and her work for themselves. In August 1941, during the worst polio epidemic Manitoba had then experienced, Canadian pathologist Bruce Chown, who had become director of the Winnipeg Children's Hospital while its regular administrator was in the armed forces, invited Kenny to visit the hospital and demonstrate her work.[113] A few weeks earlier Chown had visited polio clinics in the United States including an unscheduled trip to Minneapolis. While "the time obviously was too short... to learn Nurse Kenny's methods in detail," he told his hospital's trustees, he had been impressed by what he had seen and felt "very strongly that, if possible, we should send a member of the Physiotherapy Department... to spend three to six months under Nurse Kenny studying her methods in detail."[114]

In a dramatic move, reported in the Minneapolis newspapers, Kenny and Mary flew to Winnipeg. At the Children's Hospital Kenny "went from one bedside to another and called attention to the errors that had been made by the orthodox procedure." "Fortunately," she noted, the "orthodox procedure had not been adhered to strictly" and patients were not immobilized "to the same extent as in many other institutions."[115] Kenny's identification of previously unnoticed symptoms caught the attention of hospital staff who watched as she "showed us spasm in some of muscles of every one of our patients."[116] This act of showing and then treating was dramatic and transformative. "Sister Kenny showed us some things about poliomyelitis of which we had not been aware," Alfred Deacon, the hospital's senior orthopedic surgeon, told Don Gudakunst a few weeks later; "we had not noticed these things ourselves, nor had we seen them mentioned in [the] medical literature on poliomyelitis." Deacon was particularly struck by Kenny's ability to demonstrate the "functional nature of flaccid paralysis"; after she named and treated the new symptoms, patients began "to use muscles they had not used for days or weeks, a few times in a few minutes."[117] Here evidence of the disabled and then healed body told a memorable clinical story.

Kenny left Winnipeg after a few days, leaving Mary for 2 more weeks to oversee the work and to teach members of the hospital staff the new methods. When the Winnipeg epidemic subsided Deacon and Helen Ross, the hospital's chief physical therapist, traveled to Minneapolis to learn more.[118] They "came back convinced of two things," Bruce Chown reported to the hospital's trustees, "1, that the method *is* good and 2, that we have been carrying it out essentially as Sister Kenny does except that we have been over cautious in allowing patients out of bed." Chown also proudly told the board that he had been asked to report "on our experiences here" to the director of the national department of pensions and national health in Ottawa. "Once again," he declared, "we are in the forefront of the attack on disease as we have been in the past."[119] The doctors, nurses, and physical therapists at the Winnipeg Children's Hospital continued their clinical commitment to Kenny's work long after this early visit, and as national and international publicity around her work intensified, the hospital became known as a center for the Kenny method. When specialty committees later began to investigate her method they traveled to Winnipeg.[120]

The success of the Winnipeg trip inspired Kenny to seek out other opportunities to speak to medical groups. During the following months she addressed medical societies in Duluth, Minnesota, and in Columbus, Ohio, and was the featured speaker at the New York Hospital for Joint Diseases.[121] She also visited the Willard Parker Hospital (the city's contagious disease hospital), the Ruptured and Crippled Hospital, and New York's Orthopedic Hospital. She made sure that the NFIP's medical director Don Gudakunst accompanied her on as many of these visits as possible and listened to the praise she received.[122]

Travel enabled her to gather comments from new allies and to introduce her methods and ideas directly, not filtered through second-hand reports. Throughout her career she consistently made much of the credibility of personal observation. Ignoring her own resistance to showing her work during the physical therapists' visit, she reminded O'Connor that it had surely been unwise to have chosen therapists to evaluate her treatment that "they had never seen" and were "not even familiar" with. Fortunately the Kendalls' attacks could now be countered by her new American medical allies. "I was informed by the Senior Orthopedic Surgeon of a world famed clinic that my knowledge of muscle action was not equalled [sic] in any part of the world," she told O'Connor, and, at a recent meeting in New York that Dr. Gudakunst had attended, "a foremost orthopedic surgeon" had said "that my knowledge of muscle anatomy and function was unsurpassed anywhere."[123]

Kenny's base in Minneapolis was boosted by her first celebrity patient: Marjorie Lawrence, a soprano from the Metropolitan Opera who had become paralyzed while singing in Mexico a few months earlier. Lawrence was a fellow Australian. Born in a country town outside Melbourne, she had made her debut at New York's Metropolitan Opera in 1935 and delighted opera audiences when she became the first Brunnhilde to follow Richard Wagner's directions explicitly by riding a horse into the flames of Siegfried's funeral pyre in the final scene of the Ring cycle.[124] Lawrence became Kenny's patient in September 1941 and found her both fierce and gentle, exuding "the strength of authority" combined with "a blend of warm humanity."[125] After a month Lawrence moved out of the hospital into a nearby apartment, where Kenny therapists could visit her, and her husband, an osteopath, could continue her treatment. Although she was not able to walk Lawrence began to retrain her voice, and in 1943 she returned to the Metropolitan Opera stage as a guest artist, singing Venus in "Tannhauser" seated on a divan. She was wheeled out to take her bows. "Diva Returns, Paralysis Beaten" announced the *New York Times*.[126]

Kenny did not read a copy of the Kendall's report on their visit until after she returned from Canada. In her 8-page reply to O'Connor she explained that their attack on her work was the result of their inability to "calmly make a comparison of the two treatments and the results." Had they approached their task rationally and unemotionally instead of with professional defensiveness, they would have seen, just as "all previous critics" had admitted, that "deformities do occur despite the best efforts of the orthopedic surgeon... [and] that quite a degree of this deformity was corrected when all supporting apparatus is removed and Kenny treatment substituted."[127] Kenny also became convinced that the Kendalls were trying to turn other professionals against her. "It was rather unfortunate that Dr. Lewin had the disadvantage of several days with the Kendalls before having the opportunity of meeting myself," she complained in a letter to Fishbein, for "the Kendalls have a wrong conception of the disease, and, I am afraid, know very little about the symptoms they are undertaking to present a treatment for and would prefer the child to suffer rather than their own professional pride."[128] In later years Kenny described the January 1941 visit many times. Sometimes she attacked the Kendalls' "obstinance and prejudice," which had led them to stay away from the afternoon demonstrations; at other times she said "they were probably honest in their convictions and preferred not to see afflicted children suffer from a treatment they believed to be not only unwise and positively damaging."[129]

When Kenny later discussed the January 1941 visit in her autobiography she made it a serious professional group: "a convention of members of the American Physiotherapy Association, delegates...from Baltimore, Chicago, Georgia Warm Springs, and many other cities." She referred to the Kendalls as 2 "prominent physiotherapists," and not by name but as 2 men who "especially requested that I should not be permitted to teach my treatment of the disease." The erasure of Florence Kendall was a poignant reminder of the women physical therapists who had mocked Kenny in Australia. In ignoring the warm reception she received from local women therapists Kenny made herself the lone woman standing up against all these men. She dismissed their report as a personal and irrational attack that "appeared to be much more concerned with me personally than with my work."[130] She did not refer to Alice Plastridge's more positive reports on the visit, which she may not have seen, but she also did not recount the enthusiasm expressed by Plastridge and the other visiting therapists. Indeed, physical therapists were portrayed as unable to break out of their traditional mindset and recognize another woman professional's contribution to medicine. "It was too much for me to hope that an audience habituated to one way of thinking would turn from the opinions of indisputable authorities and embrace those of a comparative stranger."[131]

Kenny recognized that she had to provide evidence to justify her provocative claim that her work led to fewer disabilities than any other polio treatment. The testimonials she had brought with her from Australia and those she was gathering from American physicians had not impressed the visiting therapists and might not sway other skeptics. While the bodies of her patients in Minneapolis remained her most powerful living testimonials, she knew that they could be dismissed as anomalies. Although she continued to resist the necessity for detailed clinical records or muscle testing, Kenny did seek to harness the power of statistics. She was especially struck by the publication of McCarroll and Crego's article in the *Journal of Bone and Joint Surgery*, which the Kendalls had vainly sought to edit before publication. In one table the St. Louis surgeons listed the number and percentage of patients who had achieved what they called "normal" recovery: 4 patients (13 percent) who had been immobilized for 1 to 4 months with no physical therapy; 9 patients (15 percent) who had received a combination of immobilization and physical therapy, which they termed the Kendall method; and 25 patients (19 percent) who had received "no treatment."[132] While she recognized that her own methods had not been used Kenny interpreted these statistics to mean that only 15 percent of children had recovered even when treated by "the best technicians" trained in methods recommended by the Kendalls' *PHS Bulletin*.[133] The St. Louis article made a permanent impression on her. She read it as a published acknowledgment of orthodox failure and quoted its statistics for the rest of her life. The list of polio authorities McCarroll and Crego quoted—including Baltimore's George Bennett and Charles Irwin of Warm Springs—were leading orthodox representatives who had to be either converted or denigrated.[134] Partly as a result of Kenny's frequent reference to it, the St. Louis study lingered in the minds of many polio experts in the early 1940s, and, to the Kendalls' distress, it was interpreted as proving the poor results of immobilization and, worse, as an accurate characterization of the Kendalls' work as epitomizing a conservative and damaging method of polio therapy.[135]

Kenny's use of these comparative statistics ignored the problems of using quantitative analysis for a disease whose sequelae could not be solidly predicted. The credit Kenny claimed for all recoveries, the Kendalls had tried to impress on their NFIP sponsors, ignored the likelihood that many of her patients had made a spontaneous recovery. When Kenny did try to make statistical comparisons between her recoveries and those treated with orthodox methods, the Kendalls remained unconvinced, pointing out that "there are no accurate statistics in this country" for the number of polio recoveries, spontaneous or not.[136]

In fact, comparing the results of polio therapies was almost impossible. Physicians frequently commented that paralysis was an unstable symptom, sometimes intractable and sometimes swiftly ameliorated. Polio was considered such a seriously disabling disease that when Kenny showed physicians her impressive results they often told her the patient had not had polio. She had to establish polio as a disease whose clinical symptoms could be safely and predictably ameliorated (although not "cured"), yet serious enough that it required intelligently designed and executed methods of care. Physicians had long been suspicious of taking efficacy as the defining factor in assessing therapy. The controlled trial was not widely used, and talk of careful scientific study usually meant descriptive observations of patients. Behind the statistics Kenny quoted were grateful

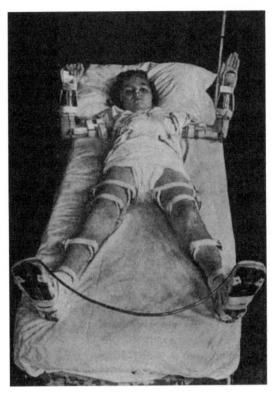

FIGURE 2.2 Image of a child patient in a splinted position "frequently used...to maintain constant muscle protection" from a 1941 guide for the care of polio patients in the home. Reprinted in 1943 from Robert V. Funston and Carmelita Calderwood *Orthopedic Nursing* (St. Louis: Mosby Co., 1943), p. 424. Courtesy of Elsevier.

parents, pain-free children, and solicitous attendants. Happy, healthy Kenny-treated patients, compared to the familiar sights on most polio wards, made a profound impression on every observer. These became the sights and sounds of therapeutic efficacy.

BOOKS AND AUTHORITY

Kenny recognized that her fleeting visits to medical societies and hospitals might intrigue physicians and other professionals but that true conversion had to come from a concerted study of her work.[137] In this era textbooks were at the heart of all medical education. Kenny noticed that 2 recent books on polio therapy mentioned her work, neither of them satisfactorily. Chicago orthopedic surgeon Philip Lewin's text *Infantile Paralysis* was "very vague about the condition of spasm" and "still presents a treatment for a soft, flabby, flaccid paralysis," a symptom she did not believed existed. She especially disliked his publisher's advertisement in *JAMA* claiming that "the technique of my work had been fully described by Dr. Lewin in his book," despite the fact that his reference to her work "scarcely covered a page."[138] She was also unhappy about the "distorted and untruthful statements" in Krusen's 1941 text *Physical Medicine*.[139] Krusen had noted that her ideas were "almost diametrically opposed to those of the Kendalls" and were "so revolutionary that, on first consideration, they would seem hardly to warrant careful scrutiny." Despite her "considerable following" he felt American physicians must rely on the "essentially fair" report of 7 British orthopedists in the 1930s, which concluded that her methods were "harmless but of unproved value."[140] Neither Krusen nor Lewin, Kenny complained to the dean of Minnesota's medical school, "know anything about my work," and both made "very sarcastic reference...to certain important principles of my method."[141] Medical publishers such as W.B. Saunders saw her work as significant and, as Lewin's *JAMA* advertisement showed, even a selling point. These books made her certain that she needed her own textbook.

Kenny recognized that her textbook would have to contain evidence that, unlike her Australian 1937 text, she intended to control closely. Her *Treatment of Infantile Paralysis in the Acute Stage* was published by a local Minneapolis company in September 1941.[142]

Its 264 pages were divided into 17 chapters and 3 appendices. The prose was repetitive and disjointed with many of its chapters simply versions of lectures Kenny had given in Brisbane in the late 1930s and then in Minneapolis. The book included 61 photographs of patients as well as several images of Kenny clinics in Australia and England. The images of the patients, Kenny explained in her preface, were "photographic confirmation" of the value of her work; the images of the buildings and wards were probably included for the same reason.[143] As the book was intended to be used as a pedagogic resource, most of its chapters were organized by body part: Chapter 9 on the neck, Chapter 10 the shoulder girdle, Chapter 11 the forearm and hand, and Chapters 13 and 14 the limbs. The remaining chapters and appendices provided an intellectual defense of her scientific contribution.

Kenny believed that this text would play a crucial role in establishing her work as a serious medical contribution as "it must be understood by all that it is impossible to teach without a book of reference." Even more crucially, the book's detailed explanations of her work would "insure its permanency."[144] Designed for those learning to be Kenny technicians, it was filled with descriptions of detailed techniques that were distinctively different from those used in standard polio care. Kenny had long ago found that skeptical professionals, especially nurses, tended to be "impressed by the authority associated...with the printed word."[145] The book would stand in for her own voice when she left America, providing both a warning and a defense for her technicians and their medical supervisors who would otherwise "have slipped back into the wrong method if it was not recorded in the book how damaging would be this procedure."[146]

Even those sympathetic to Kenny's cause were disappointed by this book. A Chicago surgeon told Gudakunst that its awkward prose meant it was "not very easily read or easily understood."[147] Still, its pictures and detailed instructions made it a useful clinical guide. Perhaps it was a bit too accessible, Cole warned Gudakunst, so "that there is great danger of this book being misused by poorly trained or irregular practitioners." Nonetheless Cole felt "that the part of the book dealing with methods has been very excellently prepared and that a lot of the stuff in the book is good."[148] In publishing this text, Kenny had gone over the head of the NFIP to reach American medical professionals directly. When professionals and members of the public asked the NFIP for a copy Gudakunst explained that the book had been written and published "without the knowledge of the Foundation" and distributed "in spite of the Foundation." Its poor quality, he told one physician frankly, was the reason "it is necessary that the Foundation prepare a pamphlet of its own describing some of the main points of her technique."[149] In 1942 NFIP produced a pamphlet based on reports by Kenny's Minnesota medical supervisors.[150]

Efforts to ensure that the textbook was not seen to have the imprimatur of the NFIP were, however, mostly in vain. Both Gudakunst and O'Connor were convinced that the book had breached the NFIP's policy that grant recipients "refrain from writing articles for public or professional magazines, lecturing or releasing information in any way except through this Foundation."[151] In his role as the head of the NFIP Committee on Information Fishbein phoned John Bruce, head of the Bruce Publishing Company, to warn him of this breach of contract.[152] Bruce knew nothing about any contract with the Foundation, and repeated Kenny's assurance that she had "entered into no contracts and made no commitments." His publishing company, Bruce emphasized to Fishbein, intended "to market this book [only] to the medical profession" and he believed that "nothing in the book or in Kenny's method" conflicted "in any way with ethical medical practices." Gudakunst asked Cole to make sure that Bruce agreed "to insert a flyleaf giving a statement to the effect that the National Foundation had no responsibility for the publication nor does it sponsor the distribution of the book."[153] "We could of course take the necessary steps to stop the publication," Fishbein reflected in a rare letter to O'Connor marked "Personal," "[but] this would, I fear, do more harm than good." Whatever Bruce claimed about marketing the book only to physicians, Fishbein could see that "it will naturally be worked over by the lay press when it published." "I shall of course arrange to have a suitable review of the book in the Journal of the American Medical Association and sooner or latter [sic] I shall write a piece about Sister Kenny to put her in proper perspective," he assured O'Connor. Perhaps, Fishbein added wickedly, Kenny should be allowed to speak at the NFIP meeting that December, maybe "a two minute presentation so that [the] audience can get the full flavor of her personality."[154]

In a haughty defense of her book Kenny protested to Fishbein that she was under control of neither her Minnesota supervisors nor her NFIP sponsors. In one phone call Fishbein told her that although he had "advised the Foundation to allow the publication . . . when we review the book, we shall call attention to such misstatements of fact as appear."[155] Kenny then "minutely examined" her book and told him she "could not find the mistakes referred to." The idea of a contract breach was nonsense, she added, as the lectures that made up the book did not deal with the results of work carried out under the NFIP grant.[156] "She was very much on her high horse," Fishbein said when he described this conversation to O'Connor, and had declared " 'Well, I don't care for America anyway. I merely came over here to get my book published, and I am going back to Australia as soon as I can.' I asked her if she would authorize me to use that statement to the press, and then I hung up on her." "She is, of course, an impossible person as far as concerns any sensible conversation," he added, "I propose to have nothing further to do with her."[157] But as Fishbein recognized, such a policy of high-minded neglect was not going to work. Privately O'Connor agreed with Fishbein's desire to have nothing further to do with Kenny but as NFIP director he had no such option. After discussing the problem of her book with Gudakunst, O'Connor decided to ignore her claim that the book established the worth of her work. He assured Fishbein that he would continue to point out to her, as he had repeatedly, that the University of Minnesota's medical school "is our grantee to evaluate her work, and we therefore look to that institution rather than to her."[158]

In a move that gained her even more publicity Kenny cooperated with Lois Maddox Miller in the writing of "Sister Kenny vs. Infantile Paralysis," the featured article in the

December 1941 issue of *Reader's Digest*. Fishbein had assured O'Connor a few months earlier that he knew Miller, "a friend of mine," was working on an article on Kenny; "however, all of the medical articles of the Digest are submitted to me and I will have the opportunity to go over that one."[159]

Miller, a freelance science journalist, deftly drew a picture of Kenny that intrigued American readers. In 5 pages her article moved from "the lonely outlands where she served as visiting nurse, midwife, and counselor to the sparsely settled families" to a "small boy, his legs strapped in splints, his face contorted from pain" to the 8 government-supported large hospital clinics in Australia where "hundreds of nurses take the two-year postgraduate course which fits them to use the Kenny method." These exaggerated claims—the hundreds of nurses, the formal 2-year course, and the 8 government clinics—were part of a story Kenny had developed since her return from Australia in June. Having "dedicated her life to extending her merciful work as widely as possible" Kenny ("the British give chief nurses the title of 'Sister'") had looked toward the United States and discovered that "the United States has maintained the most enlightened and realistic attitude toward the problem— has tried hardest to push research into polio's mysteries, has done more in after-therapy, and, through the great National Foundation of Infantile Paralysis, supported by contributions from the entire nation, has demonstrated its determination to reach out for the best and newest at any cost."[160] Such hyperbole showed Fishbein's likely hand.

In this picture, Kenny was a "tall, gray-haired, motherly woman [who] proudly refers to herself as a 'bush baby.'" Miller described her age as "some 50 years"; in fact Kenny had just turned 61. Kenny's methods were contrasted with the effects of ordinary treatment during which "there is a long, grim siege of pain—anywhere between two weeks and many months." Miller's description of the method itself was somewhat inaccurate: spasm, an important symptom "which apparently doctors had not noticed before," was relieved by hot foments, massage, manipulation, and passive exercise.[161] Kenny was usually annoyed when professionals or the press talked about "massage" (she fought for and later won a *JAMA* retraction) but here she made no comment.

The spectacular results of Kenny's work were exemplified by the miraculous recovery of Kenny's American patients. Rita N. a patient with bulbar poliomyelitis had been given last rites by a priest but after 20 days of Kenny treatment she recovered fully. Her mother said "'It seemed like a miracle—we had given up hope." Joan B., who would have been placed in an iron lung, was "completely cured" in 6 weeks. The bulk of the article dealt with Kenny's effort to convince physicians: some denied the "phenomenon of spasm, or minimized its importance"; many considered her "bold refusal to use splints or braces...unwise and hazardous." But Kenny had been victorious, proving her work was new and revolutionary.[162]

In a section that most closely showed Fishbein's editing hand, Miller tried to establish that Kenny herself, however unorthodox and shocking her methods, was not challenging the medical hierarchy. Kenny was an enthusiast, but she also knew her place. She had "devoted her life to the one crusade, demonstrating to physicians, training other nurses in her methods, spreading her influence with missionary zeal." Yet "the nurse practicing the Kenny method does not replace the doctor, but works with him. She does not cure the disease—medical science knows no cure for it. But she does make it easier to bear, and does cut down—often completely eliminates—aftereffects." Most of all, Kenny had "turned a deaf ear to suggestions that she would get ahead faster if she ignored the doctors. 'This treatment can be developed only within the medical profession,' she said, and stuck to it." Miller left ambiguous whether Kenny's contribution was simply a treatment or a new concept as well. She quoted Kenny's

Australian mentor Aeneas McDonnell, probably via Kenny herself, saying "She has knocked our theories into a cocked hat; but her treatment works, and that's all that counts."[163]

This story had something for everyone. It provided polio survivors and their families as well as other disabled readers with hope in a scientific form. Physical therapists and nurses dissatisfied with current polio practices were intrigued about this miracle healer. Readers seeking alternatives to surgery saw Kenny's work as natural, domestic, and pain-free. Here was a sympathetic picture of a middle-aged, yet still vigorous nurse who both worked within the traditional restraints of her career and gender—a physician's helpmeet, a caregiver who touched bodies and dealt with the messy stuff of pain and disability—and yet stood outside it, challenging orthodoxy in thinking as well as practice, telling doctors what to do. Miller called Kenny motherly for she cared for children, but such a designation could also call up a picture of mothers fiercely defending their young, or perhaps the kinds of characters featured in Wild West movies where the rancher's wife knew how to use a gun to warn off marauders. This nurse, readers were assured perhaps too vehemently, was committed to orthodox medicine, its culture, and its professional hierarchy. But what if she moved away from the auspices of the respected medical school? What if her patients' families began demanding that she take control of polio care instead of their doctor? What if she felt that the NFIP was not properly supporting and promoting her work?

Despite her protests, Kenny was a quick study. She began to consider writing another book with the explicit sponsorship of the NFIP and her medical supervisors. Her next textbook, as we will see, was published in 1943 with a preface from O'Connor and an afterward by Knapp, and was co-written with Pohl.

APPROVED BY THE MARCH OF DIMES

The pinnacle of Kenny's early success came on December 5, 1941, 2 days before Pearl Harbor. At the second annual meeting of the NFIP's medical advisors held in New York— to which Kenny was not invited—the Committee on Research for the Prevention and Treatment of After-Effects announced that, based on reports from Minneapolis, the Kenny method used during the early stages of polio "greatly reduced...the length of time during which pain, tenderness, and spasm are present" and prevented "contractures caused by muscle shortening during this period." The general physical condition of her patients also seemed to be better than patients treated by other methods.[164] In a dramatic policy announcement, the NFIP's medical advisors then recommended that health officials throughout the nation should promptly be given information "regarding the nature of the Kenny technique and its integration with other measures of treatment"; the NFIP should establish training programs for physicians, nurses, and physical therapists to become "fully trained in the essentials and principles of the Kenny method"; and it should produce "a concise manual providing the essential principles and details of the Kenny method and of other applications of hydropathy and physical treatment in the early stage of infantile paralysis."[165] With careful timing, Fishbein published a sympathetic editorial in JAMA arguing that recent physiology research had shown that immobilization might be harmful as normal groups of muscle fibers could become atrophic with the restriction of "the flow of these proprioceptive impulses." The editorial firmly rejected the concept of alienation, arguing, as the Kendalls had done, that "no experimental evidence" supported "the contention that single muscle units might, as a result of appropriate manipulation, be encouraged to send their nerve fibers to muscles fibers which had been rendered atrophic by anterior horn cell degeneration." In his description of Kenny's technique Fishbein deliberately provided few details, and the details he did provide were casual and inaccurate. "If all available motor units in paretic muscles are to retain their maximum physiologic capacity," Fishbein wrote, then "massage and freedom of movement" were "clearly indicated."[166] Neither massage nor free muscle movements were part of Kenny's work.

Here were explicit signs of clinical change and proposed policies for the inculcation of this work into medical practice. Defending this change in NFIP policy in promoting a kind of polio care that sounded so different from standard methods, O'Connor sought to downplay both Kenny and her clinical results. At the NFIP meeting's annual dinner at the Hotel Pierre, O'Connor emphasized that the Minnesota clinicians' conclusions were supported by NFIP-funded physiological research, including animal experiments from Iowa State University and the University of Toronto that suggested that restricted motion could delay muscle recovery. To placate skeptical orthopedists O'Connor referred to research by eminent Iowa orthopedist Arthur Steindler that had shown that shortening and distortion could be caused by contractions of severely paralyzed muscles that were allowed to remain in one place for too long.[167]

Despite these efforts to incorporate Kenny's work within serious scientific research the press delighted in the story of a crusading nurse and her revolutionary method of treatment. With headlines like "Sister Kenny's Triumph," *Time* and *Newsweek* explained that her methods, unlike standard clinical practice, stimulated rather than immobilized muscles in early cases, and that *JAMA*—"organized medicine's leading publication"—had "formally approved" her work.[168] "Kenny Paralysis Treatment Approved by U.S. Medicine" agreed the *New York Times*, quoting O'Connor's statement that her methods had been proven "superior to the present orthodox methods of treatment."[169]

In vain Fishbein prepared a further *JAMA* editorial that urged American physicians to remember that the conclusions of the NFIP's advisory committees were based on "reports from various experimental laboratories and clinics." He also sought to move the work out of Kenny's hands, describing Knapp's detailed study of the Kenny method that would enable Knapp and other physicians "to continue with the teaching after Miss Kenny and her staff return to Australia." The new method "represents an elaboration of well recognized principles in the treatment of acute paralysis" and was based on "scientific research on the physiology of the nervous system which explains the value of the technic."[170] It was, in other words, not a strange, unscientific system developed by an innovative nurse, but the practical articulation of methods that fit into mainstream medical science and were therefore worthy of funding and further study.

Annoyed at the inaccuracies of the first editorial, Kenny was irate that this second editorial portrayed her work as simply part of the progress of medical science. "It is impossible to merge any other existing treatment with the Kenny treatment," she protested to O'Connor. "All other systems have been evolved for symptoms that do not exist. Dr. Gudakunst admitted this to me when I spoke to him."[171] Urging Kenny to complain to Fishbein directly, O'Connor implied that he had little influence over the AMA's journal but Kenny would have none of it. "I quite understand the Foundation has no control over the American Medical Journal," she pointed out to him, "but I should imagine it has the power to correct the misleading statements made in connection with the Foundation's activities."[172]

Kenny was right. The NFIP was able to exert influence over *JAMA*, but O'Connor refrained from doing so until Fishbein published an anonymous review of Kenny's text-book. Mealy-mouthed in its praise and sharp-tongued in its criticism, the review by Edward Lyon Compere, an eminent Chicago orthopedic surgeon, found Kenny's book full of "infinite detail" and providing a "confusing discussion of pathologic principles." A nurse might not be expected to understand polio's complexities, he argued, but any physician "thoroughly grounded in physiology, anatomy and pathology" who had observed "the degenerative changes in the anterior horn cells . . . will find much in the Kenny theory that is absurd and unscientific." Irrespective of the author's "enthusiasm" that appeared in every chapter of the book and bordered "on religious fanaticism," Compere noted, there would continue to be patients who needed splints, those who would undoubtedly die if they were not in an iron lung, and those would never walk a step "without the aid of the braces she condemns." Still, the medical profession owed Kenny "a debt of gratitude for having made us realize that prolonged splinting without exercise, without heat and mois-ture applied to the limbs, is harmful." Compere hoped his peers would be "sufficiently liberal minded to accept the good elements of the Kenny theory without losing our bal-ance and falling head over heels into a pit which both Galen and Hippocrates succeeded in climbing out of many centuries ago."[173] This pit, *JAMA* readers could assume, was empiri-cal, symptomatic medical care, bereft of the rigor of male Western scientific knowledge.

Outraged, Kenny called Gudakunst twice, reversing the charges, to complain that the AMA's official journal had called her ideas "absurd and unscientific." If the review was not retracted, she said, she would return immediately to Australia "since there was no use trying to fight the American Medical Association." Gudakunst urged her to forget the review and go on with her work, but Kenny said she was too upset. Shifting her argument to an appeal to populism she declared that she would go on a lecture tour to appeal directly to the public for Americans had supported her more than the NFIP or the University of Minnesota.[174] She also wrote to Fishbein, accusing his reviewer of not keeping "abreast with current literature" such as "the acknowledgment of the official observers of the Medical School, University of Minnesota." It was not true that the condition of spasm was familiar to polio experts. In Kenny's experience, based on the many thousands of cases seen in different parts of the world, polio authorities had ignored "this painful and damaging condition." Trying to be both courteous and vehement, Kenny "respectfully" suggested the reviewer "come to Minneapolis as soon as possible, and I will produce the evidence to convince him that he is altogether wrong in his concept, and how unwise it is to condemn a work he knows nothing whatever about."[175] Discovering the reviewer's identity, Kenny contacted Compere directly and urged him to come to Minnesota and see her work for himself.[176]

NFIP officials were becoming familiar with Kenny's threats of leaving and her demands for public recognition. But after the NFIP's December decision to promote her work Kenny could now more confidently challenge critics with evidence that its own elite medical advisors recognized her methods as a valuable improvement to former polio therapies.

Kenny found that she was able to win over critics of her written work with the clinical evidence of her patients. In response to her letters and phone calls, Compere traveled to Minneapolis for a day's observation and returned to Chicago, he admitted to NFIP officials, "very much more sold on her methods than I had been before." His opinion of the book did not "represent my opinion of the treatment itself." While he did not "understand why she achieved some of her results" and was not "prepared to accept all of her theory" he was convinced that "her methods are definitely good."[177] Gratified that she could now count Compere among her supporters, Kenny now reminded him of his promise "to rectify the erroneous ideas you had about my work" by writing a statement that could be published in *JAMA*.[178] While Compere did not write a correction, he did invite Kenny to come to Chicago to discuss her work before an audience of doctors, nurses, and physical therapists at the Wesley Memorial Hospital. Fishbein, whom Kenny invited, did not attend.[179] Her lecture, Compere told her later, was a great success. He hoped she would return to give another talk and demonstration and he promised to explain "the advantages of the Kenny method" at the next meeting of the Chicago Orthopedic Society.[180] A delighted Kenny thanked him, but wanted to correct a comment about Cole and Knapp's skepticism that had been made during her trip. "I asked Dr. Cole and Dr. Knapp where they disagreed with me, and they said that they do not disagree with me anywhere. They did at first but not now."[181] Perhaps Compere, having met Kenny in person, could guess that Cole and Knapp had learned not to engage in debates with their Australian visitor.

Even before Compere's visit Gudakunst had also traveled to Minnesota, a visit that led him, like Compere, to change his mind. He had been appointed the NFIP's medical director only a few months before Kenny's arrival in New York in April 1940. As Michigan's state health officer during the 1930s he had survived many stormy experiences, and his position as medical advisor to O'Connor, who was a lawyer and not a doctor, gave him ample opportunities to confront and dissuade aspiring polio innovators, and to "weed out the obviously sorry applications."[182] He had organized the visits of the 5 physical therapists to see Kenny in Minneapolis and read their mixed reports. Concerned that she was a publicity seeker and perhaps a bit crazy, he had begun to caution others not to laud her too extravagantly. When the NFIP was consulted by *Parents Magazine* about the advisability of making its annual award on behalf of children to Kenny in 1941, Gudakunst had warned that "it would be unwise to have such an award made immediately." The award was not given to Kenny until the following year.[183]

When Gudakunst arrived in Minneapolis, Kenny eagerly demonstrated her work and gave a lengthy lecture during which she called on the NFIP "to correct the erroneous statements" in the first *JAMA* editorial. These mistakes, she claimed, had harmed patients by suggesting to patients and medical professionals that massage was part of her work. Further, its lack of detail had resulted in some patients having to undergo "the [unnecessary] operation of appendectomy...owing to the lack of knowledge of the true symptoms of the disease." She quoted tributes made by "all visiting doctors to this clinic," such as a group of Ohio orthopedists who told her "they could only look back with sorrow and regret at the mistakes made in the past." Shrewdly, her lecture included not only a defense of her ideas but also the claim that her work returned patients to economic independence. Thus, an 18-year-old patient who had gained "a certain amount of recovery in all muscle groups" could now wash and feed herself and stand up alone, and she had won a scholarship to study commercial art.[184]

His visit to Minneapolis convinced Gudakunst both of the value of Kenny's work and the danger of inaccurate publicity, which was hurting both the NFIP's promotion of the new method and the fund's own reputation. He became convinced that the AMA was deliberately undermining Kenny and thereby her philanthropic sponsor. After a radio program sponsored by the AMA "gave her an extensive plug but described her work as consisting of early active exercise," he suggested that someone from the AMA "should go to

Minneapolis to visit Miss Kenny and see what she is doing," and that whatever *JAMA* published about Kenny "be reviewed by such an informed individual." The ill-advised *JAMA* editorial, he added, repeating another point Kenny had made to him in Minneapolis, may even have harmed patients if physicians used "active massage in the early stage of the disease" acting "under the misconception" that they were "using at least a modification of the Kenny method."[185] To O'Connor he also wondered whether "a conference with Dr. Fishbein might not be out of order."[186]

Gudakunst began to use Kenny's explanations to defend her work. One of her objections to splints, he told one skeptic, "is that the pressure of the splint on the skin serves to stimulate the reflexes and produce additional spasm," admitting "I'm getting so I talk like Kenny."[187] When Henry Viets, an editor of the *New England Journal of Medicine*, sent him a draft of an editorial on Kenny, Gudakunst protested that "the techniques developed by Miss Kenny call for an intimate knowledge of muscle anatomy and function" and praised "the excellent end results seen in her cases" and her specialized physical therapy that treated "incoordination and alienation as well as through the proper application of heat during the stage of spasm."[188] Like Kenny, Gudakunst rejected the idea proposed in *JAMA* that Kenny's work "represents an elaboration of well recognized principles in the treatment of acute paralysis." Her view of polio was not simply part of the progression of medical science, he assured Fishbein's *JAMA* assistant Larry Salter, for nowhere in the medical literature with which he was familiar was polio described as having symptoms that were "primarily spastic contractures of the muscles." Previous medical teaching "very definitely has been that loss of function was due to paralysis and that there was no other damaging involvement of the nervous system," yet Kenny "has demonstrated that actually the paralysis of this disease is a very minor contributing factor to disability" and "the inability to use 'healthy muscles' really accounts for the disfunction creating disability." Gudakunst realized that defensive physicians might be unable to admit the extent of Kenny's innovation. "There is a revolutionary element," he told Salter, "hence, the unwillingness and even the inability to appreciate just what she has."[189] After reading Compere's report of his visit Gudakunst wrote to him agreeing that "there is much of good in the Kenny method" and the NFIP had "a tremendous responsibility" to acquaint "American physicians with her work." While Gudakunst "wholeheartedly" agreed that "Miss Kenny's book is a sad mistake," he was "in complete sympathy with your attitude and what you say—that the book does not express an opinion of the treatment itself."[190]

Gudakunst also developed a new way of looking at polio patients. When he visited patients at Cleveland's contagious disease hospital a few weeks after his Minneapolis visit, he reported that they were "in very good shape, [but] they in no way compare with those treated by the Kenny method." Indeed, Gudakunst himself was able to identify "evidence of definite spasm in the hamstrings and gastric-nemius groups in several patients," a sign, he felt, of the patients' inadequate care.[191]

But clinical results were one thing; scientific theory was another. Fishbein, Salter, and other AMA officials retained their skepticism that a nurse could use clinical experience alone to come up with any credible explanation for understanding the physiology or pathology of a disease. In "my personal opinion," Salter told Gudakunst bluntly, "when she starts to discuss anyone else's opinion of her theories—in contrast to her method—she is on controversial ground and the less she says about differing opinions, and even her own *theories* on how her *method* works, the better off she will be and the happier she will make you, me and a lot of other people who are continuously dragged into her 'fights.' "[192]

In mocking Kenny's theories Fishbein's assistant was drawing on a familiar tradition of denigrating those outside the medical establishment who could be valued perhaps for pragmatic techniques but not for theoretical contributions to medical science. The poor quality of her textbook helped to reinforce this distinction, and even supporters such as Gudakunst and Compere began to defend her work based more on its clinical efficacy than its intellectual originality. Thus, as Gudakunst admitted to one Connecticut health official, Kenny's book "is one of the worst attempts to describe a technique that I have ever encountered. But this does not mean that Miss Kenny's work is not good. I sincerely believe that she has made a real contribution to the treatment of early poliomyelitis."[193]

A BREAK AWAY FROM PRESENT METHODS

By early 1942, a year after the physical therapists' visit to Minneapolis, many things had changed. The *Reader's Digest* article had solidified Kenny's status as an exciting new figure in medicine—an exotic nurse from a distant land. She had also acquired powerful new allies. Even Gudakunst was now a proponent, willing on occasion to use the power of the NFIP. After protests by Gudakunst and a phone conversation with O'Connor, for example, Fishbein did publish a "Correction" in the mid-January issue of *JAMA*, correcting not Compere's review but his first editorial. Massage did not have any part in Kenny's procedure, the editor now admitted, and "according to her concept, the cardinal symptoms of infantile paralysis are 'muscle spasm, muscle incoordination and muscle alienation,'" a phrase from Kenny's letter to Fishbein.[194] Here was a reference, however reluctantly, to both her clinical techniques and her ideas.

As physicians began to take Kenny's work seriously they were eager to demonstrate the fair, scientific, and open-minded nature of their profession by welcoming the woman and the work. But the battle was not over. While it was obvious that Kenny's methods were becoming a central part of NFIP publicity, the question of authority over clinical care remained undecided. Kenny's textbook had been published, but despite Kenny's efforts to make the text serious and scientific, many readers saw it as the work of an overenthusiastic nurse, partly because it was poorly written and partly because it challenged the views of orthopedists who had been trained in more pessimistic, less activist therapies. Seeking to capture the cautious tone of the NFIP's medical advisors, Gudakunst began preparing an NFIP text based on the work of Cole, Knapp and Pohl.[195] His pamphlet on *The Kenny Method* and the courses that the NFIP began to set up in hospitals and health science schools outside Minneapolis suggested that wiser, more experienced polio experts were in control of this clinical innovation.

As physicians, nurses, and physical therapists began to alter their practice, they struggled to decide how significant clinical observation was and should be. Kenny had claimed to be seeking scientific explanations for the new symptoms she had identified, and initially she, like her critics, saw laboratory research by physiologists and pathologists as epitomizing scientific truth, a more reliable truth than one that clinicians could hope to establish. Even clinical experts expressed caution in judging Kenny's work solely by its clinical results. In a 3 page section on the Kenny treatment in *The 1941 Year Book of Physical Therapy* Richard Kovacs noted that although "the last word has not yet been spoken as to the most effective treatment," this method clearly was a break "away from the present method of prolonged complete immobilization." It might sound "revolutionary" to those who believed in "standard' treatment," but in mild yet hopeful words Kovacs felt its results appeared "encouraging."[196] Viets' editorial in the *New England Journal of Medicine* praised her methods and, unlike the *JAMA* editorials, argued that Kenny's method "completely revolutionizes modern ideas regarding the treatment of acute poliomyelitis" by rejecting "muscle testing, splinting, avoiding of overstretching, absolute rest and many other procedures." What his editorial did not refer to was any part of her growing articulation of a new view of polio itself.[197] To their surprise when orthopedists and physical medicine specialists turned to laboratory research to compare Kenny's claims to serious studies of the impact of the polio virus on muscles they discovered there were few such studies.

As Fishbein had anticipated, Kenny's book was indeed read by ordinary Americans, and this led to growing popular demand for her work. James Gray of the *St Paul Pioneer Press* praised her "blunt, matter-of-fact and sensible" tone and her publicized decision to work within the medical establishment.[198] Members of NFIP chapters began demanding more information about this method and urged the NFIP's national office to publicize it more extensively. A physician from Tacoma, Washington, who was a member of his local chapter, suggested to Gudakunst that "some of our publicity in connection with the Roosevelt Birthday Ball next month could be well devoted to a discussion of the present status of Sister Kenney's [sic] work" and urged the NFIP to offer "some official recognition of this nurse and her work."[199] The chair of the NFIP chapter in Magnum, Oklahoma, similarly told O'Connor that the *Reader's Digest* article was "the best article on the subject that I have ever read." Reprints of it, he believed, "should be in the hands of every Committee for Infantile Paralysis in the U.S."[200] During the NFIP's March of Dimes January campaign the link between polio and President Roosevelt inspired some Americans to insist that Kenny share this national attention. After reading about Kenny in the *Reader's Digest* and the *New York Times* Ann van Kavcren, a nurse working with polio patients at the Boston Children's Hospital, expressed herself "greatly shocked to learn that this treatment has been used for many years in Australia, and that we are just now hearing about it." Kenny, she argued, should be recognized in some public way, and the appropriate moment might be the March of Dimes' upcoming celebration of the president's 60th birthday in January 1942.[201] It was the beginning of a new moment in America's polio history with Kenny at the center.

NOTES

1. "Paralysis Sufferers' Pleas Come in Flood" *Minneapolis Star-Journal* February 5 1941; Willis M. Kimball "City May Become National Center in Study of New Polio Treatment" *Minneapolis Star-Journal* January 30 1941.

2. Paul *A History*, 312–317.

3. Kenny with Ostenso *And They Shall Walk*, 211.

4. Albert B. Sabin "Etiology of Poliomyelitis" *JAMA* (July 26 1941) 117: 267–269. On conferences funded by the NFIP in the early 1940s see Roy L. Chambliss, Jr. "A Social History of

the National Foundation of Infantile Paralysis, Inc, 1938–1948," Master of Science in Social Service dissertation, Fordham University School of Social Service, New York, 1950, Public Relations, History, MOD, 82.

5. John R. Paul "The Epidemiology of Poliomyelitis" *Infantile Paralysis; A Symposium Delivered at Vanderbilt University, April, 1941* (New York: National Foundation for Infantile Paralysis, 1941), 147–153; see also pathologist Ernest Goodpasture who admitted that many experts no longer saw polio as "essentially an infection of the central nervous system"; Ernest W. Goodpasture "The Pathology of Poliomyelitis" *JAMA* (July 26 1941) 117: 273–275.

6. *Annual Report: For the Year Ended May 31 1945* (New York: National Foundation for Infantile Paralysis, 1945), 17–22.

7. Kenny with Ostenso *And They Shall Walk*, 222. See also Kenny boasting to Chuter that she had been invited to instruct physical therapists in Minnesota, Kenny to Dear Mr. Chuter, May 28 1940, Home Secretary's Office, Special Batches, Kenny Clinics, 1941–1949, A/31753, QSA.

8. Alice Lou Plastridge "Report of Observation of Work of Sister Elizabeth Kenny in Minneapolis, Minnesota, January 1941" [read to Georgia Chapter of the American Physiotherapy Association on February 14 1941, at Warm Springs], Florence Kendall Collection, Silver Springs, Maryland, 1; Kenny to Dear Dr. Cole, September 12 1940, Public Relations, MOD-K.

9. "Muscle Reeducation" [review of Kenny *Infantile Paralysis and Cerebral Diplegia: Methods Used for the Restoration of Function] Medical Journal of Australia* (May 8 1937) 1: 713–714; R. W. Cilento "Report on Sister E. Kenny's After-Treatment of Cases of Paralysis Following Poliomyelitis," Ms. 44/109, Fryer Library, 13–14, 4; Cilento to The Minister, June 30 1939, [enclosed in] Cilento to Dear Dr. Cumpston, July 10 1939, Series A-1928, 802/17/Section, 3, AA-ACT.

10. Henry Otis Kendall and Florence P. Kendall *Care During the Recovery Period in Paralytic Poliomyelitis* (Washington, DC: Government Printing Office, 1938, revised 1939, Public Health Service Bulletin No. 242); Kenny with Ostenso *And They Shall Walk*, 207–208.

11. Carmelita Calderwood "Nursing Care in Poliomyelitis" *American Journal of Nursing* (1940) 40: 629– 630.

12. C. M. Sampson *A Practice of Physiotherapy* (St. Louis: C.V. Mosby, 1926), 20–22, 584–585; see also Harry Eaton Stewart *Physiotherapy: Theory and Clinical Application* (New York: Paul B. Hoeber, 1925).

13. Frank H. Krusen *Physical Medicine: The Employment of Physical Agents for Diagnosis and Therapy* (Philadelphia and London: W. B. Saunders, 1941), 774.

14. L. Caitlin Smith "Alice Lou Plastridge-Converse" *PT: Magazine of Physical Therapy* (2000) 8: 42–49.

15. "Mildred Elson, 87, Physical Therapist" *Boston Globe* September 25 1987.

16. "Gertrude Beard" *Physiotherapy Review* (June 1971) 51: 108.

17. Florence P. Kendall "Sister Elizabeth Kenny Revisited" *Archives of Physical Medicine and Rehabilitation* (1998) 79: 361–365.

18. On the history of hospital-schools in the United States see Brad Byrom "A Pupil and a Patient: Hospital-Schools in Progressive America" in Paul K. Longmore and Lauri Umansky eds. *New Disability History: American Perspectives* (New York: New York University Press, 2001), 133–156.

19. In the 1920s and early 1930s this department consisted only of Henry Kendall and Louise Mims, who had treated Roosevelt some years earlier; Florence Kendall, interview with Rogers, April 26 1999, Silver Springs; see also *The Children's Hospital Story* (Baltimore n.p., n.d.) George E. Bennett Papers, Box 503122, Alan Mason Chesney Medical Archives, Johns Hopkins University, Baltimore.

20. Kendall, interview with Rogers, April 26 1999; Henry Kendall regained partial vision but was unable to drive a car, and the glass eye he wore (before plastic eyes were developed in the late 1940s) had a tendency to explode with sudden changes in temperature.

21. Lucie P. Lawrence "Florence Kendall: What a Wonderful Journey" *PT: Magazine of Physical Therapy* (2000) 8: 41–42. A few years later they published their major textbook: H.O. Kendall and F. P. Kendall *Muscle Testing and Function* (Baltimore: Williams & Wilkins, 1949). Henry left to work in private practice, and retired in 1971.

22. Kendall, interview with Rogers, April 26 1999; Lawrence "Florence Kendall: What a Wonderful Journey," 36–45.

23. Henry O. Kendall "Some Interesting Observations about the After Care of Infantile Paralysis Patients" *Journal of Exceptional Children* (April 1937) 3: 107–112; see also Kendall and Kendall *Care During the Recovery Period in Paralytic Poliomyelitis*.

24. Lawrence "Florence Kendall: What a Wonderful Journey," 36–45; Maude W. Baum "Convalescent Poliomyelitis Cases: Moving Picture Demonstration of Their Examination, Protection, and Treatment" *Physiotherapy Review* (1939) 19: 31–32; Kendall, interview with Rogers, April 26 1999. The film was sent to Italy to help Benito Mussolini's daughter Maria when she was paralyzed by polio; Kendall "Sister Elizabeth Kenny Revisited," 362.

25. For critiques of the Kendalls' work see Krusen *Physical Medicine*, 592–593; K. G. Hansson "Present Status of Physical Therapy in Anterior Poliomyelitis" *Physiotherapy Review* (1942) 22: 3–5.

26. H. R. McCarroll and C. H. Crego, Jr. "An Evaluation of Physiotherapy in Early Treatment of Anterior Poliomyelitis" *Journal of Bone and Joint Surgery* (1941) 23: 856–861. They probably read F. H. Mills "Treatment of Acute Poliomyelitis: An Analysis of Sister Kenny's Methods" *British Medical Journal* (January 22 1938) 1: 168–170.

27. Kendall "Sister Elizabeth Kenny Revisited," 362–363; Henry Kendall to Henry Pope, April 2 1940, Kendall Collection. Florence Kendall became convinced that the St. Louis study had been deliberately done to discredit the Kendall method; Kendall, interview with Rogers, April 26 1999.

28. Pohl to [Henry] Kendall, January 10 1941, Kendall Collection.

29. Kenny to Dear Mr. O'Connor, October 11 1941, Public Relations, MOD-K.

30. Kenny "Data Concerning Introduction of Kenny Concept and Method of Treatment of Infantile Paralysis [1944]," Board of Directors, MHS-K; Kenny to Luddy and Cooper [Brisbane clinic], October 8 1941, Scrapbook, OM 65-17, 2/3, Chuter Papers, Oxley-SLQ.

31. Kenny with Ostenso *And They Shall Walk*, 228–229.

32. Kenny to Dr. Bennett, January 28 1941, Kendall Collection.

33. Kenny "Paper Read at the Northwestern Pediatric Conference, Nov. 14, 1940, Saint Paul University Club." Note that Lovett had died in 1924, Legg in 1939, and Jones in 1933.

34. Henry O. Kendall and Florence P. Kendall "Report to the National Foundation for Infantile Paralysis on The Sister Kenny Method of Treatment in Anterior Poliomyelitis," Revised March 21 1941, Public Relations, MOD-K, 2.

35. Kenny to Dear Mr. O'Connor, October 11 1941, Public Relations, MOD-K.

36. Kenny "Paper Read at the Northwestern Pediatric Conference, Nov. 14, 1940, Saint Paul University Club."

37. [Kenny] "Orthodox and Kenny System of Treatment of Poliomyelitis: Analysis of Principles Upon Which Systems are Founded," [1940] Series A-1928, 802/17/Section 3, AA- ACT.

38. Kenny to Dr. Bennett, January 28 1941, Kendall Collection.

39. Kendall and Kendall "Report," 6.

40. Plastridge "Report of Observation," 6.

41. Florence did not "remember seeing her smile"; Henry thought she was a quack who had "found herself a nice position"; Kendall, interview with Rogers, April 27 1999.

42. Kenny to Dear Mr. O'Connor, October 11 1941, Public Relations, MOD-K; Kenny with Ostenso *And They Shall Walk*, 230.

43. Florence Kendall and Henry Kendall "Our Notes" (January 19–21 1941), Kendall Collection; Kenny with Ostenso *And They Shall Walk*, 231.

44. Kenny to Dr. Bennett, January 28 1941, Kendall Collection. Kenny later told O'Connor that "unfortunately, Mr. Kendall took control of this demonstration figuratively and gave to the audience his own explanation"; Kenny to Dear Mr. O'Connor, October 11, 1941, Public Relations, MOD-K.

45. Plastridge "Report of Observation," 7; Kenny to Dear Mr. O'Connor, October 11 1941, Public Relations, MOD-K.

46. Kendall and Kendall "Report," 2.

47. Kendall and Kendall "Report," 3; for a recollection of Henry's outburst see Kendall, interview with Rogers, April 27 1999.

48. Kenny to Dear Mr. O'Connor, October 11 1941, Public Relations, MOD-K; Kendall and Kendall, "Report," 3; Kendall, interview with Rogers, April 27 1999.

49. C. E. Irwin "Early Orthopedic Care in Poliomyelitis" *JAMA* (July 26 1941) 117: 280–282.

50. Plastridge "Report of Observation," 1; Miss Plastridge to Dr. Irwin Memorandum: In re: Trip to Observe Work of Sister Kenny, March 15 1941, Kendall Collection.

51. Plastridge to Irwin Memorandum, 1941.

52. Henry M. Haverstock To Whom It May Concern, September 4 1940, Public Relations, MOD-K; Kenny with Ostenso *And They Shall Walk*, 225–227; and see Alexander on Pohl and Haverstock's memories of this case, *Maverick*, 118–119.

53. Plastridge to Irwin Memorandum, 1941.

54. Robert M. Yoder "Healer from the Outback" *Saturday Evening Post* (January 17 1942) 214: 18–19, 68, 70; Kenny with Ostenso *And They Shall Walk*, 227; Gould *Summer Plague*, 96–98; John F. Pohl "The Kenny Treatment of Anterior Poliomyelitis (Infantile Paralysis): Report of First Cases Treated in America" *JAMA* (April 25 1942) 118: 1428–1433.

55. Plastridge "Report of Observation," 8, 10.

56. Kendall and Kendall "Report," 7–8, 10.

57. Plastridge "Report of Observation," 7.

58. Plastridge to Irwin Memorandum, 1941; Plastridge "Report of Observation," 2, 8, 10.

59. Kendall and Kendall "Report," 1–2, 4. Plastridge had also noted that Kenny seemed to have only vague reports about her patients such as "patient could not put chin on chest" or "patient could not raise right arm"; Plastridge "Report of Observation," 7. "There may have been more to her written records," Plastridge noted, "but we did not see them." Note that physical medicine experts noted that many hospital departments of physical therapy did not keep "adequate records"; Krusen *Physical Medicine*, 782.

60. Kendall and Kendall "Our Notes," Kendall Collection. Florence Kendall later said that she and her husband had asked to see the hospital patient records, and were told that Kenny "had them at home." Other visitors, she claimed, "have become aware that S.K.'s statistics are based on selected cases. She refuses to treat those which she knows are hopeless"; [Florence Kendall] Notes for Talk to Nurses, St Agnes Hospital, April 28 1944, Kendall Collection.

61. Kendall and Kendall "Report," 12–13.

62. Kendall and Kendall "Report," 2.

63. Plastridge "Report of Observation," 2; Kendall, interview with Rogers, April 27 1999.

64. Kendall and Kendall "Our Notes."

65. Plastridge "Report of Observation," 5.

66. Kendall and Kendall "Report," 7–13.

67. "S.K.'s work should be limited to the giving [of] the heat treatments"; Kendall and Kendall "Our Notes."; Kendall and Kendall "Report," 2.

68. Kendall and Kendall "Report," 6.

69. James S. Pooler "Fishbein Denies Unfairness Was Shown Sister Kenny" *Detroit Free Press* April 2 1945.

70. Florence Kendall to Catherine Worthingham, May 13 1941, Kendall Collection; Catherine Worthingham to Florence Kendall, May 28 1941, Kendall Collection.

71. Catherine Worthingham to Director, Sister Kenny's Clinic, July 28 1941, Public Relations, MOD-K.

72. Kenny to Dear Miss Worthingham, August 4 1941, Public Relations, MOD-K.

73. Kenny to O'Connor, August 19 1941 Public Relations, MOD-K.

74. Emil Roy Rosner [president of the New York State Society of Physio-Therapists] to Dear Colleagues [at Children's Hospital School], November 24 1941, Kendall Collection.

75. Diehl to Dear Sister Kenny, January 27 1941, Dr. Harold S. Diehl, 1941–1944, MHS-K.

76. Robert M. Yoder "Healer from the Outback" *Saturday Evening Post* (January 17 1942) 214: 70.

77. "New Technique for Paralysis Cases Accepted" *Philadelphia Evening Bulletin* October 18 1942.

78. Kenny with Ostenso *And They Shall Walk*, 233–239.

79. Kenny to Dear Dr. Diehl, September 5 1941, Dr. Harold S. Diehl, 1941–1944, MHS-K.

80. Kenny to Dear Dr. Pye, June 25 1941, Kenny Collection, Fryer Library; Miland E. Knapp to Dear Doctor Diehl, March 10 1944, Am 15.8, folder 1, [accessed in 1992 before re-cataloging], UMN-ASC; see also Kenny to Chuter June 25 1941, Scrapbook, OM 65-17, 2/3, Chuter Papers, Oxley-SLQ.

81. Catherine Quealy "Foundation OK's Fund for Polio Clinic at 'U'" *Minneapolis Star-Journal* June 5 1941.

82. "Sister Kenny's Patient Gets Big Thrill in Walk to Table" *Minneapolis Star-Journal* June 12 1941.

83. Wallace H. Cole and Miland E. Knapp "The Kenny Treatment of Infantile Paralysis: A Preliminary Report" *JAMA* (June 7 1941) 116: 2577–2580; "Treatment for Polio" *Time* (June 23 1941) 37: 73.

84. "Kenny Paralysis Treatment Approved by U.S. Medicine" *New York Times* December 5 1941.

85. Frank D. Campion *The A.M.A. and U.S. Health Policy since 1940* (Chicago: Chicago Review Press, 1984), 114–130; see also Allen G. Debus "A Tribute to Morris Fishbein" *Bulletin of the History of Medicine* (1977) 51: 153–154.

86. Miland E. Knapp "Commentary" in John F. Pohl and Elizabeth Kenny, *The Kenny Concept of Infantile Paralysis and Its Treatment* (Minneapolis: Bruce Publishing Co., 1943), 344.

87. Knapp to Dear Frank [Krusen], March 11 1941, Public Relations, MOD-K.

88. Philip Stimson to Dear Joe [Stokes], December 3 1941, Box 2, Folder 2; Correspondence re Medical Talks, Philip Stimson Papers, Medical Center Archives, New York-Presbyterian/Weill Cornell, New York; Pohl "The Kenny Treatment of Anterior Poliomyelitis," 1428–1433.

89. [Preface] Cole and Knapp "The Kenny Treatment of Infantile Paralysis: A Preliminary Report," 2577.

90. Cole and Knapp "The Kenny Treatment of Infantile Paralysis: A Preliminary Report," 2578.

91. "Treatment for Polio" *Time* (June 23 1941) 37: 73.

92. Kenny to Dear Mr. O'Connor, August 4 1941, Public Relations, MOD-K. See also her comments that the report by Cole and Knapp in *JAMA* "was cut down a bit by a Dr that knows nothing about the work"; Kenny to Chuter, June 25 1941, Scrapbook, OM 65-17, 2/3, Chuter Papers, Oxley-SLQ.

93. Kenny to Dear Sir [O'Connor], June 13 1941, Public Relations, MOD-K; and see Kenny to Dear Dr. Diehl, September 5 1941, Dr. Harold S. Diehl, 1941–1944, MHS-K.

94. Kenny to Dear Sir [O'Connor], June 13 1941, Public Relations, MOD-K.

95. Kenny to Dear Sir [O'Connor], June 13 1941, Public Relations, MOD-K; and see Kenny to Dear Dr. Diehl, September 5 1941, Dr. Harold S. Diehl, 1941–1944, MHS-K.

96. "2 Nurses to Aid Sister Kenny in Treatment of Polio Cases" *Minneapolis Star-Journal* June 5 1941; "'U' Polio Nurse Back from Australia" *Minneapolis Star-Journal* May 21 1941, Kendall Collection; Catherine Quealy "Foundation OK's Fund for Polio Clinic at 'U'" *Minneapolis Star-Journal* June 5 1941; "Selected Students to Learn Sister Kenny's Polio Method" *Minneapolis Daily Times* June 6 1941.

97. Kenny to Dear Sir [O'Connor], June 13 1941, Public Relations, MOD-K; Kenny to Dear Mr. O'Connor, August 4 1941, Public Relations, MOD-K; Kenny to Dear Sir [Editor, *Minneapolis Star-Journal*], August 30 1941, Minneapolis Newspapers 1941–1948, MHS-K.

98. Kenny to Dear Sir [O'Connor], June 13 1941, Public Relations, MOD-K; Kenny to Dear Mr. O'Connor, August 4 1941, Public Relations, MOD-K.

99. O'Connor to My Dear Sister Kenny, October 7 1941, Public Relations, MOD-K; Basil O'Connor to My Dear Sister Kenny, September 8 1941, Basil O'Connor, 1940–1942, MHS-K.

100. Note to: Dr. Fishbein 6/23/41 "How should I answer this? BO'C?" [on] Kenny to Dear Sir [O'Connor], June 13 1941, Public Relations, MOD-K; Morris Fishbein to My Dear Mr. O'Connor, September 9 1941, Public Relations, MOD-K.

101. Morris Fishbein *The Medical Follies; an Analysis of the Foibles of Some Healing Cults, Including Osteopathy, Homeopathy, Chiropractic, and the Electronic Reactions of Abrams, with Essays on the Antivivisectionists, Health Legislation, Physical Culture, Birth Control, and Rejuvenation* (New York: Boni & Liveright, 1925); Morris Fishbein *The New Medical Follies; an Encyclopedia of Cultism and Quackery in These United States, with Essays on the Cult of Beauty, the Craze for Reduction, Rejuvenation, Eclecticism, Bread and Dietary Fads, Physical Therapy, and a Forecast as to the Physician of the Future* (New York: Boni and Liveright, 1927).

102. Lawrence C. Salter [*JAMA* editorial department] to Dear Don [Gudakunst], December 18 1941, Public Relations, MOD-K.

103. O'Connor had sent this manuscript to Fishbein after asking the NFIP executive secretary Peter Cusack to "check him and let me know who he is—if OK etc"; BOC to PC, [handwritten note on] Walter E. Quigley to Dear Mr. O'Connor, June 29 1941, Public Relations, MOD-K.

104. Morris Fishbein to Dear Mr. Quigley, August 9 1941, Public Relations, MOD-K.

105. Morris Fishbein to My Dear Mr. O'Connor, August 9 1941, Public Relations, MOD-K.

106. W. E. Quigley to Dear Doctor [Fishbein], August 12 1941, Public Relations, MOD-K.

107. Robert W. Potter to My Dear Dr. Don Gudakunst, June 13 1941, Public Relations, MOD-K.

108. Morris Fishbein to My Dear Mr. O'Connor, August 9 1941, Public Relations, MOD-K.

109. Morris Fishbein to My Dear Mr. Potter, July 15 1941, Public Relations, MOD-K. See also Potter to Gudakunst, June 13 1941, Public Relations, MOD-K; Potter to Dr. Fishbein, July 16 1941, Public Relations, MOD-K.

110. Robert D. Potter to Dr Don Gudakunst [telegram], June 26 1941, Public Relations, MOD-K.

111. Robert D. Potter "Sister Kenny's Treatment for Infantile Paralysis" *American Weekly* August 17 1941, 4–13.

112. James S. Pooler "Fishbein Denies Unfairness Was Shown Sister Kenny" *Detroit Free Press* April 2 1945.

113. Chown [Report], June 11 1940, Minutes, Board of Directors 1938–1955, Children's Hospital of Winnipeg MG 10B33, Box 7, Province Archives, Manitoba; Kenny "Data Concerning Introduction of Kenny Concept"; see also Christopher Rutty "The Middle-Class Plague: Epidemic Polio and the Canadian State, 1936–1937" *Canadian Bulletin of Medical History* (1996) 13: 277–314.

114. September 9 1941, Minutes, Board of Directors 1938–1955, Children's Hospital of Winnipeg MG 10B33, Box 7, Province Archives; President [O'Connor] to Dear Mr. Bell, August 4 1941, Public Relations, MOD-K; see also [anon] "Kenny Method of Treatment: Experiences at the Children's Hospital of Winnipeg" *Canadian Public Health Journal* (June 1942) 33: 275.

115. Kenny with Ostenso *And They Shall Walk*, 242; "Polio Nurse Will Tell Canadians of Her Methods" *Minneapolis Daily Times* August 22 1941; "Polio 'Wonder Nurse' Off on Winnipeg Mercy Visit" *Minneapolis Daily Times* August 24 1941.

116. A. E. Deacon "The Treatment of Poliomyelitis in the Acute Stage" *Canadian Public Health Journal* (1942) 33: 278–281.

117. A. E. Deacon to Dear Dr. Gudakunst, January 6 1942, Public Relations, MOD-K. See also Deacon "The Treatment of Poliomyelitis in the Acute Stage," 280. Deacon (1902–2004) graduated in medicine from the University of Manitoba in 1929 and trained in orthopedic surgery at Winnipeg's Children's Hospital and the Mayo Clinic, completing a Master of Science degree from the University of Minnesota in 1935. He joined the orthopedic staff at Winnipeg Children's Hospital and the Winnipeg General Hospital and later the Winnipeg Shriners' Hospital. Deacon supposedly had polio as a child and had a paralyzed leg; Harry Medovy *A Vision Fulfilled: The Story of the Children's Hospital of Winnipeg 1909–1973* (Winnipeg: Pegius Publishers, 1979), 60.

118. October 14 1941, Minutes, Board of Directors 1938–1955, Children's Hospital of Winnipeg MG 10B33, Box 7, Province Archives.

119. December 9 1941, Minutes Board of Directors 1938–1955, Children's Hospital of Winnipeg MG 10B33, Box 7, Province Archives. Chown (1893–1986) gained his medical degree from the University of Manitoba in 1922 and then studied pediatrics at Columbia, Cornell, and Johns Hopkins. He returned to Winnipeg to take a position as a pathologist at Children's Hospital and was chair of pediatrics at the Children's Hospital from 1949 to 1959; J. M. Bowman "Dr. Bruce Chown" *University of Manitoba Medical Journal* (1986) 56: 74.

120. Deacon "The Treatment of Poliomyelitis in the Acute Stage," 278–281; Helen H. Ross "Physiotherapy in the Treatment of Infantile Paralysis" *Canadian Public Health Journal* (1942) 33: 285–286.

121. Kenny to Dear Dr. Chown, August 31 1941, Dr. Bruce Chown, 1941–1946, MHS-K.

122. Kenny to Dear Dr. Chown, September 22 1941, Dr. Bruce Chown, 1941–1946, MHS-K.

123. Kenny to Dear Mr. O'Connor, October 11 1941, Public Relations, MOD-K.

124. "Paralysis Treatment Boosted" *Newsweek* (September 8 1941) 18: 62; "Rationed ho-yo-to-hos" *Time* (September 8 1941) 38: 55; Marjorie Lawrence *Interrupted Melody: An Autobiography* (New York: Appleton-Century Crofts, 1949), 182–205; "Soprano's Return" *Time* (September 14 1942) 40: 67.

125. Lawrence *Interrupted Melody*, 193.

126. Lawrence *Interrupted Melody*, 196; Robert M. Lewin "Comeback" *Los Angeles Times* June 13 1943; "Diva Returns, Paralysis Beaten" *New York Times* December 29 1943.

127. Kenny to Dear Mr. O'Connor, October 11 1941, Public Relations, MOD-K.

128. Kenny to Dear Dr. Fishbein, October 5 1941, Public Relations, MOD-K.

129. Kenny with Ostenso *And They Shall Walk*, 231; see also Kenny "Results of Evidence Presented at the Medical Conference Held in Minneapolis December 3rd to 6th [1945]," Public Relations, MOD-K.

130. Kenny with Ostenso *And They Shall Walk*, 229, 230–231.

131. Kenny with Ostenso *And They Shall Walk*, 231.

132. McCarroll and Crego, Jr. "An Evaluation of Physiotherapy," 851–861; Table 7, page 857.

133. Kenny *Treatment of Infantile Paralysis*, 42; Kenny "Data Concerning Introduction of Kenny Concept."

134. McCarroll and Crego, Jr. "An Evaluation of Physiotherapy," 852. They had also referred to Arthur Legg and Robert Lovett who were dead.

135. K. G. Hansson "Present Status of Physical Therapy in Anterior Poliomyelitis" *Physiotherapy Review* (1942) 22: 3–5; Henry O. Kendall and Florence P. Kendall "Let's Immobilize False Impressions" *Physiotherapy Review* (1942) 22: 136–137.

136. Kendall and Kendall "Report," 12–13.

137. On her feeling that her method must "be set down in the form of a text book" so it could be used "for intensive study"; R. W. Cilento "Report on The Muscle Re-Education Clinic, Townsville," Kenny Collection, Fryer Library, 4.

138. Kenny to Dear Dr. Fishbein, October 5 1941, Public Relations, MOD-K; Philip Lewin *Infantile Paralysis: Anterior Poliomyelitis* (Philadelphia: W. B. Saunders, 1941); Kenny to Dear Dr. Diehl, November 4 1941, Dr. Harold S. Diehl, 1941–1944, MHS-K.

139. Kenny to Dear Dr. Diehl, September 5 1941, Dr. Harold S. Diehl, 1941–1944, MHS-K.

140. Krusen *Physical Medicine*, 596–599.

141. Kenny to Dear Dr. Diehl, September 5 1941, Dr. Harold S. Diehl, 1941–1944, MHS-K.

142. Kenny with Ostenso *And They Shall Walk*, 245–246; Kenny *Treatment of Infantile Paralysis*. See also "If this work cannot be recorded by description and illustration no lasting benefit shall be derived from my efforts"; Kenny to Sir [Chuter], January 19 1940, Home Secretary's Office, Special Batches, Kenny Clinics, 1941–1949, A/31753, QSA.

143. Kenny *Treatment of Infantile Paralysis*, xix. The clinics shown were Rockhampton, Royal North Shore, Queen Mary's in Carshalton, Cairns, Hampton, Townsville, George Street in Brisbane, and the Brisbane General Hospital.

144. Kenny to Dear Mr. Connor [sic], September 30 1941, Basil O'Connor 1940–1942, MHS-K; Kenny to Dear Sir [O'Connor], December 4 1940, Public Relations, MOD-K.

145. Cilento "Report on The Muscle Re-Education Clinic, Townsville," Kenny Collection, Fryer Library, 4.

146. Kenny to Dear Mr. Connor [sic], September 30 1941, Basil O'Connor 1940–1942, MHS-K.

147. Edward L. Compere to Dear Doctor Guderkunst [sic], January 27 1942, Public Relations, MOD-K.

148. DWG to BO'C Memorandum, October 2 1941, Public Relations, MOD-K.

149. Gudakunst to Dear Doctor Compere, January 29 1942, Public Relations, MOD-K.

150. Wallace H. Cole, John F. Pohl, and Miland E. Knapp "The Kenny Method of Treatment for Infantile Paralysis" *Archives of Physical Therapy* (June 1942) 23: 399–418, and November 1942, *Archives of Physical Therapy*, published as a separate pamphlet by the National Foundation for Infantile Paralysis (Publication No. 40, 1942).

151. DWG to BOC Memorandum re Lectures by Sister Kenny, September 18 1941, Public Relations, MOD-K.

152. Kenny to Dear Dr. Diehl, June 21 1943, Dr. Harold S. Diehl, 1941–1944, MHS-K. In Kenny's recollection of the incident, Fishbein had phoned Bruce saying that the NFIP "had an iron bound contract with me and exclusive rights to all literature, for which they had paid $40,000. Bruce later claimed that Fishbein had also asked for proofs of the book's first few chapters, saying "he wanted to check them over"; James S. Pooler "Kenny Complaint Based on Money" *Detroit Free Press* March 31 1945.

153. J. R. Bruce to Dear Dr. Fishbein, September 19 1941, Public Relations, MOD-K. Gudakunst asked Cole to make sure that Bruce agreed "to insert a flyleaf giving a statement to the effect that the National Foundation had no responsibility for the publication nor does it sponsor the distribution of the book"; DWG to BO'C Memorandum, October 2 1941, Public Relations, MOD-K.

154. Fishbein to My Dear Mr. O'Connor, September 20 1941, Public Relations, MOD-K.

155. Kenny to Dear Dr. Diehl, June 21 1943, Dr. Harold S. Diehl, 1941–1944, MHS-K; Fishbein to My Dear Mr. O'Connor, October 9 1941, Public Relations, MOD-K.

156. Kenny to Dear Dr. Fishbein, October 5 1941, Public Relations, MOD-K; Kenny to Dear Mr. Connor [sic], September 30 1941, Basil O'Connor 1940–1942, MHS-K.

157. Fishbein to My Dear Mr. O'Connor, October 9 1941, Public Relations, MOD-K.

158. O'Connor to My Dear Dr. Fishbein, October 14 1941, Public Relations, MOD-K.

159. Morris Fishbein to My Dear Mr. O'Connor, September 9 1941, Public Relations, MOD-K.

160. Lois Maddox Miller "Sister Kenny vs. Infantile Paralysis," *Reader's Digest* (December 1941) 39: 1–2.

161. Miller "Sister Kenny vs. Infantile Paralysis," 4–5.

162. Miller "Sister Kenny vs. Infantile Paralysis," 3, 5.

163. Miller "Sister Kenny vs. Infantile Paralysis," 2, 5.

164. "Statement Relative to the Kenny Method of Treatment of Infantile Paralysis in the Early Stage" [press release], December 6, 1941, Public Relations, MOD-K.

165. "Statement Relative to the Kenny Method"; and "Kenny Paralysis Treatment Approved by U.S. Medicine" *New York Times* December 5 1941.

166. Editorial "Physiologic Anatomy of Poliomyelitis" *JAMA* (December 6 1941) 117: 1980–1981.

167. "New Infantile Paralysis Treatment Gets Approval" *Science News Letter* (December 13 1941) 40: 371.

168. "Sister Kenny's Triumph" *Newsweek* (December 15 1941) 8: 77; "Sister Kenny Endorsed" *Time* (December 15 1941) 38: 85.

169. "Kenny Paralysis Treatment Approved by U.S. Medicine" *New York Times* December 5 1941.

170. Editorial "The Kenny Method of Treatment in the Acute Peripheral Manifestations of Infantile Paralysis" *JAMA* (December 20 1941) 117: 2171–2172.

171. Kenny to Dear Mr. O'Connor, December 27 1941, Public Relations, MOD-K; Kenny to Dear Dr. Gudakunst, December 14 1941, Dr. Don W. Gudakunst, 1941–1944, MHS-K.

172. Kenny to Dear Mr. O'Connor, December 27 1941, Public Relations, MOD-K.

173. [Review of] "Elizabeth Kenny *The Treatment of Infantile Paralysis in the Acute Stage*" *JAMA* (January 10 1942) 118: 179.

174. DWG to BO'C Memorandum: Re Miss Kenny, January 19 1942, Public Relations, MOD-K.

175. Kenny to Sirs [*JAMA*] January 18 1942, Public Relations, MOD-K.

176. Compere to Dear Doctor Guderkunst [sic] January 27 1942, Public Relations, MOD-K.

177. Ibid.

178. Kenny to Dear Dr. Compere, February 16 1942, Dr. Edward L. Compere, 1942–1945, MHS-K; see also Kenny to Dear Dr. Fishbein, January 24 1942, Dr. Edward L. Compere, 1942–1945, MHS-K.

179. Kenny to Dear Dr. Compere, March 2 1942, Dr. Edward L. Compere, 1942–1945, MHS-K; Fishbein to Dear Sister Kenny, January 28 1942, Dr. Edward L. Compere, 1942–1945, MHS-K.

180. Compere to Dear Miss Kenny, March 6 1942, Dr. Edward L. Compere, 1942–1945, MHS-K; Compere to Dear Miss Kenny, March 15 1942, Dr. Edward L. Compere, 1942–1945, MHS-K.

181. Kenny to Dear Dr. Compere, March 17 1942, Dr. Edward L. Compere, 1942–1945, MHS-K.

182. J. D. Ratcliff "Minutemen Against Infantile Paralysis" *Colliers* (October 9 1943) 112: 18; "Dr. Don Gudakunst, Paralysis Expert" *New York Times* January 21 1946; "Medical Chief In Polio Drive Dies In Hotel" *Chicago Daily Tribune* January 21 1946; see also "Don Walsh Gudakunst" *JAMA* (January 26 1946) 130: 234; Benison *Tom Rivers*, 276–278.

183. DWG to BO'C Memorandum, December 10 1941, Public Relations, MOD-K; "Sister Kenny Receives Parent's Magazine Award" *Parents Magazine* (December 1942) 17: 38.

184. Kenny [paper "I wish to present to you"] "Handed to DWG by Miss Kenny, 12-16-41 in Minneapolis," Public Relations, MOD-K; Kenny to Dear Dr. Gudakunst, December 31 1941, Public Relations, MOD-K.

185. DWG to BO'C Memorandum: Re Miss Kenny, January 19 1942, Public Relations, MOD-K; Salter to Dear Don [Gudakunst], January 23, 1942, Public Relations, MOD-K; Gudakunst to Dear Larry [Salter], December 19 1941, Public Relations, MOD-K. *JAMA*, he complained to O'Connor, "has done a rather poor job of reporting her work"; DWG to BO'C Memorandum: Re Miss Kenny, January 19 1942, Public Relations, MOD-K.

186. DWG to BO'C Memorandum: Re Miss Kenny, January 19 1942, Public Relations, MOD-K; Salter to Dear Don [Gudakunst] January 23 1942, Public Relations, MOD-K; see also Gudakunst to Dear Larry [Salter], January 21 1942, Public Relations, MOD-K.

187. Gudakunst to Dear Larry [Salter], December 19 1941, Public Relations, MOD-K.

188. Gudakunst to Dear Doctor Viets, January 17 1942, Public Relations, MOD-K.

189. Gudakunst to Dear Larry [Salter], December 19 1941, Public Relations, MOD-K.

190. Gudakunst to Dear Doctor Compere, January 29 1942, Public Relations, MOD-K.

191. DWG to Files Memorandum Re Frances Payne Bolton School of Nursing Western Reserve University Kenny Method, January 15 1942, Public Relations, MOD-K.

192. Salter to Dear Don [Gudakunst], January 23 1942, Public Relations, MOD-K.

193. Gudakunst to Dear Doctor Knowlton, January 22 1942, Public Relations, MOD-K.

194. "Correction: The Kenny Method" *JAMA* (January 17 1942) 118: 241; on Fishbein speaking with O'Connor by phone see Salter to Dear Don [Gudakunst] January 23, 1942, Public Relations, MOD-K.

195. Wallace H. Cole, John F. Pohl, and Miland E. Knapp *The Kenny Method of Treatment for Infantile Paralysis* (New York: National Foundation for Infantile Paralysis, Publication No. 40, 1942).

196. Richard Kovacs ed. *The 1941 Year Book of Physical Therapy* (Chicago: Year Book Publishers, 1941), 329–332.

197. "The Kenny Method of Treatment of Infantile Paralysis" *New England Journal of Medicine* (April 23 1942) 226: 700–702. Another editorial in the same journal praised the NFIP's sponsorship of an investigation of Kenny as "outstanding," and the endorsement by the NFIP's medical advisory committee as "proof of the value of the foundation's farsighted policies"; "National Foundation for Infantile Paralysis" *New England Journal of Medicine* (April 9 1942) 226: 620.

198. James Gray "Sister Kenny's Progress: A Triumph for Modern Medicine" *St Paul Pioneer Press* [n.d.], Clippings, MHS–K.

199. Burton A. Brown to Dear Doctor Gudakunst, December 17 1941, Public Relations, MOD-K.

200. Lem H. Tittle to Dear Mr. O'Connor, December 6 1941, Public Relations, MOD-K.

201. Ann van Kavcren to My Dear Mrs. Roosevelt, January 10 1942, Public Relations, MOD-K.

FURTHER READING

On polio and American physical therapy see Glenn Gritzer and Arnold Arluke *The Making of Rehabilitation: The Political Economy of Medical Specialization, 1890–1980* (Berkeley: University of California Press, 1985); Beth Linker "The Business of Ethics: Gender, Medicine, and the Professional Codification of the American Physiotherapy Association, 1918–1935" *Journal of the History of Medicine and Allied Sciences* (2005) 60: 320–354; Beth Linker "Strength and Science: Gender, Physiotherapy, and Medicine in Early Twentieth Century America" *Journal of Women's History* (2005) 17: 106–132; Marilyn Moffat "The History of Physical Therapy Practice in the United States" *Journal of Physical Therapy Education* (2003) 17: 15–25; Wendy B. Murphy *Healing the Generations: A History of Physical Therapy and the American Physical Therapy Association* (Alexandria, VA: American Physical Therapy Association, 1995); Donald A. Neumann "Polio: Its Impact on the People of the United States and the Emerging Profession of Physical Therapy" *Journal of Orthopaedic and Sports Physical Therapy* (2004) 34: 479–492; Dorothy Pinkston "Evolution of the Practice of Physical Therapy in the United States" in Rosemary M. Scully and Marylou R. Barnes eds. *Physical Therapy* (Philadelphia: J.B. Lippincott, 1989), 2–30; Daniel J. Wilson *Living with Polio: The Epidemic and its Survivors* (Chicago: University of Chicago Press, 2005).

On medical politics in the 1930s and early 1940s see James G. Burrow *AMA: Voice of American Medicine* (Baltimore: Johns Hopkins Press, 1963); Frank D. Campion *The A.M.A. and U.S. Health Policy Since 1940* (Chicago: Chicago Review Press, 1984), 114–130; Jonathan Engel *Doctors and Reformers: Discussion and Debate over Health Policy 1925–1950* (Charleston: University of South Carolina Press, 2002); Elizabeth Fee and Theodore Brown eds. *Making Medical History: The Life and Times of Henry E. Sigerist* (Baltimore: Johns Hopkins University Press, 1997); Michael R. Grey *New Deal Medicine: The Rural Health Programs of the Farm Security Administration* (Baltimore: Johns Hopkins University Press, 1999); Rickey Hendricks *A Model for National Health Care: The History of Kaiser Permanente* (New Brunswick, NJ: Rutgers University Press, 1993); Daniel S. Hirschfield *The Lost*

Reform: The Campaign for Compulsory Health Insurance in the United States from 1932 to 1943 (Cambridge: Harvard University Press, 1970); Elton Rayak *Professional Power and American Medicine: The Economics of the American Medical Association* (Cleveland: World Publishing Company, 1967); Paul Starr *The Social Transformation of American Medicine* (New York: Basic Books, 1982); Patricia Spain Ward *"United States versus American Medical Association et. al.:* the Medical Antitrust Case of 1938–1943" *American Studies* (1989) 30: 123–153.

3

Changing Clinical Care

AMID THE EXCITEMENT around Kenny and her work came the wrenching moment of Pearl Harbor, followed by Roosevelt's declaration of war against Japan and Germany. In this new era isolationism was defeated, Roosevelt transformed from Dr. New Deal to Dr. Win the War, and a massive economic upturn ended the Great Depression. The war also remade American alliances around the world. For the first time Australian foreign policy was formally oriented toward the United States. As American troops arrived they were mocked as "dammed Yanks" but also welcomed by most Australians as they fought alongside Australian troops to push back Japan's expansion in the Pacific.[1]

In the United States polio was immediately another war at home. With the declaration of war coming just weeks before the annual March of Dimes campaign, O'Connor conferred with Roosevelt and his advisors, and announced that the president agreed that "even in time of war those nations which still hold to the old ideals of Christianity and Democracy, are carrying on services to humanity which have little or no relationship to torpedoes or guns or bombs."[2]

Caught up in the patriotic fervor of wartime America, Kenny volunteered her technicians in Minneapolis—a group she called the Australian Unit—"to give our services to any military or naval fort, camp, hospital or depot" should a polio outbreak occur in any of these centers.[3] Vernon Hart, an orthopedic surgeon who had attended her lectures and demonstrations before joining the Army, published a study of knee injuries treated by the Kenny method in *JAMA*, which showed, according to Kenny, "that this type of treatment is most satisfactory for restoring function after war wounds."[4] Hart did praise the Kenny principles as "simple and scientific," although—in an argument Kenny did not repeat—he described them as "old ones which have been salvaged from a disorganized field of physical therapy [by]...a sincere, intelligent and practical nurse."[5] As American troops arrived on Australia's east coast, bringing attention to the nation's new Pacific ally, Kenny was "always referred to as 'the Australian nurse,'" according to the *New York Daily Mirror*. "Her Australianism is part of her, and she claims it proudly."[6] "The United States has given Australia Douglas MacArthur," Chicago orthopedist Philip Lewin declared, and "Australia has given us Elizabeth Kenny."[7]

The National Foundation for Infantile Paralysis (NFIP) hoped that Kenny's work would become another element in its own propaganda. Even before she published her autobiography, local NFIP chapters used her story to enhance fundraising efforts and a Chicago radio station's March of Dimes program dramatized Kenny's life starring Ethel Barrymore as Kenny.[8] The foundation wanted to control how the work was presented and tried to restrict Kenny "from writing articles for public or professional magazines, lecturing or releasing information in any way except through this Foundation."[9] But Kenny became the story and the agent of change. She loved the limelight. She talked to reporters wherever she went, determined to spur patients and their families to demand that experts in their communities be trained in her methods. Informal AMA censor Fishbein was horrified after he had read and approved a story on Kenny in the *Saturday Evening Post* when he found that the magazine began to promote this article saying that the American Medical Association (AMA) had reversed its accepted views of polio therapy "with a bow of recognition to the nurse from down under." After Fishbein made a sharp call to the Curtis Publishing Company a salesman explained abjectly to the magazine's retailers that "the American Medical Association has never officially considered Sister Kenny in any way whatever."[10] Still, despite Fishbein's efforts to draw a line between medical practice and AMA policy, Cole and Knapp's *JAMA* article and the NFIP's subsequent announcement in December 1941 were easily interpreted as signs of AMA-approved progress in polio care.

By raising the question of clinical change, Kenny's results made physicians uncomfortable. Here was a breakthrough without a pill or surgical tool, involving the use of familiar methods based on a new reading of the paralyzed body. When Kenny quoted physicians who "thanked me most profusely and said they could only view with great sorrow the terrible mistakes made in the past in the treatment of this disease," she saw such remarks as a powerful indication of the ability of professionals to be humble in the face of an original contribution.[11] But her interpretation simplified a far more complex process. Had physicians in the past made "terrible mistakes"? What did it mean to accept the notion that previous therapies might have harmed their patients?

Therapeutic change was the most difficult part of medical progress to explain. New drugs like insulin, hormone therapy, and the sulfonamides were concrete technologies backed by the familiar trappings of laboratory research and pharmaceutical promotion; physical therapies were more difficult to evaluate. Nor was it easy to pin down the rationale for therapeutic change beyond the derogatory designation of medical fad. Elite researchers talked about "controlled trials," but this was not yet a standard practice.

In the 1940s clinical research was still an amorphous field. Many physicians were convinced that valuable evidence could still be gained from case studies of individual patients or small groups of patients, and offered these studies to medical journals. In fact most clinical research published in mainstream medical journals was, like Kenny's, based on a group of patients, usually fewer than 50. Rarely were there any formal controls, other than comparisons to patients in other hospitals or other wards or under another physician's care. McCarroll and Crego's 1941 study, for example, had simply altered elements of the care provided to their own patients over a series of years, and then compared the clinical results.

But moving from potentially useful clinical observations to an assessment of therapy based on those observations raised tricky epistemological issues, especially around the definition of scientific evidence and the idea of a clinician as a researcher. Were clinicians scientists? Did they practice scientific medicine?

The search for quantifiable evidence was especially elusory for polio. Its early clinical signs before the appearance of paralysis—pain, skin sensitivity, fatigue, a stiff neck—were frequently misdiagnosed. When clinical improvements occurred, they were often assessed by the patient or the patient's family, ignoring the evidence of muscle tests such as those codified by Robert Lovett and his physical therapists in the 1910s. Even more crucial for patients was the issue of functionality, which was even less easily standardized. Still many physicians turned hopefully to physiological research for a definitive answer. During the 1940s Kenny proponents and opponents grasped at laboratory studies seeking a concrete link between clinical practice and laboratory research, but found evidence for both sides of the Kenny debate.

The taint of psychology was also in the air, a disturbing hidden factor that threatened to mislead true scientific investigation. The enthusiasm of recently graduated Kenny technicians reminded their medical supervisors of a kind of evangelism, reminiscent of overly hopeful patients rather than the neutral professional demeanor of polio experts. Further, Kenny's strict therapeutic routine—with its distinctive terms, hand grips, positioning of hot packs, and muscle exercises—disconcerted physicians seeking to integrate only parts of her method into their regular practice. "We must be careful not to become bound by a ritual of terms and procedures which physicians and laymen think of as a magic formula," Warm Springs director Robert Bennett warned.[12]

The enthusiasm around Kenny's therapies reminded many physicians of the convalescent serum controversy. Made from the blood of patients who had recovered from polio, this therapy was introduced in the 1910s both to prevent paralysis and to lessen its severity.[13] With no formal clinical trials, physicians began to write enthusiastic papers advocating its use after trying it "on a few cases without controls," one physician observed. Then panicky parents began to demand its use in every case, making it "difficult or actually hazardous to conduct a properly controlled study," and wasting "money, time, energy and blood."[14] Medical and popular faith in the serum continued into the 1940s, despite later research, including an extensive study of New York City's 1931 epidemic, showing that it did not prevent or ameliorate paralysis.[15] The serum did not even make scientific sense for the polio virus was believed to travel through the body through nerve tissue and not through the blood. Nonetheless the serum continued to be produced and distributed by health departments.[16] "The serum treatment of polio has very little to stand on, either theoretically or from statistical results," Yale epidemiologist John Paul reflected, but "the public has become so aware of the fact that there is a serum for the disease that it is difficult not to administer it."[17]

THE INSTITUTE

Kenny had for some time been dissatisfied with her position as guest instructor: not a doctor and not a nurse; a pivotal figure in training courses yet constantly negotiating with skeptical medical school faculty; a consultant at most Minnesota hospitals yet unable to control the conditions of her work. Backed by local politicians and businessmen, she began to seek out a place where she could direct her work free of the control of university officials and hospital administrators. She visited 3 city facilities: the Glen Lake tuberculosis sanatorium, the Parkview tuberculosis hospital, and Lymanhurst, a former tuberculosis rehabilitation center on Chicago Avenue, part of which was still in use for children with chronic heart disease. Only Lymanhurst, she argued, was close enough to the city hospital to provide "easy access to all visiting Doctors and the Doctors attending the monthly classes at the Continuation Center and the University."[18] The Elizabeth Kenny Institute at 1800 Chicago Avenue was formally opened in December 1942.

When Kenny learned that some local physicians were unhappy about the eviction of their patients with chronic heart disease, she scornfully told reporters that "research has been completed regarding heart ailments, while research regarding infantile paralysis barely has started," adding (as she often did when she felt undervalued) "if it's too much trouble to move a few patients from one hospital to another...Perhaps I should go elsewhere."[19] Until this point O'Connor and the Minneapolis surgeons had seen Kenny as a visitor who would leave a new kind of clinical practice institutionalized. Kenny herself seemed to have shared this view. But with the founding of the Institute bearing her name and under her control, Kenny became firmly situated in the Twin Cities.

In an era when nurses were seen as the recipients of medical science rather than its designers, Kenny knew that her claims to new knowledge were controversial before their content was even known. But as the Institute prospered and Kenny was feted as a savior, she began to argue that her work embodied a new knowledge of polio drawn from a close reading of the body. Polio, she said, was not solely a neurological disease but also a disease of muscles and "peripheral structures." She published 2 books in 1943: her autobiography *And They Shall Walk* coauthored with novelist Martha Ostenso and a textbook entitled *The Kenny Concept of Infantile Paralysis and Its Treatment* coauthored with orthopedist John Pohl. Both books challenged medical skepticism. In *The Kenny Concept of Infantile Paralysis* she began to argue that it was impossible to teach anyone to treat the symptoms she had identified if they did not understand her concept of the disease. Indeed, she frequently added, the prognosis for a patient treated without this new knowledge would always be far poorer than for a patient treated by professionals who fully understood the Kenny concept. Both books, of course, provided the opportunity for Kenny to settle scores and to retell stories her way.

NOT JUST A NURSE AMONG NURSES

Kenny's feisty style suited a newly militarized environment as American nurses embraced the war effort.[20] Nurses praised Kenny as another heroic contributor to nursing progress. In May 1942 she was invited to the American Nurses Association (ANA) Biennial

Convention in Chicago, attended by an estimated 10,000 nurses and nursing students, where she was a featured speaker and was awarded an honorary membership as the "noted Australian nurse poliomyelitis worker." The convention was filled with nurses in military uniforms, a vivid reminder, as ANA president Major Julia Stimson pointed out, that American nurses were the only female health professionals who could claim military officer status. The Biennial's message was reinforced by Chicago department stores whose windows illustrated the contributions of nurses to the war effort.[21] Kenny was interviewed by the editor of the *Trained Nurse and Hospital Review* who praised her "poise, strength and enormous reserve" as well as the technical film Kenny showed at the meeting in which "a single finger would be raised in command, and the patient would make prodigious efforts to make his muscles comply."[22]

This appearance boosted her credibility among American nurses. Frustrated with standard methods of polio care many nurses were eager for both greater clinical responsibility and clearer guidance. Orthopedists were responsible for prescribing splints but expected nurses to deal with daily care and to follow Robert Jones' dictum that "the value of weeks of careful handling may be undone by one careless stretching of a regenerating muscle."[23]

For some leading clinicians the transformation in accepting Kenny's work was dramatic. Jessie Stevenson, a New York orthopedic nurse, was a nationally recognized polio expert whose *The Care of Poliomyelitis* (1940) was distributed by the NFIP. Intrigued by reports of Kenny's work, Stevenson spent 2 weeks in Minneapolis, and admitted, Kenny reported proudly to O'Connor, "that she had no idea that the symptoms and signs I have pointed out to her were in existence."[24] Stevenson then published a widely cited article on "The Kenny Method" in the *American Journal of Nursing* and revised her NFIP guide to include elements of Kenny's work. She accepted the basic assumptions of what she called the Kenny theory, and argued that nurses must understand how it differed from previously accepted concepts.[25] Other nurses similarly praised Kenny's work as "a radical departure from the older methods" and with outstanding results quite unlike "the extreme pain and discomfort formerly experienced."[26] Yet Stevenson and her fellow orthopedic nurses maintained a careful distance from the public enthusiasm, embracing only certain elements of Kenny's work and indicating where they thought her claims went too far. In her review of Kenny's 1941 textbook in the *American Journal of Nursing*, Denver orthopedic nurse Carmelita Calderwood praised Kenny's extremely valuable methods, but criticized her refusal to accept any modification that might allow a nurse to combine "her hot pack methods and still maintain immobilization." "The experienced orthopedic nurse feels definitely reluctant in accepting her theories *en bloc*," Calderwood argued, "until there is more solid, scientific proof of the permanent efficacy of this method."[27]

Strikingly, Kenny rarely repeated comments made by nurses. While feted as a nurse she stood apart from the profession. What was important to her was reaching the top of the American medical hierarchy. She saw nurses and physical therapists as the hands and feet of her movement: carrying the work into hospitals and inspiring their medical supervisors to change. Her vision of a Kenny technician was closer to an independent specialist nurse, not the handmaidens of Nightingale's era. Many nurses in the early 1940s similarly embraced this vision, declaring that "nurses aren't angels—and they do not like to be called angels!"[28]

The caution of many American nurses was not mirrored by the response of most physical therapists. The publicized image of Kenny as a rehabilitation expert brought welcome attention to professionals who dealt exclusively with disabled bodies. For the first time since the work of reconstruction aides during the Great War, physical therapy was news. In the early 1940s almost every issue of the *Physiotherapy Review* had articles on her work. While it was shocking to be told by a nurse—and a bush nurse—that trained therapists had missed symptoms of polio and that the standard rehabilitative methods they had relied on were harmful, her work offered exciting opportunities for clinical action. Her rejection of the Kendalls' work also appealed to many therapists who had quietly considered the Baltimore group too conservative; the Kendall method soon became synonymous with failed polio orthodoxy. Baltimore remained one of the country's anti-Kenny enclaves.

Together nurses and physical therapists created a new understanding of bodies disabled by polio. In a distinct break from clinical tradition, they began to worry less about deformities resulting from overstretching and more about those that could develop from lengthy splinting and inadequate exercise. Kenny's antagonism to muscle testing was also adopted by some who began to suggest that the muscle tests developed by Lovett indicated only "degrees of flaccidity."[29] Kenny's work, 2 nurses reflected in 1942, had done away "with the taboo against 'stretching the paralyzed muscle.'"[30] To have nurses call a standard part of polio practice a "taboo" was astonishing, a signal of a new way of thinking. Here were signs of clinical change.

TEACHING THE KENNY METHOD

Kenny poured herself into teaching. Being able to show others her methods and have them understand her reasoning would help to combat accusations that enthusiasm or maybe some kind of hypnosis explained her results.

In early 1942, appointed as a guest instructor by the University of Minnesota, Kenny was teaching 18 local physical therapists and several therapists and nurses from Pittsburgh, Los Angeles, Iowa City, Indianapolis, Des Moines, and Warm Springs.[31] She had already won over most of the region's physical therapists including those at the Gillette State Hospital for Crippled Children who were, a visiting physician reported, "enthusiastically in favor of Sister Kenny's treatment."[32] When the NFIP was initially reluctant to fund a formal teaching program Kenny found wealthy patrons Margaret Webber and her husband businessman Charles C. Webber who donated $4,500 to the University of Minnesota to be used as scholarships for 10 local nurses. Kenny delighted in these students, whom she called the Webber scholarship girls, and boasted that they would soon be "a valuable asset to any institution."[33] Members of this first generation of students became the core circle of senior Kenny technicians for the following decade.

Kenny also took her work to the people. In 1942 she traveled several times to Chicago and New York and also visited Wilmington, Cincinnati, Columbus, New Orleans, and Boston. When polio outbreaks appeared in Memphis and Little Rock she went there where a *Life Magazine* photographer caught her glistening face and unruly hair, and *Time* praised the way her technicians were showing Arkansas doctors and nurses how to use

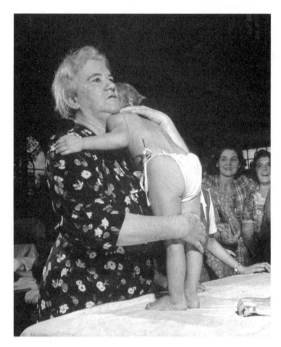

FIGURE 3.1 Photograph of Kenny and a child patient during the Little
Rock, Arkansas, epidemic in 1942, featured in *Life*; "Sister Kenny: Australian
Nurse Demonstrates Her Treatment for Infantile Paralysis" *Life* (September
28 1942) 13: 73. Courtesy of Time & Life Pictures/Getty Images.

"her gentle, natural exercises" that helped muscles regain their normal coordination
"before dangerous new behavior patterns can be set up."[34] Wealthy parents, worried that
a journey to Minnesota would harm their paralyzed child, begged her to visit their home
or local hospital. Kenny used these opportunities to speak to new audiences. "Mary and
I had our hotel expenses at the Medical Society meeting paid for us by the father of a little
girl from West Virginia who had benefited [sic] by our treatment," Kenny noted in May
1942, "so the only expense was our return fare."[35] In an era when commercial flights were
rare, Kenny flew whenever she could, explaining that traveling by air enabled her to "limit
the time away from my classes as much as possible."[36]

Courses in the Kenny method were formally institutionalized after Gudakunst and
O'Connor came to Minneapolis in February 1942 where they met with university officials
and local physicians.[37] Drawing on the model of postgraduate courses already in place at
the university, the new program was directed by Knapp and financed by the NFIP. There
were 1 week courses for doctors, 3–4 month courses for physical therapists, and 6 month
courses for nurses.[38]

Kenny was pleased that her ideas and techniques were being taken seriously by exactly
the experts she had hoped to impress, but she could see that others were trying to take
control of her teaching. While O'Connor had "asked me to present some scheme about
instructing people," she complained to Dean Diehl a few weeks later, "it is evident that
that had already been arranged before he saw me."[39] The NFIP had indeed, as Kenny
guessed, begun to discuss how to institutionalize her work not just at the University of

Minnesota but at a variety of centers.[40] At O'Connor's urging Robert Bennett, the medical director of Warm Springs, visited Minneapolis where he "talked at great length with the medical and technical personnel working with Miss Kenny."[41]

Like Kenny, Bennett recognized the power relations in polio care. Most patients with polio were cared for by hospital nurses and physical therapists who practiced under the supervision of physicians in institutions with set routines. Patients in polio's acute stage—the stage at which Kenny insisted her work must begin—were sent first to infectious disease hospitals where there were strict contagion rules. To alter clinical practice Kenny technicians had to be admitted to these hospitals and then be able to continue their work during a patient's convalescent stage whether in a hospital or a child's own home. Such changes required the support of supervising physicians, professionals who were the lynchpin between Kenny's teaching and hospital routine.

Bennett believed that the most important immediate need was "to acquaint the medical profession with all available scientific proof supporting the concepts of this system and to outline to them the treatment in their own language." Physicians who directed physical therapy schools should be sent to Minnesota so this system could be quickly incorporated into physical therapy teaching programs. Although Bennett clearly saw Kenny's work more as a clinical innovation than a radical reinterpretation of polio's pathology, he did agree that there was a need for fundamental research that would "be the basis upon which all long range estimations of the system could be evaluated." In a frank letter to O'Connor he admitted that, considering the skepticism of many of his peers, it would be "wise at present that all research should be designed to prove the merits of the system rather than to disprove them."[42] Here then was a deliberate plan to institutionalize clinical change, with an emphasis on physicians as supervisors and potential researchers. In addition to the Kenny courses at the University of Minnesota, the NFIP began funding courses at other medical and nursing schools around the country including Stanford, the University of Southern California, Northwestern, New York University, the D. T. Watson Home in Pittsburgh, and Warm Springs.[43]

Kenny's pedagogic philosophy was based on changing the minds of physicians and retraining the hands of nurses and physical therapists. She was careful to make her technician courses as formal as possible. Students attended lectures and demonstrations, worked with patients under the supervision of her Australian staff, and after experience with acute patients (something that depended on the erratic nature of polio outbreaks) sat an examination. Only then were they awarded what was called a certificate of efficiency.[44] By early 1943 more than 100 had become Kenny technicians.[45] This teaching, Kenny believed, was and should be a struggle, for her students "are taught symptoms and condition of a disease... they had no idea exists."[46] She had little sympathy when students complained about her teaching style. The Webber scholarship nurses, she reflected in 1943, "rebelled and wept and thought they were being requested to learn too much" but later came to "thank me for the knowledge given them and the way it was given."[47]

Kenny was well aware of the pragmatic difficulties of introducing her work in institutions with antagonistic health professionals. Every technician, she explained to O'Connor, should have a "duly qualified medical practitioner" who could understand the method and supervise it. Still, she added, even if her technicians were only partly trained "no doubt, whatever they did it would be an improvement on previous treatment."[48] Kenny shortened this idea to "poor Kenny is better than the best orthodoxy," and her students shortened it further to "P.K. is better than B.O."[49] With her technicians' medical supervisors, however, she argued that the complexity of her work required full training. She had hoped to be invited to Warm Springs, but instead Robert Bennett sent 3 of his physical therapists to Minnesota, assuring her that they were "particularly keen individuals who have excellent knowledge of applied anatomy and who are very sympathetic with your work." When Bennett recalled his therapists to Georgia after only 3 weeks, Kenny warned him that it had been "impossible for them to learn the work during their short stay" for, in an argument she used frequently, "the time has been so short that the ideas have not had any time to sink in and, therefore, will not be permanent."[50] Later she was annoyed to hear that Warm Springs was offering courses in the Kenny technique.[51]

For their part her graduates reveled in a method they saw as a break from older unsatisfactory practices. One New York City therapist—who described herself as still "green"—told Kenny there were "hundreds of Physiotherapists who are grateful to you for enriching their profession with your knowledge." Kenny's training had given her a sense "of Anatomy and Body Mechanics, far clearer and with a deeper foundation than all the books, lectures, and 200 hours of dissection I have had."[52] For physical therapists and nurses familiar with the careful, repetitive work necessary to rehabilitate disabled bodies, Kenny's method seemed fresh and modern, an attack on medical orthodoxy in a safe way. This treatment "has added new zest to a job I was already crazy about," one graduate admitted, "it is fun to be doing polio work when there are such bright prospects for the patients."[53]

Technicians returned to their home institutions armed with fervor, new skills, and the promise of impressive results. For some, this training made them minor celebrities; for many it provided an opportunity to become teachers in their own hospitals, instructing not only their peers but also their supervisors. At the Children's Hospital in Los Angeles Dorothy Behlow was confident that she had proved to the medical staff at her hospital that "there is a great deal more to the Kenny Treatment than just packing" and that it

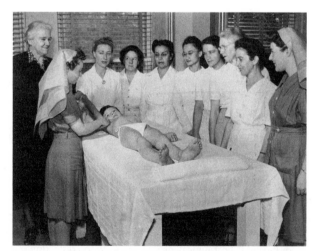

FIGURE 3.2 Kenny technician Valerie Harvey demonstrating a muscle to a group of physical therapists, flanked by Sister Kenny (left) and Mary Kenny (far right) [perhaps 1942 or 1943]. Box 11, Elizabeth Kenny Papers, Minnesota Historical Society, St Paul.

was "far superior to any other form of treatment." She proudly described how her clinical results had countered pessimistic prognoses. With one patient "the tendon work-up is wonderful. At first, no anterior tibial; 'Gone,' cried the doctors and other physiotherapists, but hear them now when it appears when working up the tendons! It is the most exciting and thrilling work I have ever done." In a postscript Behlow added that "If I lived to be 100 yrs. old I could not begin to repay you for [the] knowledge you have given me. Thank you Sister, from the bottom of my heart."[54]

Taking Kenny's course in Minnesota was also exhilarating. A cult of personality emerged, especially among the first generation of Kenny technicians. "You are the first truly great woman I have ever known personally," Adelaide Smith of Pittsburgh gushed.[55] With their minds full of the stories Kenny had told them about antagonists and converts, her students saw their own struggles to convince other professionals as part of the same narrative. One therapist was treating 27 patients and "at night, after hours and hours of work, I return home discouraged and tired, ready to quit but I seem to get a lift as I glance at your photograph and think how brave and courageous you were thru [sic] all the years with barriers all along the way."[56] The personal loyalty among Kenny technicians to their teacher occasionally pitted therapists against their supervisors. Thus, after NFIP medical director Don Gudakunst visited the Kenny technicians working in Little Rock during the 1942 epidemic and told them that there were "too many of us down here" and he would send some to other places, Ethel Gardner, one of the Webber scholarship students, let Kenny know that she and the other technicians had replied flatly that "you sent us here and here we stay until you tell us to come home. We don't pay any attention to him and will not do a thing for him without orders from you."[57]

Technicians told Kenny about their successes and failures. My "whole community is thrilled over the Kenny Method," Emily Griffin wrote from the Monmouth Memorial Hospital in Long Branch, New Jersey. Administrators at her hospital had been "wonderfully cooperative" and had turned an isolation ward into a Kenny Ward. Griffin was teaching hot pack classes to other therapists and nurses who were all enthusiastic.[58] Other graduates grew discouraged. Lorraine Paulson had come from the D. T. Watson Home in Pittsburgh to study with Kenny for 6 weeks and she left vowing "she would prefer not to treat a patient at all if she had to resort to the old method." But Paulson was not able to change polio practices in her institution, and within a few weeks Kenny received letters from the parents of patients complaining that splints had been reapplied.[59] A single physical therapist or nurse could not alter the entire routine of a hospital's entrenched practices or the views of medical skeptics. A New York therapist became so frustrated by one mocking physician that she "burst out, hurt the gentle doctor's ego" and then was reprimanded and asked to resign. In her experience physicians were inherently resistant to change. "I am surprised you are still sane after the trouble you have had dealing with the most jealous, egotistic and blind profession," she told Kenny bitterly.[60]

Kenny and her technicians fought to ensure that Kenny training remained on a strictly professional level, available only to respectable professionals and used solely for altruistic purposes. After studying with Kenny and returning to San Diego, Ruth Giaciolli complained that a local woman osteopath "thinks I will teach her your method in two easy lessons [but]...I have no intention of trying to teach your method to any persons likely to use it for personal gain. It should remain on the sound ethical basis upon which you began it."[61] Giaciolli was not the only technician to note that "many unscrupulous practitioners of massage & Chiropractory [sic] are only too willing to accept money for treating chronic polio with Kenny Hot packs."[62]

In Honolulu technician Charlotte Anderson, working at an Emergency Poliomyelitis Hospital run by the Office of Civilian Defense, was pressured to offer short training courses by her hospital's medical director who, Anderson told Kenny, was "*very* anxious to have us teach other technicians." But Anderson resisted, believing "the only place to get proper training is with you." She asked Kenny to explain to her hospital director the necessity of a formal course with high standards. He was planning to visit Minneapolis and "perhaps you can make him realize it would not be right for us to do" this training, without, she hoped, "mentioning our names."[63]

These experiences left both Kenny and her technicians more than ever convinced that supervising physicians must visit Minneapolis to learn to understand and respect the Kenny method. Miland Knapp shared this view. "It is obviously impossible for a technician to treat a case under the supervision of the doctor who knows nothing about the method being used," he reflected after a year as director of the Kenny courses. In his experience "one of the most satisfactory ways for the Kenny treatment to be established is to have the doctor come to a class first and become so enthusiastic about the method that he arranges to have a technician and nurse trained." Aware of the tensions inherent when a subordinate hospital staff member tried to institute change not understood or appreciated by senior staff, Knapp had on occasion "considered refusing the application of technicians where a physician has not agreed to take the course also."[64]

EARLY MEDICAL CONVERTS

Physicians may have been wary of the purple prose in popular magazines but they were impressed by reports in *JAMA* and other medical journals indicating that old-fashioned polio therapy was being modernized. So many researchers now admit that immobilizing limbs causes "destruction of muscle fibers as well as irreparable joint changes," one physician remarked in January 1942, that "it is hardly necessary to devote much time to the benefits derived by discarding immobilization."[65]

The first formal course for physicians began in March 1942. Led by Pohl and Knapp, with a number of lectures and demonstrations by Kenny, the courses were intended to turn the curious into converts, and to inspire them to send their nurses and physical therapists to Minneapolis for full training. Knapp's lectures on pathology and physiology were very good, one physician commented, impressed by Knapp's comments that "there has been no research yet which refuted Miss Kenny's ideas on the pathology in Infantile Paralysis" and that her work was "opening up a field of research to you doctors unafraid to face new ideas."[66] With funding from local NFIP chapters class size ranged from 10 to 34 physicians. Although Kenny and NFIP officials hoped to attract supervisors in infectious disease hospitals where acute stage patients were treated, most physicians in the classes supervised convalescent care: pediatricians, orthopedic surgeons, and physical medicine specialists.[67] By early 1943 around 200 physicians had attended.[68] A number of other physicians who could not travel to Minnesota began to use a version of Kenny's methods after reading about them.[69]

In an era when nurses were expected to defer to physicians and when women rarely taught medical or science subjects to men, it must have been a shock for these physicians to see and hear Kenny. With a style perhaps closest to the matron of a nursing school, she was uncompromising in asserting the truth and logic of her own ideas. Not interested in a middle ground, she refused to present her ideas as a development of established standards or to alter her distinctive and sometimes confusing terminology by making analogies to more familiar terms. She told the physicians in her courses, as she recalled it in 1943: "if they wished to learn what I had to teach them, they must begin by understanding that the disease they were so familiar with simply did not exist." On the other hand, "if they wished to continue treating for symptoms with which they were familiar, then my lectures and demonstrations were a waste of time."[70] She understood that she was overwhelming men and women not used to being overwhelmed.

Kenny saw doctors as supplicants who needed to be converted and many did become believers. One epidemiologist told her that "after seeing from day to day your work and results I had to admit that we were wrong and you were right. I thank you all very much for the 'conversion of ideas.'"[71] Even suspicious physicians were eager to hear from those who had seen Kenny in action. Floyd Clarke, a member of the June 1942 class, gave a talk on the Kenny treatment for the Omaha-Midwest Clinical Society to an audience of around 700.[72] Some of the doctors who attended the courses were amused; most were intrigued; and many left determined to convince their own colleagues and hospital directors that patients needed these new methods and properly trained technicians.

Still, many physicians who praised her work's clinical applications distanced themselves from her theories. Thus, pediatrician Irvine McQuarrie told everyone that although he was not convinced by most of Kenny's ideas, if his own child had polio he would want to have Kenny's method used.[73] Perhaps, Kenny hoped, this sort of endorsement was only the first step and gradually physicians would want to seek out explanations for the efficacy of her methods.

Other physicians who publicly identified themselves in favor of these new clinical practices were nonetheless careful to present their change of heart as the result of scientific skepticism.[74] Mayo physician medicine expert Frank Krusen knew he would be taken more seriously when he hesitated to affirm his belief in Kenny's work. In his "Observations on the Kenny Treatment of Poliomyelitis" published in the *Proceedings of the Staff Meetings of the Mayo Clinic* in August 1942 Krusen reminded his colleagues of how skeptical he had been from the outset. When he had been asked by O'Connor to serve on a committee to evaluate Kenny's work and had protested that he was skeptical about the whole procedure, O'Connor had assured him that "my skepticism eminently qualified me for membership on the committee." Only after he had finally visited Minneapolis himself and examined Kenny's patients did he acknowledge how impressed he was with her clinical results.[75] Kenny similarly saw that characterizing her medical allies as initially skeptical helped to demonstrate their credibility as scientific professionals. Krusen, she often pointed out, had "thought I was unbalanced when I arrived in the United States and presented my ideas."[76]

The enthusiasm of Cole, Knapp, and Pohl continued to trouble their colleagues in orthopedics and physical medicine, especially when the NFIP published their June 1942 article in *Archives of Physical Therapy* as a separate pamphlet. To prove it was not the result of being swayed by Kenny's personality all 3 physicians began to stress how skeptical they had initially been and how only the objectivity of close clinical observation had led them to change their minds. "Nothing occult is involved in her methods," they assured their peers; indeed her complex therapies required "an intimate knowledge" of anatomy and the neuromuscular system.[77] Pohl had been so skeptical of the work at first, Krusen claimed, that he had refused to have his name appear on the first publication in *JAMA* although he was now "a most enthusiastic advocate of the procedure."[78]

Another skeptical convert was prominent Chicago orthopedist Philip Lewin, who taught at Northwestern's medical school and was the chair of the NFIP's Aftereffects Committee. His 1941 polio textbook had called Kenny's methods "of questionable practical value" and Kenny had named Lewin's book as an example of mistaken old-style polio care.[79] But after Lewin came to Minneapolis to see her work in person, he "completely changed his views," as the *Saturday Evening Post* put it.[80] At the annual meeting of the Illinois State Medical Society in May 1942 Lewin argued that Kenny "has jarred the medical and allied professions out of their complacency into an immediate offensive attack on the local condition which she has proved exists." Continuous rigid splinting "is not only 'on its way out' but...it is 'out.'" Kenny's patients, he declared, were "in better condition than any similar group I have seen anywhere in the world."[81] Kenny delighted in this admission of conversion and called Lewin her first American disciple.[82]

Pediatrician Philip Stimson became another Kenny convert. Stimson came from a patrician family and had graduated from Yale (1910) and Cornell's medical school (1914).[83] An excellent public speaker, he was frequently sent by the NFIP to regional medical societies to talk about polio care.

Even before meeting Kenny in person, Stimson had begun to refer to her ideas in lectures, admitting that after reading about her work he had altered his own hospital practice by doing a little less immobilization and by putting heat on "a cramped muscle...to keep it from getting stiff."[84] Stimson first met Kenny when she visited the Willard Parker Hospital, the city's infectious disease hospital, in September 1941. Thereafter he began to use her methods systematically and with the urging of the NFIP gave numerous talks to local medical societies using her terms *spasm, incoordination,* and *alienation.* After offering a detailed description of her methods, he concluded (and this final line in his notes for one talk was underlined) "*A little Kenny is better than none.*"[85]

By the time Stimson reported on his own Willard Parker patients at an NFIP meeting in December 1941 he had become a skilled presenter who dramatized Kenny's methods using a model. He preferred "a pretty nurse...in a bathing suit of the bra and panties type [or]...a gym suit costume." On one occasion when "a male orderly in bathing trunks was provided...the audience was not half as interested in the actual demonstration."[86] In early 1942 Stimson invited Kenny to lecture to the New York Physical Therapy Society where several orthopedic surgeons agreed during the discussion that immobilization could be harmful, damaging, and crippling, that spasm was a significant symptom, and that surgeons had "concentrated...too much on the diseased nerve cells [and been]...afraid to stretch the muscles."[87] While Kenny saw such occasions as opportunities to defend her work, Stimson said privately that he had invited her mostly for entertainment. "She is a terrible talker," he admitted to a friend, "and really not worth hearing, but she is well worth seeing."[88]

As Stimson became identified as a Kenny convert, he was confronted by antagonistic opponents. After hearing him give a radio talk that seemed to be endorsing her views, one physician sent him a reprint of his own prize-winning essay on polio that had warned of "numerous quacks who thrive upon the ignorance of the unfortunate people" and proposed the use of a light corset or a well-padded splint along with massage, heat, electricity, muscle training, and hydrotherapy.[89] Charles Zacharie, another physician who heard Stimson's radio talk, felt that Stimson's training and hospital connections showed that he was educated and intelligent, which made his praise of Kenny all the worse. Zacharie was convinced that Kenny had "never studied Pathology, Histology, nor Anatomy nor Diagnosis, nor Symptoms." Mocking the doctors who had "all jumped on the Kinney [sic] Wagon," he argued that her methods could not "cure or prevent atrophy of muscles & the deformity that goes with it," and that, in any case, hot packs "were known & used way back in 1600 in many diseases before you and Kinney [sic] were born."[90] Stimson replied courteously that while he agreed that Kenny "knows nothing of histology, and very little about the central nervous system," nonetheless "she has a greater knowledge of muscle anatomy and muscle function than most doctors, obtained by many hours of study." "On the speakers' platform" she was "more apt to antagonize doctors than win them over," Stimson admitted. "But at the bedside, she is an entirely different proposition" for "practically every doctor who has seen her at work [agreed] . . . that at the present time, her methods of treatment are the best we have for minimizing the after-effects of the disease."[91]

It is difficult to say how much of the opposition to Kenny's treatment was based on actual clinical disagreement and how much was the result of resistance to change and the feeling of being under attack. "It is interesting, and if one can take it, stimulating to have one's life-long theories and teachings completely reversed," a Philadelphia orthopedist remarked to a medical audience.[92]

EVALUATIONS

In 1943 the *Journal of Bone and Joint Surgery* published the first controlled clinical study of Kenny's work. Robert Bingham, a young orthopedist and the study's author, had met Kenny in April 1941 in New York City while he was a resident at the New York Orthopedic Hospital, and had watched her infuriate the hospital's orthopedic surgeons by telling them how wrong their treatment was and what terrible results they would get. He was further impressed by her demonstration of symptoms such as muscle spasm, which his teachers had not recognized. Bingham began using Kenny treatment experimentally a few months later at the hospital's White Plains branch, and when his patients seemed significantly better he substituted it for orthodox care. He had faced a "tremendous amount of antagonism . . . [and] a great deal of ridicule," a colleague admitted privately, especially from orthopedists.[93] Based on 60 patients in the convalescent stage at the White Plains hospital, Bingham's study had compared 3 groups of patients treated between May 1941 and May 1942: Group 1 (12 patients treated by "older" methods only); Group 2 (24 patients treated using Kenny methods later in their care); and Group 3 (24 patients treated with "only Kenny"). He had found the "extent of recovery of some patients under the Kenny treatment . . . so great" that he warned readers "in studying the final results considerable careful judgment must be used in deciding which of the improvements in the patient's condition are due to the Kenny treatment and which would have followed from a mild or abortive attack of poliomyelitis." In one crucial table, 46 percent of Group 3 had excellent "functional results," compared to 8 percent of Group 1 and 25 percent of Group 2. Group 3 patients were "more comfortable, have better general health and nutrition, are more receptive to muscle training, have a superior morale, require a shorter period of bed rest and hospital care, and seem to have less residual paralysis and deformity than patients treated by older conventional methods."[94] One of Bingham's orthopedic supervisors felt his study was "unscientific and misleading" for it was not fair to compare the earlier patients whose paralysis had been much more severe to the milder ones who received the Kenny treatment.[95] Kenny, though, was delighted by Bingham's study and frequently quoted its "gratifying results."[96]

Kenny's claim that her patients had higher recovery rates than those treated by orthodox methods was refuted by critics who argued that she tended to select potential patients who could best be helped by her work. Florence Kendall had long complained, as she told a group of nurses, that "S.K.'s statistics are based on selected cases. She refuses to treat those which she knows are hopeless."[97] There were also many cases of patients who recovered, confounding their physicians. Most patients "recover no matter what type of therapy is employed," pediatrician John Toomey argued, and those patients should be excluded from "the statistical study of therapeutic results, or at least tabulated separately."[98] Kenny's constant reference to McCarroll and Crego's 1941 study was also suspect because the study could be seen as an example of treating the most seriously paralyzed patients. Orthopedist Bruce Gill had wondered whether Kenny's work had been compared to patients who had "*really* been treated in accordance with *standard* principles and methods?"[99]

Throughout Kenny's career her critics demanded "scientific" tests and questioned the evaluations that she claimed supported her. Many suggested that her results could be explained by "a psychological factor," and others mocked her "hypnotic training" and "her ministrations" as "abracadabra."[100] The false hopes Kenny created among many patients and their families were believed to have led to a kind of popular hysteria that made it even more difficult to evaluate her work.

There was a clear way to establish proper science from "cultist" claims and that was the clinical trial. This idea had been raised since Kenny's early days in Minneapolis.[101] Three factors made this kind of rational assessment almost impossible: the power of public demand; Kenny herself; and the nature of polio. Public enthusiasm, a recognized feature of Kenny's work, threatened to undermine familiar strategies of control. Thus, patients in one Minneapolis hospital were intended to be in a control group, Philip Lewin recalled, but their parents "refused to permit the withholding [of] the Kenny treatment."[102] "The whole debate might be settled by a single experiment," one science writer suggested, but "experts say such a test can never take place; no American mother would allow her child to be subjected to conventional treatment while some other child got Kenny hot packs."[103] Here the emotionality of the public—embodied in an irrational mother—was a roadblock to the pursuit of scientific truth.

Polio itself was a disease that was difficult to diagnose accurately and had wide variation in its clinical symptoms. A control study would never be possible, one orthopedist warned, "because of the variation in the effect of the disease in different individuals during the same epidemic and in different epidemics."[104] This notion became a truism, repeated by physicians into the late 1940s. A growing awareness of different types of the polio virus (finally stabilized at 3 a few years later) created an additional concern with clinical variation. Not only did the unpredictability of polio make it "difficult to compare the statistics, mortality rates, and forms of therapy of different groups of workers," Colorado physicians argued, but varying strains of the virus made it "difficult...to try to run controlled studies."[105]

THE CULT OF PERSONALITY

Recognizing that physicians were uncomfortable with a new method identified too closely with an individual—especially someone who was not a physician—the NFIP tried to separate the woman from the work. The foundation's national office, which regularly organized exhibits for the AMA's annual meetings, proposed an exhibit on Kenny's work to respond to the "tremendous demand," to "furnish sufficient knowledge to enable a physician to competently apply the treatment," and to "dispel many current bits of misinformation."[106] During the June 1942 AMA meeting an estimated 3,500 physicians, nurses, and physical therapists crowded into the NFIP corner exhibit where Cole, Knapp, Pohl, and Stimson were featured as lecturers.[107] Two of Kenny's Australian technicians were invited to be special demonstrators but Kenny herself was not to be included. Knapp warned Gudakunst that "Sister Kenny was grossly insulted by being excluded," but Gudakunst replied that "the Foundation is exhibiting Miss Kenny's method and not Miss Kenny."[108] Stimson and the 3 Minnesota physicians showed how to examine and treat a patient for muscle tenderness, muscle spasm, and other major symptoms, and, following Stimson's usual practice, used live models: a male college student and a young woman physical therapist.[109]

Outside the Scientific Exhibit Kenny's work was debated in the AMA's regular sessions. In Pediatrics, Stimson gave, as his chairman's address, a lecture on "A Rationalization of the Sister Kenny Treatment of Poliomyelitis."[110] An entire panel debated her work in a session jointly organized by the Section on Nervous and Mental Diseases and the Section on Orthopedic Surgery.[111] More ominously, the Section on Orthopedic Surgery formed a committee "to study and evaluate the Kenny treatment of infantile paralysis." The only Minnesota orthopedist chosen to be a member of this committee was Ralph Ghormley, Henderson's colleague at the Mayo Clinic who had not met Kenny or ventured any public comments about her work.[112] This was the third committee of experts to assess Kenny's work, and its composition—prominent orthopedic surgeons—suggested that it was likely to be especially critical.

KENNY'S CONCEPT AND PRACTICE

Recognizing that the AMA committee would be unlikely to complete its work for a year or so, Fishbein made sure that there was a balance between proponents and opponents when he published the 1942 AMA papers on Kenny's work in *JAMA*. As a result the overall impression was that some experts endorsed clinical change and some opposed it. Two physiologists supported her theory that immobilization was dangerous. In experiments with rats whose nerves had been crushed Harry Hines found that immobilization "definitely retarded recovery" but that forced activity like swimming or exercising in a revolving barrel had aided neuromuscular recovery.[113] Donald Solandt similarly found that decreased fibrillation and electrical excitability in rat muscles were the result of disuse rather than overwork. Making an analogy to human bodies, he suggested that "splinting should be used with caution [for] ... possibly this observation indicates the rationale for one feature of the Kenny method of therapy."[114]

The 2 orthopedic surgeons whose papers were published took opposing views of Kenny's work. Harvard orthopedist Frank Ober, who had met Kenny in Minneapolis a few months earlier, believed her treatment was "superb nursing and common sense." He was convinced by her call for treating polio's early stage and believed that "deformities in the early stages are due to pain, muscle spasm and muscle contractures." With his own patients Ober had not used "prolonged rest and immobilization in plaster" but wire splints and hot packs 2 or 3 times a day. Spasm, he argued, was a serious symptom, although how it was caused "at present is not quite clear to us." The clinical signs Kenny highlighted implied a new kind of pathology for he doubted that "pain, spasm in muscles, unexplained bone growth changes and vascular disturbances on the extremities" could all be the result merely of a lesion in the anterior horns.[115]

In contrast St. Louis orthopedist Relton McCarroll was shocked that some of his peers were taking Kenny's work seriously, especially after the publication of his and Crego's 1941 study. He dismissed her methods as yet another popular fad based on the mistaken idea that polio was "a purely local muscle lesion," an idea that could not "be reconciled to our present knowledge of the proved pathologic process in this disease." "It is easy to understand how physical therapists, enthusiastic in their work, might lose sight of this primary pathologic process," McCarroll reflected, but he found it impossible to understand how orthopedic surgeons could "wholeheartedly endorse any of these methods." He was "certain that this method in time will take its place among the others offered by the field of physical therapy as having been tried but found wanting."[116]

McCarroll was attacked by Kenny supporters whose letters were published in the next several issues of *JAMA*. Despite the "purely empiric origin" of Kenny's concept, Wisconsin physical medicine specialist Frances Hellebrandt argued, "her observations were so acute that they approached truth, as truth is revealed in nature." In any case, "newer knowledge" of polio's pathology and physiology had shown the "rationale of her physical therapeutic methods."[117] Pohl pointed out that McCarroll had completely missed the main point of Kenny's work: "that there are muscle conditions which are far more damaging to the bodily mechanics if unrecognized and untreated." Unlike McCarroll, he and other Minnesota physicians had "taken the time during the past two and one-half years to observe her work" and found that Kenny had decisively proved her point for only the methods she had developed "could have been effective in treating the disease of poliomyelitis, since it is based on symptoms which she alone discovered."[118] In her own letter, which appeared in the December 19 issue of *JAMA*, Kenny claimed that she was not "referring to the pathology of the disease but to the symptomatology." In an unusual interpretation of Kendalls' *PHS Bulletin* and McCarroll and Crego's study she suggested that both had showed that traditional physical therapy methods had "failed to achieve results." In any case, she argued, the clinical evidence quoted by Cole, Knapp, Pohl, and Bingham, who had properly treated "the true symptoms of this disease ... speak for themselves and need no comment from me."[119]

Back in Minnesota Kenny tried to design her Institute drawing on models of the Mayo Clinic and the Rockefeller Institute. She was impressed by the way that the nearby town of Rochester appeared to be run as a kind of Mayo medical marketplace and hoped her institute could combine a scientific research center like that at the Rockefeller Institute with a clinical research hospital.[120] She also deliberately designed a uniform for her Kenny technicians to make them stand out: long, light blue dresses in cotton and polyester with a full blue veil. These headdresses, which resembled Australian nursing uniforms of the early twentieth century, were scorned by nurses at the neighboring Mayo Clinic who wore small round hats that looked like donuts. For her part, Kenny considered that traditional starched collars, cuffs, and aprons were not modern and did not "appeal to young girls."[121] As Institute director Kenny did not wear a uniform. She wore a suit or a full-length dress in all black or all white, suggesting someone dependent on nothing and no one. Her over-sized accessories (hats, corsages, and dress pins) also presented the visual opposite of the ordinary nurse's outfit: dramatic, bold, the image of an assertive equal rather than a timid doctor's assistant, the sign of a respectable lady.[122]

THE QUESTION OF CREDIBILITY

Before Stimson's AMA speech appeared in *JAMA* in 1942 he and his medical staff at the Willard Parker hospital had published a study comparing 33 patients who had the "accepted" treatment with 28 treated by the Kenny method. They concluded that for patients with spasm Kenny's method should be the "treatment of choice."[123] Now Stimson argued not just for a change in therapy but in theory as well. Kenny's work along with "recent studies of many medical research workers and clinicians" should lead physicians to rethink polio's pathology and physiology. While currently many theories were available to explain the causes of spasm, spasm itself was constantly present in acute polio and could be aggravated by forced immobilization with the use of casts and splints. Stimson defined and then used Kenny's terms *incoordination* and *alienation* to try to establish them as part of the ordinary medical vocabulary.[124] Despite this confirmation of Kenny's concepts, Stimson (or perhaps *JAMA* editor Fishbein) placed quotation marks around the term *alienation*; the other 2 terms were left free of textual doubt.

Stimson's *JAMA* article reinforced a general sense among American physicians that Kenny's method was effective, especially for polio's acute stage, and that Kenny herself was reliable. Although Stimson was convinced that her ideas were original and worthy of scientific investigation, not everyone agreed. Her training—as a nurse she presumably knew nothing of tissue culture or dissected bodies—and her gender made her sound like a technical innovator who had gone too far in talking about science and theory. How much should physicians use her new terms and her ideas? Were her ideas just lucky guesses, based in ignorance or perhaps clinical acumen, or were they based on a distinctive scientific understanding of the body? If what she argued made scientific sense must previous scientific explanations be rejected? Had standard polio therapies been based on poor science?

In Canada observers of Kenny's work took on the question of credibility. Drawing on their experience during and after a serious epidemic in Manitoba in 1941, physicians at Winnipeg's Children's Hospital argued that not only was Kenny's work effective but it made scientific sense. Their arguments combined the evidence of their eyes and hands with a new understanding of the body based on Kenny's theories. Kenny had "revolutionized our ideas on the symptomatology and treatment of acute anterior poliomyelitis" said orthopedist Alfred Deacon. During her visit to Winnipeg the medical staff "could feel the spasm she demonstrated and see the effects they were producing" and had been especially impressed—indeed "astounded"—by Kenny's ability to show that some patients deemed paralyzed could indeed move "merely by restoring the patient's mental awareness of those muscles, and thus correcting their alienation." These results convinced the staff that her methods made sense physiologically and that "in most cases…the flaccid muscles are indeed alienated from their brain control." The outcome of the new therapies was equally dramatic, for they produced "better results than any method we have hitherto used."[125] These impressive clinical results were also mentioned by the hospital's administrator who, however, warned his board of trustees that the 1941 *Reader's Digest* story had been "painted in too brilliant colors," leaving the impression "that the method of treatment returns paralyzed muscles entirely to normal" with patients "returned to complete robust muscular health."[126]

"We cannot use the known pathology of the disease to justify a refusal to re-examine the clinical picture of this disease," Children's Hospital director Bruce Chown declared boldly in the *Canadian Public Health Journal*. Writing as a pathologist and a pediatrician, Chown cited recent work by Johns Hopkins virologists Howard Howe and David Bodian whose critique of the standard classification of polio, Chown argued, could explain the diverse "symptoms and signs" of temporary paralysis that Kenny called mental alienation. Speaking as a clinician, a researcher, and an administrator well aware of the routine of caring for patients during and after an epidemic, Chown was convinced that "the whole disease is in need of reassessment." "Some have found the stimulus unpleasant," he warned, "but reaction is taking place."[127]

Even more important was physiological research by University of Rochester orthopedist Plato Schwartz that established the existence of spasm through electronic analysis of muscles. In work funded by the NFIP Schwartz used the oscillograph he had developed in his Gait Laboratory to try to measure spasm. Schwartz and his colleague Harry Bouman took more than 500 records from 7 patients with acute polio and compared them to records of normal subjects and to patients without polio but with other kinds of "spastic" paralysis. Their research identified what they called "spasticity" (spasm) in patients with polio, although whether this was responsible for muscle weakening "cannot be answered at this time." They also found evidence of "spasticity" in the muscles of patients with polio "where no clinical evidence of muscle weakening can be found" as well as in weakened muscles, suggesting both that spasm did exist but also that it could not necessarily be identified by clinical observation alone. Their *JAMA* article included 4 illustrations of "oscillographic records of muscle action currents" that showed "definite evidence of muscle spasm."[128] These 4 images seemed more serious and scientific than photographs of patients sitting up or walking.

Both Kenny and the NFIP immediately saw the implications of this study. A photograph of Kenny with Schwartz at the University of Rochester was published in the *Rochester Times* and reprinted in the *National Foundation News*.[129] In her speech as the guest of honor at the university's annual alumnae dinner Kenny described Schwartz's article as the first formal academic recognition of her work showing "scientific proof for her concept of poliomyelitis and its treatment." Less effusively and without mentioning

Kenny's theory, Schwartz replied that he gave her "full credit for discontinuing methods of fixation or immobilization and for stressing early reeducation of muscles."[130] The NFIP's newsletter featured the study, noting that a "laboratory equipped with delicate electrical instruments" had picked up and magnified minute electrical currents of nerve impulses and then measured, recorded photographically, studied, and analyzed them, providing "the first real proof that Miss Kenny was treating a condition which actually did exist."[131] Gudakunst similarly assured professionals and parents that this study proved Kenny's work was not based on "wild theory and uncontrolled imagination" but "that Kenny has described exactly what does happen."[132]

Both Stimson's and Schwartz's studies were highlighted in the 1942 *Yearbook of Physical Therapy* that devoted 24 pages to studies of Kenny's work compared to 3 pages the year before.[133] At the American Congress of Physical Therapy Knapp similarly praised researchers such as Schwartz and Bouman who had begun to search for the physiological cause of spasm and referred to his own research conducted with a physiologist that supported "the fundamentals of the method." While it was true that Kenny's work was "based on radical changes in physiologic interpretations of the observed symptoms," Knapp said, there was no disagreement with known pathology. Indeed her work had made clear how little physicians did know "about the fundamental pathologic physiology of poliomyelitis."[134]

In "Sister Kenny Wins Her Fight," a follow-up *Reader's Digest* story in 1942, Lois Miller declared that the NFIP's approval of Kenny was "without precedent or parallel in medical history." Boosted by clinical results described by Stimson and physiological evidence by Schwartz at the University of Rochester, "overnight the theories and practices that had been applied to the treatment of infantile paralysis for decades became outmoded; in their place came a new treatment—opposed to the old ideas—which had in its favor only one thing: it worked!" Miller did add that it was "still too early to inquire exactly how and why the treatment achieves its remarkable results."[135]

A COMMITTEE COMES TO VISIT

In November 1942 5 members of the orthopedic committee formed during the summer's AMA meeting came to Minneapolis. Some of them, Kenny recognized immediately, "had written most antagonistically and untruthfully" about her work. This enmity was clear when "one extremely antagonistic member of the group" using the fighting word "cure" asked Kenny "what do you call a cure for this disease?"[136]

Ralph Ghormley was the committee's chair, but he was not able to come to Minneapolis, so Melvin Henderson, Ghormley's Mayo colleague who was not a member of the committee, had agreed to be its acting chair. In addition, Ghormley asked each of the visiting doctors to write his impressions of the visit. Kenny showed the visitors her patients, demonstrated her methods, and lectured on her theories, with some additional lectures from Pohl. She resented this further investigation of her work and while she was eager to prove her method's efficacy she was also quick to hear quizzical comments as attacks.

Almost all of the 5 visitors' responses showed that their previous attitudes were not changed. Henderson was pointedly neutral and in a positive tone said that the visit convinced him that "there is a good deal more to this disease than merely the involvement of the anterior horn cells."[137] Edward Compere from Chicago, already known as a Kenny ally, was far more enthusiastic. He had begun to use Kenny's methods by early 1942 and had praised them in the *Archives of Physical Therapy*. Though "not a cure," he wrote, they did reduce the "severity of the paralysis."[138] Compere recognized that the visit had not gone well and did not want personal animosities to derail a fair assessment of Kenny's contribution. While "it will not be easy to separate the personal equation," he told Ghormley, "we should not judge the method, however, or the theory, on a basis of our dislike of some of the publicity which has so flooded the newspapers or because we may have had conflicts with Miss Kenny herself."[139] Robert Funston, chair of the Department of Orthopedic Surgery at the University of Virginia, had allowed his younger colleague to attend one of Kenny's courses a few months earlier and had sent members of his hospital staff to Minneapolis for further training.[140] In a noncommittal report Funston noted that Kenny's patients had better flexibility and fewer "contractures" than other patients he had seen. As for her ideas about "the function of individual muscles," in some "I think she is right and other[s] I do not."[141]

St. Louis orthopedists Albert Key and Relton McCarroll came and left as adversaries. Key distrusted the examples of "apparently normal children" Kenny showed the committee, seeing them as very mild patients who "would have recorded normal muscles whether or not they had had the Kenny treatment." He admitted he was intrigued by X-ray films of a patient with mild scoliosis who had worn a spinal support for 3 years and then been treated by Kenny. The more recent X-rays showed curves in the lumbar and dorsal spine that "were slightly less than were those in the earlier film" and he felt that "this case would bear study."[142] Both men disliked Kenny's rejection of orthopedic apparatus and her use of Kenny (short) crutches; both felt that such patients would be better off with braces "from an economic standpoint" and "that many of these patients will later choose a brace in preference to the crutches." With no sympathy for Kenny's new definition of "deformity," McCarroll was annoyed by Pohl's upbeat predictions of a patient whose peroneal muscles were still paralyzed after 14 months of treatment. Pohl had said that even if the muscles did not regain normal power "there would be no tendency to deformity in later years. How they can be so certain of this is impossible to see."[143] Both men also found Kenny rude and inflexible. According to Key "she made numerous dogmatic and, to my mind, obviously untrue statements and when questioned said to me on three occasions, 'There are none so blind as those who will not see,' and turned her back. On other occasions she merely said that she was wasting her time trying to show us anything." Her claims of having "discovered a cure" and having "revolutionized the treatment of this disease" they saw as "nonsense," and both berated the NFIP "for fostering this publicity."[144]

Kenny had hoped to sway the committee by a demonstration of mental alienation, using a trick she had developed years earlier. She asked the visitors to examine one of her patients and, as she recalled it, all "pronounced the extensors of the leg completely paralyzed. I disagreed and stepped forward. Again, as I had done in my own wild out-back of Australia thirty years before, I taught the muscle what to do, gave back to it its motor pattern, and then linked it up with the brain path. Full use of the muscle was restored in less than twenty seconds."[145] Then she declared dramatically "that muscle is normal; it was only alienated and I have restored its power."[146] Key and McCarroll were both unimpressed and perhaps also embarrassed to have been shown up.[147] Nor did Kenny's efforts to have the surgeons feel the clinical signs she had identified with their own hands succeed. McCarroll recalled that he was asked to compare a muscle in spasm with the same muscle in the opposite limb. "I very frankly could not detect any difference in the feel or the appearance of these muscles," he reported to Ghormley. He saw no evidence that any of these muscles could return to their normal power, pointing out "they keep no detailed records on these muscles."[148]

A physician also present at this visit who openly embraced Kenny's work was Ethel Calhoun. A 1925 medical graduate from the University of Michigan, Calhoun had worked as a private practitioner in Detroit before marrying and having a child. Now in her forties she found a new direction in her life as a passionate supporter of Kenny and her work.[149] In her own letter to Ghormley, Calhoun was appalled by Key and McCarroll's "'chip on their shoulder' attitude." They had "started asking one question after the other in rapid fire order without waiting for Miss Kenny to finish an explanation" and were so "very rude" that Calhoun "could no longer keep silent." She told them that she had just finished a week's course and that as it "takes most doctors two days at least before they understand some of the basic principles of the Kenny concept" they should "stay long enough to know what she [Kenny] is talking about." One of them got "very red in the face" and retorted "you don't know what you are talking about or why we are here." Calhoun told Ghormley her own child "would never get anything but Kenny treatment, at least not until some one can show me something better." She regretted that any prejudiced physicians who felt that they "must continue their opposition as a 'face saving' method" should have been appointed to this committee.[150] Back in Michigan she introduced the Kenny method to the polio wards of the infectious disease hospital in Pontiac and gained the support of her local NFIP chapter.[151]

The one orthopedist who admitted that the visit had profoundly altered his views was Herman Charles Schumm.[152] He had come to Minnesota from Milwaukee, he admitted to Ghormley, "very anti-Kenny" but he left convinced that "our ideas as to what muscles were paralyzed were all wrong." Her method "certainly gives better results than I have seen in the past, or have been able to obtain." She also convinced him that most patients "need no type of appliance or brace whatsoever and that they do much better without it." Schumm was not put off by Kenny's manner. He found her clinical results powerful and may even have become more sympathetic watching her battle with Key and McCarroll. "I have apologized to myself several times since my trip to Minneapolis for making up my mind that her treatment was no good before I had made an adequate investigation," he concluded his report.[153]

Kenny somehow obtained a copy of these reports. While she told Ghormley she would "overlook the unkind and hateful personal reference[s]...in the interests of humanity" she did protest the therapeutic and professional attacks. She had not been discourteous or "turned my back." Her demonstrations had taken place before the opening of the spacious Institute. Forced to show her patients while her visitors stood in a circle around 2 tables, she had had to "keep turning from one table to another." Kenny was not surprised by her visitors' initial skepticism for she had shown them "a disease with which [each doctor]...was unfamiliar and had no idea existed." But she was frustrated that her demonstration of mental alienation had not altered their skepticism and that her environment, supervised by a medical school, had not effectively shielded her from accusations that her recovered patients had not really had polio. Thus, when "Dr. McCarroll had doubted the diagnosis and asked me who had diagnosed the cases," Kenny had replied with great satisfaction that "the pediatric staff was responsible."[154] At a meeting of the Academy of Orthopedic Surgeons a few months later she learned that Key and McCarroll remained antagonistic. Although during a visit to Wesley Memorial Hospital they had congratulated the hospital's Kenny technician on her patients' "splendid condition," at the Academy meeting McCarroll declared that if the patients "had belonged to him he would hang his head in shame." He later phoned the technician and "apologized for passing this remark," adding that he had been "to use his own expression, 'just mad.'" [155] A private phone call to one technician, Kenny feared, would hardly counter the profound impact of this public denigration of her work.

Key remained one of Kenny's most prominent critics. In "The Kenny Versus the Orthodox Treatment" in *Surgery* he argued that the Kenny treatment of spasm was harmful for it rejected crucial therapies such as immobilization and rest. He defended "orthodox" treatment as "the result of the accumulated experience of many physicians" and "well standardized throughout the civilized world." Not only was rest "probably the most important therapeutic measure in our armamentarium," but patients also required well-padded and fitted plaster molds or padded metal splints in order to protect paralyzed muscles from stretching and to hasten "the disappearance of hyperesthesia, muscle tenderness, and contractures." Despite Kenny's claims, such apparatus "do not interfere with circulation nor are they left in place constantly." Nor was there any evidence that the polio virus "attacks the muscles" or that the Kenny method would prevent "paralyzed muscles from stretching." In any case, Key argued, none of her claims could be properly assessed for without records "it is not possible to verify the exorbitant claims of cures."[156]

TALES OF SACRIFICE

Despite the brutal attacks of these critics, the Institute grew in public acclaim, a brick and mortar emblem of Kenny's contribution to American medicine. Kenny's methods— or at least key parts of them—were embraced by hospitals throughout the country. Publicity from *Reader's Digest*, *Life*, *Time*, and other magazines confirmed Kenny as a celebrity. The Minnesota Public Health Association gave her a plaque for Outstanding Service to Humanity and *Parents Magazine* awarded her the magazine's annual medal for Outstanding Service to Children, following former recipients such as Eleanor Roosevelt, Walt Disney, and Surgeon-General Thomas Parran.[157] The Variety Clubs of America, a group of show business philanthropies focused on the needs of poor children, gave her its Humanitarian Medal for 1942, which was presented to her in Sacramento "in the presence of Governor Earl Warren of California and other people of note." In her speech which was broadcast across the country by radio she compared her work's results to those of patients treated "under orthodox methods from the orthodox concept." Her contribution—"the result of lonely research [in] . . . the bush land of Australia"—was "an entirely new concept of the disease, with an entirely new treatment based on that concept."[158]

Kenny enlarged on these arguments in her 1943 autobiography *And They Shall Walk*, which brimmed with tales of sacrifice and justified outrage. The book described an outsider who moved from the Queensland bush to the city of Brisbane, and then from the exotic nation of Australia to the modern United States in order to obtain medical respect. Descriptions of wattle, black swans, koalas, and other distinctive flora and fauna gave this work the flavor of a travelogue. To remind readers that she was contributing to a global health problem—not one specific to Australia—there were descriptions of her extensive international traveling to treat patients. Her experiences in the United States were shown as the culmination of a life's work of struggle and sacrifice.

In the book, almost all negative examples of professional opposition take place in Australia or England. In the United States, physicians—although at first cautious and quizzical—are wonderfully open-minded and free of prejudice against either Kenny's training or gender. "Such recognition, though late in coming, did much toward healing the wounds that had been left by scurrilous criticism and by the even more humiliating experience of being loftily ignored. It helped me to forget the bitter tears I had shed in solitude."[159] Positioning herself as a female medical pioneer, Kenny stresses her impatience with orthodoxy, the restrictive conventions of gender roles, and the inflexibility of medical thinking and professional ethics. Perhaps reflecting commercial pressure to add a love interest, a few pages present the story of Dan, a local farmer. Big and bronzed with kind blue eyes, Dan believes "a woman's place was 'in the home'" and he tells Kenny she "must give up this nursing nonsense if I were to take the place for which my Creator had ordained me." When she chooses to attend a woman in labor instead of a dance, "we quarreled our last quarrel," and she delivers the baby "fighting back the tears."[160]

Nowhere, other than on the book's title page, was there a reference to Kenny's co-author Martha Ostenso. Ostenso, a prize-winning novelist, later claimed that Kenny sometimes yelled when Ostenso altered her overblown phrases, but that she was delighted with the final version. The Dodd, Mead contract gave Ostenso 5 percent of the book's profits, and she seems to have been willing to have the publisher advertise the book without highlighting her name as co-author.[161]

Despite the numerous descriptions of exotic places, *And They Shall Walk* has only 3 illustrations, all photographs of Kenny in America. The first 2 reinforce the image of Kenny as a clinician capable of training other professionals. In the picture captioned "Sister Kenny demonstrates her revolutionary treatment," Kenny is pointing to the strong legs of a boy on a treatment table as skeptical nurses look on. In "Training nurses to carry on the Kenny treatment," eager nurses and physical therapists watch her wrap a child's legs. The third photograph features Kenny with the world's most famous polio survivor. The caption "President Roosevelt greets Sister Kenny" ignores the third person in this image: Basil O'Connor, the most powerful person in polio philanthropy. Yet in her introduction Kenny thanks the NFIP along with the citizens of Minneapolis and Cole, Knapp, and Pohl, "without whose support and encouragement wider recognition might have been indefinitely postponed." She concludes with her declaration that "to the medical men of the United States of America I pass the torch."[162] But her growing stridency in response to critics belied this statement. And her new textbook published a few months later went further, arguing that only those experts who accepted her contribution would be able to guide the progress of polio science.

Physicians who adopted Kenny's work tried to express enthusiasm mixed with caution. "Our physiologists and pathologists must, and eventually will, give us the basis for these newer clinical manifestations," Robert Bennett argued in the *Southern Medical Journal*.[163] In the *Archives of Physical Therapy* he praised the patient, intelligent guidance of men such as Miland Knapp who had enabled Kenny to develop her techniques and, he was sure, equally keen and devoted researchers would now "support [or] . . . if necessary . . . intelligently alter that which she and other serious investigators have given us."[164] Importantly Arthur Steindler, one of the nation's leading orthopedic researchers and teachers, declared in the *Journal of Bone and Joint Surgery* that he and his staff had accepted many of the "Kenny technics" to treat pain and spasm. Experiments in his department at the University of Iowa using novocaine on nerves affected by polio suggested, like the Kenny concept, that the cause of spasm "is peripheral and not central." Thus, Steindler argued, "tendons, ligaments, and capsular reinforcements are involved in pathological changes, as are the muscles."[165]

These physicians were aware that many British professionals would see their support of Kenny as an unfortunate example of naive American enthusiasm. At the end of 1942, affecting the more objective perspective of a nation of great orthopedists, the editor of the *British Medical Journal* reminded readers that in the 1930s a London County committee had reviewed Kenny's methods sympathetically but had concluded that they were of unproven value. In those days, the editor pointed out, "little was heard of any revolutionary ideas about the pathology." The editor excoriated the "confusing and uncritical" ways in which physicians like Stimson, Pohl, and even the editor of *JAMA* were trying to rationalize Kenny's theories. While there was certainly room for improvement in polio treatment, American physicians did not seem to be pursuing "critical inquiry upon strictly neurological lines." Schwartz and Bouman's study did not support "Miss Kenny's theories," and Lewin was wrong to claim in the *Illinois Medical Journal* that Kenny's method was the last word in acute polio care. In any case many of Kenny's ideas were hardly new. She had given "new names for old ideas" and inspired American proponents to give "extravagant credit to her work," which was "detracting from traditional American orthopedics." Physicians should properly seek a "road of conduct, free from orthodoxy and from radicalism." Still, Kenny had "stimulated many of our American friends to favor heat" and along with "modification and development" this work would contribute to the proper understanding of polio.[166] Here Kenny's methods were not new and her ideas not good; her proponents in the United States were also sadly mistaken in their praise of her work.

Her critics in the United States were further emboldened by an attack from Philadelphia orthopedist Bruce Gill. In a 14-page commentary which he sent to all 50 members of the Orthopaedic Correspondence Club and later published in the *Journal of Bone and Joint Surgery*, Gill reminded his peers that they could draw on their clinical experience—as supervisors of polio therapy and as surgeons—and on their specialized training in anatomy, pathology, and physiology. They knew what the polio virus did and did not do inside the body, and what the appropriate and safe technologies were to treat the symptoms of the disease. Conservative, steady orthopedic surgeons, he implied, should not follow the lead of easily swayed physical medicine doctors who were not strong enough to fend off ill-informed hospital trustees, uppity therapists, and demanding parents.

Gill had retired from the University of Pennsylvania in 1942 after over 2 decades as chair of the department of orthopedic surgery. He continued his private practice and when Alfred Shands left for the army, Gill replaced him as director of the Alfred DuPont Institute, a hospital for disabled children in Wilmington, Delaware. He tried in vain to draw a line between necessary clinical improvement and slavish following of Kenny's work. At a meeting of the Philadelphia chapter of the American Physiotherapy Association, divisions deepened after Rutherford John, a prominent surgeon on the board of directors of the Philadelphia Society for Crippled Children and an associate professor of orthopedic surgery at the University of Pennsylvania, called the Kenny method "very rational" and

Gill retorted that John was "either stupid or willfully misrepresenting the truth."[167] Gill was appalled to see an advertisement for Kenny and Pohl's new textbook whose publishers had "the unblushing audacity" to declare that "orthodoxy has erred both in recognition as well as in the interpretation of the physical findings in this disease" and that Kenny's concept and treatment were "now generally accepted and approved by the medical professional everywhere." He was also annoyed that 3 recent publications on Kenny had all proclaimed that Kenny's work would be "the basis for the future treatment of infantile paralysis" and that her "original" and "revolutionary" concept was "fundamentally different from that hitherto prevailing."[168]

Kenny's method, in Gill's view, had become famous not through scientific research but "as the result of publicity designed for the public." Under the influence of this publicity parents were demanding that their child be treated by the Kenny method; "in other words, the doctor is being told by the layman how he should treat a specific disease." With an implicit jab at the NFIP Gill warned that allowing "methods of propaganda" to "outrun scientific research and clinical observations and rational analysis" was dangerous both for physicians as well as the public for it would lead physicians to be "swept away from their positions of scientific observation and rational criticisms" and they might subsequently "feel some inward embarrassment and humiliation."[169]

Gill again took up the argument that little in Kenny's work was new. Many of her "concepts of principles and methods of treatment" were the same as those published by Robert Lovett and many other physicians in preceding years and ignored "our common fund of knowledge concerning the nature and the pathology in infantile paralysis." Proud of orthopedic treatment and its results, Gill believed "if any of us treat a child from the beginning of the disease and throughout the following months and deformities develop, we know that we are not following orthodox principles of treatment." Nor did Gill believe that Kenny's results had been fairly compared to patients treated by standard methods. In any case, a control study of polio would never be possible for even during the same epidemic patients had varying symptoms and there was an "uncertain prognosis in any individual case." When the wide publicity around the Kenny movement had "run its course," he concluded, the final result "whatever it may be, will depend not upon the statements now made by Miss Kenny and her followers, but upon scientific observation and reasoning."[170] In 1944, not long after his comments were published in the *Journal of Bone and Joint Surgery*, Gill replaced Ober as president of the American Orthopedic Association, a symbol of anti-Kenny orthopedic leadership.

As Gill recognized, Kenny's work had become central in NFIP publicity, featured in the NFIP's 1942 annual report and the NFIP pamphlet *The Kenny Method of Treatment*. The *National Foundation News*, a monthly newsletter sent to all NFIP chapters, began urging local and state officials to send one or more persons to be trained in the Kenny method, explaining that "it is a wise and legitimate expenditure of funds for the Chapter." The *News* carefully listed not only the Institute but 5 other centers that offered "Kenny Method Courses."[171] While pleased with these signs of philanthropic support Kenny remained dissatisfied. She was not convinced that the NFIP had fully revised its support of previous medical practice. It continued, for example, to distribute other pamphlets whose content contradicted her understanding of the disease. *Doctor, What Can I Do?*, she complained to O'Connor, referred to "damaging" treatment and "describes the symptoms of a disease which I have proved does not exist." Both *Splints: Their Distribution and Use* and *The Use of the Respirator in Poliomyelitis* referred to "devices...for a disease that does not exist."[172]

Kenny had come to believe that her methods were being diluted in the various centers outside Minneapolis supported by the NFIP and that even sympathetic physicians were altering elements of her work when they returned to their home institutions. Where she had once bragged that treatment by even partly trained technicians would be an improvement on previous treatment, she now railed against deviation from any aspect of her method. Further, instead of her initial support for nurses and physical therapists who had trained at the Institute to work as teachers after receiving their certificates, by early 1943 she was no longer convinced that most of them were sufficiently trained to work as teachers. Kenny began to denigrate centers outside the Institute, using, as she often did, the words of others. Some of the physicians who had taken her class in early 1943, she reported, had gone to "other centers where the treatment is supposed to be taught" and stated "that the other centers have fallen far short of the standard at Minneapolis."[173] These comments contradicted efforts by the NFIP to integrate her work at diverse well-respected medical centers across the country. It also reflected her growing sense that the Institute must rank as the most important center for teaching her methods.

THE ARGENTINA FIASCO

The argument, made frequently in medical, nursing, and physical therapy journals, that Kenny had merely drawn attention to neglected, mainstream polio therapies, frustrated Kenny. She had identified clinical signs, which she argued were crucial and which had not been previously recognized; otherwise surely a physician would have developed therapies to treat them. The more that the "attention" argument was made, the more vehemently Kenny argued that her new signs could not be added onto the standard view of polio, that the success of her methods proved that she had developed a distinctive understanding of what caused polio's paralysis. Thus, her work must *replace* standard care, not complement it.

She became convinced that only her specially trained technicians could lead the national and international effort to alter polio's clinical care. Eager to provide these technicians with opportunities to showcase their work she was delighted when the NFIP agreed to send Mary Kenny and Ethel Gardner, one of Kenny's inner circle from the Institute, to travel to Argentina during a serious polio epidemic. In early 1943 the head of Argentina's national department of health had asked for help from the NFIP and also contacted the *Reader's Digest*, which had published an article on Kenny in its Spanish edition and set up a scholarship fund for South American nurses and doctors to train at the Kenny Institute.[174] In Buenos Aires an American expert at the Rockefeller Foundation's International Health Division reiterated the request for technical assistance, and, after O'Connor contacted Roosevelt, Gudakunst began working out the details.[175] Sending aid of any kind to Argentina was tricky. Argentina was the only Latin American country that had not severed diplomatic relations with Germany and Italy, and its unstable government was allowing Nazi Germany to establish a spy network there.[176] In a statement that combined U.S. foreign policy with its own philanthropic mission, the NFIP announced proudly that the trip would "not only aid those stricken by infantile paralysis but will, through that manifest assistance, further implement the Good Neighbor policy."[177]

Gudakunst had heard disturbing reports from Miland Knapp about the Little Rock epidemic in which patients had supposedly been discharged too early and the hot packing had been poorly organized, "partly due to lack of help and facilities and partly due to a feud between the nurse in charge of the floor and the nurses who had been sent to Minneapolis for Hot Pack training."[178] So as not to make "the same mistake that we made in Little Rock," Gudakunst made sure that an approved physician accompanied the 2 Kenny technicians.[179] His choice, Philadelphia orthopedist Rutherford John, had contacted Gudakunst in February proposing himself for the Argentina trip, for "the Army won't take me, and my foot itches to do some traveling."[180] John had already declared at a meeting of the state's chapter of the American Physiotherapy Association that he believed Kenny's work was "very rational" and that her ideas "dovetail[ed] wonderfully with our scientific knowledge of the disease."[181] Gudakunst considered John "a top-notch man fairly well acquainted with the Kenny method" who had traveled in South America and therefore "knows something of the customs, and has a fair ability to converse in Spanish."[182] He also asked the opinions of Mayo orthopedist Melvin Henderson and Morris Fishbein, who both gave their approval.[183]

John and the 2 technicians arrived in March 1943 and based themselves in Buenos Aires.[184] Diplomatically, John stayed at a hotel instead of the hospital where the technicians were staying. Debates among Argentinean physicians about the proper way to treat patients with polio were ferocious, so staying at a hotel helped him, he explained to Gudakunst, "not be associated with any one clique."[185] In a letter to the Secretary of State, U.S. Ambassador Norman Armour praised the "tact, patience, and persistence of Dr. John and the nurses," which had overcome obstacles such as "bureaucratic procrastination, professional rivalries, lack of trained personnel, inadequacy of material equipment, and want of a common language." The local press was all "unanimously and enthusiastically favorable," and "only the extreme nationalist and Nazi-Fascist sheets have ignored the visit."[186] John, however, was uncomfortable. He was unable to convince some of the local physicians who disliked both the Kenny method and its "wide publicity by the Argentine press."[187] He also found the federal and city polio commissions at odds and described the strain to "keep in with both." He gave a series of lectures that were well attended and widely reported by local newspapers. But the course he organized on muscle reeducation was overwhelmed by applicants, most bringing letters from physicians. Mary Kenny and Gardner told him they could not handle more than a dozen students. As a result, he told Gudakunst, "I had to be hardboiled and have probably made many enemies [although]...we are still immensely popular with the Press and the people." He recognized that many Argentineans wanted the technicians "to stay on indefinitely and teach but my feeling is that we have done what can be done in a short time and it might be wiser to leave at the height of the enthusiasm."[188] In early May John returned to Philadelphia.

O'Connor began to hear troubling reports that the demands of wealthy families for private care were diverting Mary Kenny and Gardner from their teaching work. He told Gudakunst to explain to Kenny that the technicians must return to the United States. Gudakunst reminded her of "language problems" and "some hospital quarrels" and warned that "the political situation in the Argentine" was unstable.[189] At first Kenny agreed that "with regard to Miss Gardner's and Mary's return from the Argentine, that is a matter for the Foundation to decide. They sent them down, and I think Mr. O'Connor would know more about the inside affairs than I do. If he thinks it wiser for them to return, that is all right."[190]

But she changed her mind a week or so later. "The work they are doing and the friendships they have formed through this work is [sic] doing much for the U.S.A.," she told Gudakunst in what he admitted to O'Connor was "a rather heated conversation."[191] The quarrels, she had learned, "were between the Doctor from the United States and my own technicians," and John had threatened to "have them returned to the United States before their time was up." In any case, neither technician wished "to leave an unfinished job."[192] As Kenny recollected it a few months later, Mary had asked to be allowed to stay, "as the children were so very sick and there was no one to attend to them. She also informed me that the doctors were very interested and that she was giving them lectures three times per week." Mary also described "the tears of gratitude in the eyes of the mothers."[193] Kenny's obstinate stance was fueled by her sense that John had not properly valued her work. To explain how wrong Gudakunst had been to defend John, Kenny sent him a copy of a lecture John had given to local orthopedists that she characterized as "a gross misrepresentation of my work and primarily a lecture on the value of orthopedic surgery."[194] In reassuring Argentine orthopedists about the power relations inherent in adopting the Kenny method, John had said that Kenny technicians were all "trained under orthopedic surgeons and the mechanism of the treatment itself is basically orthopedic," and that Kenny's work was a useful "adjunct to orthopedic surgery."[195] "[He] does not know how terribly sick these patients are and how much general care they need apart from orthopedic attention," Kenny retorted, adding that "my contribution is not a treatment or adjunct to anything but a new concept of the disease and treatment for this concept."[196]

Kenny responded, in effect, as the director of the technicians, ignoring what she saw as misguided advice from the NFIP. Gudakunst warned her that the NFIP would no longer fund the technicians if they remained, but, she assured him, "I shall personally take steps to see they are afforded the financial support and protection they may need."[197] She then organized a series of telegrams to the secretary of Argentina's Infantile Paralysis Commission and to the American Consul in Buenos Aires.[198]

In early June the Argentine army led by General Arturo Rawson and General Pedro Ramirez marched on the federal capital and ousted President Ramon Castillo. Kenny paid little attention to this hazardous political situation. A day after the June coup was reported in American newspapers, she sent a telegram to the technicians formally granting them 2 months extension. Finally, on June 4, Gudakunst sent Mary Kenny an explicit telegram—with a copy to Kenny—warning of the dangers of staying and making it clear that the NFIP was no longer accepting any responsibility for their safety.[199] The 2 technicians stayed in Argentina for an additional 2 months, in part so that Kenny could make the point that providing medical care could and should trump politics. A few weeks after the coup Kenny urged the secretary of Argentina's Infantile Paralysis Commission to send doctors and nurses to be trained at the Institute in order to "make Buenos Aires a center to give assistance to the rest of Spanish-speaking America," for "I presume the change of government shall not interfere with this project."[200] Gardner later recalled that during the revolution she and Mary had gone downtown and saw a mob of people, buses tipped over, and bullets whizzing around, but they had not seen the upheaval as any reason to return home.[201]

Relations between Kenny and the NFIP began to deteriorate after O'Connor withdrew the NFIP's sponsorship of the technicians. In June she met with O'Connor in his office in New York City and was shocked when he defended his actions, saying his desk was full of complaints from American doctors.[202] Kenny was outraged by what she felt was a disrespectful act, and that it was directed at Mary, her beloved ward, made it a personal attack. Mary, she pointed out in long letters to Minnesota's medical dean, "ran the risk of infection in one of the most deadly diseases where death, or worse than death, can be reasonably expected." Kenny had read the telegram as an abandonment of Mary, not an effort to get her to return to safety. "To be cast off in a foreign country that has just experienced a revolutionary change in government and told that no effort would be put forth for her safe return is, to me, an act of barbarism than even Hitler could not exceed," she argued.[203] In Kenny's opinion, the telegram had even insinuated that "the patients suffering from the disease infantile paralysis in the Argentine would be better served if she left them." Yet, she protested, the American Consul, the Argentine Ambassador, the secretary of the Infantile Paralysis Commission, and a representative of the parents were all grateful and had "thanked me most cordially for my splendid cooperation." Thus, this statement was "untruthful and malicious."[204]

The Argentina fiasco was, in her mind, a turning point, separating the NFIP leadership from her American supporters. Kenny told dean Diehl that she was unwilling to accept any further money from the NFIP, and that when Mary returned from Argentina she would not be accepting any more either.[205] In early July Kenny returned a $415 check with a letter to Diehl, noting that "the reason has already been explained to you."[206] Diehl replied quickly that he was "indeed sorry that you feel that your relations with the National Foundation for Infantile Paralysis are such that you are unwilling to accept any further support from funds supplied by them," but he was happy to hear her say that her difficulties with the NFIP would not interfere with her cooperation with the University of Minnesota.[207] That summer Kenny did not publicize her dissatisfaction with O'Connor. As she completed the last pages of her autobiography, she described the Argentina trip in glowing terms and said nothing about the telegram, noting only "how sweet the thought that the plane carrying them to this new and distant county did not bear bombs to spread death and disaster even to innocent childhood, but a message of hope and comfort to all!"[208] And that August in a radio talk she praised the assistance of C. C. Webber, the NFIP, and the *Reader's Digest* in helping "this message of healing... spread throughout the continent of the Americas."[209] Similarly, Gardner expressed no hint of antagonism when she submitted her expenses to O'Connor in August. It had been "a wonderful experience," Gardner said. "We were quite successful in setting up a Kenny unit in Buenos Aires" and "the people of Argentina will be ever grateful to the National Foundation and Sister Kenny for what was done for them."[210]

By the fall, however, local newspapers were announcing "U.S. Polio Foundation, Kenny Split." She could no longer accept support from an organization, Kenny told reporters, that "can administer or withdraw funds at the will of a few people."[211] The Argentina story became a powerful weapon in her growing arsenal. Hoping this would soon blow over, NFIP officials responded by quoting the $230,000 the NFIP had spent "evaluating and teaching" the Kenny method, pointing out that the organization was the "sole financial supporter of Sister Kenny's work" and (unwisely) terming the Argentina dispute "a local controversy over the establishment of a local clinic."[212] Later, and in vain, O'Connor's staff showed reporters copies of the letter from Kenny telling Gudakunst "that if Mr. O'Connor thought it wiser for them to return, that is all right."[213]

In Minneapolis Kenny's sense of community support was deepened when, in August 1943, the city council announced that it was buying her a house. "'I think it is about time we did something for Sister Kenny so she will have a direct connection with the city,'" explained an alderman.[214] Marvin Kline, the new mayor of Minneapolis, arranged for the city council to thank Kenny formally for having "graciously chosen Minneapolis as the place to carry on her work and the City's reputation as a center of healing has been increased thereby not only in this country but throughout the world."[215] Kenny was delighted with the "beautiful home" whose "spacious, well-furnished rooms,...green lawns and flowering lilacs and window boxes" allowed her to feel "as if I had reached a secure haven at last."[216] Her friend businessman James Henry turned to one of his civic clubs to help her financially, and in August 1943 the Exchange Club began to pay an allowance to Mary and Kenny; the club's monthly checks were, she noted, "issued promptly."[217]

IMPATIENT INNOVATOR

Kenny was beginning to see herself not as an NFIP-sponsored clinician and teacher but as a scientific innovator with a national reputation whose patience with narrow-minded critics was coming to an end. In a long letter that she sent to Gill, the Orthopaedic Correspondence Club, and the NFIP, she denied that the value of her work had been established by newspaper publicity rather than by serious professionals. Indeed, she claimed, the press had made "poor presentations" of her work compared to "the signed statements of medical men of unquestionable ability and many of international repute." Most of her letter was filled with short testimonials from a mixture of pediatricians, health officials, physical medicine experts, and orthopedists, all of whose ability to change their mind took "courage" and showed "the mind and heart of the true physician."[218]

Kenny did not try to address the physiological debates, other than remarking that "paralysis occurs from causes other than destruction of parts of the central nervous system" and that the significance of spasm was "one of the things I came to the United States to find out." Gill's references to Lovett were easy to combat. Many doctors in Minneapolis "had been Lovett trained and were just as strong disciples as yourself prior to being presented with the true symptoms." Mental alienation and incoordination were "damaging symptoms over which Lovett or anyone else could not have any control." Defending the attack on her character, she explained she did not seek fame or fortune. Indeed her national reputation had provided her increasing opportunities for both, which made her restraint even more honorable. "I have patiently, intelligently, humanely, and voluntarily presented this evidence to the medical world whom I consider are the keepers of the nation's health and well-being, denying myself the opportunity to capitalize the results of my own research, steadfastly refusing to associate myself with any of the minor branches of medicine—such as, osteopathy, neuropathy, etc.—although repeatedly invited to do so." She urged Gill and other skeptics to come to Minneapolis where "you will see and agree with all other medical men that the concept is the opposite and the treatment is the opposite."[219]

THE RED BOOK

Kenny's most powerful weapon was her new textbook, whose advertising had so incensed Gill. Boldly defending her techniques and her theories it was co-written with her ally John Pohl and framed by 2 forewords—one by Harvard orthopedist Frank Ober and the other by Basil O'Connor—and ended with a commentary by Miland Knapp, representing physical medicine. Wallace Cole, the senior orthopedist at the University of Minnesota, had no part in this effort but the text was dedicated, rather pointedly, to him "in recognition of his efforts to investigate, test and finally approve of the Kenny concept and treatment of the disease anterior poliomyelitis."[220] With its striking crimson cover and gold lettering, *The Kenny Concept of Infantile Paralysis and Its Treatment* became known as the Red Book.

Both forewords were cautiously positive. Ober, as president of the American Orthopedic Association, praised this "well-received plan" for the relief of pain and muscle spasm and "for the re-education of the neuromuscular system." He said nothing about any possible physiological explanation for spasm, remarking instead on the method's continuous superb nursing that helped patients "gain the maximum amount of recovery more quickly and much more satisfactorily than by the techniques previously employed." Moist heat, he noted, had been used by Lovett, but not in the acute stage and not for the relief of spasm. Spasm was not mentioned in textbooks yet there was "no doubt that it is present and is a great factor in the production of early deformities unless relieved."[221]

O'Connor tried to promote Kenny's work without further antagonizing orthopedists or other professionals. With the support of America's "progressive and sympathetic medical profession" and the NFIP to lead the fight against polio, Kenny was working "side by side with clinicians, scientists, [and] research workers, preparing a complete and connected picture of her ideas and methods" in order to develop a technique that could be taught to others. With an implicit critique of the dramatic demonstrations the press and Kenny loved, he noted that "in medicine it is not well to believe the eye alone." Both American physicians and the American public needed to have many questions answered before they could "be certain this was not legerdemain or mere chance." Fortunately, "those who work in the laboratories with problems on histopathology, anatomy, and physiology claim that the major concept is reasonable and rational." These researchers, he declared in a statement that awkwardly separated her techniques from her ideas, were convinced that Kenny "presents an entirely new concept and a satisfactory treatment for this concept."[222] But O'Connor's effort to dampen debate around Kenny's work and to present the controversial issues as resolved fooled no one. O'Connor's statement, especially his "reference to the sympathetic and progressive medical profession," Chuter joked to Kenny after reading the foreword, "is a corker."[223]

In her preface, Kenny told the now familiar story of the lone worker in the bush of Australia who saw painful muscles "being subjected to contraction in some way affected by the disease" and realized that "the muscle was sick and needed nursing." After her methods had relaxed the muscles she saw "the muscle which had been pulled from its normal resting length had forgotten how to contract and must be taught over again." In telling the story of her discovery of alienation Kenny dived into the murky depths of mind and memory. "Remembering that consciousness is born from the subconscious,

I endeavored to bring consciousness about by attempting to bombard this area with impulses from the surrounding muscles." But as "the normal flow of impulses" had been interrupted "the patient could not visualize in space the exact area from which an attempt to contract should [be] materialized, and the impulses ran riot as it were." The social organization of the body's neuroelectrical functioning was out of harmony, and awareness and regularity of muscle movement had to be reestablished. After she described these new symptoms she reiterated that "the treatment evolved by me is not for symptoms previously recognized, but for a different concept altogether." Despite ridicule from Australian physicians, studies by American physiologists like Schwartz had upheld her work and "proved my concept correct." Reflecting her growing uneasiness that the teaching of her work outside the Institute was being diluted, she reminded her readers of the Institute featured as the book's frontispiece. This "noble building" had been established by Minneapolis's Board of Public Welfare and "will, I hope, provide a further means of distributing this work throughout the world."[224]

In his introduction Pohl had the difficult task of both confronting and convincing his wary peers. He began with an attack on orthodox polio therapy pointing out that immobilizing techniques that allowed weakened muscles to rest had made sense, based on the orthodox concept of polio, and yet, as he and other orthopedists knew well, "deformities too frequently occurred." The Kenny concept explained why immobilization was so often unsuccessful. Orthodox therapy had ignored the possibility that "loss of control of muscle could be due to disorganization and disruption of the nerve cell connections." As a result, Pohl declared, "orthodoxy has erred both in the recognition as well as in the interpretation of the physical findings in the disease." Indeed the new concept introduced by Kenny was "so radically opposed to the old as to almost warrant considering the entity as a new disease." He speculated briefly on the physiological and pathological etiology of these new symptoms, concluding that the polio virus probably "affects muscle as well as nerve tissue."[225]

In frustratingly repetitive prose Kenny and Pohl's main text explained how to identify and treat spasm, alienation, and incoordination. Unlike the kinds of spasm seen in "other disorders of the neuromuscular or skeletal system of the body," polio spasm did not completely relax under general anesthesia and could be relieved by moist heat "treating the specific area of involvement," suggesting that a "local process is taking place in the muscle." The exact mechanism of the process of alienation was not clear, but it was possibly the result of "disturbance of the physiological continuity of the motor tracts between the conscious voluntary brain and the muscle." Incoordination was the result of "a disorganization of the regulating motor centers of the nervous system" that disrupted the "natural rhythmic and cooperative action of associated muscles."[226] Here, the body's neurological functioning had become disordered like the middle of a war or a badly organized hospital. Kenny's method could restore physiological order by bringing body memory to the conscious mind.

Crucial to the healing process was the Kenny technician, skilled in reading the body and in special techniques to help patients regain proper body awareness. So insightful were these techniques that the "contractile function [that]... occurs first in the subconscious level of the mind" could be observed by a technician "long before the patient's mind is conscious of the returning ability to perform voluntary action."[227] The text provided contradictory comments about who should care for patients. Because polio care required "extraordinary attention to detail, alertness for the interpretation of unfavorable conditions, and ingenuity in the application of methods to relieve distress" it demanded a higher degree of nursing skill, and therefore patients should be sent to a properly equipped hospital or clinic so that therapy could begin at the earlier possible moment. But because early treatment consisted not of highly technical procedures but simple nursing and the "solicitous care of sick muscles," any person could tell "by visual examination the part of the body where muscle spasm is present" and could use domestic equipment such as a common laundry wringer, woolen blankets, and hot water.[228] Thus Kenny technicians were crucial for effective muscle alignment and regaining muscle awareness but sympathetic parents could make their own hot packs and deal with the initial pain and sensitivity.

Pohl's bold claim that "deformities do not occur" made sense only if readers accepted Kenny's new definition of "deformity" as a patient without muscle strength or supple movement.[229] This definition was reinforced by 100 illustrations, including a series of 15 photographs showing Kenny overseeing a boy's exercises that demonstrated the "complete restoration of normal function to the neuromuscular system of the body." More explicitly, the caption below one photograph of a young woman using a Kenny (short) crutch noted that she "has complete paralysis of left lower extremity, and partial of right lower extremity...yet she walks well without braces. Note the absence of deformities." Surgery was mentioned briefly but as a therapy of last resort that would "aid in the rehabilitation of selected cases."[230] Fully functioning bodies were the ideal; assistive devices were signs of therapeutic failure.

A year before this text was published Knapp had protested to other polio specialists that he wanted to get rid of the idea that Kenny's methods consisted solely "of hot packs and passive motion" instead of "an attempt to treat the disease systemically."[231] Now in his concluding commentary Knapp argued that he and other Minneapolis physicians were convinced that Kenny had introduced a "new concept" that was "correct." He retreated slightly to argue that new therapies did not need to have a scientific rationale from the outset, for "clinical results are, after all, the final proof of the value of any treatment method." Still as "the medical mind requires explanations and theories" and sought to interpret results in terms of pathology and physiology, researchers should now investigate "the scientific basis for the Kenny concept" in order to improve this treatment "to its highest possible level." Some of her ideas might initially look "unphysiological" but "deeper and more detailed thought shows them to be consistent with the best of muscle physiology." In any case few studies had correlated the relationship between damaged anterior horn cells and affected muscles; in fact, he knew of "no extensive studies of pathologic changes within the muscle itself during the acute stage of the disease." Kenny's methods were based on a "radical" interpretation of polio's symptoms, which he believed was her "greatest contribution." As for her new interpretation of polio it was possible, Knapp admitted, that "inflammatory or toxic changes might be present in the muscle itself." In any case, Kenny had jolted physicians "out of our complacent groove of thought [and]...some worthwhile advance is bound to result from both her revolutionary ideas and the frantic efforts of her opponents to refute them."[232]

O'Connor sent copies of the new textbook to 2 leading scientists: neuroanatomist Howard Howe at Johns Hopkins and physiologist Walter Bradford Cannon at Harvard. Both men, neither of them clinicians, found Kenny's methods "well worked out, effective, and in many instances very ingenious," and they assured O'Connor that they were "well disposed toward the Kenny method."[233] But their assessments of the textbook differed. Howe disliked the book's "authoritarian style" and its mixing of facts "with contradictions and undocumented theorizing." He felt it showed "a very superficial knowledge of neuroanatomy and physiology." Pohl (whom Howe regarded as the senior author) regarded alienation and incoordination "as proved because he merely states them as truth," yet in reality these symptoms were "so contrary to well substantiated observations that considerable objective evidence is required." Howe drew a stark difference between pathological evidence and clinical evidence. He did not believe there was direct action of the virus on the muscle, which he called "a concept for which at the moment there is not the slightest evidence." Recent NFIP grants, he noted, were awarded to a number of projects dealing with the problems of nerve and muscle and he regretted that "that the interpretation of Miss Kenny's results" was not left to those who were "well qualified to do it." Still, he doubted that his opinion would convince "the prejudiced and uninformed," for making such scientific distinctions was "like trying to explain the difference between a steam engine and a gasoline motor to a Hottentot."[234]

Cannon, who had just retired from his position as the chair of Harvard's physiology department and was battling Bell's palsy and other ailments, was more open to the physiological challenges Kenny's concept posed.[235] He could see why it was difficult for Kenny to have the medical world understand her ideas for, in his view, her terms were poorly chosen. Alienation reminded him of "specialists in mental disease [who] are known as alienists!" As for "mental awareness" that was "the only kind there is" and a better term would be "*directed* awareness." Her use of "the subconscious mind" was "reprehensible, despite fairly common usage," and a term like "subconscious centers" would be better. From a physiological point of view Cannon was willing to consider that the polio virus might directly affect the muscle and that "testing affected muscles for the virus would be worthwhile." Spasm, he felt, "in all probability results from irritation of motor cells in the spinal cord." The phenomenon of alienation of a normal muscle "is, so far as I am aware, quite novel [and]...deserves careful investigation." In taking seriously both Kenny's concept and the evidence she used, Cannon was horrified by what it implied about past polio therapy, which he felt was one of "the grimmest mistakes in all medical history."[236]

Howe's and Cannon's comments did not provide NFIP officials with the clarity to weigh in on either side of the controversy. But the silence was filled by other voices. Illustrated by electromyographic images, studies by physiology researchers provided hints of a complicated picture of nerves and muscles that invigorated nurses and physical therapists already imbued with "Kenny enthusiasm." Although orthopedists continued to argue that patients' clinical improvements were the result of better nursing or some poorly understood pathological process, the evidence of recovered patients suggested that, whether Kenny was able to explain it or not, there was some connection with the virus and the paralyzed muscles. The press called her successes "Kenny miracles." Although she argued that any of her technicians could achieve the same results, she nonetheless enjoyed occasions when surrounded by doctors, nurses, parents, hospital trustees, and reporters she could demonstrate the efficacy of her work. In New York City, for example, as 50 other patients waited to be examined, she told one boy to "put your brain in your foot. Think of nothing except your foot and how it works." When the muscle jumped there was "an audible gasp from the circle of spectators." "I have given that muscle its sense," Kenny told her audience. "If it had been actually paralyzed, of course I could not have done what I did."[237]

We have but one weapon against the ravages of polio, *Colliers* declared: "the method of treatment devised by Sister Elizabeth Kenny, the Australian nurse." The magazine briefly mentioned orthopedic surgeons who could transplant muscle and tendon sections "from good muscles to bad ones." But more powerful was the description of a warehouse owned by the NFIP that was full of splints, for during the previous year only one physician had requested "this cruel apparatus." "If the disease does strike," the article concluded ominously, "pray that someone in your town has had the foresight to have a local physiotherapist trained in Kenny methods."[238] More cautious was the War Department whose 1943 Circular Letter No. 175 on the management of polio recommended the use of hot packs, passive movements, and other "conventional methods which have received general acceptance and are in general use" applied by physical therapists under the "careful direction of medical officers."[239]

In a fiery editorial titled "Fact and Fancy in Poliomyelitis" the *British Medical Journal* surveyed the current debate on polio therapy inspired by Kenny and Pohl's textbook. Protesting that those interested in the many problems around polio have not been unreceptive to fresh ideas, the editor pointed out that "in the realm of treatment . . . it is always most difficult to secure the dispassionate assessment of results that is so essential to rational therapy." Kenny's methods might be useful but the assessment of their value had been "adversely complicated by the intrusion of theoretical fantasies that can only prejudice the issue." In an effort to dampen down popular enthusiasm the editor argued that "it would have been better had Sister Kenny and her supporters been content to subject her methods to adequate and prolonged trial, and to have let them stand or fall by their merits." Still, physicians must scrutinize the textbook's ideas "by the proper standard applicable to all medical theories" for Pohl, an experienced orthopedist, "sponsors the concept." Without commenting further on the book's physiological and pathological speculations the editor did agree that the "problem of pain and tenderness in the affected muscles . . . calls for some explanation."[240]

When physical medicine specialists reviewed the 1943 textbook they tried to demonstrate both skepticism and authority. Richard Kovacs wrote a vaguely laudatory review, arguing that "everyone agrees that Miss Kenny deserves great credit for her original ideas." He pointed out that her ideas had "only evolved gradually" for her 1937 text had said nothing about muscle spasm or hot packs, and he praised the new textbook for its omission of "the large amount of controversy and argumentation which marred Miss Kenny's earlier writings."[241] Moist heat was not new but had been advocated by Lovett, according to an unsigned review in the *New England Journal of Medicine*, but nonetheless the book was fundamental for an understanding of Kenny's polio treatment "and should be in the hands of everyone concerned with the care of patients with this disease."[242]

In the *Physiotherapy Review* orthopedist John Coulter called the book an "up-to-date discussion of the technics now being advocated by Sister Elizabeth Kenny," quoted Ober's praise of the method's superb nursing, and declared that "this book should be read and studied by every physical therapist treating infantile paralysis."[243] Mary MacDonald, the book's reviewer in the *American Journal of Nursing*, agreed with Coulter, adding that many nurses had hoped that the book would "settle all argumentative discussions regarding the Kenny concept and the Kenny method of treatment" and the book "has fulfilled all expectations."

MacDonald was pleased to see Kenny and Pohl state that "no disease demands a higher degree of nursing skill." Overall it provided "a definite, well-organized and authentic description" of Kenny's work and should be in the library of every nursing school.[244]

The 1943 textbook did not function as Kenny and Pohl had hoped. Kenny technicians and other therapists and nurses used the red book more as a technical manual than as a scientific work. For many physicians it confused rather than clarified. "I find the book on the 'Concept' and the other literature very easily understandable," a sympathetic surgeon told Pohl, "but am sorry to say & see too many doctors of better training than I have had who still seem completely befuddled. They should come and see the work or it should be taken to them, one or the other."[245] Clinical results still remained the most impressive evidence Kenny and her technicians could provide. Nor had the textbook resolved divisions among physicians as Stimson discovered when he gave a talk on Kenny at the New York Post-Graduate Medical School and Hospital in early 1944. His host later apologized for the criticisms of one physician who "got a little out of hand and was so very emphatic."[246]

WHOSE PATIENT?

When physical medicine specialists and orthopedists debated the value of Kenny's work it was part of a broader struggle over not only the supervision of polio care but the field of rehabilitation. Orthopedic surgeons were usually the senior and wealthier colleagues, but both groups considered themselves experts in the treatment of disabling conditions.

With the growing public interest in paralyzed children, polio had come to play a major role in defining the practice of physical medicine.[247] Capitalizing on the newsworthy nature of Kenny's work the American Congress of Physical Therapy had awarded Kenny their annual Gold Key award in 1942 to honor the person who has made the greatest contribution to the field of physical therapy during the past year. The previous recipient had been Franklin Roosevelt for "his unremitting labors for the prevention and cure of poliomyelitis."[248] Kenny's award, her supporters pointed out, was "the first time in the history of the organization that a woman had been the recipient of the honor."[249] While it was difficult to assess a recent therapeutic contribution "on account of lack of perspective and the influence of personality that colors their contributions," the president of the Congress told Kenny, the group had nonetheless recognized "your devoted labors [which] have been outstanding in nature and have resulted in raising the discipline of physical therapy to a higher standard."[250]

As doctors specializing in physical medicine struggled to improve their profession's status Kenny's work was both frustrating and exhilarating. They were the first physicians to come to Minneapolis to take Kenny's courses, and most of them were directors of physical therapy programs at their home institutions.[251] In November 1942 an entire issue of their specialty journal the *Archives of Physical Therapy* was devoted to the Kenny method, and comments on the topic appeared in almost every issue during the 1940s.[252]

Robert Bennett's acceptance of Kenny's work especially impressed his peers. Although his Warm Springs staff dealt mainly with chronic patients, he had adopted Kenny's methods and integrated them in his new school of physical therapy. When Kenny complained about a placard at the 1942 AMA exhibit announcing the Kenny method was being taught at Warm Springs, Bennett supposedly retorted that as it was "the method of choice" he

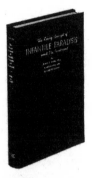
FIGURE 3.3 An advertisement for Pohl and Kenny's 1943 textbook promoting a "completely new theory" of polio. [Advertisement] *Archives of Physical Therapy* (April 1943) 24: back page.

intended to teach it whether she liked it or not.[253] In various journal articles he argued that her work did not contradict proven pathology, for her theory of a "physiologic blockage" might be part of "the central nervous system's reaction to virus invasion." In any case, the work was proving itself clinically sound and "our research men, our physiologists and pathologists must, and eventually will, give us the basis for these newer clinical manifestations."[254] He pointed to a distinct change in her ideas and practices now that she was working at the University of Minnesota. The fact that her work was "much more logical and scientific" than "just five years ago as evidenced by her book published in 1937" was, he felt, the result of the able support of the faculty of the University of Minnesota, especially the guidance of Miland Knapp.[255]

Kenny's work remained a source of tension between physical medicine specialists and orthopedists. William Stratton Clark, who directed the physical medicine department of a hospital in Dayton, Ohio, came to Minneapolis and was impressed by lectures from Pohl and Knapp, which combined "the coordination of the Kenny concept with known physiological and pathological principles and hypotheses." But back in Ohio he encountered resistance from his peers, finding it "difficult for a man in my specialty to convince our local orthopedic surgeons." Clark began to try to arrange for these surgeons to go to Minneapolis, for he felt that second- or third-hand knowledge would not convince them. "There is no doubt," he told Pohl, that "the Kenny concept, when passed through human minds, becomes opinionated and distorted, much as do certain bacteria in being passed through a series of laboratory animals."[256] Paul Carson, the director of the Wichita Children's Clinic, found that his own enthusiasm alienated rather than convinced other physicians. Even after he and his Kenny-trained physical therapist "had some very thrilling results," many of his colleagues continued to express considerable opposition and "I heard the other day that one Doctor said my middle name was 'Kenney [sic].' "[257]

Part of the problem was the issue of respect. The term *physical therapy* was generally used to refer to the work of both technicians and doctors, and orthopedists tended to consider themselves more medically qualified than physical medicine specialists. At the end of 1943 the AMA's Council on Physical Therapy renamed itself the Council on Physical Medicine. Likewise, the American Congress of Physical Therapy became the American Congress of Physical Medicine. These changes, reformers hoped, would place the specialty of physical medicine on a par with other established specialties.[258] More important than name changes were 2 major philanthropic sources of support: the NFIP, which funded physical medicine specialty training, and Bernard Baruch, the millionaire-industrialist who gave over a million dollars to establish specialized research and training centers in physical medicine.[259] The power of money was clear to some Kenny opponents. One Harvard physician suggested that many orthopedic surgeons were "falling in with the popularity of the [Kenny] method, not so much because of the genuine belief in it, but because of the possibility of getting grants."[260]

DRUGS TO TREAT SPASM

Whatever the physiological explanation for spasm, it was generally accepted as a clinical sign that required attention. Physicians began to look for ameliorative techniques less complicated and labor intensive than Kenny's methods. The drug Prostigmine (or neostigmine), first synthesized in 1931 and used to treat neuromuscular disorders like myasthenia gravis, seemed promising.[261] Prostigmine was first tested on patients with polio in Kenny's new hometown. Knapp began testing the drug with the help of Herman Kabat, a young neurophysiologist, in early 1942. Knapp and Kabat found that Prostigmine was a distinct help in decreasing spasm and pain and restoring "muscle coordination." According to science writer Paul de Kruif who had stayed away from the Kenny story but wrote about Kabat, Kabat gave his first injection of Prostigmine to a "badly spasmed woman" who, even after intensive Kenny treatment, was still unable to sit as "her back was stiffened and knifed through with pain." This patient improved as did a boy whose case of boils had meant he was not able to have hot packs; soon after the injection, he could turn over easily in bed and then do push-ups.[262] Kabat published his work in *Science* and the *Journal of Experimental Medicine* and with Knapp in *JAMA* and in the *Journal of Pediatrics*.[263] In October 1943 the NFIP gave the University of Minnesota a large grant that included this research, but after problems working with Maurice Visscher, the head of the physiology department, Kabat left Minnesota and took a poorly paid position in the U.S. Public Health Service in Washington, D.C.[264] Kabat then began to treat a variety of disabled patients with "spastic" muscles, and found that Prostigmine was astonishingly successful. One stroke victim "within 24 hours after the first injection" was able to "put a cigarette in his mouth with his right hand." His work with multiple sclerosis patients, publicized by de Kruif in the *Reader's Digest*, caught the attention of California industrialist Henry Kaiser who asked him to treat his son and later founded the Kabat-Kaiser Institute (later part of Kaiser-Permanente).[265] Even though de Kruif presented Kabat as dismissive of many of Kenny's ideas, Kabat himself promoted his "neuromuscular reeducation" techniques for multiple sclerosis, polio, and cerebral palsy that "like the Kenny treatment... [help] patients recover nerve-muscle control."[266]

Another drug was even more intriguing: curare, a muscle relaxant used as an anesthetic and to treat spastic muscles in tetanus convulsions and cerebral palsy.[267] In 1945 New Jersey orthopedist Nicholas Ransohoff added curare injections to his clinical treatment of polio to ease spasm. After a brief note in *JAMA* he offered a long paper on curare at the AMA's 1946 annual meeting, which, according to *Colliers*, "convinced some doctors it may be as important, or more important, than the famous Sister Kenny technique."[268] Despite warnings by anesthesiologists that curare could cause respiratory paralysis and death and that it was "a dangerous weapon in the hands of the inexperienced and untrained," physicians were eager to try it.[269] Ransohoff's technique promised to alter the routine of hot pack care, enabling patients to leave bed more quickly and thus, he claimed, taking a heavy burden off the nursing staff of a hospital.[270] In Pittsburgh Jessie Wright tried curare on her patients at the D. T. Watson Home and agreed that "we need to get away from packs. I think they have been very much overdone."[271]

Kenny was not convinced that any drug could work as well as her system of hot packs and muscle exercises. When she examined one of Knapp's patients whose spasm was supposed to have been corrected by Prostigmine, she found "spasm very evident." "I would not consider Prostigmine a reliable drug," she began telling medical audiences. "It may be a suitable adjunct but of itself it has not proved satisfactory."[272]

NEW CRITICAL SCIENCE

Fishbein's growing hostility to Kenny and her claims was reflected in a series of studies published in *JAMA* during 1943 on polio's physiology. The critics Fishbein published replayed the old story that much of Kenny's method was not good, and what was good was not new. The Kenny concept was inadequate as a physiological explanation, Harvard physical medicine specialist Arthur Watkins and Mary Brazier, a neurophysiologist at the Massachusetts General Hospital, argued, and in any case "muscle shortening" through spasm had been recognized for many years.[273] In "The Significance of Muscle Spasm" Plato Schwartz and Harry Bouman agreed, adding that her theory of the disease, based "solely on clinical observation," could hardly be as reliable as a "logical premise" that had been "slowly developed from the work of many men in various countries."[274]

Even more definitive was a study by Columbia neurologist Joseph Moldaver whose testing of muscles suggested that spasm did not exist, and that paralysis was the result of nerve destruction. Moldaver had attended one of Kenny's courses in Minneapolis in 1943 and, while she was away, had tested her patients, finding that a number of their muscles scored zero. Extremely annoyed to find out a visiting researcher had overridden her strict rules against muscle testing, Kenny had reminded her staff about the worthlessness of such tests before spasm had been relieved.[275] But Moldaver presented his work to the New York Academy of Medicine in May 1943, and it was reported in the *New York Times* and *Time* and published in *JAMA*. His analysis of electrodiagnostic tests of 49 patients was widely interpreted as contradicting Kenny's theory that untreated muscle spasm could lead to neuromuscular degeneration. Moldaver did not believe that spasm explained polio paralysis at all. Spasm, he argued, was a complex phenomenon involving the meninges covering the nerve roots of the spinal cord, and incoordination was the result not of the diminution of nerve impulses but "the inability of partially or totally degenerated muscles to respond to otherwise normal nerve impulses." This study, according to *Science News Letter*, reaffirmed "the century-old view of infantile paralysis as a disease of nerve destruction or damage." Thus, as orthopedists had long argued, polio had to be treated not by active exercises but with rest to avoid further nerve damage.[276] So potent were Moldaver's conclusions that even researchers who found some evidence of muscle changes resisted Kenny's explanations. In the *American Journal of Clinical Pathology*, for example, when researchers discovered "degeneration of nerve and muscle," which, they acknowledged, could be "considered to show 'spasm,'" they instead described these changes as secondary to injured nerve cells of the spinal cord.[277]

Kenny recognized that Moldaver had tried to use physiological techniques to undermine her theory while leaving the evidence of her clinical results untouched. Indeed he had told reporters that "his criticisms were in no way concerned with the Kenny treatment methods."[278] "According to Dr. Moldaver, my concept is wrong, but my treatment, which is based on that concept, works," she commented to a friend. "Are we to infer that medicine must reject good treatments because doctors disagree with the theory? If so, the practice of medicine is a farce."[279] Moldaver, Kenny assured reporters, "didn't know what he was talking about" and was "clinging to old, obsolete theories despite the fact [that] clever neurologists have proved the new theory correct."[280]

Moldaver's attack made it easier for other antagonists to dismiss Kenny as a theorist. "No one now denies that Sister Kenny is good with her hands," remarked *Time*, "but her critics insist that she does not really know how she does it."[281] Her allies saw such criticisms as additional evidence that physicians and scientists were jealous of her impressive clinical results. In his popular weekly radio program "Confidentially Yours," Arthur Hale announced that Moldaver's study demonstrated the "undercover opposition to Nurse Kenny." Moldaver had not questioned "the nature of Nurse Kenny's treatment, nor their [her] results" but had claimed that because Kenny was not a doctor she did not understand polio from a medical standpoint and therefore "her concepts of the disease are unsound."[282] The issue of whether clinical results could be judged irrespective of pathological theory continued to be raised by physicians with much heat but no resolution. One orthopedist, who praised her "excellent method of muscle re-education" and "great gift in the healing art" in the *Journal of Bone and Joint Surgery*, noted that she had reported results "which we have not yet been able to duplicate." Like Gill, he wondered how much of the Kenny concept would remain intact in the future, adding that "many of her ideas of kinesiology are still difficult to accept. Others are so simple and apparent that it seems incomprehensible that they were not recognized long ago."[283]

Clinical and laboratory investigations had shown that the principal tenets of Kenny's concepts "were found wanting," Richard Kovacs noted as he summed up advances in physical medicine at the end of 1943; thus physicians' "reluctance to accept Miss Kenny's explanation for the success of her method appears to be justified." Still "her path-finding and enthusiastic work" had led to a more effective use of physical treatment in polio's early stage.[284] Here was a narrowed sense of Kenny's contribution: her enthusiastic work had inspired research and led other professionals to reassess polio therapy and to engage in measured research.

These kinds of reports left the NFIP in a difficult position. Critics were complaining about inappropriate propaganda while supporters said that her method was not being expanded quickly enough. Although NFIP officials had effectively sidestepped many disputes within the American medical profession, the Kenny controversy was one they could not avoid. Relations between the NFIP and orthopedists began to deteriorate as reports surfaced that "physicians are being pushed into the position of having to accept the skills of nurses in this field about which they know nothing" and that the NFIP had encouraged "the use of the Kenny method by nurses without appropriate supervision by doctors."[285]

To be seen as both responsive and balanced, NFIP officials decided to tighten the standards and content of the Kenny courses offered in Minneapolis. Although physicians who came usually for only a week had praised the institutional setting whether at the university's hospital, the city hospital, or the Institute, many of the nursing and physical therapy students who stayed for 3 weeks or longer were less enthusiastic, complaining that they felt "disappointed, confused, and dissatisfied" in a poorly organized program with "inadequate supervision of experience with patients."[286] At the end of 1943, pressured by the NFIP, the University of Minnesota's medical school reorganized the Kenny courses it continued to direct. Therapists and nurses now took separate courses that included lectures on the basic nature of polio followed by clinical instruction and supervised experience in the application of Kenny's methods. To be sure that graduate technicians had the character as well as professional background to become "qualified teachers," the university introduced new entrance requirements, including a physical examination and a series of tests "concerned primarily with intelligence, manual dexterity and personal adjustments" conducted by the university's testing bureau.[287]

Although physicians had not formally complained about their course, the dean reorganized it as well, renaming it "The Management of Infantile Paralysis." The course now covered the etiology, epidemiology, pathology, and physiology of polio, followed by a presentation of the Kenny technique along with a report of investigations on its value, and finally a broader discussion of the treatment of the disease.[288] Demonstrating its approval of these changes, the NFIP's national office agreed to continue its teaching grant to the university's medical school and to keep paying the living and travel expenses of Kenny and her associates.[289]

These curricula changes reflected a shift in professional thinking whereby Kenny's work was categorized as a technological innovation rather than as a contribution to medical science. Kenny, however, had a different vision of her work. She continued to demand recognition for her concept of polio and envisioned a far more thorough training for the nurses and physical therapists who would then call themselves Kenny-trained.

She reminded Diehl that she had consistently asked for the teaching courses to be longer and that her medical supporters had said that "the details of this method of treatment cannot be learned quickly."[290] Gradually Kenny began to envision Kenny technicians as graduates of a 2-year course who would be qualified both to teach her work and to train others to become technicians. Such a course would be directed not by a physician from the university's medical school but by one of her medical allies at the Institute.

CELEBRITY

Even as medical journals were beginning to attack her concepts a few universities began to recognize Kenny as an appropriate subject for an honorary degree. In 1943 she received 2: a doctorate of humane letters from New York University and a doctorate of science from the University of Rochester.[291] New York University's vice president praised her as a "heroic daughter of the Australia bush" whose "revolutionary treatment" had "proved amazingly successful." After she had "patiently, persistently and triumphantly labored against untold opposition...today the foremost medical scientists of many lands acclaim it incomparably effective."[292] In Rochester the nursing school dean lauded Kenny as an altruistic humanitarian who had accepted no money for her work and "looked for no reward" other than as a nurse. Now, though, "leading scientists in the United States and Canada...endorse her theory" and "hundreds of nurses and physiotherapists multiply the benefits of her teachings."[293] More dramatically, Rochester president Alan Valentine declared "in the dark world of suffering you have lit a candle that will never be put out."[294]

Kenny tried to balance triple roles as clinician, teacher, and celebrity. She became more self-conscious about her appearance and began to dress like a wealthy woman, using lipstick which she once had scorned.[295] She traveled more frequently by plane, wearing jeweled pins, fancy corsages, and even larger hats. "You certainly seem to be affluent," a Brisbane friend teased her, "as it has been remarked that you have a different bonnet for every picture."[296] She also began to wear as her trademark a distinctive kind of hat with an overly wide brim she called a "digger" hat, modeled, she claimed, on the Australian Light Horse hat of the Great War.[297] She never learned to drive, but the NFIP bought her a 4-door Buick sedan and paid for a driver.[298] Her Minnesota base began to attract more celebrity patients such as Metropolitan Opera baritone Lawrence Tibbett's son Michael who had previously received "the very best treatment" at Warm Springs.[299]

In 1943 photographer Jack Delano, representing the Division of Photography of the Office of War Information, included Kenny in his travels around Minnesota. He took a series of photographs of Kenny in Minneapolis: in her apartment correcting a paper to be read at a medical meeting; relaxing while playing her favorite gramophone record; presenting 3 patients to a class of physicians and technicians; and being asked for her autograph by 2 visiting Australian soldiers.[300] In each image she looms large, a woman participating in the professional world, in many ways more than a nurse.

Journalists sometimes explained away Kenny's belligerence by citing her ethnic background and her birth in the wilds of rural Australia. "A pliant and diplomatic person might perhaps have softened some of the criticism," the *Saturday Evening Post* suggested, "but Miss Elizabeth Kenny, born on a frontier, half Irish and half Scotch, convinced she is right, is no diplomat."[301] Some used her age to justify her impatience. Perhaps she should use more tact with her opponents, but, another reporter concluded, "she hasn't time for tact."[302] Reporters liked her direct manner and made her lack of artifice a sign of sincerity. "From the quietness of her low voice to the direct gaze which looks deep into you, she is as compelling as she is unaffected," argued a *Los Angeles Times* reporter.[303] Although reporters rarely saw a relaxed Kenny telling jokes and war stories, they did see evidence of her sharp tongue. When Gudakunst introduced her at an NFIP lunch held in Philadelphia at the Ritz Carlton hotel and praised her "new treatment" Kenny corrected him, delighting reporters with her retort: "'I have not presented a new treatment...I have presented a new concept of poliomyelitis. And you should know that, Dr. Gudakunst. It would not need a medical man to see what I've been showing you. A blacksmith could see it." Her nondeferential attitude to doctors was a provocative antidote to the familiar doctor–nurse relationship. When a photographer pleaded for another picture with the words "'Please, Dr. Kenny,'" according to one reporter, "she glared at him. 'Young man...I am NOT a doctor.'"[304]

NOTES

1. See E. Daniel Potts and Annette Potts *Yanks Down Under 1941–45: The American Impact on Australia* (Melbourne: Oxford University Press, 1985); John Hammond Moore *Over-Sexed, Over-Paid, & Over Here: Americans in Australia 1941–1945* (St. Lucia: University of Queensland Press, 1981); Ray Aitchison *Thanks to the Yanks? The Americans and Australia* (Melbourne: Sun Books, 1972); Edward J. Drea "'Great Patience Is Needed': American Encounters Australia, 1942" *War & Society* (1993) 11: 121–151.

2. "Roosevelt Cites U.S. Humanity As Faith in Victory of Right" *Christian Science Monitor* January 31 1942; "Faith, Hope, Charity Still Rule World" *Washington Post* January 31 1942.

3. Kenny to Dear Mr. O'Connor, February 19 1942, Basil O'Connor, 1940–1942, MHS-K. See also Kenny's claim that she had offered her services to the U.S. government for training men in physical therapy but had not yet been called; J.M.G. [Janet M. Geister] "The Lady from Australia" *Trained Nurse and Hospital Review* (July 1942) 109: 37.

4. Kenny to Dear Dr. Diehl, April 13 1944, Dr. Harold S. Diehl, 1941–1944, MHS-K.

5. Vernon L. Hart "The Kenny Principles and Injuries of the Knee Joint" *JAMA* (November 21 1942) 120: 900; see also Ethel Calhoun to Dear Dr. Ghormley, February 15 1943, Ethel Calhoun, MHS-K; "Vernon L. Hart 1898–1950" *Minnesota Medicine* (1952) 35: 240–241.

6. Elizabeth Riddell "U.S. Swears By Sister Kenny" *New York Daily Mirror* February 4 1943.

7. Hedda Hopper "Star Nurses An Enthusiasm!" *Washington Post* July 27 1942. Lewin later recalled that he had written a paper on Kenny and at the end had said this dramatically but Fishbein had asked him to strike it out; [Cohn interview with] Philip Lewin, October 19 1954, Cohn Papers, MHS-K.

8. "Miss Barrymore Star of Playlet on W-G-N Tonight" *Chicago Daily Tribune* January 22 1942; "W-G-N Ramparts Show Salutes Paralysis War" *Chicago Daily Tribune* January 23 1942.

9. DWG to BOC Memorandum re Lectures by Sister Kenny, September 18 1941 Public Relations, MOD-K.

10. Robert M. Yoder "Healer from the Outback" *Saturday Evening Post* (January 17 1942) 214: 18, 68, 70; A. B. Hardy [Sales Promotion Department, Curtis Publishing Company] to Gentlemen, January 12 1942, Public Relations, MOD-K.

11. Kenny to Dear Mr. Connor [sic], September 30 1941, Basil O'Connor 1940–1942, MHS-K.

12. Robert L. Bennett "Discussion of Papers by Drs. John A. Toomey, Jessie Wright, and Miland E. Knapp" *Archives of Physical Therapy* (November 1942) 23: 673.

13. There were 2 kinds of polio sera: one made from the blood of patients who had recovered from polio, and another—based on evidence that adults rarely developed paralytic polio—was a "normal adult serum" collected from healthy adults; see Paul, *A History*, 190–199; Rogers *Dirt and Disease*, 96–103.

14. James E. Perkins to Dear Miss Kenny, May 15 1945, Dr. James E. Perkins, 1944–1945, MHS-K.

15. See also W. H. Park "Therapeutic Use of Anti[-]poliomyelitis Serum in Preparalytic Cases of Poliomyelitis" *JAMA* (1932) 99: 1050–1053; "Infantile Paralysis" *Time* (December 21, 1931) 18: 24; S. D. Kramer et al. "Convalescent Serum Therapy in Preparalytic Poliomyelitis" *New England Journal of Medicine* (1932) 206: 432–435; "Convalescent Serum for Poliomyelitis" *JAMA* (1941) 117: 1269.

16. For examples of convalescent serum see Richard Owen in Edmund J. Sass, with George Gottfried and Anthony Sorem eds. *Polio's Legacy: An Oral History* (Lanham, MD: University Press of America, 1996), 30–32; Philip Lewin *Infantile Paralysis: Anterior Poliomyelitis* (Philadelphia: W. B. Saunders, 1941), 122–125; see also Paul H. Clark "History of Poliomyelitis up to the Present Time" in *Infantile Paralysis; A Symposium Delivered at Vanderbilt University, April, 1941* (New York: National Foundation for Infantile Paralysis, 1941), 18; Rogers "Polio Can Be Cured: Science and Health Propaganda in the United States from Polio Polly to Jonas Salk" in John Ward and Christopher Warren eds. *Silent Victories: The History and Practice of Public Health in Twentieth-Century America* (New York: Oxford University Press, 2007), 81–101.

17. John Paul to John Bauer [Pennsylvania Hospital], August 10 1931, #1333 Series 1, Box 1, Folder 14, John Rodman Paul Papers, Yale University Library Manuscripts and Archives, New Haven.

18. Kenny to Dear Sir [Marvin Kline], August 10 1942, Marvin L. Kline, 1942–1959, MHS-K; see also Jay Arthur Myers "Autobiography" (n.d.), UMN-ASC, 97–98.

19. "Threat to Quit City Is Sister Kenny's Answer to Critics" *Minneapolis Tribune* August 25 1942.

20. See B. B. Tomblin *GI Nightingales: The Army Nurse Corps in World War II* (Lexington: University Press of Kentucky, 1996); Philip Arthur Kalisch and Beatrice J. Kalisch *American Nursing: A History* (Philadelphia: Lippincott, Williams & Wilkins, 2004).

21. "The Biennial" *American Journal of Nursing* (July 1942) 42: 754–762; "Conventions of 10,000 Nurses to Open in City Tomorrow" *Chicago Daily Tribune* May 17 1942; Janet M. Geister "Twice Five Thousand Came!" *Trained Nurse and Hospital Review* (July 1942) 109: 31; Kenny with Ostenso *And They Shall Walk*, 250. The Biennial was organized by the nation's 3 major nursing societies—the ANA, the National League of Nursing Education, and the National Organization for Public Health Nursing.

22. J.M.G. "The Lady from Australia," 36–37. At the meeting the delegates unanimously approved the proposal from the ANA's board of directors that Kenny be granted honorary membership; *Excerpts from Proceedings of the Thirty-third Convention of the American Nurses Association Chicago, Illinois May 17–22 1942*, 42–43, Box 19, Folder 1, Myers Papers, UMN-ASC.

23. Carmelita Calderwood "Nursing Care in Poliomyelitis" *American Journal of Nursing* (June 1940) 40: 624, 628.

24. Kenny to Dear Mr. O'Connor, January 13 1942, Basil O'Connor, 1940–1942, MHS-K; Jessie L. Stevenson to My Dear Doctor Knapp, February 10 1943, Technicians—Misc., undated and 1941–1949, MHS-K; Jessie L. Stevenson *The Nursing Care of Patients with Infantile Paralysis* (New York: National Foundation for Infantile Paralysis, 1940). Stevenson had graduated from the prestigious Presbyterian Hospital's nursing school and then trained in physical therapy at Northwestern.

25. Jessie Stevenson "The Kenny Method" *American Journal of Nursing* (August 1942) 42: 904–910; "Pamphlet on Polio" *Trained Nurse and Hospital Review* (September 1943) 111: 209. Stevenson's revised guide was distributed by the NFIP as *Nursing Care of Patients with Infantile Paralysis—Including Nursing Aspects of the Kenny Method* as well as a brief *Guide for Parents*. For a demonstration of the Kenny method at the opening session of the Connecticut State Nurses Association in 1942 see "400 Attend Convention of Nurses" *Hartford Courant* November 6 1942.

26. Martha K. Rains "Infantile Paralysis" *Trained Nurse and Hospital Review* (August 1943) 111: 107.

27. Carmelita Calderwood "[Review of] Elizabeth Kenny *The Treatment of Infantile Paralysis in the Acute Stage*" *American Journal of Nursing* (January 1942) 42: 121.

28. Janet M. Geister "Mr. and Mrs. Hospital Trustee—You Have a Big Job!" *Trained Nurse and Hospital Review* (September 1942) 109: 176.

29. Helen H. Ross "Physiotherapy in the Treatment of Infantile Paralysis: Kenny Method" *Canadian Public Health Journal* (June 1942) 33: 285–286.

30. Dorothy I. Ditchfield and Ethel M. Hyndman "The Nursing Procedure" *Canadian Public Health Journal* (June 1942) 33: 282–284.

31. Kenny to Dear Mr. O'Connor, February 19 1942.

32. A. E. Deacon to Dear Dr. Gudakunst, January 6 1942, Public Relations, MOD-K.

33. Kenny to Dear Dr. Diehl, June 30 1943, Dr. Harold S. Diehl, 1941–1944, MHS-K; Harold S. Diehl, "Summary of the Relationship of the Medical School of the University of Minnesota to the Work of Sister Elizabeth Kenny" May 1944, Public Relations, MOD-K; Miland E. Knapp to Dear Doctor Diehl, March 10 1944, [accessed in 1992 before recent re-cataloging], Am 15.8, Folder 1, UMN-ASC. By 1943 the scholarship class included Ethel Gardner, Vivian Hannan, Ethel Burns, Alva Lembkey, Dorothy Lovaas and Ida Kay.

34. "Sister Kenny: Australian Nurse Demonstrates her Treatment for Infantile Paralysis" *Life* (September 28 1942) 13: 73; Kenny to Dear Dr. Boines, March 19 1942, Dr. George J. Boines, 1941–1946, MHS-K; Kenny to Dear Dr. Boines, August 15 1942, Dr. George J. Boines, 1941–1946, MHS-K; Ethel Gardner to Dear Sister Kenny, [1942], Ethel Gardner, 1942–1943, MHS-K. Ethel Gardner and Alva Lembkey to Dear Sister Kenny, September 15 1942, Ethel Gardner, 1942–1943, MHS-K; Ethel Gardner to Dear Sister Kenny, September 15 1942, Ethel Gardner, 1942–1943, MHS-K; "Treatment for Polio" *Time* (August 10 1942) 40: 46.

35. Kenny to Dear Dr. McGuinness, May 13 1942, Dr. Madge C. L. McGuinness, 1941–1943, MHS-K.

36. Ibid.

37. Knapp to Dear Doctor Diehl, March 10 1944; "The only thing worse than not having a good treatment for a disease," according to O'Connor, was "to have a good treatment which the public could not obtain"; O'Connor to Diehl [1942] quoted in Kenny to Dear Mr. Crosby, November 30 1950, George C. Crosby 1943–1951, MHS-K; see also Diehl, "Summary."

38. Diehl "Summary." There were also 1-week courses for nurses to learn to apply the packs, which were discontinued in February 1943. For other medical postgraduate courses see "Courses for Continuation Study" *JAMA* (September 20 1941) 117: 1027; "Continuation Courses for Practicing Physicians" *JAMA* (January 3 1942) 118: 69–75.

39. Kenny to Dear Dr. Diehl, February 26 1942, Dr. Harold S. Diehl, 1941–1944, MHS-K.

40. Gudakunst to Dear Doctor Diehl, February 16 1942, Public Relations, MOD-K.

41. Robert L. Bennett to Dear Mr. O'Connor, January 19 1942, Public Relations, MOD-K.

42. Robert L. Bennett to Dear Mr. O'Connor, January 19 1942. To supply communities "with trained personnel capable of introducing the Kenny technique," O'Connor and Gudakunst debated whether the training for physical therapists could be shortened to 2 months instead of 6 months, and what the "minimum time" could be to teach physicians; DWG to BO'C Memorandum: Re Kenny Program, Dr. Robert Bennett's Communication of January 19, 1942, January 22 1942, Public Relations, MOD-K.

43. "Kenny Method Courses Now in 6 Centers; Chapter Participation Again Urged" *National Foundation News* (October 1942) 1: 57; Mary Morton "Action Groups On 'Polio'" *Trained Nurse and Hospital Review* (August 1943) 111: 109; A. L. Van Horn [Assistant Director for Crippled Children, Division of Health Services, Children's Bureau] to Miss Louise Reville, March 26 1943, Central File 1941–1944, Children's Bureau, Box 102, Record Group 102, Infantile Paralysis 4-5-16-1, National Archives.

44. Kenny to Dear Dr. Diehl, September 5 1941, Dr. Harold S. Diehl, 1941–1944, MHS-K.

45. Memorandum of a Conference Held May 5, 1943 on the Program and Training in the Kenny Method of the Treatment of Infantile Paralysis, [accessed in 1992 before recent re-cataloging], Am 15.8, Folder 16, UMN-ASC.

46. Kenny to Dear Dr. Diehl, June 30 1943.

47. Kenny to Diehl, July 19 1943, Dr. Harold S. Diehl, 1941–1944, MHS-K.

48. Kenny to Dear Mr. O'Connor, February 19 1942.

49. "Polio's Mortal Enemy Can't Stand 'Orthodoxy'" *Free Press (London, Ontario)*, November 6 1944, Wilson Collection; see also Ella Frances Johnson to My Dear Sister Kenny, September 27 1942, Technicians—Misc., undated and 1941–1949, MHS-K.

50. Robert L. Bennett to Dear Miss Kenny, January 24 1942, Dr. Robert L. Bennett, 1942–1943, MHS-K; Kenny to Dear Dr. Bennett, March 10 1942, Dr. Robert L. Bennett, 1942–1943, MHS-K. For the claim that Kenny "wanted so badly to go to Warm Springs and change it over to her method of working" but Irwin and Bennett decided that instead of having her go to Georgia they would send Plastridge to her for training instead see L. Caitlin Smith "Alice Lou Plastridge-Converse" *PT: Magazine of Physical Therapy* (2000) 8: 42.

51. Kenny to Dear Mr. O'Connor, June 12 1942, [accessed in 1992 before recent re-cataloging], Am 15.8, Folder 4, UMN-ASC.

52. Kamlesh Kumari to Dear Sister Kenny, September 12 1944, Technicians—Misc., undated and 1941–1949, MHS-K.

53. Charlotte Anderson to Dear Sister Kenny, March 19 1942, Technicians—Misc., undated and 1941–1949, MHS-K.

54. Dorothy Behlow to Dear Sister Kenny, April 8 1942, Dorothy Behlow, 1942–1943, MHS-K.

55. Adelaide Smith to Dear Sister Kenny, June 15 1942, Technicians—Misc., undated and 1941–1949, MHS-K.

56. Ella Frances Johnson to My Dear Sister Kenny, September 27 1942, Technicians—Misc., undated and 1941–1949, MHS-K; Ella Frances Johnson to Dear Sister Kenny, November 3 1942, Technicians—Misc., undated and 1941–1949, MHS-K.

57. Ethel Gardner to Dear Sister Kenny, July 17 1942, Ethel Gardner, 1942–1943, MHS-K.

58. Emily J. Griffin to My Dear Sister Kenny, October 9 1941, Technicians—Misc., undated and 1941–1949, MHS-K.

59. Kenny to Dear Dr. Bennett, March 10 1942; see also Lorraine Paulson to Kenny, March 11, 1942, Technicians—Misc., undated and 1941–1949, MHS-K.

60. Kamlesh Kumari to Dear Sister Kenny, September 12 1944, Technicians—Misc., undated and 1941–1949, MHS-K.

61. Ruth Giaciolli to Dear Sister Kenny, February 16 1942, Technicians—Misc., undated and 1941–1949, MHS-K.

62. Ibid; see for example R.E.D. "A Step Forward in Poliomyelitis Care" *Journal of the American Osteopathic Association* (January 1942) 41: n.p. [reprint], Public Relations, MOD-K.

63. Charlotte Anderson to Dear Sister Kenny, June 2 1943, Technicians—Misc., undated and 1941–1949, MHS-K; "A Book A Day [*And They Shall Walk*]" *Honolulu Star Bulletin* June 23 1943. The NFIP had already paid for the hospital's physical therapist Sybil Jennings Vorheis to take a short Kenny course a few months earlier.

64. Miland E. Knapp to Dear Dr. Diehl, May 21 1943, [accessed in 1992 before recent re-cataloging], Am 15.8, Folder 16, UMN-ASC. On the idea of doctor, nurse, and physical therapist "from each institution, so that they can work as a team" see Miland E. Knapp "The Kenny Treatment for Infantile Paralysis" *Archives of Physical Therapy* (November 1942) 23: 668.

65. George J. Boines "Observation of the Kenny Treatment" *Delaware State Medical Journal* (January 1942) 14: 11–14.

66. Ethel Calhoun to Dear Dr. Ghormley, February 15 1943.

67. Diehl "Summary;" Gudakunst to Dear Doctor Diehl, February 16 1942.

68. Memorandum of Conference Held May 5, 1943 on the Program and Training in the Kenny Method; see also Kenny with Ostenso *And They Shall Walk*, 255.

69. Edward L. Compere to Dear Doctor Guderkunst [sic], January 27 1942, Public Relations, MOD-K. A month after Philip Stimson described Kenny's work to a group of physicians in Buffalo, a local doctor assured him that the city's single case of paralytic polio had been "placed on a make shift Sister Kenny technique and is doing remarkably well"; Bill [William J. Orr] to Dear Phil [Stimson], June 18 1942, Box 2, Folder 3, Correspondence re Medical Talks, Stimson Papers.

70. Kenny with Ostenso *And They Shall Walk*, 223–224.

71. T. C. Kimble [M.D. Kansas state polio epidemiologist] to Sister Elizabeth Kenney [sic] & Associate, August 2 1943, [accessed in 1992 before recent re-cataloging], Am 15.8, Folder 1, UMN-ASC.

72. Esther I. McEachen to Dear Miss [Mary Stewart] Kenny, October 15 1942, Technicians—Misc., undated and 1941–1949, MHS-K; see also a description of an evening meeting in Indianapolis, Charlotte Anderson to Dear Sister Kenny, April 4 1943, Technicians—Misc., undated and 1941–1949, MHS-K.

73. F. H. Krusen "Observations on the Kenny Treatment of Poliomyelitis" *Proceedings of the Staff Meetings of the Mayo Clinic* (August 12 1942) 17: 452.

74. For examples of the claim that physicians were initially skeptical see Don W. Gudakunst "Up To Date on Infantile Paralysis" *Parents' Magazine* (June 1942) 17: 75; "New Technique For Paralysis Cases Accepted" *Philadelphia Evening Bulletin* October 18 1942; "Girl Walks Again in Kenny Cure Test" *New York Times* October 27 1942.

75. Krusen "Observations on the Kenny Treatment of Poliomyelitis," 449–460; Gudakunst to Dear Doctor Compere, January 29 1942, Public Relations, MOD-K. See also Winnipeg orthopedist Alfred Deacon who visited Kenny in Minneapolis with funding from the NFIP, and assured Gudakunst that he had also traveled to Rochester to talk with Krusen for "I also knew that he had not definitely endorsed Sister Kenny's treatment"; A. E. Deacon to Dear Dr. Gudakunst, January 6 1942.

76. Kenny, letter to editor, *British Medical Journal* (January 29 1944) 1: 163.

77. Wallace H. Cole, John F. Pohl, and Miland E. Knapp "The Kenny Method of Treatment for Infantile Paralysis" *Archives of Physical Therapy* (June 1942) 23: 399–418; Miland E. Knapp "The Kenny Treatment for Infantile Paralysis" *Archives of Physical Therapy* (November 1942) 23: 668–673. The Cole, Pohl, and Knapp paper was published as a separate pamphlet by the National Foundation for Infantile Paralysis; Wallace H. Cole, John F. Pohl, and Miland E. Knapp *The Kenny Method of Treatment for Infantile Paralysis* (New York: National Foundation for Infantile Paralysis, Publication No. 40, 1942). Typical was an editorial in the British *Lancet* that praised the University of Minnesota group as "composed of men who at the outset were sceptical [sic] of the value of the method; "The Kenny Method In Poliomyelitis" *Lancet* (January 30 1943) 241: 148.

78. "New Technique For Paralysis Cases Accepted" *Philadelphia Evening Bulletin* October 18 1942.

79. Elizabeth Kenny *Treatment of Infantile Paralysis in the Acute Stage* (Minneapolis: Bruce Publishing Company, 1941), 102; Lewin *Infantile Paralysis*, 137–138.

80. Yoder "Healer from the Outback," 18; see also Kenny to Dear Dr. Fishbein, October 5 1941, Public Relations, MOD-K.

81. Lewin "The Kenny Treatment of Infantile Paralysis during the Acute Stage" *Illinois Medical Journal* (April 1942) 81: 281–296; see also "Official Program of the One Hundred Second Annual Meeting, Illinois State Medical Society" *Illinois Medical Journal* (May 1942) 81: 366.

82. [Cohn interview with] Lewin, October 19 1954.

83. "Dr. Philip Stimson Dead at 82: Active in the Fight Against Polio" *New York Times* September 14 1971.

84. Philip Stimson "Poliomyelitis," Address before the York County Medical Society, York, Pennsylvania, Friday, August 22 1941, Box 1, Folder 16, Address by PMS to York County Medical Society, Stimson Papers.

85. Philip Stimson "Kenny Treatment & Minimizing the After Effects of Polio" [notes] September 26 1941, Box 2, Folder 1, Correspondence re Medical Talks, Stimson Papers.

86. Ibid. Stimson began using Kenny's methods with patients at the Willard Parker Hospital, and the director of New York Orthopedic Hospital Alan DeForrest Smith and his head physical therapist William Benham Snow "promised to continue the Kenny treatment"; Philip Stimson to Dear Joe [Stokes], December 3 1941, Box 2, Folder 2, Correspondence re Medical Talks, Stimson Papers. Stimson also gave a joint speech with Wallace Cole to the Medical Society of Westchester County in March 1942 where he was described as "foremost in the development and recognition of the Kenny treatment"; "Program of March Meeting" *Westchester Medical Bulletin* (March 1942) 10: 8.

87. Boines "Observation of the Kenny Treatment," 11–14; Kenny "The Technique of the Kenny Treatment: Delivered by Miss Kenny 1-7-42 at Einhorn Auditorium and Lenox Hill Hospital before N.Y. Physical Therapy Society" [attached to] Program of New York Physical Therapy Society, January 7 1942, Public Relations, MOD-K.

88. Philip Stimson to Dear Bill [William J. Orr], April 17 1942, Box 2, Folder 3, Correspondence re Medical Talks, Stimson Papers; G. B. Lal "Sister Kenny Gains in Fight On Paralysis" *Washington Post* May 3 1942; see also Kenny "Infantile Paralysis: Importance of Treatment in the Acute Stage" *New York State Journal of Medicine* (September 1 1942) 42: 1645–1650.

89. H. B. Sheffield to My Dear Dr. Stimson, January 12 1943, Box 2, Folder 4, Correspondence re Medical Talks, Stimson Papers; see also Herman B. Sheffield "Infantile Paralysis" *New York State Journal of Medicine* (1920) [reprint enclosed in] H. B. Sheffield to My Dear Dr. Stimson, January 12 1943, Box 2, Folder 4, Correspondence re Medical Talks, Stimson Papers.

90. Charles C. Zacharie to My Dear Dr. Stimson, January 11 1943, Box 2, Folder 4, Correspondence re Medical Talks, Stimson Papers.

91. Philip Stimson to Dear Dr. Zacharie, January 12 1943, Box 2, Folder 4, Correspondence re Medical Talks, Stimson Papers.

92. "Opponent Now Backs Kenny Treatment" *Philadelphia Evening Bulletin* January 9 1943.

93. [Cohn interview with] Robert Bingham May 19 1955, Cohn Papers, MHS-K; William Benham Snow to Dear Dr. Stimson, August 12 1943, Box 1, Folder 4, Stimson Papers.

94. Robert Bingham "The Kenny Treatment for Infantile Paralysis: A Comparison of Results with Those of Older Methods of Treatment" *Journal of Bone and Joint Surgery* (July 1943) 25: 647–650; see also [Cohn interview with] Robert Bingham May 19 1955, Cohn Papers, MHS-K.

95. Alan [Deforest Smith] to Dear Philip [Stimson], August 13 1943, Box 1, Folder 4, Kenny Treatment of Infantile Paralysis, Stimson Papers.

96. Kenny, "Preface" in Pohl and Kenny *The Kenny Concept of Infantile Paralysis*, 23–24, 25.

97. [Florence Kendall] Notes for Talk to Nurses, St. Agnes Hospital, April 28 1944, Kendall Collection.

98. John A. Toomey "Treatment of Infantile Paralysis in the Acute Stage" *Archives of Physical Therapy* (November 1942) 23: 651. Kansas physicians suggested that "patients classified as having a non[-]paralytic form should not be included to boost the percentage of 'good results'" in evaluating "the Kenny technic"; A. Theodore Steegmann and Kathryn Stephenson "Poliomyelitis: Differential Diagnostic Problems Encountered in an Epidemic" *Archives of Physical Medicine* (August 1945) 26: 485.

99. A. Bruce Gill to Dear Fellow Members of the Orthopaedic Correspondence Club, April 26 1943, Dr. Bruce A. Gill, 1943, MHS-K.

100. Maurice B. Visscher and Jay A. Myers [Editorial] "Sister Kenny Five Years After" *Lancet* (August 1945) 65: 309–310; Albert Deutsch "The Truth About Sister Kenny" *American Mercury* (November 1944) 59: 616; Robert V. Funsten "The Influence of the Sister Kenny Publicity on the Treatment of Poliomyelitis" *Virginia Medical Monthly* (October 1945) 72: 404.

101. See Fishbein's proposal that the NFIP fund "controlled studies on every aspect of this serious disease"; Editorial "The Kenny Method of Treatment in the Acute Peripheral Manifestations of Infantile Paralysis" *JAMA* (December 20 1941) 117: 2171–2172.

102. Lewin "The Kenny Treatment of Infantile Paralysis," 281–296.

103. Deutsch "The Truth About Sister Kenny," 616.

104. A. Bruce Gill to Dear Fellow Members of the Orthopaedic Correspondence Club, April 26 1943.

105. "Pain and Spasm in Poliomyelitis: A Symposium" *American Journal of Physical Medicine* (August 1952) 31: 333, 331; Daniel J. Wilson "Psychological Trauma and Its Treatment in the Polio Epidemics" *Bulletin of the History of Medicine* (2008) 82: 848–877.

106. Gudakunst had begun planning this in February 1942; Gudakunst to Dear Doctor Diehl, February 16 1942, Public Relations, MOD-K.

107. "Demonstrations Given Special Award at A.M.A. Session" *National Foundation News* (June 1942) 1: 33; Krusen "Observations on the Kenny Treatment of Poliomyelitis," 453.

108. Miland E. Knapp to Don Gudakunst [telegram], May 28 1942, Public Relations, AMA files, MOD; [notes on phone conversation] DWG to Miland Knapp, May 29 1942, Public Relations, AMA files, MOD; Harold S. Diehl to Don W. Gudakunst, April 30 1942, [accessed in 1992 before recent re-cataloging], Am 15.8 folder 29, UMN-ASC.

109. Philip Stimson to Dear Dr. Mitchell, December 15 1942, Box 2, Folder 4, Correspondence re Medical Talks, Stimson Papers.

110. "The Program of the Sections, American Medical Association, Ninety-Third Annual Session, Atlantic City, June 8–12, 1942: Section on Pediatrics" *JAMA* (May 2 1942) 119: 53.

111. "The Program of the Sections, American Medical Association, Ninety-Third Annual Session, Atlantic City, June 8–12, 1942: Section on Nervous and Mental Diseases" *JAMA* (May 2 1942) 119: 55.

112. "Proceedings of the Atlantic City Session: Minutes of the Ninety-Third Annual Session of the American Medical Association, Held in Atlantic City, June 8–12, 1942: Minutes of the Sections: Section on Orthopedic Surgery" *JAMA* (July 4 1942) 119: 804. The members of this committee were to be drawn from the Section, the Academy of Orthopedic Surgeons, and the American Orthopedic Association.

113. H. M. Hines "Effects of Immobilization and Activity on Neuromuscular Regeneration" *JAMA* (October 17 1942) 120: 515–517; see also H. M. Hines, J. D. Thomson, and B. Lazere "Physiologic Basis for Treatment of Paralyzed Muscles" *Archives of Physical Therapy* (February 1943) [abstract] in *Physiotherapy Review* (1943) 23: 86.

114. Donald Young Solandt "Atrophy in Skeletal Muscle" *JAMA* (October 17 1942) 120: 511–513.

115. Frank R. Ober "Pain and Tenderness during the Acute Stage of Poliomyelitis" *JAMA* (October 17 1942) 120: 514–515. Ober had given a talk to the postgraduate medical assembly of Connecticut State Medical Society on Kenny's treatment; "State Doctors Gather Today in New Haven" *Hartford Courant* September 29 1942.

116. H. R. McCarroll "The Role of Physical Therapy in the Early Treatment of Poliomyelitis" *JAMA* (October 17 1942) 120: 517–519.

117. F. A. Hellebrandt, letter to editor, *JAMA* (November 7 1942) 120: 787.

118. John F. Pohl, letter to editor, *JAMA* (December 5 1942) 120: 1157.

119. Kenny, letter to editor, *JAMA* (December 19 1942) 120: 1335–1336.

120. Kenny with Ostenso *And They Shall Walk* 214–215.

121. McCracken, interviews with Rogers, November 1992, Caloundra, Queensland; John Ralph "My Struggle By Sister Kenny" *[Britain] Sunday Graphic* May 11 1947, OM 65-17, Box 1, Folder 4, Chuter Papers, Oxley-SLQ. For images of Australian nurses in fuller, slightly longer dresses, with veils reaching down below the elbow see "On The Other Side of the Sun: Australia's Children Grow Up" *Nursing Times* (February 7 1942) 38: 88–89. For examples of American uniforms see "On The Other Side of the Atlantic: The B Hospital, New York" *Nursing Times* (July 4 1942) 38: 429–430; "New Uniforms for the Army Nurse" *Trained Nurse and Hospital Review* (March 1943) 110: 184–185.

122. See, for example, Lynn Houweling "Image, Function and Style: A History of the Nursing Uniform" *American Journal of Nursing* (2004) 104: 40–48. On the history of nursing dress see Irene Schuessler "Poplin, Nursing Uniform: Romantic Idea, Functional Attire or Instrument of Social Change" *Nursing History Review* (1994) 2: 153–169; Simonne Horwitz "Black Nurses in White" *Social History of Medicine* (2007) 20: 131–146. My thanks to Patricia D'Antonio for pointing me to these references.

123. Mary M. I. Daly, Jerome Greenbaum, Edward T. Reilly, Alvah M. Weiss, and Philip M. Stimson "The Early Treatment of Poliomyelitis with an Evaluation of the Sister Kenny Treatment" *JAMA* (April 25 1942) 118: 1433–1443; see also "Remarkable Recoveries Cited For Kenny Polio Treatment" *Science News Letter* (May 9 1942) 41: 294.

124. Philip Moen Stimson "Minimizing the After Effects of Acute Poliomyelitis" *JAMA* (July 25 1942) 119: 989–991.

125. A. E. Deacon "The Treatment of Poliomyelitis in the Acute Stage" *Canadian Public Health Journal* (June 1942) 33: 278–281. On polio in Canada see Christopher J. Rutty "The Middle Class Plague: Epidemic Polio and the Canadian State, 1936–1937" *Canadian Bulletin of Medical History* (1996) 13: 277–314; Rutty "Do Something! Do Anything! Poliomyelitis in Canada, 1927–1962," Ph.D. thesis, Department of History, University of Toronto, 1995. Manitoba had significant epidemics in 1928 and 1936.

126. December 9 1941, Minutes Board of Directors 1938–1955, Children's Hospital of Winnipeg MG 10B33, Box 7, Province Archives, Winnipeg, Manitoba.

127. Bruce Chown "The Newer Knowledge of the Pathology of Poliomyelitis" *Canadian Public Health Journal* (June 1942) 33: 276–277; see also [anon] "Kenny Method of Treatment: Experiences at the Children's Hospital of Winnipeg" *Canadian Public Health Journal* (June 1942) 33: 275–276. Chown was probably referring to Howard A. Howe and David Bodian "Some Factors Involved in the Invasion of the Body by the Virus of Infantile Paralysis" *Scientific Monthly* (October 1939) 49: 391–392.

128. R. Plato Schwartz and Harry D. Bouman "Muscle Spasm in the Acute Stage of Infantile Paralysis: As Indicated By Recorded Action Current Potentials" *JAMA* (July 18 1942) 119: 924; see also Kenny with Ostenso *And They Shall Walk*, 252–253.

129. "Grateful 'for All Mankind'" *Rochester Times-Union* May 3 1943, Folder 37, Alan Valentine Papers, Rush Rhees Library, University of Rochester, Rochester; "Sister Elizabeth Kenny Chats with Dr. R. Plato Schwartz" *National Foundation News* (May 1943) 2: 30.

130. "Sister Kenny Grateful For Recognition of Work" *Rochester Times-Union* May 3 1943, Folder 37, Alan Valentine Papers, Rush Rhees Library.

131. "The Importance of Research: The Kenny Method of Treatment" *National Foundation News* (July 1942) 1: 39–42.

132. Don W. Gudakunst "Poliomyelitis: Control and Treatment" *Canadian Public Health Journal* (August 1942) 33: 370, 372; see also Don W. Gudakunst "Up To Date on Infantile Paralysis" *Parents' Magazine* (June 1942) 17: 74–75.

133. Richard Kovacs ed. *The 1942 Year Book of Physical Therapy* (Chicago: Year Book Publishers, 1942), 267–293, 297.

134. Miland E. Knapp "The Kenny Treatment for Infantile Paralysis" *Archives of Physical Therapy* (November 1942) 23: 668–673; see also Miland Knapp to Dear Dr. Diehl, August 14 1942, Minnesota Poliomyelitis Research Committee, Box 2, UMN-ASC.

135. Lois Maddox Miller "Sister Kenny Wins Her Fight" *Reader's Digest* (1942) 41: 28–30.

136. Kenny to Dear Dr. Diehl, April 9 1943, Dr. Harold S. Diehl, 1941–1944, MHS-K; Kenny with Ostenso *And They Shall Walk*, 255. See also a reference to the committee members

"antagonized by Sister Kenny's attitude towards them"; Lois Maddox Miller "Sister Kenny vs. The Medical Old Guard" *Reader's Digest* (November 1944) 45: 42.

137. Melvin S. Henderson [Report] in "Reports on Meeting of Committee to Investigate the Kenny Method of Treatment, Sunday and Monday, November 22 and 23, 1942, Minneapolis, Minnesota," Dr. R. K. Ghormley, 1943, MHS-K.

138. Edward L. Compere to Dear Doctor Guderkunst [sic] January 27 1942, Public Relations, MOD-K; Edward L. Compere "Modern Concepts of Infantile Paralysis" *Archives of Physical Therapy* (November 1942) 23: 677–678; see also Compere "The Kenny Treatment for Infantile Paralysis" *Proceedings of the Institute of Medicine, Chicago* (June 13 1942) 14: 187–188 [abstract] in Isaac A. Abt ed. *The 1942 Year Book of Pediatrics* (Chicago: Year Book Publishers, 1943), 161–162.

139. Edward L. Compere [Report] in "Reports on Meeting of Committee to Investigate the Kenny Method of Treatment, Sunday and Monday, November 22 and 23, 1942, Minneapolis, Minnesota," Dr. R. K. Ghormley, 1943, MHS-K.

140. "Doctor Favors New Paralysis Treatment" *Washington Post* August 24 1942.

141. Robert V. Funston [Report] in "Reports on Meeting of Committee to Investigate the Kenny Method of Treatment, Sunday and Monday, November 22 and 23, 1942, Minneapolis, Minnesota," Dr. R. K. Ghormley, 1943, MHS-K.

142. J. Albert Key [Report] in "Reports on Meeting of Committee to Investigate the Kenny Method of Treatment, Sunday and Monday, November 22 and 23, 1942, Minneapolis, Minnesota," Dr. R. K. Ghormley, 1943, MHS-K.

143. H. Relton McCarroll [Report] in "Reports on Meeting of Committee to Investigate the Kenny Method of Treatment, Sunday and Monday, November 22 and 23, 1942, Minneapolis, Minnesota," Dr. R. K. Ghormley, 1943, MHS-K.

144. Key [Report] in "Reports on Meeting of Committee." McCarroll similarly felt that "lay organizations and most medical people as well" were following Kenny "blindly"; McCarroll [Report] in "Reports on Meeting of Committee."

145. Kenny with Ostenso *And They Shall Walk*, 255.

146. Key [Report] in "Reports on Meeting of Committee."

147. Kenny to Dear Dr. Ghormley [March 5 1943], Dr. R. K. Ghormley, 1943, MHS-K; see also [Cohn third interview with] Miland Knapp, August 24 1963, Cohn Papers, MHS-K. She had asked Key and McCarroll about one patient and both had agreed that the patient had a "complete paralysis of the quadriceps." "The patient in a few seconds extended her leg in mid-air and held it there." As Knapp recalled this moment, "they got mad."

148. McCarroll [Report] in "Reports on Meeting of Committee." McCarroll later recalled that the committee made 2 trips to Minneapolis to attend her clinics and examine her patients: the first trip to the General Hospital and the second trip to the Institute and the Michael Dowling School where the committee had attended a "specially arranged" part of her course given for physicians and each member of the Committee had received a certificate; H. R. McCarroll to Dear Dr. Myers, September 9 1946 [and 3 page enclosure], Box 19, Maurice Visscher Papers, UMN-ASC.

149. Calhoun received her B.A. degree from Western Reserve University in Cleveland and an M.D. from the University of Michigan. She was one of 7 women physicians graduating in 1925 out of a class of 156 doctors. She practiced medicine in downtown Detroit for 5 years, but gave up her private practice after the birth of her son; "Ethel Calhoun" Michigan Women's Historical Center & Hall of Fame http://hall.michiganwomen.org/honoree.php, accessed June

11 2013; Ethel Calhoun to Dear Dr. Ghormley, February 15 1943; see also Ethel Calhoun to Dear Miss Kenny, December 10 1942, Ethel Calhoun, MHS-K.

150. Ethel Calhoun to Dear Dr. Ghormley, February 15 1943.

151. Ethel Calhoun to Dear Sister, November 24 1943, Ethel Calhoun, MHS-K.

152. "Herman Charles Schumm 1889–1955" *Journal of Bone and Joint Surgery* (1956) 38: 714.

153. Herman C. Schumm [Report] in "Reports on Meeting of Committee to Investigate the Kenny Method of Treatment, Sunday and Monday, November 22 and 23, 1942, Minneapolis, Minnesota," Dr. R. K. Ghormley, 1943, MHS-K.

154. Kenny to Dear Dr. Ghormley, March 5 1943.

155. Kenny to Dear Dr. Diehl, April 9 1943; Gudakunst to Dear Doctor Ober, February 16 1943, Dr. Don W. Gudakunst, 1941–1944.

156. J. Albert Key "The Kenny Versus the Orthodox Treatment of Anterior Poliomyelitis" *Surgery* (July 1943) 14: 20–29.

157. Kenny with Ostenso *And They Shall Walk*, 258; Kenny "Data Concerning Introduction of Kenny Concept and Method of Treatment of Infantile Paralysis into the United States of America" [April 1944] Board of Directors, MHS-K; "Sister Kenny Receives Parent's Magazine Award" *Parents Magazine* (December 1942) 17: 38; "Medal Is Given to Sister Kenny for Child Care" *Chicago Daily Tribune* October 28 1942.

158. Kenny with Ostenso *And They Shall Walk*, 263–264.

159. Kenny with Ostenso *And They Shall Walk*, 255.

160. Kenny with Ostenso *And They Shall Walk*, 19–20.

161. Ostenso quoted in George Grim "Entertainers? Brainerd's Got Dandies" *Minneapolis Sunday Tribune* April 17 1950, 1, 5; see also Andrew Lesk "Wild Geese" *The Literary Encyclopedia* (29 April 2005; last revised 18 April 2006); http://www.litencyc.com/php/sworks.php?rec=true&UID=8791, accessed January 1 2011; Faye Hammill "Martha Ostenso, Literary History, and the Scandinavian Diaspora" *Canadian Literature* (2008) 196: 17–31, 202. Ostenso's 1925 novel *Wild Geese* had been made into a Hollywood movie, bringing its author a celebrity life filled with luxury cars, boats, and houses in Hollywood and in Minnesota. Ostenso was 20 years younger than Kenny, and, according to her recollections, she had first met Kenny as the older sister of a young man interested in Mary Kenny.

162. Kenny with Ostenso *And They Shall Walk*, ix–x.

163. Robert L. Bennett "Recent Developments in the Treatment of Poliomyelitis" *Southern Medical Journal* (February 1943) [abstract] in *Physiotherapy Review* (1943) 23: 81.

164. Bennett "Discussion of Papers," 673.

165. Arthur Steindler "Contributory Clinical Observations on Infantile Paralysis and Their Therapeutic Implications" *Journal of Bone and Joint Surgery* (October 1942) 24: 912–920; see also Steindler et al. "Recent Changes in the Concept of the Treatment of Poliomyelitis" *Archives of Physical Therapy* (June 1942) 23: 325–331.

166. "The Kenny Treatment of Poliomyelitis" *British Medical Journal* (November 28 1942) 2: 639–640.

167. Myron O. Henry to Dear Fellow Correspondent, March 6 1943, [enclosed in] O. L. Miller to Dear Mrs. Enochs [Children's Bureau], April 17 1943, Record Group 102, Children's Bureau Central File, 1941–1944, Box 102, 4-5-16-1, Infantile Paralysis, National Archives; "Opponent Now Backs Kenny Treatment" *Philadelphia Evening Bulletin* January 9 1943;

Rutherford John to Dear Dr. Gudakunst, February 23 1943, Government Relations (Foreign) Argentina, MOD.

168. A. Bruce Gill to Dear Fellow Members of the Orthopaedic Correspondence Club, April 26 1943; see also Gill "The Kenny Concepts and Treatment of Infantile Paralysis" *Journal of Bone and Joint Surgery* (April 1944) 26: 87–98.

169. A. Bruce Gill to Dear Fellow Members of the Orthopaedic Correspondence Club, April 26 1943.

170. Ibid.

171. "Kenny Method Courses Now in 6 Centers; Chapter Participation Again Urged" *National Foundation News* (October 1942) 1: 57 (2,834 compared to over 6,000 during the previous 2 years). On the 6 centers: Stanford, University of Southern California, Warm Springs, Minnesota, Northwestern, and D.T. Watson Home's School of Physiotherapy; Ida Jean Kain "Your Figure Madame!" *Washington Post* November 25 1942.

172. Kenny to Dear Mr. O'Connor, February 2 1942, Public Relations, MOD-K.

173. Kenny to Dear Dr. Diehl, June 30 1943.

174. DWG to BOC Memorandum Re Argentine Situation, February 4 1943, Government Relations (Foreign) Argentina, MOD; Mrs. Enochs to Dr. Eliot Memorandum: Assignment of specialist from U.S.A. to cooperate in efforts to control infantile paralysis epidemic in Uruguay, Argentina, etc., April 7 1943, RG 102, Children's Bureau, Central File, Box 102, 4-6-16—1, Infantile Paralysis, National Archives.

175. Don W. Gudakunst to Dear Doctor Hackett, December 23 1942, Government Relations (Foreign) Argentina, MOD; L.W. Hackett to Dr. Juan J. Spangenberg, January 11 1943, Government Relations (Foreign) Argentina, MOD; Hackett to Dear Dr. Gudakunst, February 18 1943, Government Relations (Foreign) Argentina, MOD. On a request from L. W. Hackett of the Rockefeller Foundation in Buenos Aires to the NFIP for "technical assistance"; see Basil O'Connor to President Roosevelt, February 4 1943 [abstract] FDR–OF-5188, Sister Elizabeth Kenny Institute, 1940–1944, FDR Papers. Roosevelt had supposedly suggested that the NFIP send experts to Argentina to assist in the epidemic, including instructing doctors in the newest methods of treatment, including the Kenny system; "Argentina Offered Aid Of Paralysis Experts At Suggestion of FDR" *Hartford Courant* February 5 1943; "Local Doctor Does Much to Promote U.S. Goodwill among Argentines" *Philadelphia Evening Bulletin* May 3 1943; [Cohn interview with] Basil O'Connor, June 20 1955, Cohn Papers, MHS-K.

176. Douglas B. Cornell "Views Echoed By President of Sister Nation At Historic Meeting" *Washington Post* April 21 1943; see also Max Paul Friedman *Nazis and Good Neighbors: The United States Campaign against the Germans of Latin America in World War II* (New York: Cambridge University Press, 2003).

177. "Epidemic Fighters Fly to Argentina" *National Foundation News* (March 1943) 2: 20; "3 Kenny Method Experts Fly to Argentina to Combat Infantile Paralysis Epidemic" *New York Times* March 14 1943.

178. Miland E. Knapp to Dear Dr. Gudakunst, February 5 1943, [accessed in 1992 before recent re-cataloging], Am 15.8, Folder 29, UMN-ASC.

179. DWG to PJAC Memorandum Re: Kenny Problem—South America, February 9 1943, Government Relations (Foreign) Argentina, MOD.

180. Rutherford John to Dear Dr. Gudakunst, February 4 1943, Government Relations (Foreign) Argentina, MOD.

181. "Opponent Now Backs Kenny Treatment" *Philadelphia Evening Bulletin* January 9 1943.

182. DWG to PJAC Memorandum Re: Kenny Problem—South America, February 9 1943.

183. PJAC to BOC Memorandum Re: Representative going to South America, February 15 1943, Government Relations (Foreign) Argentina, MOD; DWG to BO'C Memorandum Re: Physician for Argentina, February 19, 1943, Government Relations (Foreign) Argentina, MOD; DWG to PJAC Memorandum Re: Kenny Problem—South America, February 9 1943; "To Aid Fight on Epidemic" *New York Times* February 6 1943; "3 Kenny Method Experts Fly to Argentina To Combat Infantile Paralysis Epidemic" *Philadelphia Evening Bulletin* March 14 1943.

184. Mary Kenny and Ethel Gardner were paid $200 per month for 2 months, $200 for additional compensation for time to travel, and all travel expenses; John was paid $750 per month and $750 for the time spent traveling. See Basil O'Connor to Dear Miss Kenny, February 5 1943, Government Relations (Foreign) Argentina, MOD; O'Connor to Dear Miss Gardner, February 5 1943, Government Relations (Foreign) Argentina, MOD; O'Connor to Dear Doctor John, February 23 1943, Government Relations (Foreign) Argentina, MOD.

185. Rutherford John to Dear Dr. Gudakunst, March 19 1943, Government Relations (Foreign) Argentina, MOD.

186. [Embassy, Norman Armour] to Secretary of State Subject: Visit of Kenny Mission for the Treatment of Infantile Paralysis, March 29 1943, Government Relations (Foreign) Argentina, MOD.

187. Kenny to Dear Dr. Diehl, June 30 1943; Elisabeth Shirley Enochs [director, Inter-American Cooperation, Office of the Chief, U.S. Department of Labor, Children's Bureau] to My Dear Dr. [Oscar L.] Miller, May 8 1943, Record Group 102, Children's Bureau, Central File, Box 102, 4-6-16—1, Infantile Paralysis, National Archives; H. Keniston to Secretary from State Memorandum: Proposed Visit of Dr. Oscar Lee Miller, June 14, 1943, Record Group 102, Children's Bureau, Central File, Box 102, 4-6-16—1, Infantile Paralysis, National Archives.

188. Rutherford L. John to Dear Dr. Gudakunst, April 14 1943, Government Relations (Foreign), Argentina, MOD.

189. Gudakunst to Dear Miss Kenny, May 10 1943, Dr. Don W. Gudakunst, 1941–1944, MHS-K.

190. Kenny to Dear Dr. Gudakunst, May 11 1943, Dr. Don W. Gudakunst, 1941–1944, MHS-K.

191. Kenny to Dear Dr. Gudakunst, May 24 1943, Dr. Harold S. Diehl, 1941–1944, MHS-K; DWG to BO'C Memorandum Re Argentine, July 20 1943, Government Relations (Foreign), Argentina, MOD.

192. Kenny to Dear Dr. Gudakunst, May 24 1943; Kenny to Dear Dr. Diehl, May 26 1943, Dr. Harold S. Diehl, 1941–1944, MHS-K.

193. Kenny to Dear Mary [McCarthy] July 5 1943, Mary McCarthy, 1942–1944, MHS-K.

194. Kenny to Dear Dr. Gudakunst, May 24 1943.

195. Rutherford John "Orthopedic Aspects of the Kenny Treatment," [1943] Argentina, Misc., 1943–1945, 1949, MHS-K.

196. Kenny to Dear Dr. Gudakunst, May 24 1943; Kenny to Dear Dr. Diehl, May 26 1943.

197. Ibid.

198. Kenny to Dear Dr. Diehl, May 26 1943; Kenny to American Consul, May 22 1943, Anibal Olaran Chans, 1943, MHS-K; Felipe Espil to Kenny, June 3 1943, Felipe A. Espil, 1943, MHS-K; Kenny to Anibal Olaran Chans, June 4 1943, Anibal Olaran Chans, 1943, MHS-K.

199. Don Gudakunst to Kenny [telegram], June 4 1943, Argentina, Misc., 1943–1945, 1949, MHS-K; DWG to PJAC Memorandum Re: Kenny Problem—South America, February 9

1943; DWG to BO'C Memorandum re Argentine Situation, June 2 1943, Government Relations (Foreign), Argentina, MOD; Kenny to Dear Dr. Diehl, June 30 1943; *we are convinced that the interests of those in Argentina affiliated with infantile paralysis will be best served by your returning immediately to this country pursuant to the plans under which you were sent to Argentina by the National Foundation... If however you elect to remain in Argentina we are certain you would be the first to wish to relieve the National Foundation of any responsibility in connection with your continued sojourn or your safe return to the United States.*"

200. Kenny to Mary Stewart Kenny [telegram], June 6 1943, Mary Stewart Kenny, 1942–1947, MHS-K; Anibal Olaran Chans to Sister Kenny May 31 1943, Anibal Olaran Chans, 1943, MHS-K; Kenny to Anibal Olaran Chans, June 1 1943, Anibal Olaran Chans, 1943, MHS-K; Kenny to Anibal Olaran Chans, July 1 1943, Anibal Olaran Chans, 1943, MHS-K.

201. [Cohn interview with] Ethel Gardner, May 25 1955, Cohn Papers, MHS-K.

202. Kenny to Dear Mr. Henderson, June 25 1943, Cohn Papers, MHS-K.

203. Kenny to Dear Dr. Diehl, June 21 1943, Dr. Harold S. Diehl, 1941–1944, MHS-K.

204. Kenny to Dear Dr. Diehl, June 30 1943.

205. Diehl to Dear Sister Kenny, June 2 1943, Dr. Harold S. Diehl, 1941–1944, MHS-K.

206. Kenny to Dear Dr. Diehl, July 2 1943, Dr. Harold S. Diehl, 1941-1944, MHS-K.

207. Diehl to My Dear Sister Kenny, July 7 1943, Dr. Harold S. Diehl, 1941–1944, MHS-K.

208. Kenny with Ostenso *And They Shall Walk*, 266.

209. Kenny "Radio Talk Columbia Broadcasting System, WCCO–Minneapolis, August 18 1943", Speeches (Radio) 1942–1945, MHS-K.

210. Ethel Gardner to Dear Mr. O'Connor, August 16 1943, Government Relations (Foreign), Argentina, MOD.

211. "U.S. Polio Foundation, Kenny Split" [*Minneapolis Star-Journal*] September [1943], Scrapbooks, 1945–1952 [sic], James Henry Papers, MHS-K.

212. "Board Plans Review for Kenny Row" [*Minneapolis Star-Journal*] [1943], Scrapbooks, 1945–1952 [sic], Henry Papers, MHS.

213. Howard W. Blakeslee [science editor, AP] "Whispering Campaign" [enclosed in] Blakeslee to Dear Mr. O'Connor, February 21 1944, Public Relations, MOD-K; Kenny to Gudakunst, May 11 1943 [enclosed in] Basil O'Connor to My Dear Mr. Michaels, February 15 1944, Public Relations, MOD-K.

214. "Sister Kenny to Get House" [*Minneapolis Star-Journal*] [August 1943], Clippings, 1941–1946, MHS-K; Kenny to Dear Mary [McCarthy] July 5 1943; Kenny to Dear Mr. Bell, July 26 1943, James Ford Bell, 1942–1946, MHS-K.

215. Minneapolis City Council "Resolution" April 9 1943, Minnesota-Misc., 1942–1945 MHS-K.

216. Kenny with Ostenso *And They Shall Walk*, 267–268.

217. Kenny "Data Concerning Introduction of Kenny Concept"; see also Helen G. Hoeflinger "The Ministering 'Sister'" *The Exchangite* (December 1943) 22: 8–9, 15.

218. Kenny to Dear Dr. Gill, July 19 1943, Evidence Reports 1943–1952, MHS-K.

219. Kenny to Dear Dr. Gill, July 24 1943, Dr. Bruce A. Gill, 1943, MHS-K.

220. Pohl and Kenny *The Kenny Concept of Infantile Paralysis*, 4.

221. Frank R. Ober "Foreword" in John F. Pohl and Elizabeth Kenny, *The Kenny Concept of Infantile Paralysis and Its Treatment* (Minneapolis: Bruce Publishing Co., 1943), 7–8.

222. Basil O'Connor "A Statement" in Pohl and Kenny *The Kenny Concept of Infantile Paralysis*, 9–10. Pohl had privately thanked O'Connor for writing a foreword that he was sure would "lend authority to the work and encourage those who may have some reservations about Miss

Kenny's treatment"; John F. Pohl to Dear Mr. O'Connor, March 8 1943, Box 4, Basil O'Connor Papers, Manuscripts and Special Collections, New York State Archives.

223. Chuter to Dear Sister Kenny, June 29 1943, Wilson Collection.

224. Kenny, "Preface" in Pohl and Kenny *The Kenny Concept of Infantile Paralysis*, 11–13, 21–22, 25.

225. Pohl "Introduction" in Pohl and Kenny *The Kenny Concept of Infantile Paralysis*, 33–38.

226. Pohl and Kenny *The Kenny Concept of Infantile Paralysis*, 42–49, 51–55.

227. Pohl and Kenny *The Kenny Concept of Infantile Paralysis*, 147, 151, 185. This claim had not been accepted by the London committee; see H. A. T. Fairbanks, Macdonald Critchley, E. I. Lloyd, C. Lambrinudi, R. C. Elmslie, George M. Gray, and Henry O. West "Infantile Paralysis and Cerebral Diplegia Clinic at Carshalton" *British Medical Journal* (October 22 1938) 2: 853.

228. Pohl and Kenny *The Kenny Concept of Infantile Paralysis*, 83, 323.

229. Pohl "Introduction" in Pohl and Kenny *The Kenny Concept of Infantile Paralysis*, 37–38.

230. Pohl and Kenny *The Kenny Concept of Infantile Paralysis*, 313–314, 190, 44.

231. Miland E. Knapp in "Discussion of Papers by Drs. John A. Toomey, Jessie Wright and Miland E. Knapp" *Archives of Physical Therapy* (November 1942) 23: 675, 679.

232. Miland E. Knapp "Commentary" in Pohl and Kenny *The Kenny Concept of Infantile Paralysis*, 344–346, 347, 349, 352, 354.

233. Howard A. Howe to Dear Mr. O'Connor, June 17 1943, Public Relations, MOD-K; Walter B. Cannon to Dear Mr. O'Connor, July 9 1943, Public Relations, MOD-K.

234. Howe to Dear Mr. O'Connor, June 17 1943.

235. On Cannon retiring from his position at Harvard medical school in 1942 and suffering from Bell's Palsy, deafness, and other signs of "failing health and rapid aging" see Elin L. Wolfe, A. Clifford Barger, and Saul Benison *Walter B. Cannon: Science and Society* (Cambridge: Harvard University Press, 2000), 476–485, 503–514.

236. Cannon to Dear Mr. O'Connor, July 9 1943.

237. "Sister Kenny Exhibits Skill" *New York Journal-American* November 12 1943.

238. J. D. Ratcliff "Minutemen Against Infantile Paralysis" *Colliers* (October 9 1943) 112: 18, 80–81.

239. "Medicine and the War" *JAMA* (November 27 1943) 123 [abstract]; *Physiotherapy Review* (1944) 24: 35.

240. Editorial "Fact and Fancy in Poliomyelitis" *British Medical Journal* (July 31 1943) 2: 142.

241. Richard Kovacs "[Review of] *The Kenny Concept of Infantile Paralysis and Its Treatment*" *American Journal of Public Health* (November 1943) 33: 1360–1361.

242. Anon. "[Review of] *The Kenny Concept of Infantile Paralysis and Its Treatment*" *New England Journal of Medicine* (July 27 1944) 231: 167–168.

243. [John Coulter] "[Review of] *The Kenny Concept of Infantile Paralysis and Its Treatment*" *Physiotherapy Review* (1943) 23: 139.

244. Mary Macdonald "[Review of] *The Kenny Concept of Infantile Paralysis and Its Treatment*" *American Journal of Nursing* (July 1943) 43: 698.

245. Phil Stewart to Dear Dr. Pohl, June 16 1943, Georgia–Misc., 1942–1944, MHS-K.

246. William D. Sherwood to Dear Doctor Stimson, February 9 1944, Box 2, Folder 4, Correspondence Re Medical Talks, Stimson Papers.

247. Samuel S. Sverdlik, Donald A. Covalt, and Howard A. Rusk "Fifty Years of Progress of Physical Medicine and Rehabilitation in New York State" *New York State Journal of Medicine* (January 1 1951) 51: 90–95.

248. Disraeli Kobak [Editorial] "The 1941 Session in Historic Washington" *Archives of Physical Therapy* (September 1941) 22: 553.

249. "Amputations Without Shock Declared Achieved by Chilling" *Los Angeles Times* September 12 1942; Kenny and Ostenso *And They Shall Walk*, 257.

250. Fred B. Moor to Dear Sister Kenny [September 1942] quoted in Kenny with Ostenso *And They Shall Walk*, 257–258.

251. Kenny to Dear Mrs. Webber, April 6 1942, Mrs. Charles C. Webber, 1941–1951, MHS-K; Kenny to Dear Mrs. Webber, February 27 1942, Mrs. Charles C. Webber, 1941–1951, MHS-K.

252. Glenn Gritzer and Arnold Arluke *The Making of Rehabilitation: A Political Economy of Medical Specialization* (Berkeley: University of California Press, 1985), 90.

253. Miller "Sister Kenny vs. The Medical Old Guard," 41; see also Kenny to Dear Dr. Bennett, March 10 1942.

254. Robert L. Bennett "Recent Developments in the Treatment of Poliomyelitis" *Southern Medical Journal* (February 1943) [abstract] in *Physiotherapy Review* (1943) 23: 81; see also Bennett "The Influence of the Kenny Concept of Acute Poliomyelitis on the Physical Treatment Through All Stages of the Disease" *Archives of Physical Therapy* (August 1943) 24: 453–460 [abstract] in *Physiotherapy Review* (1943) 23: 222.

255. Bennett "Discussion of Papers," 673.

256. William S. Clark to Dear Dr. Pohl, June 23 1943, Ohio-Misc., 1941–1945, MHS-K.

257. Paul C. Carson to Dear Dr. Knapp, July 14 1943, [accessed in 1992 before recent re-cataloging], Am 15.8, Folder 1, UMN-ASC.

258. Walter S. McClellan "Physical Medicine" *New York State Journal of Medicine* (1945) 45: 1426–1428.

259. "Baruch Committee on Physical Medicine" *Physiotherapy Review* (1944) 24: 110–112. Kenny later wrote to Baruch about "a very important International matter before you" but was unable to get an appointment to see him. He replied that "I am not in a position now to do anything more than what I am doing in the field of physical medicine and rehabilitation," adding "I am quite aware of the fine work you are doing"; Kenny to Dear Mr. Baruch, January 30 1950, General Correspondence-B, MHS-K; Bernard M. Baruch to Dear Sister Kenny, January 31 1950, General Correspondence-B, MHS-K. On Baruch see also Margaret L. Coit *Mr. Baruch* (Boston: Houghton Mifflin Co., 1957); William Lindsay White *Bernard Baruch: Portrait of a Citizen* (New York: Harcourt, Brace and Company, 1950); Jordan A. Schwartz *The Speculator: Bernard M. Baruch in Washington, 1917–1965* (Chapel Hill: University of North Carolina, 1981); James L. Grant *Bernard M. Baruch: The Adventures of a Wall Street Legend* (New York: Wiley, 1997). See also "People" *Time* (May 1 1944) 43: 42. *Time* noted that most of the gift would be going to medical schools at Columbia, New York University, and the Medical College of Virginia.

260. W. Lloyd Aycock to Dear Amo [Harold L. Amoss], June 7 1943, Box 1, Folder 43, Aycock Papers, Countway Library, Harvard Medical School.

261. Leona Alberts Wassersug "Prostigmine: A New Wonder Drug" *American Mercury* (May 1945) 60: 599–605.

262. Paul de Kruif *Life Among the Doctors* (New York: Harcourt, Brace and Co., 1949), 179, 306–308; see also "Medicine: Help for Spastics" *Time* (August 5 1946) 48: 57; de Kruif "Many Will Rise and Walk" *Reader's Digest* (February 1946) 48: 79–82.

263. Herman Kabat and Miland E. Knapp "The Use of Prostigmine in the Treatment of Poliomyelitis" *JAMA* (August 7 1943) 122: 989–995; Herman Kabat and Miland E. Knapp "The Mechanism of Muscle Spasm in Poliomyelitis" *Journal of Pediatrics* (February 1944)

24: 123–137; Howard W. Blakeslee "Epidemics Offer Sound Test for Sister Kenny Treatment" *Washington Post* October 3 1943; G. B. Lal "Prostigmine Treatment Benefits Polio Victims" *Washington Post* August 10 1943.

264. Miland E. Knapp "Commentary" in Pohl and Kenny *The Kenny Concept of Infantile Paralysis*, 350; on Kabat's work discussed at the House subcommittee on aid for crippling disease see "New Drugs Used to Aid Crippled" *New York Times* November 30 1944. On the 5-year grant for $175,000 approved to study "Physiological Problems Concerned with the Mechanism of the Disease Process and the Methods of Treatment of Infantile Paralysis" see Diehl "Summary;" see also "'U' Granted $175,000 for Polio Study" *Minneapolis Daily Times* October 13 1943.

265. de Kruif *Life Among the Doctors*, 310–314.

266. "Spastic Diseases Institute Open" *Los Angeles Times* November 13 1948; see also de Kruif *Life Among the Doctors*, 306–307, 325–328; Rickey Hendricks *A Model for National Health Care: The History of Kaiser Permanente* (New Brunswick: Rutgers University Press, 1993); "Three Paralysis Victims Show Therapy Methods" *Los Angeles Times* July 5 1951. The proprioceptive neuromuscular facilitation (PNF) method Kabat later developed became popular among physical therapists and athletic trainers.

267. A.E. Bennett "The Introduction of Curare into Clinical Medicine" *American Scientist* (1946) 34: 424–431; Michael S. Burman "Curare Therapy for the Release of Muscle Spasm and Rigidity in Spastic Paralysis and Dystonia Musculorum Deformans" *Journal of Bone and Joint Surgery* (July 1938) 20: 754–756; see also Lawrence K. Altman *Who Goes First? The Story of Self-Experimentation in Medicine* (New York: Random House, 1987), 74–85; K. Bryn Thomas *Curare: Its History and Usage* (London: Pitman Medical, 1964).

268. Nicholas S. Ransohoff "Curare in the Acute Stage of Poliomyelitis: Preliminary Report" *JAMA* (September 8 1945) 129: 129–130; see also Ransohoff "Treatment of Acute Anterior Poliomyelitis with Curare and Intensive Physical Therapy" *Bulletin of the New York Academy of Medicine* (1947) 23: 661–669; J. D. Ratcliff "Poison For Polio" *Colliers* (September 28 1946) 118: 72, 76–77. Ransohoff, a 1919 graduate of Columbia's College of Physicians and Surgeons, was an attending surgeon at New York's Hospital for Joint Diseases and chief orthopedic surgeon at the Monmouth Memorial Hospital in Long Branch, New Jersey; "Nicholas S. Ransohoff 1895–1951" *Journal of Bone and Joint Surgery* (1951) 33: 817. On the special myograph machine that Ransohoff built to give a visual picture of spasm see Fred J. Cook "Walks Away From Polio Deathbed" *New York World-Telegram* April 29 1948.

269. Scott M. Smith, letter to editor, *JAMA* (November 3 1945) 129: 707.

270. Ratcliff "Poison for Polio," 72, 76–77.

271. Fred J. Cook "New Polio Treatment Waits Tests" *New York World-Telegram* April 30 1948. See also Kenny's comment that "It will be rather amusing, as it is today, when I see all the arguments about the better way to treat spasm and remember how I was ridiculed when I said the condition of spasm existed"; Kenny to Dear Mr. Chuter, November 9 1945, Box 3, Folder 12, OM 65-17, Chuter Papers, Oxley-SLQ.

272. Kenny [Paper May 1943], Louisiana 1943–1944, MHS-K; Kenny to Dear Mr. O'Connor, January 21 1944, Public Relations, MOD-K.

273. Arthur L. Watkins, Mary A. B. Brazier, and Robert S. Schwab "Concepts of Muscle Dysfunction in Poliomyelitis Based on Electromyographic Studies" *JAMA* (September 25 1943) 123: 188–192.

274. R. Plato Schwartz, Harry D. Bouman, and Wilbur K. Smith "The Significance of Muscle Spasm" *JAMA* (November 11 1944) 126: 695–702.

275. Kenny [Paper May 1943].

276. "Research Reveals 'Anxiety Chemical'" *New York Times* May 28 1943; Joseph Moldaver "Physiopathologic Aspect of the Disorders of Muscles in Infantile Paralysis: Preliminary Report" *JAMA* (1943) 123: 74–77; "Kenny Theory Doubted" *Science News Letter* (September 18 1943) 44: 183; "Medicine: Polio Polemic" *Time* (September 27 1943) 42: 60.

277. W. B. Dublin, B. A. Bede, and B. A. Brown "Pathologic Findings in Nerve and Muscle in Poliomyelitis" *American Journal of Clinical Pathology* (May 1944) 14 [abstract] in "Current Medical Literature" *JAMA* (September 16 1944) 126: 192.

278. "Medical Professor Backs Kenny Method" [*Minneapolis Star-Journal* [1943], Scrapbooks, 1945 [sic]–1952, Henry Papers, MHS.

279. Kenny to W. C. Higginbotham, November 22 1943 W. C. Higginbotham, 1942–1946, MHS-K.

280. "Sister Kenny Makes Reply: Answers Criticism in AMA Article" *Minneapolis Morning Star-Journal* [reprinted in] *The A-V* (October 1943) 51: 137.

281. "Medicine: Polio Polemic," 58.

282. W. C. Higginbotham to Dear Sir [Basil O'Connor], September 24 1943, Higginbotham File, Thomas Rivers Papers, American Philosophical Society, Philadelphia.

283. Nicholas S. Ransohoff "Experiences with the Kenny Treatment for Acute Poliomyelitis in the Epidemic of 1942, Monmouth and Ocean Counties, New Jersey" *Journal of Bone and Joint Surgery* (January 1944) 26: 99–102.

284. Richard Kovacs ed. *The 1943 Year Book of Physical Therapy* (Chicago: Year Book Publishers, 1944), 265.

285. Dr. Eliot to Dr. Van Horn Memorandum, June 2 1943, Record Group 102, Children's Bureau, Central File, Box 102, 4-5-16-1, Infantile Paralysis, National Archives.

286. Harold S. Diehl to Dear Doctor Knapp, June 15 1943, Dr. Harold S. Diehl, 1941–1944, MHS-K; Diehl to Dear Doctor Knapp, October 12 1943, Dr. Harold S. Diehl, 1941–1944, MHS-K.

287. Diehl to Dear Sister Kenny, December 1 1943, Dr. Harold S. Diehl, 1941–1944, MHS-K; William A. O'Brien to Dear Dr. Diehl, February 9 1944, Public Relations, MOD-K; see also O'Connor to My Dear Dr. Diehl, June 21 1943, Dr. Harold S. Diehl, 1941–1944, MHS-K.

288. Diehl to Dear Sister Kenny, December 1 1943, Dr. Harold S. Diehl, 1941–1944, MHS-K; Diehl to Dear Doctor Knapp, October 12 1943.

289. Diehl "Summary."

290. Kenny to Dear Dr. Diehl, June 21 1943.

291. In 1942 officials at the University of Minnesota had floated the idea of Kenny speaking at the university's convocation, pointing out that "she is certainly a striking figure to see" and that "the students would be interested in her story." Harold Diehl asked Cole and Knapp "their opinion," and nothing came of it. Indeed Kenny was never given an honorary degree by that university. Malcolm M. Willey to Dear H. S. Diehl, Memorandum, June 2 1942, [accessed in 1992 before recent re-cataloging], Am 15.8, Folder 4, UMN-ASC; Diehl to Gentlemen [Cole and Knapp], June 4 1942, [accessed in 1992 before recent re-cataloging], Am 15.8, Folder 4, UMN-ASC.

292. Unnamed article, *New York Times* June 10 1943, Chuter Scrapbook, OM 65-17, Box 2, Folder 3, Chuter Papers, Oxley-SLQ.

293. Clare Dennison "Citation: Elizabeth Kenny for the Honorary Degree Doctor of Science, The University of Rochester, May 2 1943," Folder 37, Alan Valentine Papers, Rush Rhees Library, University of Rochester.

294. Alan Valentine "Citation: Elizabeth Kenny for the Honorary Degree Doctor of Science, The University of Rochester, May 2 1943," Folder 37, Alan Valentine Papers, Rush Rhees Library, University of Rochester; C. Chuter to Dear Mr. Smith, November 13 1944, Box 3, Folder 12, OM 65-17, Chuter Papers, Oxley-SLQ.

295. Kenny altered her earlier prohibition of lipstick; Mary Kenny recalled that she had "teased her, and she said well, I photograph better"; [Cohn interview with] Mary and Stuart McCracken, April 14 1953, Cohn Papers, MHS-K; see also [Cohn interview with staff of Queen Mary's Hospital for Children, Carshalton] Richard Metcalfe, August 29 1955, Cohn Papers, MHS-K.

296. Chuter to Dear Sister Kenny, June 29 1943.

297. "Sister Kenny" *[Sydney] People Magazine* June 20 1951, 4; [Cohn interview with] Valerie Harvey, March 19 1953, Cohn Papers, MHS-K.

298. Joe Savage to Dear Mr. Dayton, August 29 1947, Public Relations, MOD-K.

299. "Tibbett's Son a Kenny Patient" *New York Times* May 6 1943; Kenny to Dear Dr. Diehl, June 21 1943. For the claim that Tibbett contributed funds to the Institute and later the Kenny Foundation see Hertzel Weinstat and Bert Wechsler *Dear Rogue: A Biography of the American Baritone Lawrence Tibbett* (Portland: Amadeus Press, 1996), 165–169; Tibbett's wife Jane was later involved in fundraising for the Kenny Foundation; see "Norma Heads Kenny Appeal" *New York Times* November 19 1945.

300. Kenny to Dear Mr. Stryker, April 7 1943, Government-Misc., 1943–1951, MHS-K; Jack Delano, Farm Security Administration, Office of War Information Photograph Collection, Library of Congress: http://www.loc.gov/pictures/search/?q=jack%20delano%20kenny, accessed June 12 2013.

301. Yoder "Healer from the Outback," 68.

302. John B. Davies "Sister Kenny Triumphs in America" *Australian Women's Weekly* (March 6 1943) 10: 9.

303. Margaret Buell Wilder "Noted Nurse Gives Hope To Stricken" *Los Angeles Examiner* [March] 1943, Clippings, MHS-K.

304. Jean Barrett "Her 30 Years War Made Sister Kenny Belligerent" *Philadelphia Evening Bulletin* April 22 1943.

FURTHER READING

On the use of the media by government and philanthropic groups in the early and mid-twentieth century see Allan M. Brandt *No Magic Bullet: A Social History of Venereal Disease in the United States since 1880* (New York: Oxford University Press, 1985); Georgina D. Feldberg *Disease and Class: Tuberculosis and the Shaping of Modern North American Society* (New Brunswick: Rutgers University Press, 1995); Evelynn Maxine Hammonds *Childhood's Deadly Scourge: The Campaign to Control Diphtheria in New York City, 1880–1930* (Baltimore: Johns Hopkins University Press, 1999); Bert Hansen

Picturing Medical Progress from Pasteur to Polio: A History of Mass Media Images and Popular Attitudes in America (New Brunswick: Rutgers University Press, 2009); Philip D. Jordan *The People's Health: A History of Public Health in Minnesota to 1948* (St. Paul: Minnesota Historical Society, 1953); James T. Patterson *The Dread Disease: Cancer and Modern American Culture* (Cambridge, MA: Harvard University Press, 1987); Suzanne Poirier *Chicago's War on Syphilis, 1937–1940: The Times, the "Trib," and the Clap Doctor (with an Epilogue on Issues and Attitudes in the Time of AIDS)* (Urbana: University of Illinois Press, 1995); Richard H. Shryock *National Tuberculosis Association, 1904–1954: A Study of the Voluntary Health Movement in the United States* (New York: National Tuberculosis Association, 1957); John W. Ward and Christopher Warren eds. *Silent Victories. The History and Practice of Public Health in Twentieth-Century America* (New York: Oxford University Press, 2007); Jacqueline H. Wolf *Don't Kill Your Baby: Public Health and the Decline of Breastfeeding in the Nineteenth and Twentieth Centuries* (Columbus: Ohio State University Press, 2001).

On the history of therapeutic change see Erwin H. Ackerknecht *Therapeutics from the Primitives to the 20th century* (New York: Hafner Press, 1973); Sydney A. Halpern *Lesser Harms: The Morality of Risk in Medical Research* (Chicago: University of Chicago Press, 2004); Harry M. Marks *The Progress of Experiment: Science and Therapeutic Reform in the United States, 1900–1990* (Cambridge: Cambridge University Press, 1997); Morris J. Vogel and Charles E. Rosenberg eds. *The Therapeutic Revolution: Essays in the Social History of American Medicine* (Philadelphia: University of Pennsylvania Press, 1979); John Harley Warner *The Therapeutic Perspective: Medical Practice, Knowledge and Identity in America, 1820–1885*, 2nd ed. (Princeton, NJ: Princeton University Press, 1997).

Of the history of drugs see Robert Bud *Penicillin: Triumph and Tragedy* (Oxford: Oxford University Press, 2007); Jeremy A. Greene *Prescribing By Numbers: Drugs and the Definition of Disease* (Baltimore: Johns Hopkins University Press, 2007); John E. Lesch *The First Miracle Drugs: How the Sulfa Drugs Transformed Medicine* (Oxford: Oxford University Press, 2007); Elizabeth Siegel Watkins and Andrea Tone eds. *Medicating Modern America: Prescription Drugs in History* (New York: New York University Press, 2007).

PART TWO

4

Polio and Disability Politics

WORLD WAR II invigorated the politics of disability in the United States. As able-bodied workers joined the armed services, groups such as the Disabled Persons Association of America exhorted employers to hired disabled workers. The term "crippled"—still used in charity campaigns—was replaced by "handicapped" with its implications of a dynamic, although inferior, relationship with the able-bodied world. Empowering disability-rights terms such as "crip" were far in the future, but disabled adults began to claim the rights of able-bodied adults and to resist infantilizing medical care, especially in rehabilitative institutions. In April 1943 newspaper reports that the wife of wealthy polio survivor Fred Snite, Jr. was pregnant with the couple's second child made concrete the idea that survivors—even men in iron lungs—were sexually potent.[1] A survey of 45 factories by the National Association of Manufacturers a few months earlier found that 35 had hired "physically handicapped workers" including those who were blind, deaf, or disabled by polio or by the loss of a limb or an eye. Here performing a patriotic duty was mixed with the display of the disabled in a way to humiliate other workers into being more productive. Thirteen blind aircraft workers were called "pace-setters" by their employers, as "without exception, they have stimulated the sighted people around them to increased production." Similarly, the manager of a New England machine tool factory praised 15 "deaf mutes" who were "among our most able and respected employe[e]s."[2]

The link between polio and the war was made tangible by stories of young men who had "overcome" polio and joined the armed forces, the ultimate sign of manly citizenship and therapeutic success.[3] The February 1944 issue of *True Comics*—where "Truth is stranger and a thousand times more thrilling than FICTION"—had a 4-page spread on the "Fight Against Infantile Paralysis" in which a young man overcomes the disabling effects of polio to become a member of the United States Army.[4] The story begins as

149

fellow soldiers tell Philip Hawco "we can't believe you've ever had infantile paralysis! Why you're just like us!" "A few years ago," Hawco explains, "I could hardly move. I sat in a chair all day reading books." Avoiding controversy, the comic does not mention Hawco's specific therapy in the "special hospital" where he is treated, but his therapy is successful enough for him to be able to return "to school and play games." Another soldier says "Gosh, Phil, I thought infantile was hopeless!" "Things have changed since the 1916 epidemic [when]... there was no central agency to which the people could turn for aid," the narrator explains. On the third page Basil O'Connor appears, a man who "serves without pay, giving willingly of his time and his keen intellect to guide the crusade." The following panel (11 out of 18) shows Kenny, her hands around the knee of a patient, being watched by a doctor and a nurse. Reflecting the popular link between the National Foundation for Infantile Paralysis (NFIP) and Kenny, the narrator says: "The Foundation sponsors unending research work and new experimental methods. In 1940 it introduced the Australian nurse Sister Kenny, and her revolutionary treatment into the United States." On the last page one panel shows a pie chart divided in half, indicating the division of NFIP funds: help for patients and providers in local communities and "special grants" to "scientists seeking the cause, prevention and cure of infantile paralysis." The story concludes with a quote from Franklin Roosevelt as able-bodied children run over grassy hills: "While we fight the global war we must see to it that the health of our children is preserved and protected [and]... help them win their victory over disease today."[5] Here the global war abroad is on par with the war on polio at home.

Not until near the end of the war, when disabled veterans became a political force, were government-funded rehabilitative services expanded as alternatives to charity "homes" and orthopedic hospitals. Ironically, the infrastructure created by New Deal programs made access to services even more difficult. As one polio survivor noted bitterly, the new "churches, libraries, colleges, post offices, courthouses, city and state federal buildings [and]... railway stations" funded by the Works Progress Administration and built in the neoclassical style, had flights of steps and stairways "which are either impossible or very difficult for people of faulty locomotion." "I used to dream that when I grew up I'd make a lot of money... and put stout hand railings on all the steps in the world," she declared. A magazine writer and not a millionaire, she could not see any "single good reason" why these buildings should not have ramps and railings.[6]

Despite a growing emphasis on older polio sufferers, the problem of "crippled children" remained prominent in public and philanthropic policy. New Deal funding for children with disabilities codified in Section V of the 1935 Social Security Act had been one of the least controversial parts of Roosevelt's expansion of government services. The Act had expanded the federal Children's Bureau and provided funds to welfare and public health divisions of state governments to survey the numbers of disabled children and the facilities for them, and then to expand those services.[7]

The harsh edge of living with a disability in the 1930s and 1940s was heightened by a widespread acceptance of eugenics. Americans who discriminated against the disabled made no distinction between people born with a disability and those who had become disabled through injury or illness. Mothers, fathers, doctors, and physical therapists knew—in ways disabled children slowly recognized—that physical disability was associated with the eugenically unfit who were placed outside the possibilities of a future with love, fulfillment, and economic independence. Not only were disabled children and adults stereotyped as "defective," but many lived in family homes dependent on the physical assistance of their relatives. Speaking from bitter experience, a nurse whose legs were paralyzed by polio appealed to all family members who agreed to help the disabled to try not to approach this task as a "grim duty."[8] The despair of the physically disabled was often hidden but well understood. When one physician who worked at the Children's Hospital in Cincinnati developed polio and was put in an iron lung he begged his fellow residents to kill him with morphine because he was convinced that if he survived he would have a "tortuous" future.[9]

Indeed, the disabling consequences of polio were frequently raised to explain why public funds and attention should be directed to polio rather than other diseases with high mortality but not "the grim wreckage it [polio] leaves behind."[10] In a *Washington Post* column soaked in pity, Mal Stevens, a physician and college football coach, reminded readers not to forget to "help the boy who keeps the score." His image of this boy was the opposite of a happy, athletic American boy: "sports develops grace and stamina and strength—This disease destroys those very things."[11] Similarly, a March of Dimes radio spot asked "Have you been grumbling because you have to walk more, ride less, these days? Then think for a moment of those who cannot even walk...the children crippled by infantile paralysis."[12]

KENNY AND DISABILITY

Rehabilitation in the 1940s was based on 2 assumptions, one old and one new. The first was that survivors must embrace the work ethic as hard work (like exercising muscles) inevitably brought results (with the concomitant idea that lack of improvement was the patient's own fault for he or she had been lazy and not worked hard enough). The second was the idea of psychological adjustment. Rehabilitation was intended to "normalize" people with disabilities to accommodate them to society. Disabled people were expected to develop especially strong egos to cope with the prejudice and discrimination they would experience in the world outside the hospital. Such "therapy" was predicated on personal transformation, not on social, cultural, or political change.

Writing in the *Johns Hopkins Nurses Alumnae Magazine*, Lucy Chase Woods advised other disabled "comrades" to "hold on to whatever physical independence you have with every ounce of strength you possess." She urged them to "release yourselves from sensitiveness" for "in the long run it matters very little how you get up from a chair! What matters is your attitude toward it."[13] Here she was asking them to ignore their anger at the pity and horror they experienced and to cope by adjusting themselves as individuals to the discriminatory, able-bodied world.

Americans associated assistive devices such as wheelchairs with old or sick people, and braces and crutches were feared symbols of social inadequacy.[14] Parents sometimes removed such apparatus when their disabled children went to the movies or to church or for some other social occasion. Above all, walking, as disability activists have pointed out, was the "Holy Grail of recovery," proof that a patient had worked hard and overcome his or her disability.

Born in the 1880s and coming of age during the eugenics era, Kenny believed that some disabling conditions made people less deserving of citizenship and respect. She shared a prejudice against people with mental disabilities. To mock her critics, for example, she referred to facts "that can be proven to the most feeble minded lay person."[15] But she stressed the aptitude and resiliency of people with physical disabilities who were able, she believed, to combat paralysis with intelligent cooperation. Indeed, she argued, the efficacy of her work with cerebral palsy patients showed that—despite widespread assumptions—such patients were not mentally disabled. After all, she told Australian physicians in the 1930s, "imbeciles cannot be treated successfully."[16]

Like all promoters of rehabilitative work, Kenny highlighted the social indignities faced by anyone visibly disabled, arguing that her work could prevent "a lifetime of disability and the humiliation of being an object of pity."[17] During the Great War she had worked with soldiers disabled by meningitis and battle wounds and since the 1920s with children disabled by polio and cerebral palsy. In her experience patients termed "incurable" could be helped to gain flexibility, muscle strength, and, sometimes, significant functional power. Her work therefore challenged some of the widely held assumptions about the rehabilitative prospects of the disabled and helped to bring patients with polio out of family back rooms and "crippled children's homes."

Kenny's work made extraordinary transformations of paralyzed bodies routine by redefining "normality" and "deformity." In the 1920s and 1930s orthopedic nurses had defended the use of plaster splints and casts as crucial to spare patients "the mental and physical pain of a hideous deformity."[18] But this was not how Kenny saw it. A deformed body, in her view, was a stiff, ungainly, weak body; in her work, recovery was measured by flexibility and strength, not the response of a particular muscle in a muscle test. She was proud of the number of her patients she had discharged "with a trace of restricted movement" whom she termed "fully recovered" as well as those who left the Institute "handicapped but not crippled."[19] A determined and optimistic clinician, she did not believe, as one orthopedic nurse pointed out, that "true paralysis" could be "distinguished from mental alienation until spasm of the opponent has been completely released and persistent muscle re-education given a satisfactory trial."[20]

Medical observers noted that many of Kenny's "recovered" patients had "flail" arms or legs and atrophied muscles. Such conditions were "certainly deformities," the editor of *Archives of Physical Therapy* noted, yet the patients had "no contractures or misalignments of joints" or common signs of weakened muscles such as scoliosis.[21] The Kenny treatment created a new dialectic of ability, combining functionality with a redefinition of normality within a disabled form. Her patients, Kenny argued, left her care no longer "deformed" although their muscles did not always have fully recovered function. When she referred to "the cruel aftermath of the dwarfed, deformed body so frequently seen in the crippled children's schools," she was identifying bodies that were visibly inflexible and not functional, leaving a child segregated from ordinary educational and social experiences.[22] To identify the success of her own work, she pointed to evidence of the new kinds of bodies it allowed polio survivors. She made much of the fact that no child in Minneapolis diagnosed with polio from 1940 to 1943 had been admitted to the city's "crippled" children's school. The majority of her patients at the Institute, she reported in 1943, had "returned to normal life"; some had left "to live a normal life slightly handicapped"; and the "remaining 2 percent" with more severe paralysis were nonetheless able "to earn their own living" at home and were "living active, normal lives."[23]

The bodies of her recovered patients also countered orthodox fears of overstretched muscles without proper resistance and reflexes, for "none have developed deformities."[24] Kenny's medical supporters shared this view. "We have not seen one deformity, not even a foot drop, develop in patients under treatment despite the fact that no splints have been used," Alfred Deacon reported in 1942.[25] During an outbreak of polio in San Antonio, 2 physicians noted, only 2 patients who had refused Kenny treatment developed "considerable muscle contracture and beginning deformity."[26]

The iron lung was another controversial polio technology that had been introduced during the 1930s to be used for severely ill patients with paralyzed respiratory muscles but it often had disappointing results.[27] Kenny argued that iron lungs were usually unnecessary and "of very doubtful value." She was not frightened of respiratory (or bulbar) paralysis, believing that patients could learn to breathe again with careful nursing and properly placed hot packs. "In many instances," she claimed, the iron lung could "debar the patient from making a satisfactory recovery."[28] Her decision to take selected patients out of the iron lung and use hot packs to treat the spasm in their neck and chest muscles shocked and impressed many hospital staffs. Unlike many polio experts who continued to rely on the iron lung, despite many unsuccessful experiences, Kenny made it another symbol of harmful orthodox practice.

Kenny's dislike of assistive supports fit with the widely popular view that braces, crutches, and wheelchairs were horrific marks that would relegate a patient to a life of discrimination. When she took off her patients' braces, this action threatened not just the stability of orthopedic authority but also the patient's physical autonomy. She promised an alternative stability based on supple and strong muscles. This was a new kind of body—a healthy body that was nonetheless disabled. She taught her technicians, further, to handle patients not as china dolls but as feeling, pliant bodies. Opera singer Marjorie Lawrence recalled how horrified she had been at Kenny's initial examination in which "she laid me face downwards on the bed and grasping me by either ankle bent my legs as far as they would go. Then she rolled me over and endeavored to push my legs up and over until my big toes nearly touched my forehead." At hospitals in Mexico City and Hot Springs, Arkansas, Lawrence had been handled "as though I would fall apart" and "doctors and nurses were forever cautious not to 'stretch' my muscles."[29] Kenny's procedures demanded patient involvement, and although polio care continued to be medicalized, her methods were performed by technicians and sometimes family members in conflict with the wishes of supervising physicians.

In other ways, however, Kenny's work reinforced conventionality, especially in her acceptance of traditional gender roles for her patients, roles that she rejected in her own life. Like many antisuffragists who took to the lecture stage in order to convince the public that a woman's place was in the home, Kenny encouraged parents to see functionality for their daughters as the ability to marry and look after a house, while getting a job was the sign of success for their sons. Her own career choices were starkly different. She had not become a farmer's wife like most of her sisters in Australia, and in the United States her work enabled her to achieve a middle-class life far from bush nursing in rural Australia.

During the 1940s the power of Kenny's view of disability was enhanced by her emerging reputation as a celebrity. Her 2 1943 books provided stories of her life and work as struggles against orthodoxy for the transformation of disabled polio survivors. Both books challenged medical skepticism and both sought to remake polio as a disease in which families and patients were crucial proponents in shaping medical care and defining scientific truth. Like First Lady Eleanor Roosevelt, who was a politically engaged and outspoken activist, Kenny was combative and authoritative.[30] In 1942 women seniors at Hunter College were asked to identify the "greatest living women." Thirty percent chose Eleanor Roosevelt and the remaining votes were split among Kenny, Chinese nationalist Madame Chiang Kai-shek, Anne O'Hare McCormick (a *New York Times* reporter who was the first woman to win the Pulitzer Prize in 1937 as a foreign correspondent), and Dorothy Thompson, known as the "First Lady of American Journalism."[31] When Kenny began to make friends in Hollywood and RKO announced it would make a film of her life starring Rosalind Russell, her celebrity status grew even further.

KENNY, ROOSEVELT, AND THE DISABLED

The most prominent polio survivor was Franklin Roosevelt, the man who had battled his paralysis and been elected governor of New York in 1928 and President in 1932. After he had bought Warm Springs in the 1920s and turned it into a polio rehabilitative center, he was fondly known as "Doc Roosevelt" for his efforts to show other polio survivors how to exercise their muscles under water. As president he regularly attended Thanksgiving dinners there and continued to use Warm Springs as a place of retreat, staying in his specially built "Little White House." At Warm Springs he was feted as a success yet also recognized as a disabled man, an identity that he strove in every other part of his life to finesse.

Roosevelt was the first American president to make a disease "his disease." His advisors made much of his transformation from polio victim to polio patron and featured his name, voice, and body in NFIP publicity. In 1943, for example, the *National Foundation News* showed Roosevelt seated, surrounded by Hollywood stars who had written, directed, and acted in a movie whose profits were to be donated to the NFIP.[32] As a symbol of polio recovery, we know now, Roosevelt was a fraud. He had managed to gain the highest political office, but at the cost of having to pretend, at least in public, that he could walk and stand like an able-bodied man. Reporters typically praised his physical ability and love of sailing.[33] A crippled body, a crippled mind, and a crippled life—this was the cultural equation that every polio survivor had to fight.

Kenny recognized how important Roosevelt was to the NFIP, to her patients and their families, and to polio politics nationwide. She had written to him several times in the early 1940s, explaining her work and reminding him that polio paralysis was "of national importance to your country."[34] In May 1943 Kenny asked the president's secretary whether she could dedicate her autobiography to him. In the wake of the arrival of General MacArthur in Australia and the alliances between Australian and American forces fighting the Japanese expansion through the Pacific, Kenny and her "fellow Australians" considered Roosevelt "the saviour [sic] of our country." She suggested a meeting in order to receive his permission in person.[35] The answer to this request, O'Connor advised the president's secretary firmly, "by all means should be 'NO.'"[36]

Nonetheless O'Connor recognized that if he did not organize an opportunity for Kenny to meet Roosevelt it would seem like a snub. Reporters sometimes said that Roosevelt had taken a deep personal interest in Kenny's work, and, while there is no evidence that this was true, the White House did receive a number of letters urging the president to recognize Kenny and allow her to introduce her methods at Warm Springs.

Finally, on June 8 1943 Kenny met the President in a carefully choreographed lunch with O'Connor, who had asked for 5 minutes to see Roosevelt beforehand for "there are some things about Sister Kenny that I should tell him."[37] Photographers took official pictures of the 3 of them: Roosevelt seated, Kenny standing over him, and O'Connor nearby. These pictures were used by Kenny and by sympathetic reporters for the rest of her life.[38] She was unable to boast about the content of her meeting. In most other situations Kenny refused to take O'Connor's advice but after this meeting she headed his warnings, perhaps because they were reinforced by the Secret Service. "I could not write and tell you anything about my visit with the President," she told a friend a few weeks later, "O'Connor cautioned me that I was not to do so."[39] Still, although she dedicated her autobiography to the "Mothers of Mankind" rather than to Roosevelt, her book made much of her visit to the White House. She praised the president's "deep humility" and "personal charm," and recalled how she had been "inordinately excited at the prospect of sitting down to luncheon with President Roosevelt."[40]

As for the President, we know little about what Roosevelt thought about Kenny and her work. O'Connor had advised Roosevelt not to agree to allow Kenny to dedicate her book to him, adding that she "writes awful stuff."[41] Warm Springs became a training site for physical therapy and incorporated aspects of Kenny's work but not to her satisfaction—and she was never invited there. Only after Roosevelt's death did Kenny, on

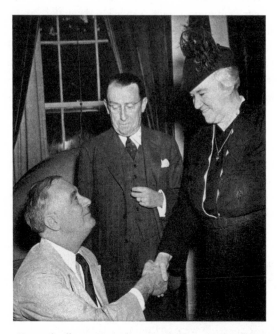

FIGURE 4.1 Kenny finally met President Roosevelt in 1943, photographed here with Basil O'Connor carefully positioned between them; Elizabeth Kenny with Martha Ostenso *And They Shall Walk: The Life Story of Sister Elizabeth Kenny* (New York: Dodd Mead & Co., 1943, 1960), opp. 256.

occasion, refer to this 1943 meeting to defend her distinction between her work and standard physical therapy. "In conversation with the late President Roosevelt," Kenny remarked in October 1945, "I explained my approach to this disease. He (Mr. Roosevelt) drew my attention to the fact that my work was not physiotherapy as he had experienced it, but was a more advanced science and therefore should not be confused with present day physiotherapy."[42] Roosevelt may well have noted how different her methods were from the ones with which he was familiar. Perhaps he had agreed that hers was a "more advanced science," perhaps he was just being polite, or perhaps she made this remark up.

NOT JUST CHILDREN

A sentimentalized picture of "crippled children" had long defined the public image of polio, leaving adult polio survivors invisible. As the children of the polio outbreaks of the 1910s and 1920s became adults, and as new epidemics targeted teenagers and adults, the popular term "infantile paralysis" came to be seen as a misnomer. By 1943 U.S. army officers recognized polio as a problem among adult soldiers, not only their children, and demanded guides to managing the disease. During the 1940s the term "polio" was used to designate polio survivors and later as a shortened form for the disease itself.[43]

A growing number of teenagers and adults began to articulate how liberating Kenny's work was. (Although the loin cloth she required her patients to wear, which looked uncomfortably like a diaper, continued to infantilize patients of all ages.) Survivors such as Henry Haverstock, known as Kenny's "first" American patient, were quoted in national magazines and shown standing without crutches.[44] Haverstock and Kenny's other older patients spoke of how impressed they were with this new kind of clinical encounter: her refusal to treat patients as fragile, her willingness to perform tests that might be initially painful or demand significant muscular strength, and her matter-of-fact attitude, offering hope without pity.

"Crippled children" looking adorable and pathetic never left center stage in polio philanthropy. But letters from hopeful and sometimes angry teenagers and adults struck by polio found that Kenny's methods fit their identities well as they confronted a world that rejected them in their efforts to gain economic independence and personal happiness. Adjustment was considered their task, not the responsibility of those who made them feel inferior and unwelcome. Buildings were impossible to enter, schools unwilling to accept them, employers unwilling to hire them, and "shut-ins" seen as a legitimate role.[45] In December 1943, for example, 54-year-old Phil McGrath, a basket-chair maker, celebrated his fiftieth Christmas at the Home for Incurables in Washington, D.C., where he had been brought as a 4-year-old child with polio and "never since left."[46] An identity as a disabled activist was possible, but it was a heavily constrained role. In the early and mid-twentieth century the adult Helen Keller fought for the rights of those who were blind and deaf, but, as her biographer Kim Nielsen has shown, whenever Keller ventured to discuss topics outside disability, she found able-bodied audiences suspicious, convinced that those speeches were written by others because she, as a disabled woman, was easily manipulated and politically naive.[47]

The NFIP made much of polio survivors who surpassed the ordinary. The January 1942 March of Dimes campaign featured Nancy Merki and Jean White, "two girls who fought their way back from infantile paralysis affliction." Merki, 15, from Portland, Oregon, had won the world freestyle record, and was later an Olympic swimmer; White, 19, from New York, was a roller skating champion.[48] But the NFIP seems to have been unclear about how these examples related to the majority of survivors whose recovery was less complete. At a reception at the Waldorf Hotel reporters were shown "a 5-year-old boy, hobbling along merrily on crutches" and behind him "tall, strong, good looking Nancy Merki" who looked "like the popular conception of the American high school girl." "Someday, if all goes well and money keeps coming into the great fight against this bone-wrecking disease," NFIP officials explained, "Jerry and kids like him will be as straight and as strong as Nancy."[49] But the discrepancy was not explained. Was it the right therapy? Or luck? Or hard work?

Like many adult survivors, Marjorie Lawrence discovered that, despite her celebrity reputation, her disability left her unemployed. In what newspapers called a "poignant scene," Lawrence returned to the stage of the Metropolitan Opera to sing at a special testimonial concert "in tribute to the courageous spirit of Marjorie Lawrence."[50] Reporters described the "steps" she was taking and her belief that "I will walk again," but this story of "a dramatic and successful 'come back'" was never achieved.[51] Once it became clear that she would be unable to walk, Lawrence lost her position at the Metropolitan although she continued to sing in concerts and on the radio. She entertained troops during World War II, and later taught opera at Southern Illinois University and the University of Arkansas at Little Rock, but she never again appeared in an opera.[52] Neither the director of the Metropolitan Opera nor of any other opera company believed audiences would be comfortable with her visible disability.

NFIP officials recognized that their work shaped the public's views of disability. While they did little to counter popular misconceptions about polio and did not lobby for greater access for the disabled to the working world, some chapters did use polio survivors as volunteers. The NFIP's New York office employed a few survivors on the staff, although with no fanfare.[53] The NFIP defined polio rehabilitation in strictly medical terms, boasting of the myriad crutches, braces, and other equipment it provided, a view reinforced by the orthopedic surgeons on its medical advisory committees. Indeed, officials were suspicious of all recovery tropes, whether by Kenny or anyone else. When a young man in a wheelchair was featured on a page of the *National Foundation News*, one Minnesota donor asked "what courage and hope any afflicted person can get from viewing a crippled-for-life person" compared to a fully recovered patient like a girl recently discharged from the Kenny Institute? "Now that would be a real example to hold out to others, but not if she would have come out crippled for life."[54] Attention to the disabled was as legitimate as extolling the recovered, Don Gudakunst replied. "Do not forget that the National Foundation holds forth a great deal of hope even for those who are permanently crippled by the disease," and "even those who have been so severely crippled can have and are entitled to have our help." While Gudakunst continued to believe that Kenny's work offered the greatest possibility of recovery, he also tried to distinguish the serious work of medical science from the unrealistic optimism of her supporters. "There is no cure and there are no miracles that will completely restore loss of function when large amounts of the central nervous system have been destroyed."[55]

One rare example of an explicit programmatic effort by the NFIP to promote new ways of thinking about disability appeared in 1943. "Infantile Paralysis Patient," a poem published in the *National Foundation News* and widely reprinted, presented 3 ages of attitudes toward the disease: the dark ages of revulsion; the recent past of scorn; and today's era of medical intervention and recovery. In grandfather's day, a polio survivor was mocked and pitied: "poor wretch," he was a "neighborhood curiosity," "his crippled bones barred him from 'polite' society,'" and it was seen as a waste of time and money to educate him. In father's day, the "poor fellow" was seen by his family as a burden, by his community as a necessary evil, "society tolerated him with ill-concealed disfavor," schoolteachers "humored" and sometimes "abused" him, while girls "tittered" and boys "jeered." Today, experts recognize the first symptoms of polio, "modern surgery performs miracles on his distorted limbs," "hot baths and X-ray treatments revitalize his tortured body," "psychologists brighten his future and broaden his outlook," "his mother and father weep with joy, his friends cheer him on," and "at last through God's mercy and Man's skill he is cured." Instead of pity, "We HELPED. Lucky Boy! He HAD infantile paralysis."[56] Here, starkly, the polio survivor is fully medicalized, as the work of medical and psychological experts help him overcome his disability so that society will not discriminate against him. And as a result, his family and friends can joyfully welcome a survivor whose body is no longer marked by the disease.

PATIENTS AND PARENTS

The public had always had a say in polio therapy: whether to take a paralyzed child to a hospital or clinic, whether to follow the advice of the doctor or nurse, whether to remove braces and other apparatus after the child had been released from the hospital, and whether to take the child to follow-up orthopedic visits and allow orthopedic surgery. Family resistance had long been reviled by professionals and explained as the result of ignorance. When polio expert Robert Lovett argued for the necessity of rest, he admitted "in nothing is it harder to secure the cooperation of the parents." So firm were these refusals to cooperate that Lovett saw these other children as useful trial subjects. To assess his methods he had "a fair number of controls in the children of unintelligent parents who have refused to follow the prescription of rest."[57] In his view, only the children treated by his prescription of rest and splinting were able to recover to the fullest possible extent.

Kenny's work, recognized by physicians and sponsored by the NFIP, offered a respectable way to counter a doctor's advice. When one young man who was paralyzed in both legs was told he needed a plaster cast, his father refused, telling the doctors "no son of mine will ever be put in plaster to make him a cripple for life." The parents then contacted Kenny who sent one of her technicians.[58] Similarly, 2 tenacious, "hard-to-convince" parents were outraged when a neurologist told them that their son "would never walk again," a comment "that, in our opinion, was merely his opinion." They insisted that the hospital call a consultant who advised "using the Kenny treatment for which the hospital had to order packs and other equipment." After a month the parents agreed to move their son to another hospital but found it provided only "stringent, run-of-the-mill, assembly-line treatment" that they believed "did our boy more harm than good." Finally the specialist "admitted he had made a great mistake," and the parents took their son to the Kenny Institute in Minneapolis.[59] Unfortunately we have no record of whether he was ever able to walk.

From the outset Kenny's work demanded a major role for her patients' family care-givers, which in most cases meant the mother.[60] In 1943 Georgia Fischer came to Minneapolis from her home in New Orleans to learn "the treatment" for her son Phil who was a patient at the Institute. After they returned home, the mother was "besieged with telephone calls and letters" from other parents with paralyzed children. "We will ever sing your praises," Mrs. Fischer assured Kenny, and "it is a great satisfaction to be able to con-tinue his treatments."[61] Kenny's publicized experience with improving the lot of chronic patients left many families determined to continue her methods for years. In 1941 Mr. and Mrs. Howard Allen of Glencoe, Minnesota, had talked with Kenny and had their son examined by Pohl. Two years later they were still "putting on hot packs and doing correc-tion exercises daily" but wanted to bring him to the Institute to be sure that they were "doing the exercises etc in the correct manner so that they will really do him some good."[62] Involving parents in this physically demanding work was difficult, especially since most assumed that doing it properly would ensure a full recovery.

Kenny's textbooks left a certain ambiguity about the level of professional training nec-essary for her work. Although her training courses were targeted to professionals, polio survivors and their families saw them as a potential resource. In January 1943 when newspapers announced that Kenny was coming to teach a course to physical therapists at New York University, letters from parents with disabled children flooded in asking to take it as well.[63] Although Kenny stressed the professional nature of her technicians when talking with doctors and physical therapists and bemoaned the level of teaching at centers other than the Institute, she did not discourage members of the public from thinking they could apply her treatment at home. When she visited Los Angeles in 1943, for example, she not only met with physicians and nurses at local hospitals but also gave a public lecture illustrated with projected pictures and answered questions from moth-ers.[64] The problem of the improper use of the Kenny method was as much a "result of popularization through Kenny's own publicity as anything else," a NFIP publicist com-mented. Kenny did not stress properly "WHO gives treatment…how can she blame people from thinking anybody can do it, and that doctors aren't necessary?"[65] Journalists also featured success stories of parents who used the Kenny method without special-ized training. In its February 7 1944 issue *Newsweek* ran a story about a mother of 8 from Warrenville, Illinois, who heard about Kenny's methods and took them into her own hands. She "prepared steaming, sterilized packs" and after 3 months her son Dwight could do farm chores.[66]

When Kenny decided to dedicate her autobiography to "The Mothers of Mankind" she was characterizing patients with polio as children and their mothers as their primary caregivers. Her emphasis on mothers also reflected her tendency to sentimentalize her work, ignoring the fact that she and her technicians worked almost exclusively in institu-tions and that she believed hospitals were the best places to provide both acute and reha-bilitative polio care. By the mid-1940s Kenny talked more often about teaching mothers to continue the exercises and hot packs she recommended *after* the child had left the hospital.

In their search for the best care for their child, parent after parent wrote to Kenny, tell-ing her how they had disregarded the doctor's orders, and all reported that they were glad they had. One 4-year-old girl had spent 2 years in the Eastern New York State Orthopedic Hospital in Schenectady. When she was discharged in 1942 her doctors told the parents that her muscles had improved as much as possible and advised an operation to stabilize her ankles and then a spinal fusion when she was older. She came home wearing a body corset and 2 full-length braces, unable to sit up without support and allowed only a half an hour each day to try. After 3 months without much improvement the parents "disregarded the doctor's orders, took her braces off during the day, and let her play on the floor as long as she wished." Before each day's exercises they gave her a hot bath followed by a cold shower. Now, the parents reported proudly, with casts only on her feet to keep them from turning inward, she was crawling and pulling herself up by holding onto a chair.[67]

BODIES ANEW

The promise of functionality and the hope of counteracting the psychological and social trials of living with a disability attracted teenage and adult survivors and their families. Paralyzed by polio in 1931 Betty Adler was treated at the Baltimore Children's Hospital-School and then at Warm Springs. Adler wondered whether Kenny's methods would give her "the possibility of recovering sufficient muscular power to enable me to again walk and resume a normal existence." She had "read almost everything by and about you, I have so much hope in what you have to offer."[68] A Jersey City woman requested treatment for her 22- year-old son who had both hands paralyzed because he was "so sensitive about his condition—especially when friends about his age visit him for while and then leave hurriedly for a dance, date or other social activities."[69]

A determination to conquer paralysis and to ignore the pessimism of doctors pervaded the letters Kenny received. In 1934 doctors had told Dorothy Meissner that she was a hopeless case and would never walk again. Eleven years later Meissner, now a high school student in Morristown, New Jersey, wrote to Kenny. After the doctors gave up on her, she and her mother had devised special exercises even though "the hospital which I attended every day did not know I was doing this." She then demonstrated her new-found strength to the hospital staff who "were greatly pleased and thought it wonderful but warned me not to try and stand." She ignored this advice, "thinking that if I did not ever walk again I would not want to live." After a year and a half Meissner walked into the hospital "and all the doctors gathered around and, Sister, they couldn't believe their own eyes." Her picture and story were in the newspapers. She was now one of the best tennis players in her school, and could also swim, ice skate, roller skate, and ride horses.[70]

Others wrote asking advice after they listed in detail what they had done for themselves. Charlotte Birch, a 23- year-old woman from Brooklyn, had spent almost 2 weeks when she was 19 years old in the Kings County Hospital with the left side of her body paralyzed. "I begged to be taken home and at home my parents had a nurse give me massage and hot applications to my hand and foot." She also "practiced walking when no one was watching." Within a year she had been able to return to work and was satisfied that now "few people can tell that there is anything wrong with any part of my body," although her hand was "still not right." For Birch, her search for therapeutic help made Kenny's expertise crucial. "I was determined to walk and I did and I have the same determination for my hand but I can't remedy it with just determination."[71]

A DIFFERENT KIND OF POLIO

Kenny's version of polio care—with cheerful, comfortable and active patients—was an inversion of standard institutional care. It also challenged the pervasive fear of polio infection. In dramatic stances she stood next to her patients, usually without any mask, touching their bodies, completely unafraid.[72] Patients with polio and their families were used to being stigmatized. Some neighbors were so frightened that they would not raise the windows on the side of their house next to the home of a stricken patient; people living in the same block would walk on the other side of street to avoid passing close to a patient's house, even after the patient had been taken to the hospital. Many rooming houses and hotels refused to rent rooms to anyone who had been exposed to polio.[73] "Years after I had polio," a survivor recalled, "when adults saw me coming they would say out loud to their children to stay away from me because they could 'catch' it."[74]

Inside hospitals the staff also stayed away from those who worked with polio patients. One hot packer learned she was "in the 'dread ward'" when she went into the hospital's kitchen and "the negro woman almost swooned in terror, saying that so long as I wore that robe, I mustn't go near anyone, nor into any part of the hospital, other than the rooms where the polio was confined."[75] During an epidemic in Florence, Alabama, polio nurses at the Eliza Coffee Memorial Hospital, sitting in the hospital's dining hall, were shunned initially, and "ate hurriedly feeling as miserable as a person who has failed to don a conspicuously necessary article of wearing apparel."[76] By the late 1940s, however, the courage of Kenny technicians as well as a substantial increase in the numbers of patients led to a decline in such strict contagion rules, and even masks were not used on many polio services.

Kenny's work, unlike standard care, made much of the pain of polio—its clinical significance as well as its emotional toll, and the relief that hot packs could provide. For Kenny pain was central to the disease, not an unfortunate side effect of best care, and she spoke of the "tragedy" of orthodox care that left patients with "a look of pain and fear."[77] This pain, which she argued most doctors could not explain, suggested to her that supposedly normal muscles were in fact directly affected by the polio virus and must be treated. For her pain was a diagnostic sign. She began treatment almost at once "while the patient was still in great pain," arguing that if technicians waited until the end of the 3-week isolation period, stiffness would have started, "deformities have begun to develop, [and] precious time has been lost."[78] Skeptical orthopedists mocked her highlighting of this symptom, arguing that this was the kind of thing an emotional, poorly trained woman would do.[79]

The popular press loved this debate. The "old treatment" was "painful" and "produced miserable results," *Colliers* reported, but with Kenny's methods, "pain disappeared in two to three days—instead of lingering for as many weeks."[80] A Buffalo supporter described the faces of the children: "I saw no eyes deeply gouged with pain; I saw no foreheads lined with agony; I saw no lips thinned with suffering. Everywhere was a spirit of optimism, confidence, cheerfulness."[81]

Some physicians, such as the editor of the *British Medical Journal*, admitted that they had frequently denied the significance of pain in polio, and it was a "matter of reproach that we have so long evaded the questions raised by this striking symptom."[82] Those physicians who already disliked Kenny and her claims to have transformed the management of polio, however, discounted this emphasis on pain. "In spite of the fact that Sister Kenny harps on the idea that the disease is accompanied by excruciating muscle pain, this

has never in the experience of most of us been an outstanding symptom," Virginia orthopedist Robert Funsten declared in 1944. Pain was usually present only "when movement
is a factor" and was always relieved by immobilization.[83]

Kenny and her patients saw the neglect of polio pain as a sign that physicians did not
listen to their patients. Many of her medical opponents, Kenny argued, believed that
"pain is not an important feature of the disease [but]...this is not the opinion of the
patients."[84] Mary Lou Drosten, who "endured four weeks of hell on earth" during her
hospital stay, recalled that the staff did nothing to relieve her "pain and discomfort."
She had "no hope in my heart until I learned of the Kenny treatment."[85] William Foote
Whyte recalled his "constant and intense pain" in his paralyzed legs in the early 1940s,
and the hot packs used at the Massachusetts General Hospital, which "relieved my pain
and helped me relax, at least temporarily."[86]

Doctors, nurses, and physical therapists found that the use of Kenny methods made the
task of maintaining their patients' morale much easier. Kenny's attention to ameliorating
pain also led patients to be more cooperative in muscle training. Indeed many child patients
saw muscle reeducation as a game. If Kenny's methods were more "generally employed,"
one New York physician argued, "there will not occur so many of the emotional and physical wrecks that we see even now, in spite of much of the expensive orthodox treatment."[87]
Kenny's focus on alleviating physical pain was also linked to physiological health. Patients
who had not had Kenny treatment, according to Ethel Calhoun, a Michigan physician who
was a strong Kenny ally, "had severe atrophy and impaired circulation, with blue extremities,
dripping with perspiration, and often with ulcers present," while the skin of Kenny-treated
patients was "soft and pliable" with good circulation and "very little atrophy." Such clinical
signs meant that patients could hope for a kind of visible normality. "These patients often
remark that they are very thankful they do not look deformed."[88]

In both the Kenny treatment and in orthodox polio care, however, muscle stretching to
try to achieve full motion was still required, and even with muscles relaxed by heat it was
still painful. Polio care had long been based on a fear of stretching muscles improperly,
but Kenny was confident that "no muscle is being stretched as long as it is within its normal arc of motion." In one of Kenny's bold analogies, she argued that to overstretch a del-
toid, "a hole would have to be made in the side of the body and thigh and the arm drawn
into the hole toward the center of the body."[89] "Most people find the stretching very painful," Kenny told Ray Gullickson, a Minneapolis patient, but he could manage this pain
by recognizing that "pain is just a signal from your body that something is wrong. Once
you recognize why it is happening, you don't need to feel the pain anymore." Her advice
"sounded really sensible" to Gullickson, who recalled thinking " 'Hey, if it means I'm making progress, I don't need to feel the pain.' And that's really how I felt about it. I've been
able to manage persistent pain ever since that day."[90]

A DIFFERENT KIND OF PATIENT

Kenny's techniques demanded that patients themselves, even toddlers, be active and
knowledgeable participants in muscle exercises and learn the location of muscles and "the
resultant action of the joint and parts when the insertion of a muscle is pulled upon by
the contraction of the muscle."[91] Orthopedist Wallace Cole said that Kenny's patients were

given a simple course in muscle anatomy and shown "with the aid of medical illustrations, the position of the muscle and how it works."[92] "Sister Kenny explained to me exactly what they were going to do and how they were going to accomplish it," one patient recalled. "She took my right hand in hers and pointed to a muscle in my wrist. As she tapped the muscle with her finger tip, she told me that muscle was the one we were going to start with, and when that muscle started to work, we'd do another and another until we got them all working...she told me to repeat the exercise until I was too tired to continue."[93]

Making a patient "muscle conscious" was quite contrary to standard rehabilitative work with children.[94] Indeed Kenny and her technicians exhibited child patients to show the efficacy of the techniques. "Boy how I hated being wheeled out in front of a bunch of poking and prodding doctors," Clemson Griggs wrote to Kenny, recalling his experience in the early 1940s as a patient for 9 months in the university hospital in Minneapolis. Kenny would tell the audience "'Now, Mr. Griggs you tell your story!' You don't realize how hard it is to make a speech with no clothes on when you are lying flat on your back and looking at the ceiling...I consider that 9AM performance my small contribution to your work." He remembered that he had learned "a lot of about muscles and their work. I can still rattle off quite a few of them, but they are getting hazier all the time." Griggs was now the head of a hacksaw factory in Middletown, New Jersey, had 3 children, and enjoyed ice skating, and concluded "I bless you and your 'quack treatment' more and more every day of my life."[95]

Warm Springs physical therapist Alice Lou Plastridge had been "very much impressed with the way Sister Kenny teaches the exercises." Patients were made "muscle-conscious" to such a degree that "even little six year old children would put their fingers on the outside of their hip if you asked them what pushed the leg sideways."[96] Even 2- and 3-year-old children were taught the Latin terms for their muscles. A favorite story during Kenny's early years in Minneapolis—repeated by Lois Miller in the *Reader's Digest*—concerned Suzy, a 3-year-old girl who named each individual muscle of her thighs and calves "by its long Latin name."[97] A New York physician mocked the idea that paralysis could be improved "by hot packs and finger manipulation, or by educating 4 or 5 yr old children by

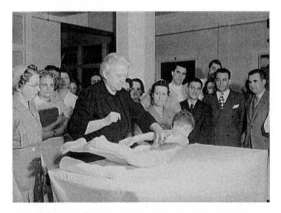

FIGURE 4.2 Jack Delano, a New Deal photographer, depicted Kenny demonstrating an acrobatic move by an Institute patient during a class for nurses and physicians, February 1943. Courtesy of the Library of Congress, Prints & Photographs Division, FSA/OWI Collection, LC-USW3- 017586-D [P&P] LOT 768.

talking." In particular, the idea of telling Suzy, identified by the *Reader's Digest* as a "colored girl," to "flex her Gluteus Maximus & she did" was "absurd."[98] In reply pediatrician Philip Stimson protested that this element of Kenny's work was effective and rational. "As for teaching little children to know the names of muscles, I myself have heard the four year old colored girl name and flex 8 or 10 of her muscles."[99] That Kenny's methods gave even young patients the psychological confidence to talk back to skeptics was a delightful example of Kenny's lack of deference to medical authority; that the girl in question was identified as "colored" made it for contemporaries even more shocking.

Her muscle exercises worked, Kenny argued, because they helped patients reconnect a "physiologic block." Initially even sympathetic medical observers assumed that she was simply using different language to talk about ways to teach patients to avoid muscle substitution (the use of a strong muscle to substitute for a weak or paralyzed one). Winnipeg orthopedist Alfred Deacon, for example, praised the way patients were taught the normal action of muscles to prevent "attempts at muscle substitution." Deacon was not sure that Kenny's methods really enabled patients to reestablish a pathway between nerves and muscles, but he did find that teaching patients "to think of and gradually to achieve motion in the affected muscles" showed impressive results, whatever the mechanism.[100]

The connection between mind and body, and the faith that the mind could—with proper training—address faulty neurological connections was, however, fully accepted by many of Kenny's patients. Haverstock recalled in 1942 that Kenny had showed him "exactly what a muscle does." "Miss Kenny would ask me to concentrate while she trained a muscle, and after a lot of training, I could move it myself."[101] Kenny's treatment depended on patient participation. She had trouble dealing with a patient who "was not cooperating with his treatment and just lying in bed, feeling sorry for himself," another patient recalled. "I could tell that she had very little patience left [for] ... it was obvious that she'd rather work with people who were willing to try and get well."[102]

Professionals unwilling to believe that Kenny's methods had any neurological effect argued that teaching patients muscle knowledge and giving them an active role in physical therapy was simply a useful psychological tool. After Toinette Balkema, head physical therapist of the Children's Orthopedic Hospital in Seattle, returned home at the end of her Kenny course, she reflected "your method of reeducation is completely reasonable, very satisfying and successful. The children express great liking for the stimulation, probably because it tends to release tension. They also show interest in the passive exercises and are pleased when their cooperation warrants active work."[103] Army psychiatrist Charles Bohnengel saw Kenny's muscle training methods as "chiefly a psychotherapeutic measure" based on reassurance and suggestion, which were "well-established methods of psychotherapy." In "An Evaluation of Psychobiologic Factors in the Re-Education Phase of the Kenny Treatment for Infantile Paralysis" published in *Psychosomatic Medicine*, Bohnengel argued that the "cheerful, hopeful, confident atmosphere" of hospital wards using Kenny's methods exerted "a strong influence over emotional forces within the individual," especially compared to the "general environmental and sociologic attitude of gloom and dread" typical of hospitals practicing "older methods of treatment." Patients who "learn to identify by name and physiologic action all of the important muscles of the body ... derive pleasure from this accomplishment." Unlike surgery and splinting in which patients were expected to subject themselves "passively to mechanical manipulation," here the patient played "an intrinsic and active role in the treatment." Bohnengel was also impressed by Kenny's attention to the grace of muscular activity, which he compared to older methods which often resulted in "awkward and ungraceful muscular movement."[104]

As newspapers and popular magazines described—in exaggerated ways—this new polio therapy that promised so much and depended on a patient's active participation, polio survivors, especially teenagers and young adults, began to criticize the institutions that did not offer this kind of care. After graduating from the Johns Hopkins nursing school, Kathryn Holman joined the Army and, while waiting for her call, worked with patients at the Baltimore Children's Hospital-School during a polio epidemic. When Holman herself was struck by polio—an unusual but not unknown consequence of caring for patients with polio—she became a patient at the Hospital-School under the care of Henry and Florence Kendall. "Fed up" with the way she was being treated, Holman wrote to the *Washington Times-Herald*, saying, according to the newspaper, "I know that Sister Kenny will be able to cure me...I want to get well so that I can devote my life to fighting this dire disease."[105] She arrived in Minneapolis a month later, and, as a reporter's purple prose phrased it, "the doors of the Kenny Institute in Minneapolis and the arms of the white-haired crusader will open as a healing haven for the stricken young girl."[106] A few weeks later Holman's father told Kenny that "Kathryn's improvement since she has been under your care has been so great as to be almost unbelievable." He added that he wished "our own government [would] endow the Kenny Institute with millions, and set up branches all over the country to take their training from you before you went back to Australia."[107] Holman's mother added that her daughter "is so happy and writes often of what an inspiration you are to her."[108]

THE DRAMA OF RECOVERY

Embolded by Kenny's work, polio survivors spoke out, defining what they considered best care and reasonable expectations as a disabled person. But another group, usually the most articulate and authoritarian in polio care, was increasingly demonized and silenced. Orthopedic surgeons, especially in the letters that Kenny received, were disliked and feared. Perhaps it was their stock in trade—the operation and the knife.[109] Kenny herself frequently argued that her work would prevent the necessity for surgical operations.[110] Many times parents wrote to Kenny telling her how they had refused to allow their child to undergo surgery, and, against the orthopedist's advice, had removed leg braces, stomach corsets, or other apparatus. Jean Renel of Detroit had spent 2 weeks in the hospital with casts on both legs. The hospital doctors then took the casts off and gave her braces for the next 16 months and a few "lamp treatments." Her family doctor told her parents she needed surgery "but we refused an operation and then the doctor said [it was] no use [to] give her lamp treatments any more because that will not help her." At home Jean's parents removed the braces and took her to a chiropractor. Jean now had "no deformation" of her legs and could walk, but her parents hoped that Kenny's methods would stop her from being "a toe walker."[111] When Kenny removed braces and stomach corsets it was dramatic because she did it in a clinical setting, in front of physicians and nurses, as a public show of rejecting the machinery of orthodoxy. Parents' quiet removal of such apparatus in their own home was no less of a rejection.

To show the extent of her patients' recoveries, Kenny developed a dramatic final demonstration. Her recovered patients were taught a series of acrobatic techniques, showing not only physical flexibility but impressive strength and balance. "These are no merely acrobatic stunts," Kenny and Pohl's 1943 textbook explained, "but an examination of paramount importance in safeguarding the future welfare of the patient."[112] It was regrettable, Kenny told one Associated Press reporter, that a short film produced for the 1943 March of Dimes campaign had shown children walking with crutches. "If the picture had been presented from the Institute we could have shown cases who were helpless in bed, unable to lift their heads, could not sit up, stand or walk [and] . . . months later could turn somersaults backwards."[113]

When Alice Plastridge saw such a demonstration she was amazed. The children were asked to walk on tip toes and on their heels, hop on each foot, squat on one foot and come to standing without touching the other foot to the floor, come to a sitting position lying on a table without using their arms, bend forward putting their foreheads on their knees, and lying on their backs bring both legs over their heads to let their toes touch the table. The exercises, Plastridge thought, "seemed pretty drastic and severe . . . but surely proved there could be no stiffness or spasm there."[114] The Kendalls had also noted examples of "extraordinary flexibility" among Kenny's patients. Their notes listed the exercises Kenny asked one boy to do:

1–Legs over head
2–Trunk rais[e] & legs supported
3–Knees to nose—sit on bottom
4–S[i]t—Knees legs
5–S[i]t on toes, on heels
6–Ly—Turn ft in—all
7–Face lying—rocking on abdomen.[115]

This kind of flexibility and strength was dramatic, but it did not always inspire the kind of awe Kenny hoped for. After their visit to Minnesota, for example, the Kendalls began a series of studies to see whether such acts were developmentally normal for young children.[116] In evaluating results of polio therapy, Cleveland pediatrician John Toomey observed dourly, a patient "does not have to have acrobatic litheness, and his muscles do not have to be trained to the point where he doubles himself into a knot, for he is a plantigrade animal [and] as soon as he start[s] to walk again he begins to have some contraction of his muscle arcs and some slight limitations."[117] Orthopedist Albert Key similarly agreed that Kenny's patients were "very limber and are able to do certain gymnastics which normal patients would have difficulty carrying out [but that] . . . this is merely a matter of training and practice."[118]

Most of all, physicians were uncomfortable about the ways that Kenny used her patients' bodies to reinforce her claims about the harm that "orthodox" treatment could cause. Assessing progress was considered the province of the supervising orthopedist, although physical therapists were the daily judges of muscle strength. Kenny looked at the bodies of polio survivors and saw not destroyed neurons or patients who had not followed the instructions of professional supervisors but improper care by medical professionals. Of course the context mattered: Kenny made these statements in front of patients and their families. Key was therefore outraged that Kenny had announced in front of 4 patients she had called "hopeless cripples" that "had they had the Kenny treatment they would now be normal." "This was a cruel statement to make before the patients," Key remarked, "and there was no evidence that it was true."[119] "The remark made by me would have had no effect upon the patient," Kenny retorted after she read Key's complaints, for "as, unfortunately he had been painfully aware of the truth. He was also aware of the improvement that change of treatment had brought about."[120] Patients, she claimed, well understood the limitations of their bodies and the kinds of therapy they hoped would transform them.

Her frank prognoses disturbed professionals trained to hide not only diagnoses they considered too psychologically difficult for patients to handle—like the likelihood of a lifelong disability or a terminal illness—but also the incompetence of a fellow professional or their disagreement with a colleague. Patients and their families frequently shopped among physicians, but they usually heard dissension only from practitioners outside orthodoxy, reinforcing the sense of physicians as members of an exclusive club. Polio experts frequently refused to admit the extent and permanence of a patient's disability. Miland Knapp, for example, said that he "always withheld a poor prognosis. Such information depressed the patient and usually discouraged cooperation with the program of rehabilitation."[121] "On my husband's insistence," Marjorie Lawrence recalled in 1949, "the verdict [diagnosis] was kept from me." When Lawrence was finally told, she became, just as many physicians feared she would, very depressed.[122]

Toomey was also appalled by Kenny's cavalier optimism. "The public unfortunately has come to believe that certain methods will definitely cure paralysis despite the fact that each patient is an individual problem," he told a meeting of physicians. She claimed that if patients had been treated a certain way "they would have made a better recovery." "It is cruel to encourage the patient or his family in such a thought because it is utter nonsense...Why not be honest and face the unpleasant, yet obvious fact that some people will be paralyzed despite any type of treatment?"[123]

Yet here was Kenny in the ward of a hospital in Minneapolis or Little Rock or Wilmington, talking about hope and the possibility of change. Truth-telling to patients— even in the context of therapeutic optimism—was a striking break from mainstream medical norms, and, like Kenny's physical examinations, felt authentic to many patients and their families who disliked the evasion common in therapeutic encounters.

A HERO?

For many disabled Americans and their families Kenny became a hero. "She is worshipped by former paralysis victims who owe their recovery to her courage and selfless devotion," said one Los Angeles journalist with typical hyperbole.[124] Polio survivors and their families were impressed not just with the results of her work but also its provocative challenge to standard medical assessments. Kenny "miracles" were usually performed in front of reporters and parents along with medical staff and members of hospital trustees. In such performances she was shown teaching doctors things they did not know. At Brooklyn's Adelphi Hospital, while reporters and the medical staff watched, 8-year-old Jerry Silverman "smiling confidently, climbed upon the clinic table." Doctors had said his leg would always remain paralyzed. "Under the soothing hands of the nurse the child relaxed. Slowly she manipulated the child's thin, left leg. In a few minutes it began to twitch. She turned to the boy's doctor and advised him to continue the procedure."[125]

As a source of inspiration, Kenny stood as a complicated lesson. "I am a crippled girl, only one of the many who are cripples today because the American Medical Association would not recognize your method when you first started it 32 years ago," Clara Hulberg of North Dakota wrote in April 1943. She was going to frame Kenny's picture "as you deserve that much honor from any Cripple," and she would remind the head of the AMA "never again to make a similar mistake in regards to other ailments now considered incurable but which may someday be cured by a simple method found by someone like you."[126] "This great woman," an Iowa mother declared, "has given to the world a new concept of this much dreaded disease." She wished every polio survivor "could see me use my 'paralyzed' legs to keep my house and go to market, or see me use my 'paralyzed' arm to hoe tomatoes and spank my babies."[127]

PAIN?

It is striking that absent from all the letters, memoirs, and articles written in the 1940s and 1950s by and about polio victims treated by Sister Kenny and the Kenny method are negative comments about the treatment patients received.

In its early stages acute polio was a painful disease, and the hot packs and exercises used by Kenny, even in the hands of the best trained technicians, must have increased this pain. The packs were made of pieces of woolen blanket cut to size, boiled in a sterilizer, picked up with forceps, and passed through a tight wringer twice to get rid of every drop of water to avoid burning the patient. They were supposed to be covered with a piece of a rubber sheet, then a dry piece of blanket and another dry towel to preserve the heat of the hot packs. It was complicated and exhausting work, and initially the NFIP had paid for nurses to take a special short course in "hot packing." But later much Kenny treatment was delivered by untrained volunteers supervised by often overworked technicians, especially during epidemics, and by parents who had only a sketchy knowledge of how the treatments should be given. The Los Angeles Orthopaedic Hospital had a shortage of packers, Kenny technician Ruby Green reported in 1943, "and those we have aren't too good, Sister, but they have been very cooperative with me in my wishes and are becoming more observing and conscientious."[128] What is clear, as Daniel Wilson has shown in his recent analysis of polio survivor memoirs, is that there were also many sadistic therapists and nurses. It took skill and care to apply hot packs in a way that did not hurt or burn a patient, and sometimes there was neither skill nor care.[129] Sometimes even kindly packers applied packs carelessly and without awareness of clinical counterindications. In the early 1940s a New York physician mentioned during a discussion of polio therapy that he had heard about a patient "with a temperature of 106 F. being treated with fomentation. They about burned him to death and he died."[130]

In light of all this and the painful graphic memories recounted in the memoirs of polio survivors published in the 1980s and 1990s it is amazing that virtually all of the accounts by polio survivors written in the 1940s and 1950s as well as letters to newspapers and magazines articles were so positive. Psychiatrist Charles Bohnengel spoke of wards of smiling children, and reporters described children "laughing and treating their exercises as a game."[131] Many polio survivors clearly tried to forget or explain away their bad experiences with polio therapies. If they mentioned discomfort, they blamed themselves for not having adjusted to the problems of paralysis or not having the mental and physical stamina to work hard enough to gain the necessary muscle strength.

It was not until the 1980s and 1990s that survivors began to recount painful graphic memories of their months of treatment. The only records from the 1940s we have that describe the negative side of Kenny's method are the complaints of overworked nurses. A pediatric nurse at Mount Sinai Hospital in the 1940s recalled a visit from Kenny when "we had no air conditioning. To use hot, steam packs on a hot, steamy day was very trying. We had to run those hot packs through those wringers and then wrap them in a waterproof covering so that that [the] bed wouldn't get too wet."[132]

ALTERNATIVE OPTIONS

When families avoided doctors or ignored their advice, St. Louis surgeons McCarroll and Crego referred to the result as "no treatment." But, in fact, families seeking polio care chose from a range of treatments outside the orthodox health system. Alternative practitioners ran health spas and other facilities that offered services that orthodox medicine provided poorly, such as care for chronic and disabling conditions. The character of these practitioners varied considerably. Some, like chiropractors, osteopaths, and naturopaths, identified themselves as members of an alternative profession critical of orthodox medicine. Some were medical entrepreneurs who directed private rehabilitation centers that accepted referrals from hospitals and private physicians, some promoted a particular medical system or technique, and others were outright health profiteers. Indeed, the growing visibility of polio epidemics along with "the wide publicity of your birthday parties," as one alternative therapist told Roosevelt, had "brought into being a new vocation" as many patients fell "into the hands of inexpert persons...with semi-medical experience."[133] Techniques such as hydropathy, manipulation, and massage, as orthopedists, physical medicine physicians, and physical therapists recognized unhappily, were "exploited by poorly educated technicians or adherents of cults."[134] All were practitioners who, one orthopedist admitted ruefully at an AMA annual meeting in 1944, "the man in the street" often confused with the orthopedic specialist.[135] Beyond debates about medical practice and professional legitimacy were even more destabilizing issues around what constituted proper evidence to drive medical progress. Naturopaths, antivivisectionists, and other long-standing critics of medical science hailed Kenny as one of their own. When she spoke of doing clinical research at the Institute, antivivisectionists heard her promote research outside the experimental laboratory, a "medicine without monkeys." When she spoke of hot packs and muscle exercises developed in the isolated Australian bush, naturopaths heard her talking about natural, drugless healing that should be available to every man and woman.

Kenny sought to tread a narrow path. She continued to attack elements of medical orthodoxy, including leaders of organized medicine who, she claimed, sought to hinder the expansion of her work. But she also argued that her work was scientific and deserved the respect of elite scientists. She complained that the NFIP, the U.S. Public Health Service, and the Rockefeller Foundation had not sent a research man to the Institute and she began to call her work (awkwardly) "the newer science of dermo-neuro-muscular therapy." Her proposal to make the Institute a research center was intended to attract basic scientists such as her old ally Queensland anatomist Herbert Wilkinson. At the same time she was careful not to attack unorthodox healers. When she refused to ally herself publicly with particular groups who sought her allegiance, she explained that she had promised her

Australian mentor that she would "stick to the orthodox path." This sounded like a choice made as a personal vow rather than a decision to denigrate practitioners outside organized medicine. The letters she received from naturopaths, chiropractors, and others suggested that many did not see her as antagonistic to the alternative path, just politically savvy.

THE BERRY SCHOOL

The best known alternative polio therapist in the 1920s and 1930s was Milton H. Berry, director of the Berry School for Paralysis and Spastic Correction. Born in San Francisco in the 1880s, Berry had worked as a newspaper and shoe-shine boy, a "rub-down" assistant for college football players, the manager of a Turkish bath, and began working as a paralysis specialist in the 1920s.[136] Located on 2 acres in Encino, California, the Berry School was "completely surrounded by orange, lemon and walnut groves," a secluded location "ideally adapted to the concentration necessary in the work." The School, which Berry promoted as "the most famous paralytic correction center in the world," was intended to be "a clinic as famous in its way as the Mayo Brothers' sanitarium [sic] in Rochester, Minn."[137] Its practice was based on Berry's "unique field of Patho-kinesiology," a distinctive method of muscle re-education. Berry claimed distinctive professional ethics to distinguish him from other kinds of healers for he was willing to turn away prospective patients who he felt he could not "cure."[138]

Although Berry did not work solely with polio survivors, his institution, clinical practice, and attitude to orthodox medicine were strikingly similar to Kenny's. "Patho-Kinesiology," a term Berry said he had coined, was "the science of bodily motion and locomotion as it concerns the individual who is physically sub-normal." Like Kenny's work, it involved a special way of reading the body that linked muscle action and brain function, it claimed scientific accuracy, and it relied on careful muscle training and the active participation of patients. The school's use of systematized rehabilitation in a beautiful setting set it apart from most children's homes and orthopedic hospitals. His patients were "not ill," he said, "only physically handicapped. They should be taught, not treated." Almost all his patients, Berry estimated, had been seen by orthopedists or other doctors, and been told that nothing more could be done for them.[139] Well versed in California's strict medical practice laws, he used no drugs and performed no surgery, but instead "locates the trouble with his fingers, parts adhesions of the muscles, freeing cords and nerves and veins, then brings the power of the patient's mind into play." Like Kenny he emphasized functionality. He promised his patients they would "walk better, farther, faster, with less limp and gait conspicuousness, with more ease and assurance, and with less crutch apparatus" and that the use of such devices as a single-bar leg brace, "from a front or side view almost completely hides the brace from the calf down... [and] can hardly be seen on older girls who wear the proper skirt length."[140]

Berry's fundamental principles were, he claimed, "not understood or taught by any one other than myself," and his methods were "radically different and superior to any of the orthodox methods used by orthopedic hospitals or by orthopedic surgeons." Like Kenny, Berry sought not to market or patent his work but to have it integrated into mainstream medical practice so that "the extensive teaching of my methods" could lead to "a very grave and lasting benefit to the world." And, he also claimed, his work was "no secret" and "no doctors or scientific men have been denied the privilege of witnessing my work."[141]

He wrote to President Roosevelt several times asking that his method of treatment "be embraced" by the newly established NFIP and reminding him that besides research the NFIP's chief aim was "to combat the after effects of polio."[142] Berry also began a campaign "to enlist the support of the physical education departments of universities of America." His 1939 pamphlet *A Challenge on Behalf of Crippled Children to the Universities of America: Victims of Infantile Paralysis Need Not Hospitals...But Muscle Training; Not Doctors...But Trained Teachers* asked for "an unprejudiced committee of the heads of the Physical Education Department [to]...investigate my method and my records, and compare them with the record of Orthopaedic Institutions." Doctors, he explained, unlike physical educators, were not taught "kinesiology (bodily movement)" and therefore did not understand the action of muscles in live bodies.[143] Recognizing that he had to demonstrate that his methods did not depend on himself, Berry pointed out that he had trained his 2 sons, which proved "that the work can be transferred to others." Any man or woman with a full knowledge of anatomy could "acquire proficiency in the use of my methods, under my instructions in a term of, say, two years."[144]

The most powerful source of evidence proving the value of this work was, Berry believed, its efficacy. He had worked "personally upon the bodies of some three thousand crippled victims." Three-quarters had returned to normal and more than 20 percent of the remaining group "returned to physical independence."[145] The dramatic effect of his clinical skills allowed him in 9 seconds to diagnose one boy's foot in which "muscles had adhered, grown together. The cord was imprisoned, and tightened. It had drawn the foot up on one side, twisted it grotesquely." Telling the boy, "'this may hurt you a little, but it will make a new boy out of you,'" Berry "parted" the muscles with "a loud 'pop' that could be heard in the next room," and the following day the child was able to place his foot flat on the floor. Comparing the "forty years of failure of orthopedic doctors" to "my forty years of success," Berry was confident that "there can be no other method except the one I use that can bring about these results."[146]

In December 1939 Milton Berry died and his son Milton Berry, Jr. took over the direction of the Berry School.[147] Berry Jr. considered Kenny an interloper and a competitor. He and members of his school's board of directors contacted her several times during the 1940s. At first he wished her success, noting that "the Berry Organization...had pioneered in a somewhat similar method as early as 1915" and agreed with most of her principles "in dealing with Poliomyelitis in its early stages." Kenny's reply, in Berry Jr.'s view, was "rather caustic." She stated that she "alone had pioneered this theory" and declined a series of invitations to visit the Berry school.[148] He began to warn Kenny that publicity around her work, including newspaper articles stating that "you have a cure for Spastic Paralysis" and that "you made it possible for a veteran to walk alone, without crutches, after only one Kenny treatment," were instilling "false hope into the hearts of paralyzed individuals." As president and national medical director "of the largest paralysis correction...organization in the world," Berry Jr. challenged Kenny "to a demonstration of your technique in the correction of post-polio and Spastic Paralysis conditions." "If you can prove that you have a method of paralysis correction superior to ours" then the hundreds of his patients "should have the opportunity of knowing about it." He proposed that members of the press should be present "so that thousands of others may know of the results of this demonstration."[149] Kenny ignored this offer.

It may have been Berry Jr.'s frequent invitations that Kenny had in mind when she was quoted a few months later in the *New York Post* saying "if the legitimate medical professional doesn't want my method, osteopaths and chiropractors and practitioners of that sort will be glad to get it."[150] Kenny intended this statement as a threat to orthodox physicians, reminding them of the appeal of alternative therapies and the potentially greater challenge of Kenny as an explicit antiorthodox clinician with impressive public support.

DISABILITY CHANGES

World War II veterans played a major role in shaping disability care during and after the war, laying the groundwork for the disability rights movement of the 1960s and 1970s. During the war when there was a lack of able-bodied workers physical disability was not considered a reason to limit employability; as one magazine article noted in 1944, "there are no cripples in wartime."[151] But after the war ended and thousands of able-bodied veterans returned to the workforce, it grew more difficult to argue that a disabled body was not a defective body. While occasional popular films such as *The Best of Our Lives* depicted physically disabled actors who were themselves veterans, the wider public continued to see physical "normality" as a sign of civic "normality."[152] Numerous civic groups continued to urge employers to hire disabled veterans but less as a gesture of patriotic pride than as a kind of patriotic pity. Although, as one veteran who had been paralyzed by polio in 1942 reflected, "disability is mainly in the eye of the beholder," there was, he added, often "a gap between a disabled person's view of his own disability and other people's view of it."[153] And this view affected more than employment. Disabled veterans, even those whose disability was the result of combat or a disease contracted while in the military, were less likely to marry than able-bodied veterans.

During the war military physicians redesigned hospital rehabilitation care to enable disabled soldiers to return to battle more rapidly. At the Fitzsimons General Hospital in Denver, Colorado, for example, there was a special convalescent ward where patents were "not pampered" or "permitted the lax discipline of the usual hospital ward, but are rehabilitated under a strict military regimen under the direction of army sergeants." These patients supposedly "revel[ed] in this type of management."[154] Howard Rusk, who became one of America's main spokesmen for what came to be called vocational rehabilitation, set up convalescent training programs in air force hospitals to get men into physical condition to return to full duty in the shortest possible time. In these programs a soldier was "taught what he was doing and why he was doing it." Rusk found this kind of care reduced the period of convalescence for soldiers with many infectious diseases, including pneumonia, measles, and scarlet fever. When veterans entered these programs the aim was "to restore them to active participation in their communities" and "to return to their daily lives as self-respecting, self-sustaining, dignified citizens with a definite community contribution to make."[155] The term "handicapped" developed as a positive term for recognizing restrictions in functioning but not as an indication for the inability to be educated or employed. Thus, the Handicapped Persons Industries of Buffalo, a toymaker that employed only disabled people, noted the "innate desire of self-respecting men and women to earn an honest livelihood and live a life of usefulness, despite physical handicaps."[156] In Rusk's popular text *New Hope for the Handicapped* (1946) he argued that "one of the great social values of the war was a more widespread social acceptance of physical disability."[157]

Physicians in civilian hospitals began to experiment with active rehabilitation even for postsurgical patients. In maneuvers that would have seemed familiar and perhaps ironic to Kenny, proponents began to talk about the benefits of postsurgical ambulation. Medical journals such as *JAMA* published articles warning of the danger of prolonged periods of bed rest as "anatomically, physiologically and psychologically unsound and unscientific."[158] Even *Time* devoted a feature to the topic, noting that specialists in obstetrics, abdominal surgery, arthritis, and heart disease all agreed on "The Evil Sequelae of Complete Bed Rest."[159]

In an even more striking moment proponents began to describe standard postoperative practice in a way that conveyed both the ordinariness of the hospital ward and also its unseen dangers, much as Kenny had often done. Thus, Kristian Hansson noted in the *New England Journal of Medicine* that "it has become familiar to all to see wards full of patients lying flat in bed, absolutely quiet and guarded against moving by nurses." This kind of medical practice, he warned, led to painful necks, aching backs, and stiff knees; lost muscle tone that could lead to atrophy; disturbed blood circulation that could result in congestion, edema, and perhaps thrombosis; and irritated skin that might lead to ulcers and bedsores. While Hansson did not want to propose any "radical" changes, he did make an analogy to Kenny's methods compared to previous polio care. Her methods may not have cured more patients but they had led to patients "in better general health and with better circulation and muscle function than the old immobilization treatment produced."[160]

Immobilization in polio care—and increasingly for other medical conditions as well—came to be mocked as a practice of the sadly mistaken medical past. Thus, in a photo essay on polio's 100-year history *Hygeia* contrasted a naked girl crawling with "helplessly distorted limbs" to 4 photographs depicting modern polio care of 1947. "Today's young polio patient," the magazine explained, did not "experience the immobilization that was endured by the child of a century ago."[161]

The notion of an independent, self-respecting disabled person spread slowly into wider medical and popular culture. A 1945 nursing article entitled "The Disabled Can Be Independent" reminded nurses about patients with disabilities "of long standing" where "little or nothing has been done to prevent or repair the havoc caused by wasted muscles, faulty posture or inactivity." Such patients could gain confidence with the use of short training crutches (such as Kenny used) to accustom the body to a gradual change of position and shift in weight bearing and help develop the muscles of the upper body.[162] Polio survivors played a crucial role in this transformation. Able-bodied Americans recognized the hard-working, overachieving attitude of many survivors. Thus, one school classroom had a contest to see who could do the most sit-ups and pushups. According to a New York reporter, when one boy did so many that nobody could beat him the other children said "Aw, what ya expect? He had polio."[163]

A few physicians began retrospectively to blame patients for the continuing use of braces and crutches. Joseph Molner argued at a postgraduate course on physical medicine and rehabilitation in 1946 that such apparatus had "long been recognized by the medical profession as capable of producing what virtually amounts to addiction among patients, or an obsession on the part of the patient to the effect that he cannot get along without the crutch or brace. Some of this is mental, some physical, some physiological, and mechanical."[164] On occasion, professionals recognized their own part in this problem. Warm Springs orthopedist Charles Irwin admitted in 1947 that "splints often produced more deformities than they prevented" and that too often in the past physicians had "made a superficial examination of an infantile paralysis patient and simply telephoned the brace maker to go by the isolation ward and fit him with the necessary braces."[165]

NOTES

1. "Fred Snite, Jr., Again to Be Dad" *Washington Post* April 11 1943. Snite contracted polio in Beijing in 1936.

2. "13 Blind Workers Are Pace-Setters In Aircraft Plant" *Washington Post* December 27 1942.

3. See "Surgery Made Polio Victim Fit for Army" *Washington Post* February 21 1942.

4. "Fighting Against Infantile Paralysis" *True Comics* (February 1944) 32: 26–29. For an additional analysis of this comic see Bert Hansen "Medical History for the Masses: How American Comic Books Celebrated Heroes of Medicine in the 1940s" *Bulletin of the History of Medicine* (2004) 78: 148–191.

5. "Fighting Against Infantile Paralysis," 26–29.

6. Reinette Lovewell Donnelly "Watch Your Steps" *The Polio Chronicle* (February 1933) 2: 3.

7. See Ralph M. Kramer *Voluntary Agencies in the Welfare State* (Berkeley: University of California Press, 1981), 58–61.

8. Lucy Chase Woods "A Traveled Road" *Johns Hopkins Nurses Alumnae Magazine* (January 1943) 42: 21.

9. James Yamazuki, quoted in Julie Silver and Daniel Wilson *Polio Voices: An Oral History from the American Polio Epidemics and Worldwide Eradication Efforts* (Westport, CT: Praeger, 2007), 21. Yamazuki was paralyzed by polio in 1949 and was in an iron lung.

10. J. D. Ratcliff "Minutemen Against Infantile Paralysis" *Colliers* (October 9 1943) 112: 18.

11. Mal Stevens [guest columnist] Considine "On the Line" *Washington Post* January 14 1942.

12. "Radio Spot" January 20 1943, National Foundation for Infantile Paralysis, Box 96, Folder 1943, George L. Radcliffe Papers, MS 2280, Maryland Historical Society, Baltimore.

13. Woods "A Traveled Road" 20–21.

14. See, for example, C. L. Lowman "The Use of Splints and Brace: Part 1" *Physiotherapy Review* (1943) 23: 57.

15. Elizabeth Kenny to Ladies and Gentlemen, [July 1944], Am. 15.8, Folder 23 [accessed in 1992 before recent re-cataloging], UMN-ASC.

16. R. W. Cilento "Report on Sister E. Kenny's After-Treatment of Cases of Paralysis Following Poliomyelitis," Ms. 44/109, Fryer Library, 4.

17. Elizabeth Kenny to Ladies and Gentlemen, [July 1944].

18. Jessie L. Stevenson "After-Care of Infantile Paralysis" *American Journal of Nursing* (1925) 25: 729; and see "Infantile Paralysis" *American Journal of Nursing* (1931) 31: 1142.

19. Jean Barrett "Her 30 Years War Made Sister Kenny Belligerent" *Philadelphia Evening Bulletin* April 22 1943; see also Kenny to Dear Sir [O'Connor], June 13 1941, Public Relations, MOD-K; Kenny with Ostenso *And They Shall Walk*, 218.

20. Jessie Stevenson "The Kenny Method" *American Journal of Nursing* (1942) 42: 904–910; Editorial "The Kenny Treatment for Poliomyelitis" Archives of Physical Therapy (June 1942) 23: 366.

21. Editorial "The Kenny Treatment," 364–367.

22. Elizabeth Kenny to Ladies and Gentlemen, [July 1944].

23. Kenny to Dear Dr. Gill, July 19 1943, Evidence Reports 1943–1952, MHS-K.

24. Ibid.

25. A. E. Deacon "The Treatment of Poliomyelitis in the Acute Stage" *Canadian Public Health Journal* (1942) 33: 281.

26. Walter G. Stuck and Albert O. Loiselle "The 1942 San Antonio Poliomyelitis Epidemic" *JAMA* (July 24 1943) 122: 853–855.

27. See David J. Rothman *Beginnings Count: The Technological Imperative in American Health Care* (New York: Twentieth-Century Fund and Oxford University Press, 1997); Daniel J. Wilson *Living with Polio: The Epidemic and its Survivors* (Chicago: University of Chicago Press, 2005).

28. Kenny *Treatment of Infantile Paralysis*, 215.

29. Marjorie Lawrence *Interrupted Melody: An Autobiography* (New York: Appleton-Century Crofts, 1949), 194.

30. See Blanche Wiesen Cook *Eleanor Roosevelt: A Biography* (New York: Viking, 1992); Cook *Eleanor Roosevelt: Volume II: The Defining Years, 1933–1938* (New York: Penguin, 2000).

31. "Hunter Girls Hope To Join Air Force" *New York Times* February 8 1942.

32. "'Forever And A Day' To Help Tomorrow's America" *National Foundation News* (1943) 2: 19.

33. See Hugh Gregory Gallagher *FDR's Splendid Deception* (New York: Dodd, Mead, 1985); Davis W. Houck and Amos Kiewe *FDR's Body Politics: The Rhetoric of Disability* (College Station: Texas A & M University Press, 2003); Theo Lippman, Jr. *The Squire of Warm Springs: F.D.R. in Georgia 1924–1945* (Chicago: Playboy Press, 1977); Turnley Walker *Roosevelt and the Warm Springs Story* (New York: A. A. Wyn, 1953). For an argument that the American public may have been aware of Roosevelt's disability, see C. Clausen "The President and the Wheelchair" *Wilson Quarterly* (2005) 29: 24–29.

34. Kenny to Dear Mr. President, September 2 1940, Public Relations, MOD-K; Kenny to Roosevelt, September 2 1940 [abstract], FDR-OF-5188, Sister Elizabeth Kenny Institute 1940–1944, FDR Papers; Kenny to Dear Mr. President, September 6 1940, Public Relations, MOD-K; Kenny to Roosevelt, September 6 1940 [abstract], FDR-OF-5188, Sister Elizabeth Kenny Institute 1940–1944, FDR Papers.

35. Kenny to Major General Edwin Watson, May 6 1943, FDR-OF-5188, Sister Elizabeth Kenny Institute 1940–1944, FDR Papers.

36. E. M. W. [Edwin M. Watson] Memorandum for the President, May 10 1943, FDR-OF-5188, Sister Elizabeth Kenny Institute 1940–1944, FDR Papers. He also wrote to Kenny saying that the president "hopes very much that he will have a chance for a visit with you, but that the appointment should be arranged through Mr. Basil O'Connor"; Edwin M. Watson to My Dear Sister Kenny, May 12 1943, FDR-OF-5188, Sister Elizabeth Kenny Institute 1940–1944, FDR Papers.

37. Basil O'Connor to Dear Grace [Tully], June 4 1943, FDR-OF-5188, Sister Elizabeth Kenny Institute 1940–1944, FDR Papers; "The Day in Washington" *New York Times*, June

9 1943. O'Connor had proposed a lunch meeting with Kenny and the president several times; Basil O'Connor to Roosevelt, January 12 1943, FDR-OF-5188, Sister Elizabeth Kenny Institute, 1940–1944, FDR Papers. See also O'Connor [memoranda of] February 1 1943 and April 1 1943, FDR-OF-5188, Sister Elizabeth Kenny Institute, 1940–1944, FDR Papers.

38. "President Roosevelt Greeting Sister Kenny Yesterday" [Associated Press Photo] *New York Times* June 9 1943. Roosevelt told reporters later that they "discussed plans to train more Americans in the use of Sister Kenny's method."

39. Kenny "Report of Activities: June, 1940–1943," FDR-OF-5188, Sister Elizabeth Kenny Institute, 1940–1944, FDR Papers; Kenny to Dear Mary [McCarthy], July 5 1943, Mary McCarthy, 1942–1944, MHS-K.

40. Kenny and Ostenso *And They Shall Walk*, 268.

41. E.M.W. [Edwin M. Watson] Memorandum for the President, May 10 1943, FDR-OF-5188, Sister Elizabeth Kenny Institute, 1940–1944, FDR Papers.

42. Kenny to Dear Doctor Stimson, October 8 1945, Public Relations, MOD-K.

43. Edward Compere "Management and Care of the Infantile Paralysis Patient" *Archives of Physical Therapy* (December 1943) [abstract] *Physiotherapy Review* (1944) 24: 80.

44. Robert M. Yoder "Healer from the Outback" *Saturday Evening Post* (January 17 1942) 214: 18–19, 68, 70; anon. "Sister Kenny: Australian Nurse Demonstrates Her Treatment for Infantile Paralysis" *Life* (September 28 1942) 13: 73–75, 77; Kenny with Ostenso *And They Shall Walk*, 227. See also Alexander *Maverick*, 118–119.

45. Seth Koven has pointed out that the role of "shut in" was restricted to the disabled members of wealthy families; Seth Koven "Remembering and Dismemberment: Crippled Children Wounded Soldiers, and the Great War in Great Britain" *American Historical Review* (1994) 99: 1167–1202.

46. "Still in Wheel Chair: Polio Invalid Inmate For 50 Years" *Washington Post* December 18 1943.

47. See Kim E. Nielsen *The Radical Lives of Helen Keller* (New York: New York University Press, 2004).

48. "Mr. Smith Again Will Come To Washington—for Jubilee" *Washington Post* January 18 1942; "Nancy Merki, Girl Tank Star, Gets Bid to White House" *Washington Post* January 11 1942.

49. Considine "On the Line" *Washington Post* January 22 1942.

50. Lawrence *Interrupted Melody*, 219–226; "Marjorie Lawrence Real Star of 'Tannhauser' at Metropolitan" *Christian Science Monitor* January 23 1943.

51. "Diva Returns, Paralysis Beaten" *New York Times* December 29 1943; "Singer Wins Over Paralysis" *Hartford Courant* January 10 1943.

52. Lawrence *Interrupted Melody*, 227–230, 247–263.

53. See one example of an NFIP scholarship for an orthopedic nurse, who was a former polio patient; "Professional Advancement Expedited by Polio Treatment Scholarships" *Archives of Physical Therapy* (November 1944) 25: 687. See also the head of Nebraska's Scotts Bluff County NFIP chapter who was a polio survivor; Mr. Stone to Mr. Wear, Memorandum: Re Scotts Bluff County, Nebraska, August 17 1945, Public Relations, MOD-K.

54. F. P. Sahli to Gentlemen, December 12 1944, Public Relations, MOD-K.

55. Gudakunst to Dear Mr. Sahli, December 21 1944, Public Relations, MOD-K.

56. Neil M. Tasker "Infantile Paralysis Patient" *National Foundation News* (March 1943) 2: 20.

57. Robert W. Lovett "Orthopedic Problems in the After-Treatment of Infantile Paralysis" *Journal of Bone and Joint Surgery* (1917) 2: 693. See also Fishbein warning of public "ignorance"

as the cause of both popular fears and also the use of "quack practitioners"; Morris Fishbein "The National Foundation Reports" [radio address], Columbia Broadcasting System, November 8 1940, Public Relations, Fishbein, MOD.

58. Lewis L. Clarke to Dear Mr. President, February 7 1944, Public Relations, MOD-K. See also a father who "studied everything I could find and believe I knew as much and more about the disease than does the average doctor"; Frank P. Fischer to Dear Sister Kenny, May 17 1943, Case Files-Misc., A-K, 1943–1946, MHS-K.

59. A Parent, "Our Son Has Polio" [1945], Ray of Light Letters, 1944, MHS-K.

60. Nurses had long recognized the importance of providing mothers with concrete instructions; see Jessie L. Stevenson *The Nursing Care of Patients with Infantile Paralysis* (New York: National Foundation for Infantile Paralysis, 1940), 23–24. For other examples of mothers as primary rehabilitative caregivers see Ruth Esau, quoted in Silver and Wilson *Polio Voices*, 42; Katherine Pappas, quoted in ibid, 46.

61. Kenny to Mrs. Frank P. Fischer, March 3 1944, Case Files-Misc., A-K, 1943–1946, MHS-K; Georgia Fischer to Dear Sister, May 17 1944, Case Files-Misc., A-K, 1943–1946, MHS-K.

62. Mr. and Mrs. Howard Allen to Dear Sister Kenny, November 4 1943, Mrs. Howard Allen, 1944 [sic], MHS-K.

63. "Sister Kenny To Speak" *New York Times* February 4 1943; "News for Nurses: Sister Kenny in N.Y." *Trained Nurse and Hospital Review* (February 1943) 110: 127.

64. Clarence R. Newman "Sister Kenny Here to Aid Polio Victims" *Los Angeles Examiner* [1943], Clippings, MHS-K. Her 1943 textbook, she proudly told lay supporters, "would be of tremendous help to all mothers and fathers on whom the burden of this work is thrust in many cases"; Elizabeth Kenny to Dear Mr. Harris, August 18 1944, Calvin Harris, 1944–1945, MHS.

65. Dorothy Ducas to P. J. A. Cusack Memorandum on *Reader's Digest* article by LMM 'Sister Kenny vs. the Medical Old Guard', December 5 1944, Public Relations, MOD-K.

66. "Kenny Way" *Newsweek* (February 7 1944) 93.

67. Mr. and Mrs. Steven Hotinska to Dear Sister Kenny, January 28 1943, Requests for Treatment 1942–1945, MHS-K.

68. Betty Adler [Baltimore] to Dear Sister Kenny, January 28 1943, Requests for Treatment 1942–1945, MHS-K.

69. Mrs. Clara Conte to Dear Sister Kenny, January 31 1943, Requests for Treatment 1942–1945, MHS-K.

70. Dorothy Marie Meissner to Dear Sister Kenny, January 24 1943, Requests for Treatment 1942–1945, MHS-K.

71. Charlotte Gruber Birch to Dear Miss Kenny [1943], Requests for Treatment 1942–1945, MHS-K.

72. This attitude was shared by other polio experts; see also Florence Kendall's view that people who worked with polio patients "can't afford to be afraid or just couldn't do their job"; Kendall, interview with Rogers, April 26 1999.

73. Marion Williamson "Review of a Polio Epidemic" *Public Health Nursing* (June 1945) 37: 312; Robert D. Blute, Sr., father of Margaret Marshall, quoted in Silver and Wilson *Polio Voices*, 54; William Foote Whyte *Participant Observer: An Autobiography* (Ithaca: ILR Press, 1994), 133; Marian Williamson "Review of the Current Poliomyelitis Epidemic" [November 13 1944] Central File 1944–1945, Children's Bureau, Box 103, Record Group 102, Infantile Paralysis 103-4-5-16-1, National Archives.

74. Patient quoted in Richard L. Bruno *The Polio Paradox: Understanding and Treating 'Post-Polio Syndrome' and Chronic Fatigue* (New York: Warner Books, 2002), 83. Even years later a polio survivor might face this. "Sometimes people would look at me like I had some kind of contagious disease," one survivor recalled; Robert Gurney in Edmund J. Sass with George Gottfried and Anthony Sorem eds. *Polio's Legacy: An Oral History* (Lanham, MD: University Press of America, 1996), 28.

75. Lora M. Lee "I Contact Polio" *Dr Shelton's Hygienic Review* (July 1945) 6: 255. A physical therapist in Massachusetts recalled that she "had to scrub, before I went in, [and] after I came out, change my shoes"; Irja Hoffshire, quoted in Silver and Wilson *Polio Voices*, 23–24. See also a recollection of ward nurses wearing masks and floor length isolation gowns at Columbia University's Babies Hospital in 1944; William A. Silverman *Where's the Evidence? Controversies in Modern Medicine* (Oxford: Oxford University Press, 1998), 1.

76. Myra G. Lehman "Poliomyelitis Problems: The Alabama Epidemic" *American Journal of Nursing* (October 1946) 46: 690.

77. Kenny with Ostenso *And They Shall Walk*, 204.

78. Helen H. Ross "Physiotherapy in the Treatment of Infantile Paralysis: Kenny Method" *Canadian Public Health Journal* (June 1942) 33: 286.

79. See, for example, Charles J. Frankel and Robert V. Funsten "Use of Neostigmine (Prostigmine) in Subacute Poliomyelitis" *Southern Medical Journal* (June 1946) 39: 483.

80. Ratcliff "Minutemen Against Infantile Paralysis," 80.

81. "A Date with the Future" [Buffalo], November 2 1949, Buffalo, NY, MHS-K.

82. Editorial "Fact and Fancy in Poliomyelitis" *British Medical Journal* (July 31 1943) 2: 142; "The Kenny Method In Poliomyelitis" *Lancet* (January 30 1943) 241: 148. Yet the editor felt it was necessary to refer to other sources of authority. The results of the new method had "been observed by other workers outside the Minneapolis group" and "spasm" had been "demonstrated and photographed."

83. Robert V. Funsten "The Influence of the Sister Kenny Publicity on the Treatment of Poliomyelitis" *Virginia Medical Monthly* (October 1945) 72: 404. His speech was given in 1944 and published the following year.

84. Elizabeth Kenny to Ladies and Gentlemen, [July 1944].

85. [Mary Lou Drosten] A Layman's Report, "Evaluation of the Kenny Treatment for Poliomyelitis" [July 1944], Ray of Light Letters, 1944, MHS-K.

86. Whyte *Participant Observer*, 132–133.

87. Richard Kovacs in "Discussion of Papers by Drs. John A. Toomey, Jessie Wright and Miland E. Knapp" *Archives of Physical Therapy* (November 1942) 23: 674.

88. Ethel Calhoun "A Report On The Use of The Sister Kenny Concept and Method of Treatment for Poliomyelitis Patients at Oakland County Contagious Hospital, 1944–1949" [1949], Minnesota-Hospitals, 1944–1961, Sister Kenny Institute, Walter H. Judd Papers, MHS. See also Edward L. Compere "Modern Concepts of Infantile Paralysis" *Archives of Physical Therapy* (November 1942) 23: 677; Dorothy I. Ditchfield and Ethel M. Hyndman "The Nursing Procedure" *Canadian Public Health Journal* (June 1942) 33: 284.

89. Plastridge "Report," 9.

90. Ray K. Gullickson in Sass with Gottfried and Sorem eds. *Polio's Legacy*, 44–45.

91. Pohl and Kenny, *The Kenny Concept of Infantile Paralysis*, 152.

92. "Nurse's Paralysis Therapy Endorsed" *Los Angeles Times* May 7 1942.

93. Gullickson in Sass with Gottfried and Sorem eds. *Polio's Legacy*, 44.

94. See the assumption that a patient must be motivated and able to understand the goals of therapy; "Recovery is slow and difficult in the patient who does not understand what is

wanted, in the lazy person and in the spoiled, pampered child"; John A. Toomey "Observations on the Treatment of Infantile Paralysis in the Acute Stage" *Canadian Medical Association Journal* (January 1946) 54: 1–6.

95. Clemson Griggs to Dear Sister Kenny, September 1 1951, Personal Correspondence and Related Papers, 1942–1951, MHS-K. J. Philip Kistler, a child from California, was another Institute patient who was also taken to a big auditorium "where she would demonstrate"; J. Philip Kistler, quoted in Silver and Wilson *Polio Voices*, 43–44.

96. Plastridge "Report," 7.

97. Lois Maddox Miller "Sister Kenny Wins Her Fight" *Reader's Digest* (1942) 41: 27–28; see also Irene F. Shea, "Notes on Kenny Method of Hot Foments Taken at the University of Minnesota, September 28 to October 4, 1942," Sydenham Hospital Collection, MS C 243, Box 82, History of Medicine Division, National Library of Medicine. My thanks to Janet Golden for showing me this source. See also Janet Golden and Naomi Rogers "Nurse Shea Studies the 'Kenny Method' of Treatment of Infantile Paralysis, 1942–1943" *Nursing History Review* (2010) 18: 189–203.

98. Charles C. Zacharie to My Dear Dr. Stimson, January 11 1943, Box 2, Folder 4, Correspondence re Medical Talks, Philip Stimson Papers, Medical Center Archives, New York-Presbyterian/Weill Cornell, New York.

99. Philip Stimson to Dear Dr. Zacharie, January 12 1943, Box 2, Folder 4, Correspondence re Medical Talks, Stimson Papers.

100. Deacon "The Treatment of Poliomyelitis in the Acute Stage," 278–281; "New Infantile Paralysis Treatment Gets Approval" *Science News Letter* (December 13 1941) 40: 371.

101. Yoder "Healer from the Outback," 70.

102. Gullickson in Sass with Gottfried and Sorem eds. *Polio's Legacy*, 47.

103. Toinette Balkema to Dear Sister Kenny, November 10 1942, Technicians—Misc., undated and 1941–1949, MHS-K.

104. Charles Bohnengel "An Evaluation of Psychobiologic Factors in the Re-Education Phase of the Kenny Treatment for Infantile Paralysis" *Psychosomatic Medicine* (1944) 6: 83–86.

105. Richard H. Todd to Dear Sister, January 8 1945, District of Columbia-Misc., 1944–1946, MHS-K; Rita Fitzpatrick "Polio Stricken Nurse to Get Aid Of Sister Kenny" *Washington Times-Herald* January 31 1945.

106. Fitzpatrick "Polio Stricken Nurse to Get Aid Of Sister Kenny."

107. William G. Holman to Dear Sister Kenny, March 23 1945, Case Files-Misc.: A-K, 1943–1946, MHS-K.

108. Mrs. W. G. Holman to Dear Sister Kenny, [1945], Case Files-Misc.: A-K, 1943–1946, MHS-K.

109. In Krusen's 1941 text he warned that polio patients usually within 2 years of fixed deformities must be relieved by an operation such as arthrodesis or tendon transplantation; Frank H. Krusen *Physical Medicine: The Employment of Physical Agents for Diagnosis and Therapy* (Philadelphia and London: W. B. Saunders, 1941), 595.

110. Kenny "Preface" in Pohl and Kenny *The Kenny Concept of Infantile Paralysis*, 23. Typically, operations were tendon lengthening, ankle fusion, bone stapling, and muscle transplantation.

111. Mr. and Mrs. Louis Renel, August 7 1944, Case Files-Misc. I-Z, 1943–1946, MHS-K.

112. Pohl and Kenny, *The Kenny Concept of Infantile Paralysis*, 314.

113. Howard W. Blakeslee [June 1944], Public Relations, MOD-K.

114. Plastridge "Report," 6–7.

115. Kendall and Kendall, "Our Notes."

116. Henry O. Kendall, Florence P. Kendall and George E. Bennett "Normal Flexibility According to Age Groups" *Journal of Bone and Joint Surgery* (1948) 30: 690–694.

117. Toomey "Observations on the Treatment of Infantile Paralysis," 5.

118. H. Relton McCarroll [Report] in "Reports on Meeting of Committee to Investigate the Kenny Method of Treatment, Sunday and Monday, November 22 and 23, 1942, Minneapolis, Minnesota," Dr. R. K. Ghormley, 1943, MHS-K.

119. J. Albert Key [Report] in "Reports on Meeting of Committee to Investigate the Kenny Method of Treatment, Sunday and Monday, November 22 and 23, 1942, Minneapolis, Minnesota," Dr. R. K. Ghormley, 1943, MHS-K.

120. Kenny to Dear Dr. Ghormley, [March 5 1943], Dr. R. K. Ghormley, 1943, MHS-K.

121. Wilson *Living with Polio*, 77 [quoting Knapp (1953) *Journal of Iowa State Medical Society*].

122. Lawrence *Interrupted Melody*, 185, 189.

123. Toomey "Observations on the Treatment of Infantile Paralysis," 5.

124. Margaret Buell Wilder "Noted Nurse Gives Hope To Stricken" *Los Angeles Examiner* [March] 1943, Clippings, Box 5, MHS-K. For an example of Kenny as a model for some disabled veterans, see disabled servicemen gathered around Kenny when she came to a party at the Evalyn Walsh McLean's Friendship House in Washington, D.C., waiting their turn for an autograph; "Disabled Vets Meet Famed Sister Kenny" *Washington Times-Herald* May 7 1945.

125. "Sister Kenny Tests Paralysis Methods" *New York Times* November 13 1943.

126. Clara Hulberg [White Earth, North Dakota] to Dear Miss Kenny, April 13 1943, Board of Directors, MHS-K.

127. [Drosten] A Layman's Report "Evaluation of the Kenny Treatment."

128. Ruby M. Green [Orthopaedic Hospital, Los Angeles] to Dear Sister Kenny, [October 1943], Los Angeles- Misc., 1942–1951, MHS-K.

129. Wilson *Living with Polio*. For other examples of cruel nursing care see Judith Leavitt "'Strange Young Women on Errands': Obstetric Nursing Between Two Worlds" *Nursing History Review* (1998) 6: 3–24; and Julie Fairman "Not All Nurses Are Good, Not All Doctors Are Bad..." *Bulletin of the History of Medicine* (Summer 2004) 78: 451–460. For other examples of sadistic health professionals see Beatrice Yvonne Nau and Ted Kellogg, quoted in Silver and Wilson *Polio Voices*, 46–47; see also Hugh Gregory Gallagher *Black Bird Fly Away: Disabled in an Able-bodied World* (Arlington: Vandamere Press, 1998) who recalled his experience in Bryn Mawr Hospital in 1952 and "the cruel, vicious, and inhumane manner" in which one of his physical therapists weaned him from the iron lung and stretched his muscles; she was "the only true sadist I have ever known," 43–44.

130. K. G. Hansson in "Discussion of Papers by Drs. John A. Toomey, Jessie Wright and Miland E. Knapp" *Archives of Physical Therapy* (November 1942) 23: 675.

131. Bohnengel "An Evaluation of Psychobiologic Factors" 83–86; "Sister Kenny" *London Illustrated* [reprinted in] *Hospital Magazine* [Australia] (June 1943) 17, Wilson Collection.

132. Sylvia M. Barker quoted in Silver and Wilson *Polio Voices*, 29.

133. Milton H. Berry to My Dear Mr. President, January 22 1939, FDR-OF-1930, Infantile Paralysis 1934–1942, Box 1, FDR Papers.

134. Richard Kovacs "Progress in Physical Medicine During the Past Twenty-Five Years" *Archives of Physical Medicine* (August 1946) 27: 473.

135. Guy A. Caldwell "The Postwar Challenge to Orthopedic Surgery" *JAMA* (September 30 1944) 126: 270.

136. Edward J. Doherty *The Saint of Paralytics* (Los Angeles: Times-Mirror Press, 1925, 2nd. ed.), 25–33.

137. *A New Life: The Milton H. Berry School for Paralysis and Spastic Correction, Encino, California* (n.p., [c.1937]) [pamphlet enclosed in] Mrs. Nevada Gates [Baldwin Park, California] to FDR, February 8 1945, FDR-OF-1930, Box 2 (Infantile Paralysis 1943), Infantile Paralysis 1943–1945, FDR Papers [1-2, 6]; Doherty *The Saint of Paralytics*, 7–10. For a brief discussion of Berry's work see Tony Gould *A Summer Plague: Polio and Its Survivors* (New Haven: Yale University Press, 1995), 95.

138. [Advertisement] "Constipation: Banished Without Drugs, Diet or Exercise" *Los Angeles Times* July 10 1921; [Advertisement] "A School for Paralysis and Spastic Correction: Milton H. Berry School, Encino, California" *Los Angeles Times* January 2 1940; *A New Life* [2]; Doherty *The Saint of Paralytics*, 7–10.

139. *A New Life* [3–4]; Milton H. Berry *A Challenge on Behalf of Crippled Children to the Universities of America: Victims of Infantile Paralysis Need Not Hospitals . . . But Muscle Training/ Not Doctors . . . . But Trained Teachers* (Milton H. Berry Foundation, [1939]) [enclosed in] Milton H. Berry to My Dear Mr. President, January 22 1939, FDR-OF-1930, Infantile Paralysis 1934–1942, Box 1, FDR Papers; *A New Life* [2].

140. Doherty *The Saint of Paralytics*, 15, 34; *A New Life* [3, 5].

141. Berry *A Challenge on Behalf of Crippled Children*; *A New Life* [2]; Berry to Doherty, October 19 1925, [letter reprinted in] Doherty *The Saint of Paralytics*, 148.

142. Berry to My Dear Mr. President, January 22 1939; O'Connor to My Dear Mr. President, June 27 1939, FDR-OF-1930, Infantile Paralysis 1934–1942, Box 1, FDR Papers.

143. Berry to My Dear Mr. President, January 22 1939; Berry *A Challenge on Behalf of Crippled Children*.

144. Berry *A Challenge on Behalf of Crippled Children*. His son Milton Jr. was supposedly studying medicine at the University of California; Doherty *The Saint of Paralytics*, 10; Berry to Doherty, October 19 1925, letter reprinted in Doherty *The Saint of Paralytics*, 146.

145. Berry to My Dear Mr. President, January 22 1939; Berry *A Challenge on Behalf of Crippled Children*.

146. Doherty *The Saint of Paralytics*, 98–99; Berry to My Dear Mr. President, January 22 1939.

147. Rosemonde Rae Wright "A Great Humanitarian," letter to the editor, *Los Angeles Times* December 12 1939.

148. "Milton Berry Jr." *New York Times* April 13 1954; Milton H. Berry and G. Stanley Gordon to Dear Sister Kenny, March 30 1944, Los Angeles-Misc., 1942–1951, MHS-K.

149. Berry and Gordon to Dear Sister Kenny, March 30 1944.

150. Peter Cusack to Basil O'Connor [telegram], June 15 1944, Public Relations, MOD-K.

151. Margaret Stedman "There Are No Cripples in Wartime" *Hygeia* (October 1944) 22: 750–755.

152. David Serlin *Replaceable You: Engineering the Body in Postwar America* (Chicago: University of Chicago Press, 2004), 28–39; David Gerber "Anger and Affability: The Rise and Representation of a Repertory of Self-Presentation Skills in a World War II Disabled Veteran" *Journal of Social History* (Fall 1993) 27: 5–27.

153. "Disabilities: Infantile Paralysis" *Lancet* (July 24 1948) 252: 155–157.

154. Editorial "Physical Therapy and the Problem of Rehabilitation" *Archives of Physical Therapy* (May 1943) 24: 299–300.

155. Howard A. Rusk "Convalescence and Rehabilitation" in Morris Fishbein ed. *Doctors at War* (New York: E. P. Dutton & Company, 1945), 303–318.

156. "Toymakers" *National Foundation News* (May 1945) 4: 25, 28.

157. Howard A. Rusk and Eugene J. Taylor *New Hope for the Handicapped: The Rehabilitation of the Disabled from Bed to Job* (New York: Harper & Brothers, 1946, 1949), 220. Howard A. Rusk (1937–1991), a member of the Army Air Force Corps, was chief of medical services at Jefferson Barracks in St. Louis, Missouri where he developed a convalescent training program that became a model program for the entire Army Air Force Corps. After the war he opened a medical practice with emphasis on rehabilitation in St. Louis, and then moved to New York City where he worked at Bellevue and Goldwater Hospitals to rehabilitate civilians, and directed the Department of Physical Medicine and Rehabilitation of New York University and in 1950 the Institute of Rehabilitation Medicine at Bellevue Medical Center.

158. William Dock "The Evil Sequelae of Complete Bed Rest" *JAMA* (August 19 1944) 125: 1083–1085; [abstract] John H. Powers "The Abuse of Rest as Therapeutic Measure in Surgery: Early Postoperative Activity and Rehabilitation" *JAMA* (August 19 1944) 125 in *Physiotherapy Review* (1944) 24: 217; Bernhard Newburger "Early Postoperative Walking: Collective Review" *Recent Advances in Surgery* (July 1943) 14: 142–154.

159. "On Bed: Abuse of Rest" *Time* (September 11 1944) 44: 90; "Use and Abuse of Bed Rest" *New York State Journal of Medicine* (April 1 1944) 44: 724–730; Dock "The Evil Sequelae of Complete Bed Rest," 1083–1085.

160. K. G. Hansson "Physical Therapy in Wartime" *New England Journal of Medicine* (November 2 1944) 231: 619–620.

161. "Infantile Paralysis [1847–1947]" *Hygeia* (June 1947) 25: 439.

162. "The Disabled Can Be Independent" *Trained Nurse and Hospital Review* (August 1945) 115: 110–111.

163. Fred J. Cook "Lead Belt Helps Polio Victim Walk" *New York World-Telegram* April 28 1948.

164. Joseph G. Molner "The Kenny Method" [paper presented at] Post-Graduate Course in Physical Medicine and Rehabilitation, University of Texas, Medical Branch, Galveston, March 7 1946, Public Relations, MOD-K.

165. C. E. Irwin "A Brief Resume of the Kenny Method of Treating Infantile Paralysis" [1947], European Trip 1947, MHS-K.

FURTHER READING

On disability history and politics in early to mid-twentieth-century U.S. see Emily K. Abel *Hearts of Wisdom: American Women Caring for Kin 1850—1940* (Cambridge, MA: Harvard University Press, 2000); Edward D. Berkowitz *Disability Policy: America's Programs for the Handicapped* (Cambridge: Cambridge University Press, 1987); Edward D. Berkowitz *Rehabilitation: The Federal Government's Response to Disability, 1935–1954* (New York: Arno Press, 1980); Helen Deutsch and Felicity Nussbaum eds. *'Defects:' Engendering the Modern Body* (Ann Arbor: University of Michigan Press, 2000); David Gerber "Anger and Affability: The Rise and Representation of a Repertory of Self-Presentation Skills in a World War II Disabled Veteran" *Journal of Social History* (1993) 27: 5–27; Glenn Gritzer and Arnold Arluke *The Making of Rehabilitation: The Political Economy of Medical Specialization, 1890–1980* (Berkeley: University of California Press, 1985); Wendy Kline *Building a Better Race: Gender, Sexuality, and Eugenics from the Turn of the Century to the Baby Boom* (Berkeley and Los Angeles: University of California Press, 2001); Seth Koven "Remembering and Dismemberment: Crippled Children Wounded Soldiers, and the Great War in Great Britain" *American Historical Review* (1994) 99: 1167–1202; Paul K. Longmore and David Goldberger "The League of the Physically Handicapped and the Great Depression: A Case Study in the New Disability History" *Journal of American History* (2000) 87: 888–922; Paul K. Longmore and Lauri Umansky eds. *New Disability History: American Perspectives* (New York: New York University Press, 2001); David T. Mitchell and Sharon L. Snyder eds. *The Body and Physical Difference: Discourses of Disability* (Ann Arbor: University of Michigan Press, 1997); Kim E. Nielsen *The Radical Lives of Helen Keller* (New York: New York University Press, 2004); Ruth O'Brien *Crippled Justice: The History of Modern Disability Policy in the Workplace* (Chicago: University of Chicago Press, 2001); Martin Pernick, *The Black Stork: Eugenics and the Death of "Defective" Babies in American Medicine and Motion Pictures since 1915* (New York: Oxford University Press, 1996); David Serlin *Replaceable You: Engineering the Body in Postwar America* (Chicago: University of Chicago Press, 2004), 28–39; Tom Shakespeare, Kath Gillespie-Sells, and Dominic Davies *The Sexual Politics of Disability: Untold Desires* (New York: Cassell, 1996); Joseph Shapiro *No Pity: People with Disabilities Forging a New Civil Rights Movement* (New York: Times Books, 1993); Christopher R. Smit and Anthony Enns eds. *Screening Disability: Essays on Cinema and Disability* (Lanthan: University Press of American, 2001); Barbara Waxman and Anne Finger "The Politics of Sex and Disability" *Disability Studies Quarterly* (1989) 9: 1–5; Frieda Zames and Doris Zames Fleischer eds. *The Disability Rights Movement: From Charity to Confrontation* (Philadelphia: Temple University Press, 2001).

On experiences of polio, including at Warm Springs, see Richard L. Bruno *The Polio Paradox: Understanding and Treating 'Post-Polio Syndrome' and Chronic Fatigue* (New York: Warner Books, 2002); Lynne M. Dunphy "'The Steel Cocoon:' Tales of the Nurses and Patients of the Iron Lung, 1929–1955" *Nursing History Review* (2001) 9: 3–34; Amy L. Fairchild "The Polio Narratives: Dialogues with FDR" *Bulletin of the History of Medicine* (2001) 75: 488–534; Hugh G. Gallagher, *Black Bird Fly Away: Disabled in an Able-Bodied World* (Arlington, VA: Vandamere Press, 1998); Hugh Gregory Gallagher *FDR's Splendid Deception* (New York: Dodd, Mead, 1985); Tony Gould *A Summer Plague: Polio and Its Survivors* (New Haven: Yale University Press, 1995); Robert F. Hall *Through the Storm: A Polio Story* (St. Cloud, Minnesota: North Star Press, 1990); Daniel Holland "Franklin D. Roosevelt's Shangri-La: Foreshadowing the Independent Living Movement in Warm Springs, Georgia, 1926–1945" *Disability & Society* (2006) 21: 513–535;Davis W. Houck and Amos Kiewe *FDR's Body Politics: The Rhetoric of Disability* (College Station: Texas A & M University Press, 2003); Leonard Kriegel *Flying Solo: Reimagining Manhood, Courage, and Loss* (Landham, NY: Ballantine: 1998); Theo Lippman, Jr. *The Squire of Warm Springs: F.D.R. in Georgia 1924–1945* (Chicago: Playboy Press, 1977); Janice Flood Nichols *Twin Voices: A Memoir of Polio, the Forgotten Killer* (Bloomington, IN: iUniverse, Inc., 2007); Naomi Rogers "Polio Chronicles: Warm Springs and Disability Politics in the 1930s" *Asclepio: Revista de Historia de la Medicine y de la Ciencia* (2009) 61: 143–174; Naomi Rogers "Silence Has Its Own Stories: Elizabeth Kenny, Polio and the Culture of Medicine" *Social History of Medicine* (2008) 21: 145–161; Edmund J. Sass with George Gottfried and Anthony Sorem eds. *Polio's Legacy: An Oral History* (Lanham, MD: University Press of America, 1996); Marc Shell *Polio and Its Aftermath: The Paralysis of Culture* (Cambridge: Harvard University Press, 2005); Susan Shreve *Warm Springs: Traces of a Childhood at FDR's Polio Haven* (New York: Houghton Mifflin, 2007); Julie Silver and Daniel Wilson *Polio Voices: An Oral History from the American Polio Epidemics and Worldwide Eradication Efforts* (New York: Praeger, 2007); Turnley Walker *Roosevelt and the Warm Springs Story* (New York: A. A. Wyn, 1953); William Foote Whyte *Participant Observer: An Autobiography* (Ithaca: ILR Press, 1994); Daniel J. Wilson "Braces, Wheelchairs, and Iron Lungs: The Paralyzed Body and the Machinery of Rehabilitation in the Polio Epidemics" *Journal of Medical Humanities* (Fall 2005) 26: 173–190; Daniel J. Wilson *Living with Polio: The Epidemic and Its Survivors* (Chicago: University of Chicago Press, 2005); Regina Woods *Tales from Inside the Iron Lung (and How I Got Out of It)* (Philadelphia: University of Pennsylvania Press, 1994); Heather Green Wooten *The Polio Years in Texas: Battling a Terrifying Unknown* (College Station: Texas A&M University Press, 2009).

5

The Polio Wars

1943 HAD BEEN a bad year for polio, and 1944 was worse. With a total of 19,272 reported cases, it was the second-largest epidemic year yet recorded in U.S. history. Impossible to predict or prevent, polio epidemics followed Americans as they moved around the country seeking jobs in the wake of wartime industries, especially in the mid-Atlantic region and the South.

During the early 1940s Kenny, the National Foundation for Infantile Paralysis (NFIP) and the American Medical Association (AMA) had worked as uneasy allies. But in the mid-1940s, this alliance turned into a fierce battle over medical orthodoxy and professional self-interest. In February 1944 Kenny announced that the NFIP had refused her Kenny Institute the $150,000 it needed to expand its training program and to hire anatomists and physiologists to pursue research. She did not make clear how she or the Institute had requested this amount, but she did claim that Fishbein and O'Connor continued to treat her with skepticism and hostility. Recently Fishbein had told her to "leave the United States because other countries need my assistance."[1] This was the opening salvo of the polio wars between Kenny and the NFIP.

The polio wars were medical culture wars, played out in the popular and professional press with a feisty, uncontainable woman at the center. As they escalated, Kenny accused the NFIP of never having supported or respected her and of funding worthless polio treatments recommended by antagonistic physicians. Even its support of research was wrong-headed, she complained, because scientists working under NFIP grants ignored the insights of her work. By this time Kenny had behind her supporters in business, politics, and the press, along with expansive public good will. Despite a frantic effort to contain the fight the NFIP found itself on the defensive, and by 1945 it was losing allies among the wealthy, many women, and even Hollywood moguls.

The AMA's lock on power began to unravel as well, as the conservative policies of its leaders—especially Morris Fishbein—fell out of favor with policymakers, patients, and many physicians. While the AMA had been successful in lobbying to keep federal health insurance out of the 1935 Social Security Act, it suffered a major public humiliation in 1943 when the Department of Justice won an antitrust suit against the AMA and its affiliated medical society in Washington, D.C. The society, backed by the AMA, had sought to deny hospital privileges and membership to doctors associated with a prepaid health insurance plan.[2] Sensing weakness, Congress began debating new health insurance programs. Meanwhile, Fishbein became an easy target for discontent within the association. At the AMA's June 1944 annual meeting California delegates tried to oust him as general secretary and editor of *JAMA*. Their resolution was defeated 144 to 9 but each year the vote became closer. It was the beginning of the end for Fishbein, whom the *Saturday Evening Post* characterized in 1946 as "the best-known and least-liked doctor in the United States." Grudgingly, the AMA's House of Delegates formally approved limited group medical practice and voluntary insurance plans sponsored by medical societies (later called Blue Shield).[3] In the mid-1940s, however, Fishbein still held the reins, and he continued to see Kenny as an annoyance who would be easily controlled.

The polio wars were invigorated in July 1944 when the Kenny Institute boldly applied for a large research grant from the NFIP, an application O'Connor managed to thwart by asking yet another group of experts to assess and reject the Institute as a site for clinical research. Frustrated, Kenny tried to expand her clinical practice at the Institute by accepting patients with other neuromuscular conditions such as cerebral palsy, but a combination of city and professional politics ended that effort. Kenny's claim that her work was being undermined by an "organized opposition" was taken up by a few national politicians who saw a way to attack both the AMA and President Roosevelt. And in Minneapolis the Institute's board reorganized itself into a fundraising corporation known as the Kenny Foundation. But after Roosevelt's death in April 1945 polio politics shifted into a competition between 2 polio philanthropies both trying to convince the American public of social and financial support.

MUST KENNY LEAVE?

In February 1944 Kenny announced that because the NFIP was not willing to provide the Institute with funding, although her work in America was not done, she would have to return to Australia. At the same time, recognizing the role that research breakthroughs played in the March of Dimes publicity, she announced a new diagnostic sign, a distinctive muscle condition to help professionals begin treatment even before the first signs of paralysis appeared. The misdiagnosis of polio had continued to be a serious problem for families and health professionals, with a number of patients admitted to already overcrowded polio wards who were later diagnosed with, for example, diphtheria and meningitis.[4] Earlier treatment, she claimed, would improve every patient's chance of recovery, ameliorate polio's symptoms, and reduce pain "almost entirely." This would be "the greatest contribution that has yet been given to the medical world in connection with this disease." The sign was a peculiar rubbery sensation in the muscle that could be felt by a technician rotating a patient's joints. It indicated, Kenny said, that the muscle would soon go into spasm and would probably become paralyzed. But, she added, although many physicians had begged her to teach them, without the support of the NFIP and the AMA she would be unable to do so. "I am loath to leave this country," she told reporters dramatically, "but there is not much use in me staying unless I get greatly increased support."[5]

"Must Sister Kenny Leave?" asked the *Chicago Herald-American*, the *New York Journal-American*, and other newspapers. Fishbein quickly told the press that he had meant only that "her work needs dissemination throughout the world."[6] But his antagonism to Kenny was widely known. A few weeks earlier in a *JAMA* editorial entitled "Physiologic Nonsense and Poliomyelitis," he had quoted with relish the assessment of the eminent neuroscientist Stanley Cobb who praised "qualified investigators" like Joseph Moldaver and warned that "new and empirical methods of treatment backed by uncritical enthusiasm may produce many cures but much physiologic nonsense. The treatment may be good, but the ex post facto conclusions of the therapeutist are usually bad."[7] A "therapeutist" was obviously far from a scientist.

Seeing this at first as a minor skirmish, O'Connor and his staff defended the NFIP with a few brief statements. There was no "controversy between the National Foundation and Sister Kenny," O'Connor told reporters. "We have put [up] all money ever requested to evaluate and teach the Kenny method. Our reports and all our public statements show that." He recognized that Kenny had expressed her dissatisfaction with continuing investigations of her work, but declared that the NFIP would "continue to evaluate the Kenny method...in the hope of finding greater values in it."[8]

These denials were not effective. Amplified by the Hearst newspapers and later the *Reader's Digest*, they became weapons in a nascent populist movement. Here was a woman wronged, a selfless nurse devoting her life to healing children, yet being given no respect or honor by the men of the medical profession. Americans sent letters of outrage to Kenny, Roosevelt, O'Connor, their congressmen, and their local newspapers. They formed campaigns to raise money for the Kenny Institute, and warned local and national NFIP officials that the March of Dimes would receive no further support from them if its policy did not change. Most of all, Americans debated the nature of professional authority and research priorities, and the role that gender, social status, and character played in determining who received the respect of the medical establishment and the funding of powerful philanthropies. To its great surprise the NFIP found itself forced to defend and define what constituted scientific evidence, how medical expertise was and should be determined, and the purpose of research. Inspired by Kenny's struggles, the media campaign rapidly became a wider forum for the public to express long-standing frustration with unresponsive physicians and hospitals, autocratic public officials, the dismissal of strong women, the neglect of chronic disease, and enforced medical orthodoxy.

This was a new moment in American medical politics. Although on other occasions Kenny had threatened to leave, accused the NFIP of not supporting her work, and mentioned her early diagnostic sign, the story had always faded quickly. This time it caught fire. In the fervor of this battle, Kenny succeeded in challenging the public to rethink the medical establishment's claim to a monopoly on scientific truth and medical authority, and forced a powerful philanthropy to defend its research funding policies. She made the battle personal—about respect for herself and proper care for the disabled—as well as political. Her accusations that a medical cabal was attacking her and denying proper care to patients rang true to many Americans. How did the NFIP decide who to give money to? Was it just a club of elite physicians, funding each other? The NFIP, once able to command the public's unlimited faith, now encountered every philanthropy's worst nightmare: the suspicion of its donors. In pulling the powerful down to the level of public debate Kenny revived and expanded a medical populist movement that had previously been restricted to male entre-preneurs such as John Brinkley and female evangelists such as Aimee Semple McPherson.

PUBLIC OUTRAGE

The March of Dimes campaign in January 1944, like earlier campaigns, had featured Kenny. But now it looked as if the NFIP had falsely claimed her as a symbol of its commit-ment to the battle against polio. "To the millions of Americans who contributed generously to the 'March of Dimes' a week ago" the news that the NFIP "will not give $150,000 for the budget of the Kenny Institute...will come as a shock," said the editor of the *Tulsa Tribune*. "She doesn't get a nickel from it."[9] With headlines like "After 10 Years of Giving America Begins to Wonder" newspapers made this a story about money and arrogant medical men. A *New York Journal-American* editorial described Kenny's "discouraging and unhappy experi-ence in the United States" as she "faced the skepticism and even the active hostility of some sections of the medical and scientific professions." As a result, her work "has never had adequate financial support." Yet leaving "is the very last thing Sister Kenny wants to do."[10]

The NFIP had always said it spent the "people's money"; now Americans began to demand accountability. Although he had "always supported the drives for funds," one supporter warned NFIP officials, "if she leaves this country because of lack of funds to continue her work I will definitely refuse to continue to contribute funds."[11] "I have been a contributor to the 'March of Dimes' ever since it was started," an executive at a Tulsa oil company similarly told the chief surgeon at Warm Springs, "but I can assure you that if this editorial is true there will be no more contributions from me."[12]

In March 1944 nurse supporters in Chicago launched a movement to "Keep Sister Kenny in the USA" and to raise the $150,000 her Institute needed. Unusually, this group of nurses allied themselves with a group of disabled adult activists and a joint meeting was chaired by Harvey Church, president of the Disabled Persons Association of America. The meeting also featured Noreen Linduska, who had been disabled by polio during the 1943 Chicago epidemic and was a proponent of Kenny's work. "It is we who are disabled who know what a blessing the work of Sister Kenny is," Church told reporters. "There is a place for her in America and a great need for her."[13] Reports of this meeting in local papers featured the usual picture of recovered child patients, but in this case it was a fierce-looking group, holding a "Keep Sister Kenny Here" banner.[14] The *Sunday Mirror* reprinted this image juxtaposed with a photograph of Kenny lying in what looked like a hospital bed in a white hospital gown. "Bewildered and discouraged by apparent neglect of her method in America," the caption read, "Sister Kenny manages to smile while recov-ering from a cold in Los Angeles. Her comment: 'If America had taken heed when I first arrived I could return to Australia today—my work ended.'"[15]

Kenny's story of being rejected by the AMA and the NFIP reinforced what many Americans saw as a complex dynamic: the impotence of orthodox physicians to heal com-bined with their arrogance in attempting to monopolize legitimate health care. "You have found a way to relieve the suffering and tortuous crippling of our little children, while our great, scientific medical specialists stood by helpless, hand on chin, brow wrinkled," a man from Chino, California, told Kenny.[16] Could "professional jealousy" explain the antagonism of American physicians, asked a *Washington Post* editorial.[17] This hostility was a combination of prejudiced orthodoxy and professional exclusion, others suggested. "Where Sister Kenney [sic] made her mistake," argued the *Citizen's Health News* of San Diego, "was in trying to get the 'medical trust' to admit that a drugless method was superior to a medical method." Kenny's struggle against "medical monopolists" was part of a wider fight for what the magazine called "Health Freedom." "We are fighting all over the world for democratic principles but still have a totalitarian health set-up here at home."[18] Physicians who were already jealous of Kenny were further motivated by the fear of economic competition, others assured her. "We must realize that anyone who cures anything, seriously jeopardizes the fee-splitting system of medicine," wrote one man to Kenny. "Just think of the millions of dollars that have already been lost by you showing the world how to cure these little tots."[19] Gender, money, and professional jealousy were at the root of her trouble, one woman reflected. "Just realize what is against you," she told Kenny. "First the fact you are a woman, second anyone giving your treatment can't capitalize on it and get

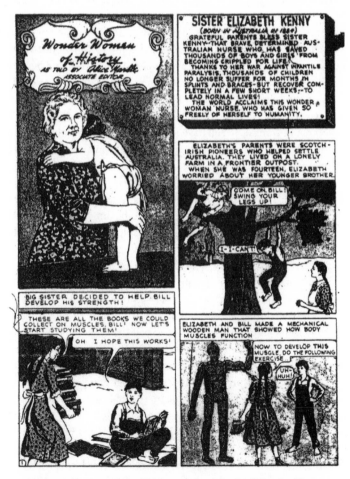

FIGURE 5.1 First page of a 1944 comic book in the "Wonder Women of History" series. From Alice Marble, *Wonder Women of History: Sister Elizabeth Kenny* (Spring 1944) no. 8. Courtesy of D.C. Comics.

rich, third you lack a college degree and all that rot. (Just remember the greatest healer of all Jesus Christ wasn't an M.D.) And fourth the money interests who are reaping a harvest from the manufacture of braces etc are against you."[20] A few supporters went further by suggesting that the corrupting power of the AMA was robbing Americans of the ability to choose providers. "Without the Kenny treatment," Robert Gurney, the father of Kenny's first acute patient in Minneapolis, told the St Paul Pioneer Press, "our son would have either passed away, or been a horribly deformed boy for the rest of his life." Now he not only attended school but he could "shoot pool, kick a football, walk by himself, goes to shows with other boys and walks alone to a store over a block away." "Has it come to pass that the doctors of this nation are going to say who will or will not treat us?"[21]

Supporters believed accusations about Kenny's personality were in fact veiled attacks on Kenny for acting in a way doctors found unfeminine. NFIP officials had said that Kenny was "hard to get along with," the Tulsa Tribune mocked, but in fact she had simply refused to cooperate with certain doctors and NFIP officials. Was the NFIP unhappy because "she refused to leave the United States as soon as she arrived, as Mr. O'Connor suggested?" or because "she was not overawed by high medical authorities who did not want to be disturbed in the practice of letting sick muscles die in splints?" In fact her altruism proved she was not a charlatan, the paper noted. She had come to Oklahoma during the 1943 epidemic and asked for nothing but the travel expenses of herself and her assistant. The paper praised her as the epitome of the wholesome older woman untainted by the suspicious morals of the celebrities featured in March of Dimes publicity: "How different her attitude from the tearful pleas of mascara-ed Hollywood in the high-pressure campaign for the March of Dimes!"[22] "You have fought your way through thus far with all the courage of a pioneer," one letter-writer assured her in similar tones, placing her in the pantheon of American frontierswomen, "you have that fortitude and courage that never quits and never gives up, especially when the going is the toughest."[23]

And why did the NFIP not publicly attack these antagonistic doctors? Was it because its medical advisors were all part of the same elite establishment? The news that Fishbein had told Kenny to leave was "a most outrageous insult to every thinking American citizen," a woman from New York City declared. "I represent 'the public' and am not known," she told O'Connor; "You, however, are prominently known and I call upon you to make adequate reply to Morris Fishbein in the press."[24]

Underlying some of this populist support was a broader dislike of Roosevelt and the New Deal. The NFIP had long battled public suspicions that it was too closely tied to Roosevelt and the Democratic Party. "It was too bad that you did not explode that news before the panhandling got under way for the President['s] Birthday," one man told Kenny, "however the American people are at long last awakened to that fact that the National Foundation was nothing but a private affair."[25] A number of newspapers pointed out that O'Connor was "Mr. Roosevelt's former law partner," and began to demand accountability of "the prodigious amount of money that has been collected during the past ten years."[26] The NFIP's close relationship with the AMA further horrified people who already disliked Fishbein. One man assured Kenny that "America needs you more than it needs the Morris Fishbein Tripe and his ilk." "For years," he argued, "well informed" Americans have known "that the American Medical Association, dominated by these Alien Shysters, was but a racket, it took a visitor to these shores to get that into the public press."[27] Similarly the Chicago Associate Nurses, a small group that had organized pro-Kenny rallies, argued that attacks on Kenny were efforts "to break-down Nurse morale" and were instigated by "the Communist-Atheistic combine."[28] Fishbein knew a little about this organization and, he told O'Connor privately, "I am, of course, not troubling to notice this."[29]

Such responses were clearly on the fringe of American politics. They illuminate some of the darker sides of American medical populism, especially its longstanding antisemitic strain, which, ironically, was shared by the AMA and America's leading medical schools. Although Fishbein never raised the issue publicly, antisemitism had tainted his own career making it impossible for him to ever be elected president of the AMA.

POPULAR CULTURE

The Hearst papers, which had long been critical of the medical establishment, had from the outset seen Kenny as an opportunity to stir public outrage. During March and April 1944 a 5-part series in the *American Weekly*, the Hearst Sunday magazine, told Kenny's story with dramatic sentimentality. Drawing partly on the model of fighter pilot Robert Scott's best-selling autobiography *God Is My Co-Pilot* and partly on Kenny's 1943 autobiography, "God Is My Doctor" made her a courageous, religiously inspired nurse able to heal children and convert doctors and other nurses. The series compared "54 straight little bodies" without "a twisted or deformed limb" to children treated without the Kenny method "who walk with halting, tortured steps" or with "medieval contraptions of leather and steel." Reporters had long implied that Kenny achieved her results through a combination of God and medical science, calling her successes "Kenny miracles." Here Kenny was similarly chosen by the "Great Power" as an "instrument to ease pain and straighten little bodies and make them walk again."[30]

The newspaper's images, even more striking than the colorful prose, intermingled recent photographs of Kenny and her Institute with sketches characterizing the tragic and hopeful moments of her life. A photograph of the Institute, captioned "Monument of the Australian Back Country Nurse's Faith in a Revolutionary Cure That Has Given Back to Hundreds of Little Victims the Ability to Walk," was overshadowed by a sketch of angry-looking men in old fashioned collars, pointing at a young nurse looking up to the heavens with a baby in her arms, captioned "Medical Die-Hards, Refusing to Believe a Woman Could Succeed Where They Had Failed, Called Her a Quack, Charlatan—and Worse." The story moved from Australia to the United States with Kenny looking proudly at a map on the wall of her office "studded with hundreds of red and blue pins marking the spots where there are Kenny technicians and where the treatments are being given." A photograph of Kenny leaning over an infant, watched by the mother and a male doctor, was captioned: "Their Skepticism Wiped Out by Her Near-Miraculous Results, Doctors and Nurses Crowd Around While Sister Kenny Shows How to Re-educate Paralysis Damaged Muscles."[31]

Kenny was also featured in the *Wonder Women of History* comic book series, although with a less evangelical edge. Kenny is first shown teaching her brother Bill muscle exercises; she then chooses the "dangerous vocation" of bush nursing and faces a paralyzed child in the bush. From this point until she comes to America in the final 2 panels she is depicted wearing a nurse's white uniform. Amazed that her patients have recovered, her Australian mentor tells her "Sister Kenny, you've knocked our theories for a loop!" After World War I she finds that "few of the doctors were as willing as Dr. McConnell [sic] to fight the disease her way." A doctor standing over a child patient whose legs are in uncomfortable-looking braces asks Kenny: "Nurse, are you trying to tell me what to do?" and another doctor comments "it seems to work but it is against scientific theory!" She is then shown shaking hands with official-looking doctors in dark suits (perhaps health officials) who promise to "publicly endorse your method." She gradually wins over "nearly the whole medical profession—except a few conservatives" whose 1935 commission "denounce[s]" her methods. While Kenny leaves for London hoping "maybe English doctors will listen," Australian patients begin to demand that their doctors use "the Kenny treatment in all Australian hospitals." Later Kenny, now in a large black hat, thanks young American physicians who offer "to devote a floor of the Minneapolis General Hospital to a demonstration of your method."

All these images fit nicely into Kenny's portrayal of herself although the comic book was careful not to enter too closely into the polio wars. Thus, in the final panel, the Kenny treatment is "endorsed by the American Medical Association" and "inspired by the splendid achievements of this wonder woman, the American people show increasing determination—through the March of Dimes—to finish the magnificent work to which she has dedicated her life." Kenny in a large hat and black jacket reaches out to a young boy while a nurse and doctor in white uniforms look on in the background.[32] Here America physicians are her solid allies compared to skeptical Australian physicians who are forced by public pressure to adopt her work. The American people are offered a similar opportunity to donate to the March of Dimes as a way of supporting Kenny.

THE MARCH OF DIMES RESPONDS

The public furor over Kenny's threat to leave forced NFIP officials to defend their organization on many fronts: the issue of O'Connor's personal rudeness toward Kenny, whether he and the NFIP had shown poor judgment in not recognizing true innovation, and whether the NFIP practiced miserly and misguided funding priorities. If 50 percent of what was raised from March of Dimes campaigns was not returned to the local community but sent back to NFIP headquarters in New York City to be spent on education and research, donors wanted to know how it was divided up. Who were the recipients and how was their merit determined? And to what extent did NFIP's funding priorities simply replicate those of elite medical interests?

Throughout 1944 the NFIP public relations staff was busy producing press releases, radio scripts, and responsive letters that tried to defend the NFIP and counter Kenny's claims without being aggressive or nasty. Trying to defend American physicians without appearing craven to organized medicine was especially difficult, given the publications of critical articles and editorials on Kenny's work in *JAMA*.

The effort to balance defense and offense appears in this extract of a scripted radio "interview" between O'Connor and an announcer, produced in a Louisville, Kentucky, radio station in February 1944:

ANNOUNCER: Tell us this, Mr. O'Connor. Just how does the National Foundation make these grants for scientific research?

O'CONNOR: Each request for financial assistance is carefully studied by the Medical Advisory Committees of the National Foundation, composed of 39 eminent medical authorities. These men consider the possible value of the proper work—the ability of the men who will do it. If they think the project is sound and shows some promise of helpful results, they recommend to our Board of Trustees that the necessary amount of money be granted.

ANNOUNCER: Have the scientists studying the Kenny Method come to any conclusion about it, Mr. O'Connor?

O'CONNOR: Yes, they have. The University of Minnesota studied the Kenny Method under grants from the National Foundation...Treatment of cases by the Kenny Method during the early stages of infantile paralysis seemed to lessen the duration of the disease and increase the chances of recovery without crippling after-effects...There are some cases that can't be helped, at the present time, by any known method of treatment—the Kenny Method or any other...It's for these cases particularly that our research program to find out how to prevent the disease and even better methods of treatment must go on.[33]

In this description of research and clinical progress, the public relations staff was able to turn the story away from Kenny's threatened departure and toward the positive achievements of the NFIP. *The Story of the Kenny Method*, a new pamphlet, similarly explained the role the NFIP "played and is playing...in evaluating this technique and in making it available to every infantile paralysis victim." It enumerated the ways public donations had helped to expand the Kenny method: they had provided over 15 tons of wool, hundreds of washing machines and wringers, and the training of 900 people at the University of Minnesota who had graduated "with the approval and certification of Sister Kenny." Kenny's treatment, which the NFIP "wholeheartedly espoused," represented "an important step forward in our treatment of this disease."[34] The pamphlet painted a distinctive picture: a flexible, responsive philanthropy eager to hear from even those outside the medical establishment and to use their insights to help paralyzed American children.

Kenny's work and ideas had been taken seriously by the NFIP from the outset, NFIP publicity assured the American public. In fact, she had "never requested financial support from the National Foundation without receiving it." NFIP publicity introduced a new element in this narrative. "As a matter of fact," it claimed, "we had been interested in her work before her visit." In 1938 the NFIP had given a grant to physicians at the James Whitcomb Riley Hospital for Children in Indianapolis "to examine her work."[35] The idea that a polio philanthropy and American physicians were already aware of Kenny's methods before she had even arrived made Kenny less a visitor bringing unique information than a promoter of methods already under study by American polio experts.

However, NFIP publicity made clear, Kenny was not a scientist. Treatment and diagnosis, explained a pro-NFIP editorial in the *Hartford Courant*, were "two separate and distinct factors."[36] Unlike Kenny, the NFIP could draw on expert advisors who could recognize who was a scientifically trained expert and who was not. Her demand that the Institute in Minneapolis become the only center for teaching the Kenny method was, thus, misguided and "not sound," and perhaps even a sign of proprietary promotion. A professional philanthropy such as the NFIP had a breadth of knowledge about Americans' national health needs and therefore "knew that the task of teaching the number of technicians needed to serve the whole country was too great for any one school." Indeed, the aim of the NFIP was to ensure "that the Kenny method eventually becomes part of the regular curriculum of every medical and physical therapy school, thereby removing the need for a Kenny

Institute anywhere."[37] Both Kenny and the public needed to understand that skepticism and constant reevaluation were not personal attacks but part of the proper scientific process. The NFIP therefore regretted the "unprecedented publicity" given to Kenny's work, which had led to "exaggeration" and "in the minds of many a miraculous cure."[38]

NFIP officials could see that Kenny's accusations could easily move into an attack on money wrongly or corruptly spent, dollars and dimes that had been donated by ordinary Americans, including children. In a break from the secrecy it had practiced to date, the foundation began to argue that its mechanism for giving grants was both democratic and meritocratic. In a radio speech in March 1944 O'Connor explained "how we make financial grants for scientific research." No single individual made the decision, for not even the president of the NFIP or his medical director "could have at their command the necessary knowledge or sufficient wisdom to pass upon the broad research program called for by this program." Instead, a medical advisory committee was made up of "eminent men—all volunteers" including "orthopedic surgeons, pediatricians, neurologists, physiologists, internists, laboratory workers and specialists in medical education." These advisors considered the many applications carefully, weighing "the merits of the problem, the capabilities of the investigator, [and] the integrity of the institution."[39]

In this story of scientific progress, skeptical clinicians, just like laboratory scientists, worked cautiously to test therapeutic techniques. Their scientific integrity enabled them to remain deaf to sentimental calls for "quick cures" to stem the cries of children in pain and meant they could not ignore the possibility that many patients might have recovered spontaneously. Thus, various "qualified institutions" funded by the NFIP, including centers in Pennsylvania, Illinois, Indiana, Georgia, and New York, continued the process of evaluation.[40] A place like the Kenny Institute, which practiced a single therapy provided by a single group of clinicians, was not, NFIP officials stated, an appropriate location for such clinical research, for "best results" to improve polio care had to take place "in well organized medical centers where advantage can be taken of the manifold specialties that are concerned."[41] And, *The Story of the Kenny Method* argued, therapy was only a stop-gap measure for, to achieve the "final and complete conquest of infantile paralysis," the NFIP "will not be content with any method of treatment... no matter how good." True victory over polio had to come from the laboratory. The NFIP, the pamphlet declared, "will continue to carry on the most ambitious research program ever marshaled against any disease, until it is able to cure and prevent the disease and thus eliminate entirely the necessity of any after-treatment."[42]

Despite these defensive maneuvers, the relationship between the NFIP and some of its prominent donors began to falter. Hollywood celebrities, for example, recognized the dangers of tangling with a popular figure like Kenny whose accusations of discrimination and medical elitism were gaining public credence. Singer and comedian Eddie Cantor, who had long been associated with Roosevelt's polio charities and had just produced a movie for RKO, notified O'Connor "strictly off the record" that he had been asked by RKO "to help Sister Kenny." Uncertain of the right reply, Cantor assured him he would not do anything "that would interfere with our own drive for the Foundation."[43] Former silent picture star Mary Pickford, now a Hollywood producer, also wrote to O'Connor, warning that as national chair of the NFIP's Women's Division, she was "deeply concerned" that Kenny's attacks on the NFIP were tainting the reputation of the charity she and her Hollywood friends publicly represented and "doing the Foundation irreparable injury." On a recent hospital tour Pickford had noticed the Kenny method in use everywhere, yet other members of the Women's Division had told her that the NFIP refused to fund the Kenny Institute. Further, she reminded O'Connor of a cocktail party they had both attended at the Waldorf where "Dr. Fishbein was very outspoken in his criticism of [Kenny]."[44] Peter Cusack phoned Pickford and sent her "material containing accurate information regarding the Kenny Method and its relationship to the National Foundation," which, he assured her, would provide "an entirely different picture from the one presented in certain [Hearst] newspapers." Pickford's letter also spurred the NFIP's New York office to realize that sending copies of *The Story of the Kenny Method* to every NFIP chapter chairman was not enough. Men might function as a chapter's titular head but women were often its backbone and brains, and also frequently from well-connected families. The NFIP began to make sure they received NFIP publicity directly.[45]

The network of Kenny supporters included some influential people. In the third week of February, for example, W. C. Higginbotham, a Dallas railroad company director whose son Harry had been treated at the Institute, wrote to all the NFIP trustees. The recent March of Dimes campaign, Higginbotham pointed out, had "capitalized in many ways on the hard won fame and prestige of Sister Kenny." He argued the NFIP "should give Sister Kenny anything she asks" and that "the public who sustain it [the NFIP] should certainly be advised of the reasons she is being denied assistance."[46] The trustees who replied to Higginbotham were equally prominent. Automobile magnate Henry Ford and William Clayton, Roosevelt's assistant secretary of commerce, told Higginbotham they had "complete confidence in Mr. O'Connor."[47] Railroad owner Frederick Adams noted that he was a trustee of many organizations and knew "none that has been administered by its heads more unselfishly or with more scrupulous regard for its great responsibilities to the public." "In the Foundation," Adams reminded Higginbotham, executive to executive, "we are used to projects and budgets, and I fear Sister Kenny is not."[48]

Higginbotham had little influence outside Texas, but James Ford Bell was a different story. Bell was the founder of General Mills, chairman of its board, and the only NFIP trustee living in Minneapolis.[49] Kenny's local supporters and especially the women, Bell warned O'Connor in March 1944, saw him as "a target of dissatisfaction." They had "generously contributed to the work of the Institute" and were now "unreasonable and unreasoning," but "you cannot argue with sentimental women." While Bell admitted that Kenny "has a difficult personality" and "her demands and attitude are extremely hard to cope with," he did not believe that the NFIP had been "over generous" to her or properly recognized that "the treatments she offers have done good." In any case, the polio wars were leading to "a rising tide of unfavorable sentiment developing toward the Foundation, which is most unfortunate and undesirable."[50]

Bell suggested that the NFIP use Kenny as a figurehead in the upcoming campaign, pointing out the public's "hero worship of football players, baseball players, pugilists, etc." as well as Kenny's own enjoyment of "the limelight." The NFIP needed to be cautious of an emerging Kenny movement that it might not be able to control for neither O'Connor nor the NFIP, in Bell's view, "can command the publicity or the sentiment that she possesses."[51] O'Connor recognized that Bell was placing the NFIP in a precarious position but he did not agree with Bell's assessment. He saw more clearly than Bell that Kenny would not be amenable to being used as an NFIP figurehead and that it would not appease her.[52] Still, he did recognize that her accusations were hurting the regional and national standing of the NFIP. His staff sent lengthy notes to individual wealthy donors declaring "the

National Foundation is the *people's* Foundation...we have no secrets. There is nothing the public cannot and should not know."[53]

THE MINNESOTA PROBLEM

When Kenny complained to reporters that the University of Minnesota was not supporting her work, this created a serious public relations problem for the university. From the outset the university had put itself in her camp, using the growing reputation of Kenny and her work to establish its medical school and hospital as major polio centers. Relations between the university and city officials—who controlled the city hospitals where most of the medical school's teaching took place—had often been strained. When the Institute was incorporated as a nonprofit company with its own board of directors, its administration moved further away from the medical school. Yet the Institute maintained a connection with the city; its board was headed by Mayor Marvin Kline and included other city officials.[54] The University continued to seek good relations with these local politicians and to continue the medical school's interdependence with city hospitals.

Not only had the citizens of the Twin Cities adopted Kenny as a civic hero, but Kline, a Republican city councilman who was elected mayor in 1941, had firmly linked his career to Kenny, using her, as one NFIP official complained, "as a vehicle to popularize himself with the people of Minneapolis."[55] Kline had graduated from the University of Minnesota in architectural engineering and had worked in an architectural firm before being elected mayor. During the war he combined city and federal funds to sponsor housing, victory gardens, and salvage projects and set up a child care center and a veteran's referral center.[56] When he successfully ran for reelection against Democrat Hubert Humphrey in 1943, he boasted that "the work of Sister Kenny has taken the name of Minneapolis around the world" and that he considered "the establishment of the Elizabeth Kenny Institute as one of the major accomplishments of my administration." During the campaign Humphrey had vainly protested that it was the Mayo Clinic and not Kline who deserved credit for bringing Kenny to the Twin Cities, and that her initial work at the city hospital had been welcomed by the city's previous administration.[57] Kenny was aware of some of the pitfalls of immersing herself in local politics, but she found it impossible to ignore the Republican stance of many of her friends. She told reporters that although she had "no wish to be involved in a political argument" she was pleased to note that "Mayor Kline has supported my work most wholeheartedly."[58]

Medical school Dean Harold Diehl, to his consternation, became a central player in the polio wars when Kenny demanded that the school endorse her method publicly, threatening that otherwise "it will be unnecessary for me to prolong my stay in the U.S.A."[59] At a genial but unproductive meeting with representatives of the university, the Institute and the city's Board of Public Welfare Diehl explained that this demand was a sign that Kenny misunderstood academic etiquette. The University "does not and cannot officially endorse any method of treatment for infantile paralysis or any other disease. Things just are not done that way."[60] After the meeting Diehl stated publicly that while "the Medical School is interested in further investigation and development of this method" it did not endorse it. As for Kenny's new method of early diagnosis, Diehl had not had it demonstrated to him but "when Sister Kenny reveals her new diagnostic theory, the University will cooperate fully in a study of it."[61]

Local physicians began to take sides. Wallace Cole "declined to serve" on the Institute's new board.[62] John Pohl in contrast confirmed his loyalty to Kenny and her work by joining the board and praising her work in the local press as "the finest and best treatment known at the present time." He continued to supervise Kenny technicians at the city hospital and the Institute. After what observers later called "a hurriedly called meeting" that a number of board members were unable to attend, Pohl, aided by Kline, began to write a grant application to ask the NFIP to continue to fund the Institute's teaching program and also to allow it to function as a research institute.[63] Miland Knapp, who no longer directed the Institute's teaching program, agreed to join the new board but publicly distanced himself from some of Kenny's more controversial claims. In May 1944 in the *Journal-Lancet*, the state's medical journal, he offered his "own opinion," which was, he clarified, different from the opinion "of Sister Kenny." While hot packs were "most valuable" in "the stage of acute spasm," he conceded, on the basis of his clinical observations and recent physiological research, he could find no correlation between the appearance of spasm and the "severity or distribution" of muscle weakness. He also believed that Kenny's concept of mental alienation was "probably only a minor factor" and was in any case an "unfortunate term," for it implied "a physiologic cause of loss of function which is not justified by the clinical observations."[64] That fall as the newly elected president of the American Congress of Physical Therapy, Knapp reiterated his view that Kenny's concept of mental alienation was wrong and that the location of spasm did not in any way correlate with the location of weak muscles.[65]

After Diehl refused to endorse Kenny publicly, she began to tell a different story of her reception in Minneapolis. Instead of the enthusiastic acceptance she had described in her autobiography, she now claimed that physicians in nearby Rochester had been far more welcoming than those in the Twin Cities.[66] She also began to speak more frankly about the crucial financial support she received from local businessmen, especially her friends in the Exchange Club. In this new story the NFIP's grant in her early months in Minnesota had barely enabled her to survive. "Had I been absolutely dependent upon this assistance [from the NFIP]," she told Diehl, "the only value to the teaching profession would have been a presentation of my cadaver to the Anatomy Institute for teaching purposes, for I would have starved to death."[67]

THE AMA REPORT

In June 1944 the war got hotter. The AMA held its first annual meeting during wartime. Physicians heard lectures on the use of penicillin for syphilis, gonorrhea, and meningitis, and the use of thyroid extracts for sterility. The AMA's new president reminded them that "every physician in this country...[should] devote at least two hours a day to educating the people in his community" on the dangers of national or state health insurance legislation. There was also a symposium on the abuse of rest in treating disease. Los Angeles internist William Dock warned that it could lead to blood clots, bone atrophy, muscle wasting, and other disabilities.[68] Such warnings sounded much like Kenny's own rejection of immobilization in polio, but no one drew the analogy. Importantly, a group of orthopedic surgeons presented a harshly critical report, which Fishbein made sure was published simultaneously in *JAMA*.

The committee of "seven university professors," as the *New York Times* called them, had spent 2 years visiting 16 clinics in 6 cities (including Kenny's Institute) and had examined 740 patients.[69] St. Louis orthopedists Albert Key and Relton McCarroll both disliked Kenny. Key had published 2 articles defending "orthodox" care, and McCarroll, one of the authors of the 1941 study that had provided Kenny with dramatic statistics about the ineffective results of orthodox therapies, had attacked her work in *JAMA*.[70] At the other end of the spectrum was Chicago orthopedist Edward Compere who had introduced Kenny's methods into Wesley Memorial Hospital as early as 1942 and Herman Schumm, a Milwaukee orthopedist who had been convinced of the veracity of her ideas after his visit to Minnesota. Robert Funsten from the University of Virginia had originally been supportive but had become uncomfortable with the ways Kenny technicians threatened to disrupt hospital power relations and now believed that Kenny's "dynamic personality" had led her "to further her ideas and spread her theories."[71]

Neither Compere nor Schumm's views were represented in the final report. Instead, it retained Key and McCarroll's distaste for her style of practice and her claims, especially the idea that her work was revolutionary. Beginning treatment "as early as possible is desirable," the committee agreed, yet in the "acute febrile stage the handling necessitated by the Kenny treatment can be detrimental." The AMA committee reminded doctors, nurses, and physical therapists that therapy during this stage "is primarily a medical problem."[72]

The report rejected Kenny's claim that her work bettered "orthodoxy." In fact, there was "no satisfactory evidence," the committee stated, "that the institution of early local treatment will alter the course or the extent of the paralysis." The committee also attacked the significance of the signs and symptoms Kenny claimed to have identified and the methods she had developed to treat them. While it was true that pain could be relieved by "hot foments," the committee argued, in fact, "pain is not an important feature of the disease in most instances and when present, can be relieved also by other measures." Uncomfortable with Kenny's word "spasm," the committee used it only with quotation marks. Recovery from spasm, in any case, occurred in most patients spontaneously. Hot packs were not "a panacea in this disease" and her "rigid technique" was "neither important nor essential." As orthopedists the committee members especially disliked Kenny's cavalier rejection of standard orthopedic apparatus. Splints and braces remained "beneficial for some patients," and "respirators saved many lives."[73]

The committee also found that those parts of Kenny's work that were valuable were not original. This argument was succinctly summed up by Key, quoting the Australian reviewer of her 1937 textbook, that "what is good in the Kenny treatment is not new and what is new is not good."[74] Citing eminent polio experts who had written standard orthopedic textbooks and had taught at least a generation of surgeons and physical therapists, the committee noted that "proper positioning in bed" was standard orthopedic practice and "hot wet packs" and "moist heat" had been discussed by Lovett and Legg decades earlier. The idea of reeducating muscles and the warning that physicians should not use braces "unnecessarily" could be found in Lovett and Jones' 1929 text *Orthopaedic Surgery*. Further, "stiffness, muscle tenderness and early contractures have been long recognized and considered an integral part of the acute phase of the disease."[75]

Her theory of polio as primarily a disease of muscles and skin was, the report said, simply wrong. The surgeons argued, as had McCarroll and Crego in 1941, that the "amount of residual paralysis" was dependent not on the physical therapy used but "on the amount of destruction in the central nervous system," which varied "tremendously in different epidemics." There was only one area in which Kenny could be correct, according to the committee. Perhaps there were, as Kenny claimed, "local changes in isolated muscles during the acute stage," but the nature of such changes "must be studied further." Mental alienation had already been described by Jones in 1911, but her statement "that the flaccid muscles are normal is obviously not true." The concept of incoordination was "merely another term for the condition of muscle substitution," a term used by Ray Lyman Wilbur in 1912, but it was "of relatively little importance." Even Kenny's much publicized new diagnostic sign was not new or revolutionary but had been described by William Aycock in 1928 and George Draper in 1931.[76]

Most of all the committee condemned "the wide publicity which has misled the public and many members of the medical profession," even though it may have "stimulated the medical profession to re-evaluate known methods of treatment of this disease and to treat it more effectively." This was the old argument that Kenny so disliked.[77] Echoing Bruce Gill's arguments in his 1943 letter to the Orthopaedic Correspondence Club, the committee warned that her promises of recovery were false and accused her of "a deliberate misrepresentation of the facts of treatment by other methods." "Despite reports in the medical literature that around 50–80 percent of patients paralyzed by polio had a 'spontaneous recovery,'" she attributed "all improvement...to the treatment." Her use of McCarroll and Crego's statistics was drawn from a study that "dealt entirely with severely paralyzed patients," yet she had "been told repeatedly that this is not a fair comparison to make." Accurate statistics also did not support her claim that 80 percent of her patients recovered. Despite the caveat that "this we attribute to her overzealous desire to promote adoption of the Kenny treatment," the committee was clearly accusing Kenny of deliberate exaggeration.[78]

The surgeons who wrote the "Evaluation of the Kenny Treatment of Infantile Paralysis" hoped their report would end the debate around the worth of her work. But the report's reception at the AMA meeting showed how mistaken they were. Far from being defining, it instead became a catalyst for a breakdown in physician unity. Its explicit attacks on both the work and its promoter were written in a way that cried out for quotation by newspaper reporters. Commentators noted that the report read "more like a prosecutor's brief than a scientific document."[79] Kenny's fight was now with the medical establishment. Patients, families, and ordinary doctors could support the high-handed AMA or take the side of an altruistic nurse trying to help crippled children.

The popular press took sides. Albert Deutsch in *PM* found what he called the AMA's "scathing attack" on Kenny's work "a strangely unconvincing document, charged with emotional bias against Miss Kenny and her claims." He guessed that at the base of the disagreement was money. He sharply contrasted "private orthopedic specialists who might be cut off from a lucrative source of income if Miss Kenny's method should be generally adopted" to public health officials with "no axe to grind" who found her work valuable despite "some serious flaws in her concept."[80] "Paralysis Method Held Overpraised" argued the *New York Times* in contrast, quoting with approval the NFIP's 1943 annual report that expressed regret at the "unprecedented publicity" given to the Kenny method, which had led to "exaggeration."[81]

On the first page of that month's *National Foundation News* NFIP officials placed a special notice saying that the report "by a group of distinguished orthopedic surgeons" had resulted in "numerous inquires regarding the National Foundation policy." Cautiously treading a path between Kenny and the AMA, the NFIP argued that "the somewhat controversial situation as to the exact merit of each phase of the Kenny method" did not alter the NFIP's policy "in any way." Many physicians "feel that a contribution has been made in the Kenny method and use various phases of the technique in their practice." "The National Foundation is interested in only one thing—determining the value of the various phases of this technique by scientific study in laboratories of physiology and in clinics with a view to retaining such merit as it may possess."[82] Recognizing the upheaval this report had caused, O'Connor also began an extensive tour visiting chapters in 12 states and 21 cities in the West and Northwest to try to calm the waters and to present a rational, unflustered face to a philanthropy under siege.[83]

Wily enough to know that the report would work best left on its own, Fishbein offered a brief editorial comment in *JAMA*, drawing on a study by Kabat and Knapp that argued that muscle spasm was "a reflex phenomenon" and that "there appears to be no direct relation between it and motor paralysis."[84] His editorial in *Hygeia* fulsomely praised the work of this "distinguished committee" whose members had "nothing to gain personally by their report," and reiterated that continuous hot packs were of "questionable value" and "a waste of manpower and hospital beds." "Unfortunately people in general do not read as carefully as they should the reports that appear in the press regarding medical technics," Fishbein added, and it was best to "get a competent doctors and to leave to his decision the method of treatment to be followed." He praised Kenny's "enthusiasm" and concluded that "she has acted like an enzyme or a ferment to hasten study and to encourage the earlier appearance of important facts."[85] Surgeon General Thomas Parran refused to get involved, explaining to Kenny by telegram that no action by the United States Public Health Service (USPHS) was indicated since the AMA report "points out [how] important your contribution [is] in stimulating scientific re-evaluation of various known methods of treatment."[86] The report, as its authors had hoped, provided a vocabulary and way of thinking that helped physicians distance mainstream medicine from Kenny's work. A doctor at Chicago's Michael Reese Hospital, one Kenny supporter noted, said to patients "we aren't calling it the Kenny system any more. We have made a few changes and have our own system."[87] Similarly a prominent physician at Northwestern's medical school claimed Kenny "hasn't shown doctors anything that they didn't know before. These nurses who get ideas over-value themselves because they don't know the whole picture."[88]

In Minnesota Diehl's effort to find a quiet middle ground was undermined by antagonists within his medical school led by physiologist Maurice Visscher who had been at the University of Minnesota since the 1920s. A researcher with a national reputation, Visscher was the recipient of several large research grants from the NFIP.[89] In June 1944 he helped to organize a "Symposium on the Management of Infantile Paralysis" that, as one of the editors of the *Journal-Lancet*, he then published as a special issue the following month.[90] Along with articles by neurologists and physiologists from the university, the July issue contained an editorial on "The Present Status of Poliomyelitis Management" written by Visscher and 3 other faculty members.[91] The editors praised the "energetic use of hot packs" as certainly better than "rigid immobilization" and the "highly expert" use of physical therapy that had brought attention to "an altogether too frequently neglected aspect of poliomyelitis after-care." But in pointed but not vitriolic prose, they argued that medical research had not demonstrated that any single polio therapy had "superiority over all others," so physicians had to "continue to search for better ones." More sharply, they stated that there was no proof to justify Kenny's theory of the centrality of muscles in polio pathology or that her methods minimized early paralytic damage. Further, her terms spasm and alienation were "ill-defined" and "awkward" and her attention to these clinical signs was probably not original.[92] The *Journal-Lancet* issue received strong praise from neurologists and physiologists around the country who particularly liked the editorial for having, as one man saw it, "the courage to bring out the good side of the Kenny method...against certain belligerent and reactionary groups who have acted as if their precincts in medicine were being taken from them."[93]

Members of the public in Minneapolis were not convinced. Many saw the AMA report as further evidence of jealous physicians trying to hinder the expansion of Kenny's work. A small group of Minneapolis businessmen assured Kenny that "the People on the street" were "going to bat for you."[94] The owner of the Emrich Baking Company of Minneapolis excoriated "the ridiculous and monstrously unfair attack made on you by Dr. Ghormley" and assured her that "your many admirers, including myself, are aware of the splendid contributions you have made to medical science."[95] A lumber company official was "disgusted...that an intelligent group of men, such as A.M.A. is made up of, should under rate and make such statements about one who is giving so much to Humanity."[96] Another local supporter reminded Kenny of "the secret opposition and jealousy and pride of the 'established' order."[97] Kenny needed no such reminder.

A NEW MOVEMENT?

At first Kenny fought this new level of the polio wars with familiar weapons: telegrams, letters, reports, and interviews with reporters and science writers. She told Diehl that as her work had been "discredited" she and her staff would stop participating in the University's teaching courses, but after Diehl's tactful negotiation, she agreed to continue teaching the physicians' classes and the 20 technicians who were already enrolled in her courses.[98]

The public continued to support Kenny passionately. That summer Washington experienced a serious polio epidemic. With the backing of the *Washington Times-Herald*, Kenny and the local health department decided to transfer a small group of children to the Institute, despite protests by pediatricians that sending patients to Minnesota was a "wasteful, unnecessary expenditure of time, money and manpower." With funding from Eleanor Patterson, the owner and publisher of the *Times-Herald* and a controversial socialite, Kenny traveled 3 times to the nation's capital between July and October 1944, meeting civic leaders, local physicians, diplomats including Australian ambassador Sir Owen Dixon, and a sprinkling of Congressmen and senators.[99] When parents begged to see Kenny for advice about their paralyzed children, city health officials, warning that "miracles must not be expected," organized a special event at the Statler Hotel, which they called a Forum Against Fear, a reference to one of the 4 freedoms Roosevelt had proposed as fundamental in his 1941 State of the Union address: freedom of speech, freedom of religion, freedom from want, and freedom from fear. One mother wept saying, according to the *Times-Herald*, "I just know something good will come...that she has come at all is a miracle."[100]

To some members of the public, the upheaval around the polio wars looked like the making of a new movement. The word itself was used by a Georgia Congressman who told reporters in October 1944 of his "intense interest in the Kenny movement."[101] James Hulett, a young sociologist at the University of Illinois, suggested that "the campaign carried on by Miss Elizabeth Kenny and her supporters [had]...begun to assume the proportions of a cult." "Of course," Hulett assured NFIP officials, "I use the word 'cult' objectively as a name for a particular type of social movement, and not as an epithet."[102]

In this movement, the usual power relationships between physician and parent were disrupted. Would this movement engage with national medical politics as well? Would Kenny's attack on organized medicine become a battle about the inadequacies of New Deal welfare services? Would it be a spiteful populist crusade like Father Charles Coughlin's attack on Roosevelt, Jews, capitalists, and Communists?

Kenny had only limited control over the character and direction of this nascent movement. She enthusiastically joined with politicians who expressed their sympathy with her fight, but when anyone began to talk about coordinating Kenny centers or setting up other funding groups, she clung fiercely to her Institute. Her advisors in Minneapolis, similarly, sought to ensure that all coordination came from the Institute's board. The board began to plan a regional fundraising drive. Drawing on the March of Dimes campaigns, they also began to set up a new pro-Kenny philanthropy. Instead of the March of Dimes posters showing children in braces, making their way awkwardly out of wheelchairs, Kenny's campaign would feature children joyously walking and playing.

Kenny sought to make this new populist movement less explicitly anti-doctor. A Chicago public relations man urged her to "avoid any sweeping criticism of the American Medical Association, the Warm Springs Foundation, groups of doctors, etc, to avoid alienating physicians who can be won to our side."[103] Kenny was already aware of the dangers of being the figurehead of an anti-doctor movement. Her own medical allies, she frequently declared, were all "members of the American Medical Association," and the AMA report, therefore, represented only the views of a few antagonists.[104] In her 16-page response to the AMA report addressed to the Institute's board, she pointed out that the same *JAMA* issue had published a "favorable" paper on her work "given by Doctors who had listened and learned." As for the AMA committee's complaint that she had told patients "who had received treatment at other Centers that disability would not have occurred if they had received the Kenny treatment," the Committee members were acting "like a group of petulant school boys rather than a scientific body." These patients "were well aware of this fact without me telling them." All nuance disappeared when she expressed her outrage at the claim that she had made a "deliberate misrepresentation." Such statements, she declared, were motivated by "[a] deliberate intention to belittle me and accuse me in the eyes of the public."[105]

In dramatic theater a few days after the AMA report reached the newspapers, Kenny invited a group of reporters and around 50 visiting physicians to the Institute. She showed a short film of a young paralyzed patient who "had been given up by doctors and was expected to die." Then the girl was presented to the audience alongside a boy who had been treated by orthodox methods. "The contrast was appalling," said the *Minneapolis Star-Journal*.[106] To an audience in Washington a few months later she offered the same demonstration but entirely on film. Telling the crowd "my picture will speak for itself," she showed patients transformed by care at her Institute, standing straight and sturdy beside 4 children treated by the orthodox method and "hopelessly crippled for life." While it was certainly dramatic, this scenario also posed an uncomfortable ethical dilemma: had some children been left disabled so as to stand as exemplars of bad treatment? No, Kenny assured her audience, these 4 had "volunteered" their services, and in return she had provided them with scholarships and medical assistance.[107]

Despite her efforts not to attack the entire medical community, the polio wars began to unravel some of Kenny's medical friendships, including her prized alliances with orthopedic surgeons. Her patients' families had frequently told her how they hoped that her methods would obviate the need for a surgical operation, and Kenny had often said that surgery was usually unnecessary if her methods were used early enough. Now she developed a more forceful antisurgery stance. Relations between Kenny and Chicago orthopedist Edward Compere deteriorated when the press quoted Kenny as saying that orthopedists disliked her work because if patients were treated by her methods the surgeons would lose 40 percent of their practice.[108] This "rather strong statement is completely untrue and I am sure you know it is not true," Compere told Kenny in exasperation, and he deplored her attack on the integrity of physicians whose motives for helping polio sufferers were "quite similar to your own." The AMA report, he argued, "was in no sense intended as either an attack on you or upon your methods as some of the newspapers, and I think you yourself, interpreted it to be." Compere reminded Kenny of the ways he himself had taken her work seriously, including the separate unit for acute patients he had just organized at the Wesley Memorial Hospital to enable his Kenny-trained staff to treat patients "from the time that the diagnosis can be made." At the end of his letter he announced that he would no longer engage in private debate with her. "I have refused to accept long distance telephone calls from you because I have become convinced that nothing can be accomplished by them except perhaps further misunderstandings."[109]

Kenny had no patience with obscuration. In sorrow and anger she agreed that the AMA report did not represent Compere's own opinion for "you are too honest, I hope, to be a double-dealer." But she was "surprised to think you signed your name to it," especially as it "accused me of perjury," which was "poor thanks to give to one who came from afar to give to you the greatest gift you and your people have yet received with regard to this disease and many others." Compere should be well aware that the committee had not "made a close study of this work for two years" but instead had wasted time "visiting other Centers where a crude, mongrelized treatment is given." As for her claim that orthopedists resented losing surgical patients, "an Orthopedic Surgeon from Kansas City informed me that the average work of the Orthopedic Surgeon was 40 per cent the after-effects of infantile paralysis. Whether it is correct or not I do not know."[110] She did not comment on the ethical implications of her statement, which had angered Compere, but defended herself from what she saw as accusations of fraud and deception. This was not a letter that could be answered in any calm way and Compere did not try. Instead he quietly moved away from his prominent stance as a Kenny ally and began to rebuild allegiances with his specialist peers. "My interest in any particular method for the treatment of infantile paralysis, has been over-estimated," Compere told a man seeking his support for an invention to standardize heating hot packs a few months later; "I have used hot packs, as recommended by Miss Kenny, but have found them far less curative than Miss Kenny herself."[111] Compere continued as the chair of the orthopedics department of Northwestern's medical school until 1949 and in the 1950s edited a well-known volume on orthopedics and traumatic surgery, but—perhaps as the price he paid for supporting Kenny in the early 1940s—he was never elected to a senior position in any national orthopedic society.[112]

By comparison Robert Funsten and Charles Frankel, his junior associate at the University of Virginia, remained important orthopedic authorities, speaking frequently about the dangers of Kenny's version of polio care. At the Southern Medical Association in 1945, for example, they warned that a "rigid" use of the Kenny method, which they had tried in 1943, had been "expensive, illogical and unsatisfactory." Perhaps Kenny had "stimulated a great deal of investigative work," but much research had now "disproven

many of her statements and claims." They also condemned her "bitter determination... to force her theories upon the medical profession and the public regardless of
pathological data."[113]

In July 1944, Marvin Kline, as head of the Institute's board of directors, wrote to
O'Connor to apply for a 3-year $840,000 grant. In what was clearly another move in the
polio wars Kline said boldly that this large NFIP grant would be used to continue funding the Institute's technician teaching programs in the Kenny method—"the only treatment based on sound physical medicine"—and to establish a clinical research center at
the Institute to be "devoted to clinical investigation of the disease of infantile paralysis
and the application of the Kenny principles to other neuro-muscular diseases" including arthritis, cerebral palsy, and postoperative care.[114] Gudakunst asked Diehl to find out
more about this request. Diehl checked but found that neither Knapp nor the current
coordinator of the Kenny courses at the medical school knew "anything about it."[115]

The NFIP wanted to handle this grant application as carefully as possible. The decision to turn the Institute into a center for clinical research would represent a major
shift in power relations between the NFIP and Kenny's supporters. The NFIP, further,
had consistently argued that the Institute was an inappropriate site for polio research.
Twelve months earlier Kline and 2 city aldermen had traveled to New York to discuss the
Institute's budget and had promised O'Connor "that the purpose of the Kenny Institute
was for the teaching of the Kenny method" and that NFIP funding for the Institute was
to be handled between Diehl and O'Connor.[116] But now a group of Institute officials was
acting without having consulted Diehl or even most of the physicians in its own facility.

It was here that John Pohl, superintendent of the Kenny Institute, made a decisive
move away from other Institute physicians. He had written the grant application in con-
sultation with Kline and other members of the Institute's board, and he recognized that
calling the Institute a potential research site was a defining step. Krusen at the Mayo
Clinic and Lewin in Chicago may have been able to express their support of Kenny while
holding onto the respect of their specialist peers, but Pohl was working in the eye of the
storm without a senior teaching position at the medical school.[117] His polio work had
rapidly become an inseparable part of Kenny's sphere.

Pohl was a shy man, uncomfortable with the cocktail parties and formal dinners that
Kenny adored. Yet he had increasingly linked his own career to Kenny. He admitted that
she could be difficult but he began to feel that his contribution was translating her ideas
for other doctors to understand.[118] Kenny's work with Henry Haverstock had impressed
him mightily, and in 1942 this patient (H.H.) was the first of a series of 26 patients he
described in a report on the Kenny method published in JAMA.[119]

Kenny saw Pohl as one of her most attentive and helpful supporters. He had, she noted
in early 1942, "attended every session and was present at the bedside of every acute case
when examined by me and took particular care to watch all phases of the signs and symptoms and the especial treatment for each sign and symptom."[120] Pohl's promotion of Kenny,
however, made him less reliable as an objective medical observer.[121] But he deeply believed
that the worth of her work should stand above petty politics, whether among city officials,

the Institute's staff and directors, or the medical school faculty. Immediately after the AMA report he had told the local newspapers that her work was "the finest and best treatment known at the present time" and that "antiquated methods which allow children to suffer deformities from infantile paralysis should be abolished."[122] University physicians, in Pohl's view, had allied themselves with the NFIP ostensibly for scientific reasons but really because the NFIP was one of the nation's richest sources for medical research funding. It was an expression of his personal and professional faith in Kenny's work that led him to take this provocative new step of trying to expand the Institute's mission.

O'Connor decided that the opinion of a group outside the NFIP was needed to assess this new grant application and turned to the National Research Council (NRC) to advise the NFIP on whether to fund it or, more accurately, how least problematically to reject it. Founded during World War I as a scientific advisory body for the military, the NRC had taken on this function again during World War II, establishing a series of committees offering expertise on topics ranging from foot fungus to dengue fever.[123]

In August 1944, in response to O'Connor's request, the NRC's Division of Medical Sciences set up a special subcommittee to investigate the Institute's grant application.[124] The coordinators of the subcommittee, George Darling, the vice-chairman of the Division, and O. H. (Perry) Pepper, head of the Division's Committee on Medicine, were careful to frame this investigation as the arbitration of what constituted an appropriate place to conduct scientific research and professional training based on national standards and the NFIP's already established policies. The new subcommittee, they reiterated, was not going to "get drawn into any of the pros and cons concerning the Kenny treatment itself."[125]

Pepper was a senior faculty member at the University of Pennsylvania and a member of a socially prominent Philadelphia family.[126] The rest of the NRC subcommittee consisted of 2 medical school deans (Milton Winternitz of Yale and Wilbur C. Davison of Duke), a physiologist (Philip Bard of Johns Hopkins), a virologist-epidemiologist (Thomas Francis Jr. of the University of Michigan), an orthopedist (Guy Whitman Leadbetter from George Washington's medical school), a physical medicine expert (George Morris Piersol of the University of Pennsylvania), and George Darling himself.[127] Francis, who later coordinated the Salk vaccine trials, was the only member with research expertise in polio. Neither Piersol nor Leadbetter, the 2 clinicians interested in polio therapy, had been to Minnesota or played any part in the polio wars.

In September Darling wrote a careful letter to Kline, letting him know that the committee would be traveling to Minneapolis "to make recommendations on the suitability of the Kenny Institute as a proper place to receive large grants for research, teaching, and so forth—not to study or evaluate the Kenny Treatment, as such." The visitors would want to see facilities and equipment and to talk with the Institute's medical staff, business administrator, and others responsible for the proposed research and training programs. They "will, of course, hope to see Sister Kenny," but "they will not be particularly interested in patients except incidentally, nor in demonstrations of the treatment methods."[128] This letter, Pepper told Darling in a private note, "hit the exact note which I had hoped you would."[129]

Although the NRC members tried to frame this investigation as an unbiased institutional review, it was impossible for any conciliatory letter to assuage the suspicions of Kenny and her supporters that yet another group of elite physicians was coming to Minnesota to disparage her work. Kenny shrewdly understood that the NRC could act independently of the NFIP. In a letter addressed to "Gentlemen" she presented herself cautiously as a clinical innovator without emotionality or overreaching claims. She asked for several hours to present to the committee the results "of my clinical research" and also invited the group to the Ray-Bell Studios in St. Paul where she would show her "documentary film." But then, moving from the cooperative to the brash, she added that she would like the committee to forward their "findings...with regard to this presentation" to British Medical Association branches in London, Sydney, Cape Town, Canada, and India, and to the health departments of these countries. In an unfortunate phrase that turned scientists into amanuenses rather than investigators, she noted that there was an "urgent need of a detailed description of my research in muscle anatomy and physiology and bodily mechanics."[130]

On September 24 5 committee members began their trip to Minneapolis, arriving by train the following day. They dined that evening with 6 members of Minnesota's medical school faculty who were "most concerned with the teaching and research in the field of polio" and who represented its varied views.[131] Knapp and Cole worked closely and quite effectively with Kenny; Dean Diehl and William O'Brien, the coordinator of the university's postgraduate courses, were the mediators between the university and the Institute; John McKinley, professor of neuropsychiatry, and Maurice Visscher, professor of physiology, were firmly in the anti-Kenny camp. The group had "a very free discussion" and was later joined by Mayor Kline and Fred Fadell, the Institute's new public relations manager.[132]

The next morning the NRC committee went to the Institute where they met Kenny and the business manager of the Institute, some technicians and nurses, and Pohl and a recent medical graduate who was the Institute's resident physician. After lunch the visitors watched Kenny's film and then visited the city hospital's laboratories, which they considered inadequate and poorly equipped.[133] Kline was the host of that night's dinner, and the guests included Kenny, Pohl, Henry Haverstock (father of Kenny's first patient and secretary of the Institute's board), and 2 of Kenny's wealthy local supporters.[134]

It was a short visit but the NRC committee met all the major players, saw the facilities at the Institute and city hospital, watched Kenny demonstrate her methods, and socialized with her proponents and antagonists. In November, after 2 months of discussion, the NRC committee finished its 21-page report and sent it to O'Connor.

The committee members identified a number of significant problems in the Institute's organization. The first was politics. They disliked the power exercised by Kline, who they believed was too closely connected with the Fadell agency, which was not only running the Institute's upcoming fundraising drive but also planning Kline's 1945 mayoral reelection campaign. Just what the public funds raised in the upcoming Institute drive would be used for seemed to be unclear, even to members of the Institute's board. In an early draft of its report, the NRC committee had warned that any NFIP funding policy of the Institute might increase "power in the hands of the political interests with obvious dangers of graft and still lowered standards."[135] The committee removed this comment, along with other intemperate phrases, from the final report.

The committee tried to take the idea of the Institute as a research facility seriously but it was difficult for its members to conceive of research without proper laboratory space or to imagine patient care alone as sufficient for a research program. Even the grant's proponents seemed unable to explain how laboratory evidence would be integrated with clinical observation. The committee was not impressed with the Institute's facilities or its professional structure. There were, the committee pointed out, few actively involved physicians. Knapp, neurologist Joseph Michaels, and pediatrician Alfred Stoesser, all chiefs of staff at the city hospital and at the Institute, were "largely inactive in the Institute proper" although they did examine patients before they were admitted to the city hospital and were available on call at the Institute. The Institute's disturbingly close relationship to the local medical community outside the university also suggested inadequate professional supervision. Unlike the university's teaching hospital, which restricted patient care to physicians on the medical school faculty, the Institute, like most community hospitals, welcomed outside physicians who were allowed to "continue in professional charge" of their patients. The committee noted with disapproval that these physicians had to agree to "cooperate with Kenny procedures." As for the Institute's full-time staff, the number of doctors was "grossly inadequate for the number of patients present," a situation that probably explained the inadequacy of the Institute's clinical records, which detailed "chiefly Kenny treatment and its results."[136]

The committee's skepticism turned to suspicion in describing John Pohl. During the NRC visit Pohl had not hidden his frustration with both the NFIP and the medical school. He was, the committee noted, the physician most directly involved in policymaking at the Institute, although he worked there only part time, visiting for about an hour on some days. What was clear was that the committee members neither liked nor trusted him. The early report draft noted that when he had been offered the post of Institute superintendent he had asked for a $20,000 salary, an amount that seemed high. While Pohl and other local physicians associated with the Institute might "honestly believe in the technique," the early draft noted, "the Committee has reason to believe that the motive of personal gain may enter into this picture."[137]

"Today the University, Sister Kenny and the students all seem to be dissatisfied," the committee concluded in its final report. There was "deep and serious disagreement[s] and personal dislike and distrust not only between the groups but also between many of the individuals within each group." The university wished to continue courses on polio's treatment "but on a broader basis and with complete academic freedom." The medical faculty of the University of Minnesota had been "enthusiastic at first" and "impressed in various degrees with the theory and the practice of the Kenny method," but many were "now hesitant to go along with the movement." Kenny rejected the idea of broadening the Institute's courses and instead wanted to teach courses that would "be limited strictly to the Kenny concept and method of treatment." She also felt the present courses were too short and should be lengthened to 2 years. Yet physical therapists and nurses studying at the Institute expressed wide dissatisfaction with the current courses "as too long for the content."[138]

Politics, the committee's report concluded, were at the heart of these divisions. City officials were "sincerely enthusiastic" but also not "blind to the incidental benefits to Minneapolis, to the Minneapolis General Hospital and to political careers." Local physicians benefited from an association with the Institute "either directly or indirectly." Most believed "that the method is productive of some good results" although "some may frown on the dogmatic position of Sister Kenny" and "some doubt the theory." The public support on which Kenny and her allies relied was, the committee believed, genuine but naive. Citizens "in favor of anything which will increase the use and spread of the Kenny method not only in Minneapolis but in the United States and throughout the world" were "not aware of existing scientific doubts" and did not "appreciate the complexities of the situation."[139]

Finally the committee turned to Kenny herself. She had been hospitable and patient. But she also "revealed certain very significant attitudes to the problem under study."

Not only had she expressed great disapproval of the NFIP and its president but she had "belittled additional research," stating that "30 years ago she had done all the research necessary." Yet, notwithstanding such a statement, the grant application had requested funding for "Clinical Research" and "Neurological Research." The committee was not convinced that Kenny grasped the complexities of polio science. It praised her knowledge of the anatomy involved in her treatment but warned that she lacked "fundamental information of scientific medicine." As an example the committee cited her statement in the film she showed them that "the muscle is the host to the virus." Most of all, the committee disliked Kenny's prominence at the Institute. "Her unusual personality dominates the whole scene," its final report warned. "She *is* the Kenny Institute and there is no possibility of the control of anything by anyone else for she controls everything and everybody. Her statements are empiric and final; there is no argument."[140]

The NFIP, the committee concluded, should not dissociate itself from the Institute, partly in order to protect "what is good in the Kenny method" from being "lost through unfortunate associations," and partly because the committee feared that if the Institute's fundraising campaign expanded "the duplication of nationwide drives" it would have "an effect upon public confidence." The Institute, in the NRC committee's view, was not and could not be a proper site for scientific research. The NFIP should promote Kenny's work only in the narrowest sense: as a useful method that should be available to American patients treated by properly trained technicians. The NFIP should continue to fund courses for technicians, but it should make sure that all applicants were qualified physical therapists, not nurses without physical therapy training. No money should be given to the Institute for the maintenance of patients used solely as teaching or research subjects. And, most important, there should be no grant for either basic or clinical research unless the Institute, at some time in the future, could provide "conclusive evidence of a competent investigative staff and adequate laboratory facilities."[141]

The NFIP thanked the NRC committee for their work but did not immediately respond to the Institute. It kept the NRC report secret, as the NRC committee had requested, and continued to watch the responses in Minnesota.

PENNIES FOR KENNY

In November 1944 the Institute's board of directors, confident that a public movement was behind them, organized the first separate Kenny campaign. The NRC was just finishing its report and it seemed likely that it would lead to a rejection by the NFIP, but nothing had been publicly announced. The Kenny campaign was coordinated by a public relations firm based in Minneapolis, and its slogan was "Pennies for Kenny." Kenny reigned as the campaign's celebrity.[142] Although the drive was restricted to Minnesota, she went on tour, taking with her a new technical film demonstrating her work at the Institute. Dressed in black lace with orchids on her shoulder and accompanied by Mary Kenny, Kenny entered auditoriums and ballrooms to low murmurs of "there she is," "look, there is Sister Kenny," "here she comes."[143]

She used this tour not only to attack the NFIP and laud the Institute but also to reposition herself in race politics. During the late 1930s the NFIP had scrambled to respond to civil rights activists who pointed to the neglect of black polio survivors. Convinced by Warm Springs' white trustees that the center should remain a whites-only institution, the NFIP had established a small polio hospital at the Tuskegee Institute that opened in 1941. It was designed to be both a treatment center and a place to train African American orthopedic physicians, nurses, and physical therapists unable to gain access to specialty training programs in hospitals around the country.

During the war an emerging African American middle class helped to make problems of polio care visible, especially the racist policies implicit in almost all hospital care. Some municipal public hospitals such as the Minneapolis General Hospital admitted both white and black poor patients; most private hospitals were restricted to white paying patients. Initially affiliated with the city hospital, Kenny had accepted African American patients from the outset, as the *Reader's Digest*'s depiction of Suzy had shown.[144] With the founding of the Institute, a city building under the supervision of the city's board of welfare, Kenny continued to accept both black and white child patients and also a few African American nurses for training, such as Chicago nurse Lulu Boswell who later worked at the Tuskegee polio hospital.[145] In other cities indigent black patients with polio received the Kenny method in public infectious diseases hospitals such as the Isolation Hospital in Memphis.[146] References to Kenny and her work began to appear more frequently in the black press. The *Chicago Defender* featured a photograph of a grinning 11-year-old Jean Andrews on her way to Minneapolis to receive treatment at the Institute, and one of its health columns praised the Kenny treatment as "undoubtedly helpful in lessening the paralytic deformities."[147] Before the end of the war there were only a few black celebrities involved with polio fundraising. But in 1943 African American boxer Ray Robinson, an enthusiastic supporter of March of Dimes campaigns, was featured in the *New York Amsterdam News* in a story about a black girl who "was among the first to be benefited by the Kenny treatment at the Minneapolis General Hospital."[148]

The racist assumptions Kenny had grown up with were clearly visible in her autobiography where she portrayed Australian Aborigines as savage and comic.[149] In other remarks publicized in 1943 Kenny had referred to the limited number of black patients she had treated by noting the possible shielding affects of "pigment."[150] Such views were not challenged by the white businessmen and professionals she worked with in Minnesota. During the 1944 drive, however, perhaps pressured by the Fadell firm, Kenny became more aware of the importance of race politics in polio. After she showed her film in Washington, D.C. she proudly quoted a statement from John W. Lawlah, the dean of Howard University's medical school, that "there is no mistaking the results which we have seen in this picture ... it is up to us as scientists to follow the lead Sister Kenny has given."[151]

In Minnesota the organizers of the 1944 campaign sought the support of local African Americans. Milton G. Williams, the black publisher and editor of the *Twin City Observer*, agreed to work as the campaign's state chairman of "Negro participation." The *Observer*, a Republican paper for black Minnesotans, set up a campaign committee and published pictures of Kenny and her Institute. Williams' editorials noted that the Institute had treated "a number of Negro children" and that in Minneapolis her treatment had "been given to all and sundry regardless of race and creed."[152] Kenny appeared at a meeting at the St. James A.M.E. Church in St. Paul where she "held the audience spellbound as she reviewed her struggles to initiate her treatment of polio." She asked that "a Negro physician" come to her Institute "to learn her system" and showed part of her film featuring a black girl treated at the Institute.[153]

Despite its entry into race politics, the campaign's most successful appeal was to white Minnesotans, especially white Republicans. Cans bearing the slogans "Pennies for Kenny" and "Give, and Be Thankful They Shall Walk" appeared at private bridge parties, movie nights, and society teas. Funds were raised at a wrestling show, a boxing match, bowling lanes, and the annual Gopher football dinner. The state's Republican Party made the campaign part of its annual charitable program, and the Minneapolis Association of Manufacturers donated the proceeds of its annual trade dinner at the Radisson hotel to the Institute.[154]

Earlier that month Mayor Kline had been accused of ignoring the "open flaunting" of the city's gambling and liquor laws and had appeared before a Hennepin County grand jury where he declared that he would not "tolerate any type of pay-offs."[155] Kline's connections with liquor dealers, nonetheless, helped him convince Earl Haskin, the state liquor commissioner, to become honorary chairmen of the Kenny campaign's liquor industry division. When the campaign organizers declared November 21 as Sister Kenny Day, liquor dealers in the state agreed to donate 25 percent or more of their gross receipts for the day.[156]

During the November campaign *Reader's Digest* published "Sister Kenny vs. The Medical Old Guard" by Lois Miller. There was no effort to balance this story with statements from skeptical physicians: here were unambiguous heroes and villains. Kenny's work was "revolutionary," Miller announced confidently, for "it discards previous concepts and treatments." And it was more than a departure from clinical practice: it threatened the hierarchy and complacency of the medical profession, for "it was developed not by a doctor, but by a nurse." Kenny, "a strong-minded woman" with "no time for politics" did have, Miller admitted, "an unfortunate faculty for treading heavily on sensitive toes." Miller retold the AMA report as part of Kenny's "long struggle against stubborn and reactionary elements in the medical profession." The AMA committee, Miller argued, had urged physicians to reject the Kenny treatment but offered "nothing in its place other than a return to the old method of using splints and braces." In fact, Kenny's methods were in widespread use although—in phrases that sounded just like Kenny—"not always used properly" as many technicians and nurses "have not had sufficient training or experience." The minority who continued to decry the Kenny treatment admitted that "they had no firsthand knowledge of it" and "had never tried it clinically." During heated debates at the 1944 AMA meeting, one doctor said "I wonder what we have on trial here—Sister Kenny's personality or the Kenny treatment."[157] Miller did not repeat Kenny's comment about the economic basis of orthopedists' antagonism, but she did use evidence Kenny often quoted: the closing of 2 classrooms by the Michael Dowling School in Minneapolis, a school for physically disabled children unable to attend public schools. The rooms were no longer needed because all 91 patients with polio paralyzed between 1940 and 1943 were able to return to their regular schools.[158] It was a powerful comparison between an ordinary schoolroom filled with able-bodied children and empty classrooms where despondent crippled children were once confined.

Simultaneously the *American Mercury* published its own story of Kenny by muckraking journalist Albert Deutsch. In "The Truth About Sister Kenny," Deutsch reveled in "the Amazonian figure of the gray-haired, steely-eyed, strong-jawed Elizabeth Kenny." Money was at the heart of this new fight, Deutsch guessed, noting that Kenny had turned down "many tempting offers of financial reward," and that the NFIP had "given but niggardly financial support to her activities while cashing in handsomely on the publicity she has received." Orthopedists, Deutsch believed, saw Kenny as a competitor and were angered by her claims that her methods used early enough "could have saved many patients." "This deep personal resentment" was manifest throughout the AMA report whose "bias is so obvious that it succeeds only in weakening the impact of certain criticisms which are not without merit."[159] Deutsch noted that Kenny was "a difficult person," although she showed her child patients "consummate tenderness, inspiring courage and rare devotion." But he also guessed that many of the doctors who "call her arrogant, arbitrary and domineering" resented "the reversal of their authoritarian role toward the nursing profession, with a lowly *nurse* telling the doctors where to get off!" Deutsch defended Kenny's belligerence as the unsurprising result of her experiences with refractory physicians. "Can the medical profession justly expect only sweet reasonableness from a woman who, after years of personal sacrifice, feels that its blind opposition has cost the lives or health of thousands who might have been saved had she been given a chance to demonstrate her method in time?" He did not, however, agree with Kenny's complaints that physicians had refused to assess her work. He had spent much of his career exposing the cruel and neglectful care of patients in state mental institutions and was no fan of organized medicine, having "occasionally crossed swords with Dr. Fishbein myself," but he did believe that *JAMA* had "thus far provided a balanced forum for Kenny controversialists."[160] These articles magnified Kenny's voice in response to the AMA report, critiquing both the NFIP and AMA orthopedists.

The "Pennies for Kenny" campaign enhanced Kenny's presence as a civic celebrity, and not long after it ended Kenny was chosen as both the Minneapolitan and Minnesotan of 1944, according to a poll conducted by the *Minneapolis Star-Journal*.[161] The Institute's board proudly announced that the campaign had raised more than $350,000. These funds would be used for training programs in which "true Kenny methods will be taught in their entirety" and for clinical research on "neuromuscular disorders."[162] Not coincidently, the January 1945 March of Dimes campaign, just a few months later, made much of the effective patient care the NFIP had funded during the previous year's epidemics, especially in Hickory, North Carolina. A short film starring Greer Garson, best known as MGM's *Madame Curie*, dramatized the NFIP's work during the Hickory epidemic as a battle against polio that brought people together, an implicit criticism of the divisive polio wars.[163]

In an effort to dampen antagonism in the Twin Cities and lay out a middle ground, Miland Knapp and 3 other physicians who headed departments in the city hospital published a brief analysis of patients with polio in the *Journal-Lancet*. They carefully described some of the "points in which we disagree with Miss Kenny's methods and theories" and sought to balance this with their conclusion that her methods had led to a definite decrease of "deformities." They praised patients' improved general condition, the successful management of muscle shortening or "spasm," and the overall "decreased incidence of deformity," especially scoliosis and pelvic obliquity. Such results confirmed their decision to accept "some of the methods which appeared to be of the greatest value." But they agreed with the AMA report's criticism of the unfortunate publicity around Kenny's "enthusiastic assertions" and reiterated that she had made "inaccurate comparisons of patients treated by her methods and by other methods." In a muted critique of the AMA committee, they pointed out that to assess her methods required a close study of every patient paralyzed during a series of epidemics "after sufficiently long intervals," for only then would there be "a fair and trustworthy set of facts...upon which a truly scientific evaluation can be based." Thus, they concluded hopefully, "open-minded" physicians would continue to "study and observe the work of Miss Kenny" and "judge her efforts fair-mindedly," for "full appraisal must await the passage of time."[164]

Kenny saw the similarities between this analysis and the AMA report and complained to the Institute's board that she deserved an apology from the AMA, Knapp and the other local physicians for "the accusation that I have made inaccurate comparisons has cost me much grief and humiliation."[165] Pohl began to prepare his own study of Institute patients. He was coming to share Kenny's sense that the NFIP was part of a conspiracy to denigrate Kenny's work and urged the board to publicize "the untruths, deceit, misrepresentation, and racketeering in human misery practiced by the National Foundation."[166] He was not surprised, however, when *JAMA* and the *British Medical Journal* rejected his paper. He was able to publish it in Minnesota's *Journal-Lancet* the following year where it was countered by a series of antagonistic articles carefully choreographed by Maurice Visscher and the journal's other editors.[167]

Former allies such as Gudakunst no longer supported Kenny's "concept." In an internal NFIP memorandum on "Questions Frequently Asked" Gudakunst noted that physicians had accepted the value of her method of treatment but not "her explanation as to the nature of the disease, her ideas as to pathology, or her ideas as to why her form of therapy is good."[168] In *Parents Magazine* he praised her "now famous method of treatment" but warned that the Kenny method was not a cure and would not "save a single nerve cell from death." After all, he added, using a well-honed NFIP line, "treatment is not enough": only through "research" could polio "eventually be brought under control."[169] In the *American Journal of Nursing* he also warned that despite "the exaggerated claims made in some lay publications" there was no "miracle cure for the paralysis caused by the disease." Professionals, he added, needed to distinguish "between the Kenny treatment and Sister Kenny's interpretation of the disease," for her interpretation was "still under careful scrutiny."[170]

Pressed by Kline, Gudakunst refused to concede that Kenny's work had led American physicians to develop a new concept of polio. "Based on our knowledge of the pathology and its resultant symptoms," he told Kline, polio was "a virus infection in which the princip[al] lesions involve the cells of the central nervous system." Such pathological changes must be accepted for "the rational development of any reasonable and acceptable system of therapy." In any case medical practice was more complicated. The therapeutic regime of most physicians was "not based upon any one [disease] concept [but was]...the result of years of experience and study in many parts of the world on the part of many professional persons and is continuously being modified and improved as the result of further scientific investigation and clinical experience."[171]

In another scripted radio interview O'Connor reminded the public that the best polio care was provided not just at one center but at centers all over the country where hundreds of doctors and nurses trained under NFIP grants "stand ready to administer the Kenny treatment to all patients in their area." Reiterating the image of Kenny as an insightful clinician O'Connor agreed that her work "completely reverses the old theory previously held by many doctors." But, he claimed with a rhetorical twist, this "theory" was her rejection of immobilization.[172] Even President Roosevelt, immersed in fighting the last stages of the war, was drawn into this other fight. In a fundraising statement, phrased as a letter to O'Connor, Roosevelt described the work of the NFIP "as one of the brightest pages in the history of how a nation of free people, working together, seeks to assure for its children the priceless gift of health," and particularly praised the NFIP's research program. "Treatment, no matter how adequate, cannot win this war against a disease aggressor," Roosevelt declared, but scientific research "will unquestionably conquer this disease."[173]

MORE THAN POLIO

In March 1945 the NFIP finally sent the Institute's board an official letter informing them that the NFIP's board of trustees, advised by the NRC, had rejected the Institute's grant application.[174] By this time, many of the things that the NRC committee had feared had come to pass. Seeing themselves under attack, the Institute's directors had reconstituted themselves formally as a nonprofit philanthropy, with the provocative name the Kenny Foundation (KF), and had begun to plan a national fundraising campaign. The new KF began to rely exclusively on professional publicity firms, and its board ignored the dangers of escalating administrative costs or the temptation for misuse of funds inherent in poorly supervised fundraising schemes. NFIP national officials, though, felt a sense of freedom. "For the first time, we are not supporting Kenny or her work," Peter Cusack reflected in an internal note to Gudakunst.[175]

With the NFIP grant formally rejected, Kenny made a bold move: she accepted 6 patients who did not have polio to the Institute. After 2 of them were sent home "apparently normal" she began to teach her staff "the extra treatment for these special disabilities" for the remaining 4 who had cerebral palsy, transverse-myelitis, and arthritis. But Kenny made 2 missteps: only doctors were allowed to admit patients to city hospitals, and the Institute had been designated as a polio facility. Pediatricians on the hospital staff, appalled that Kenny had stepped over the bounds of her position, ordered her staff not to treat the new patients and told the Institute's superintendent to expel them.[176] This incident was immediately reported in the local press, and, according to a reporter, "touched off the long pent-up resentment felt by Sister Kenny against those who have denied her recognition." Once again Kenny threatened to resign from the Institute and to return to Australia, claiming that she was facing an "organized opposition" to her work. Showing a sharp understanding of local politics, Kenny told the *Minneapolis Morning Tribune* that groups in Washington and New York had offered her "complete facilities" for research, treatment, and teaching if she would establish an institute in those cities.[177]

Kenny had treated patients disabled by cerebral palsy in rural Australia and her first textbook had described the way her techniques could aid both *Infantile Paralysis and Cerebral Diplegia*.[178] She had continued to treat a few such patients in England in the late 1930s, and her methods with such patients were praised by the medical officer in charge of the Queen Mary's wards in a *British Medical Journal* article.[179] Although Kenny's autobiography *And They Shall Walk* was mainly about her polio work, she did describe treating a child who was "a victim of that horrible disease, cerebral diplegia" as an example of "the cases the medical world turns its back upon."[180] In 1944 the Institute's NFIP grant application had proposed pursuing clinical research in both polio and "Spastic Paralysis."[181]

In a world where social and medical neglect of the disabled was common, cerebral palsy therapy was particularly poor. The term *cerebral palsy* was used to indicate a combination of genetic, fetal, and birth trauma disabilities, and most physicians assumed that people with these disabilities were also mentally disabled. There were few organized facilities or cerebral palsy specialists other than those at the multidisciplinary clinic at Children's Hospital in Boston and the Children's Rehabilitation Institute for Cerebral Palsy in Reisterstown, Maryland.[182] There was some interest in the use of antispasmotic drugs to treat the condition, but so far their effectiveness was doubtful.[183] On occasion an exceptional individual with cerebral palsy, such as Earl Carlson, was featured in the popular press. Carlson, a 1931 graduate of Yale's medical school, began treating cerebral palsy patients like himself at the New York Neurological Institute and published his autobiography *Born That Way* in 1941.[184]

Cautiously Minnesota Republican Congressman Walter Judd praised Kenny's methods for treating cerebral palsy patients as "definitely most helpful in many cases that I have seen personally."[185] Marvin Kline called a meeting of the city's Board of Public Welfare to hear the "pleas of sorrowing parents." The Johnsons of Salisbury, North Carolina, and the Coplans of Livingston, Montana, whose children had been expelled from the Institute, assured city officials "we aren't interested in medical technicalities...we just want our babies to be normal." Mrs. Coplan said she had shoveled sand in a Minneapolis foundry for more than 8 months to be able to pay for her daughter to have the Kenny treatment.[186] Under this pressure the city's welfare board ordered these 2 children readmitted to the Institute, although it did not amend its regulations to permit "spastic paralysis" patients to be treated at the Institute in the future.[187] Back at the Institute, the *Minneapolis Daily Times* reported, Carol Lee Coplan "not only sits up but walks around her crib and even ruffles a book" while Allen Johnson's parents—who were told by an expert that "nothing could be done for him"—"hope he will make the same progress."[188] City officials refused Kenny's resignation and promised that they would "do everything humanly possible" to obtain the clinical research facilities she demanded.[189]

Kenny's brief public foray into the field of cerebral palsy excited parents of children who had neuromuscular disorders other than polio. A mother from Chicago who was a member of a Parents Association for the Handicapped contacted other mothers of "handicapped" children and they "got busy." "We are keeping our fingers crossed in the hopes that you will continue your research for all neuro-muscular diseases," she told Kenny.[190] A few of Kenny's medical allies were also eager to pursue this new direction of her work. Orthopedist Alfred Deacon urged the director of the Winnipeg's Children's Hospital to send a physician to the Institute to study "cerebrospastic" therapies "which would be of great benefit to the Children's Hosp[ital]."[191]

Kenny continued to see herself as an independent clinician not bound by institutional restrictions. Even after the Institute's board refused to open its door to additional cerebral palsy patients, she assured an Illinois mother that "my dermo-neuro-muscular therapy is definitely not for infantile paralysis alone." Although she was restricted to polio at the Institute she would be happy to examine the child privately and advise the mother "as to the treatment."[192]

"ORGANIZED OPPOSITION"

It was not Kenny's effort to expand her work to other diseases, however, but her claim that her work was hindered by organized medicine that made it a national story. In March 1945 Congressman Donald O'Toole, a Democrat from New York, introduced a resolution calling for a House committee to investigate the "organized opposition" against Kenny.[193] Within 2 weeks 1,500 letters were sent to O'Toole's office in support of Kenny from doctors, nurses, chiropractors, builders, businessmen, housewives, and mothers. Only one letter written by a nurse from Virginia was critical, O'Toole claimed.[194] He also wrote to Roosevelt deploring the "lack of cooperation and a degree of intimidation practiced upon [Kenny]...by the medical profession." As a hearing could not be set up before Congress returned from Easter recess, he respectfully asked the President "to use your great office in an effort to detain Sister Kenny in this country for...a word from you would give new faith and hope to Sister Kenny and would insure her remaining in this country to continue her splendid work."[195] O'Toole, one reporter noted sardonically, was an independent Tammany Democrat who had been elected without support from Roosevelt's New Deal administration and was "not adverse to starting a move calculated to embarrass the President."[196]

To reinforce and broaden such populist support Kenny made it clear that when she spoke of "organized opposition" she was referring to the leading officials of the AMA, not the nation's "hundreds of fine and conscientious doctors."[197] She urged her supporters to pressure their local congressmen to set up a special committee to investigate her claims "in the interests of humanity," assuring reporters she would consider as a command any suggestion from Roosevelt that she remain in the United States.[198] She heightened the populist outrage by hinting that she would reveal contents of potentially explosive telegrams between herself and O'Connor to such a committee. Some of her supporters who had gained access to the telegrams were unwilling to wait for the formation of a congressional committee. The "All American Christian Auxiliary" of the Chicago Nurses Committee, which Fishbein had identified as an eccentric antisemitic group, urged the public to write to their congressmen and senators "demanding a full congressional investigation into the problems of Sister Elizabeth Kenny." The group quoted a telegram from O'Connor that was supposedly written during the Argentina fiasco in which he had defended his actions in withdrawing NFIP support for the 2 Kenny technicians. The telegram supposedly read "I have given you HELL and you have paid for it in your Health."[199]

It was at this moment that Fishbein chose to break his silence on Kenny. The idea that *JAMA* had suppressed any scientific evidence about the Kenny methods was, he told the national press, a "preposterous untruth."[200] He gave a lengthy interview to James Pooler of the *Detroit Free Press* who was writing an investigatory series on the Kenny controversy. Pooler's first 3 articles, NFIP staff had noted, had been rather pro-Kenny, but Fishbein knew what he was doing.[201] In April 1945 Pooler presented Fishbein as a sympathetic character, bemused by the uproar around his efforts to uphold scientific standards. Seated in his office, Fishbein "had the air of a man who would be glad to put his head sadly between his hands." "We have leaned over backward to give her every break, but we also must save the American people from exploitation," he explained, for "when people insist they are the only one who can teach something, the doctor is wary." As the "voice" of organized medicine and the editor of *JAMA* he presented himself as a judicious assessor of other experts' views. The critical orthopedic report published in

JAMA had been an "honest appraisal from top men in their field"; neurologist Stanley Cobb and most other "nerve-muscle doctors" agreed that her theories were "physiological nonsense." In a calculated breach of secrecy Fishbein quoted from the NRC committee's 21-page study that had concluded that the Institute did not have adequate laboratory resources or competent enough staff to handle a research program. To show his own clinical objectivity, Fishbein agreed that her methods lessened pain and psychological fright in the early stages of polio and were therefore "scientific and valuable." But his attack slid easily to Kenny's character as he drew a picture of an old-fashioned and inflexible nurse from the Australian bush who refused to deviate from her "ritual of treatment." At one point, he claimed, she had insisted on using hand wringers to prepare hot packs and refused to use electric wringers. Nor could she adapt herself to scientific confirmation. "It is part of the scientific method that facts shall be published and interpretations based on fact shall be subject to analysis and criticism," Fishbein reminded newspaper readers, yet Kenny "doesn't consent to either analysis or criticism."[202] Of course Fishbein's own well-publicized attacks on any critic of the AMA's policies suggested that he did not apply this process to medical politics. This denigrating picture of a nurse resisting modern technologies was reinforced by *Time* later that month. Kenny's forthright disposition and her insistence that doctors accept her theories, which "many experts say lack proof," according to *Time*, had "earned her the nicknames 'The Duchess' and 'Madam Queen.'"[203]

On April 12 1945 Franklin Roosevelt died at his Little White House in Warm Springs. His death shocked the nation and refigured the politics of polio. Polio lost its presidential patron and briefly medical politics seemed petty and irrelevant. When Kenny sent the *Detroit Free Press* a long response to Fishbein's comments she found the controversy was no longer considered news. Pooler replied that he and his editor were grateful to have her reply but "the death of President Roosevelt has altered things." Perhaps, he suggested weakly, there could now be a "reconciliation between the National Foundation and the Elizabeth Kenny Institute."[204]

After Roosevelt's death the attention of Congress shifted. Kenny's attack on the AMA had initially spurred Congressman Arnold Sabath, an Illinois Democrat who chaired the House Rules Committee, to say that he would invite her to appear before his committee, for he had "long been aware that some members of the medical profession are extremely high-handed."[205] But when Kenny returned to Washington in early May Sabath explained that the Rules Committee did not want to break its precedent of allowing only House members to testify before it and, in any case, Congress had no jurisdiction in a "private medical fight."[206] Flexibly, Congressman O'Toole now requested a national institute to be built in Washington devoted to the study, treatment, and research of polio and similar diseases as a postwar memorial for Roosevelt, but this project also died.[207] Disappointed at not being allowed to speak to Congress, Kenny told the sympathetic *Times-Herald* that "I want America to help me spread my methods for the good of children everywhere."[208] She did participate in the press coverage of Roosevelt's funeral ceremonies and was thanked by the owner of ABC's Blue Network for her efforts "at this tragic time" when "the public was groping, I believe, not only for a government leadership, but for spiritual guidance [from those] . . . who had been in close contact with the President."[209]

Denied the platform of a Congressional hearing, Kenny took her message to the Illinois legislature in Springfield. An enthusiastic group of nurses from local hospitals met Kenny at the train and arranged for her to lay a wreath on Lincoln's tomb, following "the custom of all distinguished visitors here." Springfield's mayor, at the nurses' urging, provided a motorcycle police escort and several state cars to take the delegation from the train to the tomb and then to the state house.[210]

To the state legislators Kenny spoke forcibly about the "organized boycott" by NFIP officials and Fishbein who had both denied her "the facilities for research into the further presentation I have to make of which they are entirely ignorant." She mocked Fishbein's statement in the *Detroit Free Press* that he was trying "to save the American people from exploitation" by noting that her technical film had not exploited anyone. She also tried to step away from the personality politics that had led O'Connor to refuse to meet with her or answer her calls and telegrams. It was not true, she told legislators, that "I was annoyed because I was denied funds by the foundation [for] . . . I, personally, have never made any request for funds"; it was the Institute's medical committee and the board of directors who had requested funds and were refused. Nor, she argued, had she "emerged from the Australian bushland with some unknown and untried idea." Instead, she stressed her familiarity with Australian medical journals and her clinical experience in Australian hospitals. Her care of "spastic" patients had occasioned a certain amount of publicity, she admitted, but she proudly claimed that experience for "I was not experimenting with these children" and "the reports of my work with this very sad disease are, to a degree, most encouraging."[211]

Horrified to see that the AMA report and the NFIP's grant rejection were reported in Australian newspapers, Kenny organized a letter to be written to Sir Owen Dixon, Australia's ambassador to the United States.[212] Pohl and 2 other Minneapolis physicians assured Dixon that despite the publicity around the AMA report, most American doctors "are in accord with her views [which are] . . . now quite generally accepted throughout America and applied wherever possible." Publicized excerpts from the AMA report in Australian newspapers may have created "an impression . . . that casts doubt upon the personal integrity of Miss Kenny as well as her success in America." In fact the AMA committee had spent only 2 and half days with Kenny and made little effort to examine patients or records. As physicians who had watched her work carefully Pohl and his colleagues were certain that "she has made a great contribution to the knowledge of infantile paralysis" and helped to open "new pathways of thought . . . in dealing with other neuromuscular disorders." Medical resistance remained, but that was not surprising for "old ideas firmly rooted in tradition" did not "fall easily."[213]

"SOCK POLIO WITH DOLLARS:" THE VICIOUS 1945 KF CAMPAIGN

As the new Kenny Foundation (KF) began to organize its first national campaign, previously silent Americans found an opportunity to express their dislike of changes in American society they linked to Roosevelt and the New Deal. Social welfare programs established in the 1930s were increasingly seen as Democratic-inspired, anti-American socialism rather than necessary for a nation fighting the Depression and then the Axis powers. In postwar America a new kind of populism emerged, combining strains of anticommunism, antifederalism, antisemitism, and antimedical orthodoxy. The KF also benefited from a group of right-wing Catholics, including Hollywood studio executives, actors, and directors, who had felt constrained from expressing pro-Republican sentiments during the 1930s and now saw Kenny's cause as a way of articulating this antagonism.

Bing Crosby was a superstar in 1940s America. A crooner with a golden voice and a jaunty smile, he sang with Frank Sinatra, acted with Ingrid Bergman, was a straight man to comic Bob Hope, and owned golf courses, racing tracks, and radio stations. He was also a prominent Irish Catholic family man with a squeaky clean public persona.[214] Thus, when the KF announced in July 1945 that Crosby would be its first national chair for its "Sock Polio" campaign, it was a stunning coup.[215] The NFIP had pioneered the modern celebrity fundraiser, using Hollywood singers and actors in dramatic and sentimental short films and radio programs as part of its March of Dimes events. With chapters around the country headed by prominent professionals and business leaders, and with Women's Divisions headed, frequently, by their wives, the NFIP was a popular Hollywood charity.[216] As recently as January 1945, Crosby along with Judy Garland and Frank Sinatra had been featured on "America Salutes the President's Birthday," an NFIP-sponsored show that was part of its March of Dimes campaign and was broadcast on the 4 national radio networks.[217] Yet now Crosby was bringing his celebrity power to a fledgling philanthropy whose figurehead spoke frequently against the NFIP. Crosby's decision to act as the KF campaign chairman put a powerful imprint of Hollywood approval on Kenny's work and its fundraising arm. It also reflected Kenny's growing prominence in Hollywood circles as well as a shared connection among Catholics in a society in which anti-Irish-Catholic jokes were as prevalent as antisemitic and racist ones.[218] The ambiguity of Kenny's title "Sister" also helped, as NFIP officials admitted, for "a lot of good, warm-hearted Catholics all over the country associate her with their church."[219] During the 1945 campaign an editorial cartoon in the *Los Angeles Herald-Examiner* showed Crosby dressed as a priest with his hand outstretched next to an older-looking Kenny in a long white veil that made her look like a nun.[220]

The 1945 KF campaign was nationwide with no holds barred. In its first national fundraising effort, the KF turned to proven tactics from the NFIP and the National Tuberculosis Association, using bright orange Kenny Cans to collect money, miniature boxing gloves to "Sock Polio," and fundraising stamps featuring Kenny and a happy child.[221] Relying on the winning combination of fear and hope, the campaign centered on children at risk for "deformities" and the amazing results Kenny's methods had achieved in Minnesota and elsewhere. Instead of a pathetic crippled child there was a healed, able-bodied child; in one poster the slogan "They Shall Walk" was next to the image of a young girl standing, her hands in the air, crutches at her feet.[222] And now there was a satisfying villain: the undemocratic, elitist, and disgruntled medical establishment, embodied in such professional groups as the NFIP and the AMA whose leaders were denying communities access to Kenny care and denying Kenny herself proper respect for her innovative work. The campaign tried to turn public outrage already visible from the bitter polio wars into public good will and generosity.

The KF campaign opened with an article in the Hearst family magazine *Cosmopolitan* in October 1945. In a sign of the breakdown of censorship, staff writer Harry Brundidge had not consulted the NFIP before writing his article.[223] Illustrated with a somber full-page photograph of Kenny in a scalloped black dress and leaf-shaped pin, Brundidge began with a quotation from a friend saying that if his child had polio "I'd rush her to Sister Kenny. Ethics, American Medical Association, sanction or no." Brundidge described Kenny facing veiled hints and a hostile reception from physicians, reactions that "recall[ed] . . . the martyrdom of other scientific pathfinders and discoverers." In a harsh description of her first meeting in New York O'Connor told her "nobody is interested in your theories. You had better return to Australia." The instigation of a boycott against her by O'Connor and Fishbein was inexplicable, according to Kenny, "unless it is that I have no M.D. behind my name." Mocking the idea that scientific discoveries require modern, well-equipped buildings, Brundidge quoted Kenny saying "I wonder if Dr. Fishbein knows the building that yielded the evidence that revolutionized the concept of this disease was a small bark-roofed hut in the Australian bush."[224] Bing Crosby then sent out a fundraising letter "Are You Going My Way?" (referring to his recent Oscar-award-winning movie) to remind potential donors of the need for money to train Kenny technicians. The KF, Crosby noted, "receives no financial assistance from any other National Infantile Paralysis Foundation."[225]

Here were the elements of the 1945 campaign: a selfish philanthropy (the NFIP) supported by public donations unwilling to extend its money and reputation behind important new work, an antagonistic AMA hiding behind false claims of scientific standards, prejudiced physicians suspicious of an assertive and confident woman who was a nurse and not a physician, and potentially important new knowledge about polio left unexplored. Members of the public responded just the way the KF hoped. "The stand that the Foundation, and you as its Director, has taken amazed and disgusted me," a Bloomfield, New Jersey, man told O'Connor. Unless the NFIP "recognizes and aids Sister Kenny it will receive no more contributions from me or my friends who have children."[226]

Efforts by the NFIP's national office to tell a different story were mostly unsuccessful. In an internal memo about the *Cosmopolitan* article marked "Not For Publication," the director of NFIP's publicity staff reflected that advising parents to rush their sick child to the Institute was "completely impractical," for it assumed that the Kenny method

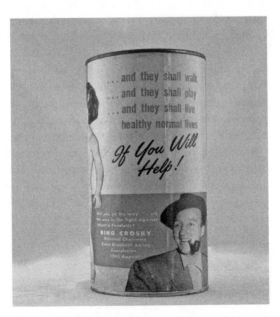

FIGURE 5.2 "Sock Polio" fundraising container for the Kenny Foundation's first national campaign, 1945, featuring Bing Crosby, the campaign's spokesman; author's possession.

was available only in Minneapolis. There was no medical boycott; her Institute's grant application had been "referred to the National Research Council for advice" and been rejected as the Institute "had neither staff nor equipment to carry on such research." As for the confusion around her methods, Kenny "has advanced certain theories…not in conformity with known facts of normal body function and the pathological picture found in poliomyelitis."[227] A public statement signed by Gudakunst argued further that there had never been an "orthodox" method. Long "before Miss Kenny came to this country," he argued, physical therapy was widely used as a method of treatment in many diseases. While physicians now used what is good in the Kenny method, they did not accept Kenny's theories about "the cause and the relative importance of symptoms of the disease," for Kenny had no specific knowledge of physiology, histology, or pathology and thus "her speculations" although "interesting…are not in conformity with the facts."[228] Thus, physicians and other thoughtful professionals used therapies based on science and not speculation; the Institute's request for research funds was rejected for fair, scientific reasons; and Kenny's theories had to be separated from her therapies. These became the NFIP's talking points, but they were not successful at derailing the KF's campaign.

The "Sock Polio" campaign attracted former NFIP volunteers who brought with them civic influence. In Schuylkill County, Pennsylvania, the campaign was supported by a local mayor.[229] In Montana the editor of a local paper who had been "a [NFIP] friend of many years" agreed to direct the KF drive.[230] Hubert Humphrey, mayor of Minneapolis, agreed to act as one of 3 co-chairs of the Minnesota KF mayors committee, and urged other mayors to declare December 8 Kenny Day.[231] Even more influential was Chester LaRoche, a wealthy advertising executive married to Rosalind Russell's sister Clara. Head of the board of directors of Young and Rubicam, an influential advertising agency in New York, LaRoche was an enthusiastic KF organizer. He identified men who had "allowed their name to be used [by the NFIP] because of President Roosevelt's personal interest" but were now turning to the Kenny campaign. Some, such as aviation entrepreneur Harold Talbott, were quiet allies, unable to join the KF's New York committee formally as the result of their business connections with physicians. But, LaRoche assured Marvin Kline, "we have some of the best people on our committee for…no drive of this sort in New York seems very important unless it is promoted by people who are well known socially."[232]

At first the NFIP urged its chapter officials to turn a blind eye. In Arizona, for example, after the Kenny people announced that there was only one nurse in the state capable of treating patients with the Kenny method, the NFIP's director of organization told the Arizona chairman to keep quiet and not "start any newspaper arguments."[233] But in most cases following this advice proved impossible. In fact, some NFIP officers actively tried to contain the 1945 campaign. "I am in hopes that I can stop the drive entirely in Oakland" as "it has been stopped in several other counties," one California organizer announced.[234] Local NFIP organizers said frequently that that the Kenny method was already used to treat every acute patient with polio in their community. Nonetheless, they complained, they had to field many questions from "certain quarters where we have some very good friends."[235] One sticky point was explaining why the Institute's $840,000 grant proposal had been rejected. Another was the "duplication" of polio fundraising campaigns.[236] Dallas was now "pretty well covered with colorful [pro-Kenny] placards" put up by the Texas KF state chairman, a wealthy oil man who had sent his daughter to the Institute 2 years before. Working in such a pro-Kenny environment was not easy, a local NFIP official reflected. "They have a perfect right to put it on. Kenny has done a wonderful work. We have no feud on with her drive." But, she commented to the New York headquarters, even if the KF "get[s] a little money...we aren't worried—we're a little powerful ourselves—now ain't we?"[237]

NFIP officials tried to convince the public that the KF was allied with profit-seeking promoters instead of civic-minded volunteers but this was a difficult argument to make for, despite its image as a voluntary organization, the NFIP had a paid organizational staff and its own publicity department. Nevertheless, angry NFIP organizers such as Arthur Reynolds of Minnesota consistently warned the New York office about the KF's considerable promotional expenses and urged the head office to publicize them.[238] According to the Portland Better Business Bureau Inc., the KF's new public relations firm ran a percentage drive campaign whereby the firm was paid a set amount (estimated in 1945 to be $48,000) and additional commissions, based on the funds raised. The Bureau also noted that members of Bing Crosby's family were involved in the campaign, although it did not state whether they were paid.[239]

Influential newspapers backed the KF campaign, especially the Hearst Corporation. In northern California there was "terrific pressure" from the Hearst interests to convince the NFIP's chapter treasurer to accept the chairmanship of the KF's northern California campaign.[240] In Los Angeles, despite the local NFIP chapter's studious avoidance of any controversy about Kenny or her treatment, "the flamboyant sensationalism of the stories in the Hearst press" had led many people to "labor under the delusion that Elizabeth Kenny has been persecuted."[241] A number of other influential papers also turned to the Kenny cause. The Hamilton County NFIP chapter in Cincinnati had already lost "one or two of our very best workers" to the Kenny campaign, along with the support of the city editor of "our largest daily paper."[242] In northwestern Minnesota, one mayor took the position of KF county chair, and the editor of a weekly paper resigned from the NFIP local board and devoted most of his paper to the KF campaign.[243]

The mixture of charity, religion, and politics was another quagmire. Although KF publicity pointed out that "In Australia, Chief Nurses Are Called Sister," the notion of this as a Catholic crusade remained potent.[244] Working amidst the New York Protestant elite O'Connor had been able to rely on his connections with Roosevelt to open doors for him despite his Irish Catholic background, and many Catholic Democrats had helped to reelect Roosevelt and had supported the New Deal and the NFIP. But by 1945 new alliances between Catholics and Republicans presaged a movement away from the Democratic Party that would alter national politics a decade or so later. Crosby had always been a staunch supporter of the Republican Party.[245] Now a few influential Catholics tried vainly to pressure him not to work with the KF. An industrialist who headed Chicago's Cook County NFIP chapter assured O'Connor that he would talk to Bishop Bernard Shiel to "get the Bishop's disapproval of this ill-advised effort of Crosby and Sister Kenny."[246] This effort failed; Crosby continued to be the KF's campaign chairman, adding respectability to Catholicism and Republican politics.

The 1945 campaign led many NFIP volunteers to express their dissatisfaction with the NFIP's national policy, especially O'Connor's argument that any effort at conciliation would be used by Kenny "as the basis for further damaging newspaper attacks."[247] Some volunteers went further. "I can't help but feel, however, that a lot more could have been done in the National office" to block the KF, wrote one organizer.[248]

The New York office rang with telephone calls from various county chairmen seeking the correct, satisfying response to local defectors.[249] A few suggested that the national office come up with "a settlement that would meet the minimum needs of the Institute and eliminate the necessity of a campaign." "You are already spending considerable money" on training nurses and doctors in the Kenny methods, one Michigan official pointed out, suggesting the NFIP take "this money and a little more . . . [and] buy off the other group."[250]

The NFIP was a popular charity in Hollywood. It had a sound reputation and caring for victims for polio was unquestionably a worthy cause. The short movies that the NFIP produced for each March of Dimes campaign were frequently tied in with current Hollywood productions.[251] The NFIP relied on the cooperation of cinema owners to show their trailers and allow ushers to carry March of Dimes cans down the aisles. Indeed, during the war years O'Connor had turned to Roosevelt to add some presidential pressure when cinema owners protested that there were too many requests for fundraising and that communities resented donations that were "sent out of the state for charities elsewhere."[252]

With Crosby as the KF campaign's chair, the link between the NFIP and Hollywood was breaking down. "Crosby can really do a job with his radio show, movie contacts, etc.," the head of NFIP's Public Relations noted in an internal memo in July 1945.[253] "If Sister Kenny is successful in securing the co-operation of the theatres in making an audience collection, it will kill our audience collection next January," warned the head of Ohio's state chapter.[254]

The efforts of NFIP officials to dampen the effect of Crosby's efforts and the possible defection of other Hollywood figures began with a *Motion Picture Herald* article that claimed that 85 percent of March of Dimes funds had been used for Kenny treatment during 1944–1945. These funds had been used to train over 1,000 physicians, nurses, and physical therapists in the Kenny technique at the University of Minnesota and many professionals who had studied the method at other teaching centers set up by the NFIP.[255] The NFIP's national office sent a copy of this article to Nicholas Schenck, the head of the Loews theater chain.[256] Behind the scenes a California official appealed to Joseph Schenck, Nicholas's brother and the head of Twentieth Century Fox, to urge him and other studio owners "who have done so much for us" to help discourage Crosby's efforts.[257]

Bing Crosby did indeed ask theatre owners to show pro-Kenny trailers. "The Motion Picture Industry has always been deeply concerned with the plight of the victims of this dread disease," he reminded the California industry's board of governors, and he believed Nicholas Schenck would agree that "due consideration and help be given Sister Kenny to carry on her great work."[258] This message, NFIP organizers feared, would be reinforced by the KF's good relationship with William Hearst. Nicholas Schenck, a Los Angeles NFIP official warned, "is close to Mr. Hearst and every once in a while goes to San Simeon [Hearst's California retreat]."[259] Many officials were aware of the fragility of the link between the NFIP, the press, and the movie industry, which had previously been so strong. "Perhaps you could contact Walter Winchell," one California official suggested, as "his friendship with our late President . . . may be instrumental in discouraging the Sister Kenny drive."[260] Meanwhile newspapers reported the celebrities Crosby had attracted who were signing on as division chairmen: singer Guy Lombardo, band leader Harry James, Frank Garnetts of Garnetts Newspapers, Thomas J. White, publisher of the

Chicago Herald-American, sports writer and author Damon Runyon, and RKO movie star Johnnie Weissmuller.[261]

The New Jersey campaign was especially vicious. The NFIP's headquarters began receiving frantic phone calls from chapter chairman, reporting rumors. Supposedly, during a recent Mercer County epidemic the NFIP had not provided either Kenny technicians or equipment; the Catholic Church was going to "fully support Sister Kenny because she was a nun"; and all the funds collected by the NFIP in New Jersey were "sent out of the state to the Georgia Warm Springs Foundation."[262] NFIP organizers were appalled when former Governor Harry Moore, a Democrat, announced that he would act as state KF chair.[263] Some of the NFIP's New Jersey allies assured the New York office that they would try to make Moore see reason.[264] Dr. George O'Hanlon, the director of the Jersey City Medical Center who also led the Hudson County NFIP chapter, refused to direct the KF's medical advisory committee.[265] Many local politicians tried valiantly to express broad charitable loyalties. "I like both foundations," a Republican state senator from Paterson announced during the KF campaign. But he was "particularly fond of the Kenny Appeal" for the Kenny method had created "great advances in medical science for the cure or aid of polio cases."[266]

The most disturbing revolt was by the women. The NFIP had relied on women volunteers as fundraisers since the 1930s, and in 1944 officials had responded quickly after Mary Pickford, then head of the NFIP's Women's Division, warned that many of her Hollywood women friends were uneasy about attacks on Kenny. During epidemics NFIP women volunteers collected blankets, safety pins, and electric fans; worked as clerical helpers, chauffeured parents, found lodging for nurses sent to epidemic areas, prepared food for hospital patients and staff, and in some places even accompanied doctors on their rounds, learning to keep medical charts so nurses could stay in hospitals to do their more important work.[267] In June 1945 the NFIP had organized these women formally into the Polio Emergency Volunteers.[268]

But the KF offered women volunteers what the NFIP had never done: power and seniority. Mary Roebling, the campaign director and vice chair of the Mercer County NFIP chapter, accepted the position of chair of the New Jersey state KF campaign. Associated with one of Trenton's outstanding families, Roebling was the first woman president of a major bank and an influential Republican businesswoman and philanthropist. The NFIP chapter head tried to convince her not to accept the position as the KF state chair but Roebling remained adamant.[269] In Pennsylvania, Mrs. Edward (Charity) Martin, the wife of the Republican governor, agreed to work as that state's KF chair, and when her husband was elected senator, Martin continued her work as a member of the KF's national executive.[270] Clearly the KF's claim that the leaders of the NFIP and the AMA refused to give Kenny proper respect because she was an outspoken woman fell on receptive ears. The turning of the women was an explicit KF campaign strategy. KF officials had urged each county organizer to find "a woman to interest other women and clubs in giving Sister Kenny Teas, Bridge Parties and Fashion Shows."[271] The ability to organize civic events and thereby raise interest and money was not, as Kenny and the KF directors recognized, an insignificant skill.

After the 1945 campaign Kenny organized a conference, inviting public health officials from every state. As well as refuting the accusations of the AMA report, she trod a careful line between praising America's many conscientious technicians and warning that few of them knew enough about her concept to be able to practice the work "in its entirety." The lack of this knowledge among physicians and medical students was especially disturbing.[272] She also sent a letter warning O'Connor and every NFIP trustee that "an inadequate presentation" of polio's symptoms was likely to "retard research and prevent the conquest of this disease."[273] The NFIP's national office, which had pointedly sent no representatives to the December conference, made sure each trustee received a statement by Gudakunst in response.[274] Kenny also began to prepare a new book she provocatively titled *Physical Medicine: the Science of Dermo-Neuro-Muscular Therapy as Applied to Infantile Paralysis*. Although its title suggested she was claiming authority in rehabilitative medicine its content and short length was more modest, and it provided clear, detailed instructions for nurses and physical therapists. Like her 1943 textbook, this book was published by the Bruce Publishing Company and it became known as the Gray Book.[275]

The 1945 KF campaign did not achieve its stated goal of $5 million, and raised only an estimated $516,000. Its poor showing was, in part, the result of givers' fatigue by Americans who felt worn out by calls for war bonds, Red Cross, the USO, and other wartime charities.[276] A confidential report by the National Information Bureau, a watch-dog assessor of charities, warned that the KF campaign had created a competitive and antagonistic relationship between the 2 Foundations. The geographic distribution of the KF board was too narrow, its fundraising costs in 1945 were excessive, and the national office had not adequately supervised the activities of state chapters. Although the KF board began to plan the 1946 campaign with the more modest goal of $2,000,000 and promised to control expenses, it nonetheless signed a contract with the same publicity firm.[277]

Crosby became a member of the new national executive committee, singer Kate Smith was named national 1946 campaign chairman, and Rosalind Russell became head of the KF's national women's division. Along with Crosby, the executive committee included Governor Frank Lausche of Ohio (the state's first Catholic governor), Governor Earl Warren of California, Charity Martin of Pennsylvania (the wife of Senator Edward Martin), Eleanor Patterson (editor of the *Washington Times-Herald*), and various business owners and union officials.[278] The growing uneasiness in Hollywood around the link between the NFIP and the studios was reflected, to O'Connor's dismay, by a decision by the studios in 1946 to end individual theater collections and thus stop showing NFIP trailers. Forced to rethink its fundraising strategies, the NFIP began to promote a new campaign of the poster child, who appeared eager and well-dressed, seeking public support to be assured of a bright future.[279]

The 1945 campaign helped to clarify a number of new policies. First, the NFIP began to expand its funding of physical therapy, acknowledging physical therapists as crucial professionals in polio care, and producing a number of technical films devoted entirely to this practice.[280] Indeed, polio and the Kenny method became crucial parts in the professionalizing of physical therapy in America.

In other ways NFIP policies shifted away from polio therapies. Senior officials no longer sought to assess polio methods of any kind. In a form letter issued to chapters the NFIP announced that it did not "establish standards for medical care or treatment of infantile paralysis" or "interfere in the patient–physician relationship [for] ... the type of treatment prescribed is entirely up to the doctor." The letter added that "as an organization we have no viewpoint toward the Sister Kenny treatment."[281] The NFIP continued to pay for any system of polio treatment if recommended by a licensed physician, even controversial therapies such as Herman Kabat's use of Prostigmine. The NFIP did boast that it funded what it called "modern treatment," which exemplified the best in polio care, not a single treatment "bearing the name of one person or one idea."[282] Indeed, officials began to argue, this policy was a sign of a flexible philanthropy, responsive to requests by medical professionals to alter therapies. "The National Foundation, being a progressive organization, is not wedded to any type of treatment."[283]

In a continuing effort to delegitimize Kenny as a medical authority, the NFIP also began to remind its own staff, as well as science reporters and others writing about Kenny, to "wherever possible use the title Miss Kenny instead of Sister Kenny."[284] At the same time the 1945 KF campaign had reinforced the importance of making women feel valued as fighters against polio, both as volunteers and as potential donors. Thus, in the 1947 NFIP film *In Daily Battle* women were prominently featured: as mothers, the secretary of a local chapter's medical advisory board who takes notes, nurses and physical therapists, and a chapter official.[285] Still, compared to bolder efforts by the KF, such depictions continued to suggest that women were participants in subordinate positions, not philanthropic leaders. It was not until 1951 that the NFIP turned a Mother's March organized by its Phoenix, Arizona, chapter into a national program. According to one historian, "the portrait of mothers marching against polio became one of the indelible images of postwar America."[286]

The NFIP relied on science writers such as Roland Berg to reiterate the "many years of careful study" it would take "to evaluate properly [Kenny's] her place in medical history." While today "physical therapy is used by nearly all doctors . . . based on Miss Kenny's methods or . . . modifications," Berg argued in *The Challenge of Polio*, Kenny's lack of medical knowledge had meant that many physicians rejected her "entirely new concept of the disease" based on ideas with no scientific basis. Kenny, after all, had no training in medical school anatomy and had observed only living patients. Physicians, who had "seen the actual damage in the brains and spinal cords of experimental monkeys and fatal human cases," knew that polio was "primarily one of the nervous system and that the muscles are only indirectly and symptomatically involved." Berg also suggested that "had she not demanded that physicians also discard the scientific facts of the pathology of the disease and accept a brand new malady based merely on her observations of certain symptoms," it was possible that her methods "would have received earlier and wider acceptance." "Her work has been recognized and supported," he concluded firmly. "Whatever is good in it has been salvaged and made available to all."[287] A reviewer in the *New Republic* called *The Challenge of Polio* a well-written, honest book with "a sober appraisal of the work of Sister Kenny," and praised the author's "keen sense of the responsibility so necessary in those who write on medical subjects for the people."[288]

Most of all, the NFIP's national office began to articulate clearly "Why Chapters Cannot Sponsor Research." Chapters were given the sole responsibility for providing for the medical care of patients with polio, the NFIP's director of research reminded an audience at the Hotel Roosevelt in April 1946. To engage in research activities "would serve only to dilute the energies and resources now devoted to medical care." Further, chapters were directed mostly by volunteers who were "not familiar with problems of research." To support a research program, an agency needed to be able to say whether the question was important, whether the institution had sufficient staff and equipment, and whether the research program proposed fit appropriately with the entire scope of the research activities. Only the NFIP's national office, relying on its network of advisory committees, could handle such issues "satisfactorily."[289]

By 1947 the KF was one of the nation's 2 polio foundations. Chester La Roche turned down O'Connor's offer to be head of the NFIP's advertising division, explaining that "more and more people of influence and means" were becoming interested in Kenny's work, which had "tremendous popular appeal."[290] The Massachusetts KF field director reported that physicians remained torn in their assessment of Kenny, but antagonists told him "she receives too much publicity and also that a nurse is not supposed to tell a doctor what to do about illness."[291] A New Jersey Kenny supporter asked O'Connor whether Kenny's treatment was going to be discussed at a NFIP symposium to be held at Warm Springs in 1947, and whether Pohl or any other physician connected with the Institute would be invited to attend. "Why is it apparently impossible for the National Foundation, with all of its vast financial resources, to merge [with] the Sister Elizabeth Kenny Institute[?]."[292] No one representing the Institute had been invited to participate, O'Connor responded, for the list of speakers had been "selected on the basis of their specific contributions, rather than from the institution which they might represent." But the papers read at Warm Springs, O'Connor assured the donor later, referred to "Miss Kenny's work" including the use of moist heat, early physical therapy, muscle reeducation, and other measures "endorsed by Miss Kenny."[293]

The polio wars exacerbated political and public pressures to expand polio researchers' attention to patient care and decreased believability about claims by orthopedic surgeons that only surgery could fix "deformities." There was a new focus on questions of efficacy and the authority of expertise. What was the meaning of clinical results? If a treatment worked did it therefore challenge previous theories on which older, less efficacious therapies were based? If not, why not? What was the relationship between therapy and theory? And how could the tools of medical science help to resolve this dispute?

NFIP national officials began to rethink their constant defense of caution when assessing new ideas in polio. Perhaps the many scientists funded by the NFIP were some of the most brilliant scientists in the world who did slow, painstaking work that "eventually...like a slow-moving glacier, will crush and conquer infantile paralysis."[294] But perhaps these scientists needed more direction and coordination, despite their professed desire for professional independence. Unlike the well-publicized model of coordinated research and testing for the new drug penicillin, polio research, Gudakunst reflected, was not achieving any headway because too many scientists were "satisfied to work over and over again those fields of exploration that have been covered by their contemporaries."[295]

Quietly, some NFIP chapters began to use the term "Kenny" in their own fundraising. In Delaware the NFIP chapter sent out a fundraising letter assuring supporters that their donations had "sent 26 children to the Kenny Clinic [at the Wilmington General Hospital] for hospitalization and medical treatment" and all but 2 had "returned to school or to their play pens minus the deformities and twisted bodies that were so prevalent in the days when Polio was thought to be unconquerable."[296] The growing influence of the Kenny method was visible in polio care everywhere.

NOTES

1. "Keep Sister Kenny Here" *New York Journal-American* February 17 1944; "Sister Kenny Irate, May Leave Country" *New York Times* February 4 1944; "Sister Kenny Expects To Leave Soon" *Hartford Courant* February 4 1944; "Polio Funds Short, Kenny May Leave U.S." *Washington Post* February 4 1944. This amount was probably prompted by the news that the NFIP was providing a 5-year grant of $150,000 for a physical medicine center at the Graduate School of Medicine at the University of Pennsylvania; "The Scientific Study and Development of Physical Medicine" *Science* (January 7 1944) 99: 10–11.

2. Frank D. Campion *The A.M.A. and U.S. Health Policy since 1940* (Chicago: Chicago Review Press, 1984), 129–130; Patricia Spain Ward *"United States versus American Medical Association et al.*: The Medical Anti-Trust Case of 1938–1943" *American Studies* (1989) 30: 123–153.

3. Greer Williams "Medicine's India-Rubber Man" *Saturday Evening Post* October 19 1946, 26; see also "Docs Flock" *Time* (May 22 1944) 43: 46; "A.M.A. Meeting" *Time* (June 26 1944) 43: 50; "Remedy for Fishbein" *Time* (July 15 1946) 48: 94. The vote in 1944 was 144 to 9 and in 1945 it was 106 to 60.

4. See, for example, Ida M. Kay to Dear Dr. Knapp, February 2 1943, [enclosed with] Miland E. Knapp to Dear Dr. Gudakunst, February 5 1943, Am. 15.8, Folder 29 [accessed in 1992 before recent recataloging], UMA-SC.

5. Kenny to Dear Sir [Editor, *Minneapolis Star-Journal*], February 1 1944, Minneapolis—Newspapers, 1941–1945, MHS-K; "Help Me, or I Quit U.S.—Sister Kenny" *Chicago Herald-American* February 4 1944; [editorial] "Must Sister Kenny Leave?" *Tulsa Tribune* February 8 1944; "Sister Kenney [sic] Withholds New Polio Discovery" *Hartford Courant* February 5 1944; "Early Diagnosis of Polio Claimed by Sister Kenny" *Washington Post* February 6 1944. Note that Miland Knapp told visitors to Minneapolis that although he had tried he could not feel what she was describing; Knapp quoted in Draft of Report of the Committee [enclosed with] Pepper to Darling, September 29, 1944, Committee to Review Request of Elizabeth Kenny Institute to National Foundation for Infantile Paralysis: General, Medical Sciences, 1944, National Academy of Sciences, Washington D.C. (hereafter Review Committee, 1944, NAS).

6. "Keep Sister Kenny Here" *New York Journal-American* February 17 1944; "Sister Kenny Expects To Leave Soon" *Hartford Courant* February 4 1944; "Sister Kenny Says Fishbein 'Asked' Her to Leave Country" *New York Times* February 4 1944; "Sister Kenny Irate, May Leave Country" *New York Times* February 4 1944.

7. "Physiologic Nonsense and Poliomyelitis" *JAMA* (January 22 1944) 124: 236. Fishbein referred to Joseph Moldaver (*JAMA* 1943), Watkins, Brazier, and Schwab (*JAMA* 1943) and Stanley Cobb (*Archives of Medicine* 1943).

8. Memorandum re: [transcript] Telephone Conversation between BO'C and Mr. Coniff of the *Journal-American*—11.23 A.M., February 4 1944, Public Relations, MOD-K; "University Willing To Aid Sister Kenny" *New York Times* February 5 1944; "O'Connor Denies Foundation Break with Sister Kenny" *Hartford Courant* February 6 1944.

9. [Editorial] "Must Sister Kenny Leave?" *Tulsa Tribune* February 8 1944.

10. "Keep Sister Kenny Here" *New York Journal-American* February 17 1944; see also "Keep Sister Kenny Here" *Baltimore News Post* February 15 1944.

11. Roy J. Bergstrom to Gentlemen, February 4 1944, Public Relations, MOD-K.

12. Arthur Mitchell to Dear Doctor Irwin, February 12 1944, Public Relations, MOD-K.

13. "Launch $150,000 Drive to Keep Sister Kenny Here" *Pictorial Review* March 11 1944, *Chicago Herald-American*, Clippings, 1944, MHS-K; "Laud Work of Sister Kenny" *Chicago*

Herald-American March 7 1944; see also Philip Leslie Shutt [Boone County, Illinois NFIP chapter] to My Dear Sister Kenny, March 23 1944, NFIP-Misc., 1941–1944, MHS-K. A featured participant was writer Noreen Linduska who had experienced 2 kinds of polio during the 1943 Chicago epidemic and whose autobiography *My Polio Past* later enthusiastically praised Kenny's methods; Robert D. Dinsmore "Happy Victory [review of *My Polio Past*]" *New York Times* October 26 1947; Lloyd Wendt "Polio Victim Writes Story Full of Hope" *Chicago Daily Tribune* August 1 1947; see also Noreen Lunduska *My Polio Past* (Chicago: Pellegrini & Cudahy, 1947). The Disabled Persons Association of America tried to ensure its members employment in war industries.

14. "Launch $150,000 Drive to Keep Sister Kenny Here" *Pictorial Review* March 11 1944, *Chicago Herald-American*, Clippings, 1944, MHS-K.

15. [No caption] *Sunday Mirror* March 12 1944, Clippings, 1944, MHS-K.

16. H. Spencer Jordan to My Dear Sister Kenny, October 28 1944, Complimentary Letters of Support 1944–1949, MHS-K.

17. [Editorial] "Sister Kenny" *Washington Post* February 5 1944.

18. "Sister Kenney [sic] Requested to Leave U.S." *Citizens' Health News* (February 1944) 2: 2; "Who's Fighting for What Freedom?" *Citizens' Health News* (February 1944) 2: 1, Clippings, 1944, MHS-K.

19. H. Spencer Jordan to My Dear Sister Kenny, October 28 1944, Complimentary Letters of Support 1944–1949, MHS-K.

20. Cosette Drew Dexter to Dear Sister Kenny, February 2 1944, Complimentary Letters of Support 1944–1949, MHS-K.

21. R. A. Gurney, letter to editor, *St Paul Pioneer Press* February 1944, Case Files- Misc., A-K, 1943–1946, MHS-K.

22. [Editorial] "Must Sister Kenny Leave?" *Tulsa Tribune* February 8 1944.

23. L. L. Oeland to Dear Sister Kinney [sic], February 5 1944, Board of Directors, MHS-K.

24. Edna V. Paul to Dear Mr. O'Connor, February 4 1944, Public Relations, MOD-K.

25. Edward James Smythe to Dear Sister Kenny, February 4 1944, Complimentary Letters of Support 1944–1949, MHS-K.

26. Editorial, "After 10 Years of Giving America Begins to Wonder" *Seattle Times* February 13 1944; see also [editorial] "Must Sister Kenny Leave?" *Tulsa Tribune* February 8 1944.

27. Edward James Smythe to Dear Sister Kenny, February 4 1944, Complimentary Letters of Support 1944–1949, MHS-K.

28. C. E. Conway to Dear Sister Kenny, July 24 1944, Chicago Associate Nurses, 1944, MHS-K; Chicago Nurses Committee "We Urge You Now To Write or Wire Your Congressman . . ." [notice] March 27 1945, [enclosed with] Morris [Fishbein] to My Dear Basil, March 30 1945, Public Relations, MOD-K.

29. Morris [Fishbein] to My Dear Basil, March 30 1945, Public Relations, MOD-K. Note orthopedic nurse Carmelita Calderwood warned the NFIP that it was "a non-professional group" that had "hitched up with Hearst papers" and had "been a cause of disquiet in nursing circles in Chicago; [Notes on conversation between] Mr. Cusack and Miss Calderwood, April 24 1944, Public Relations, MOD-K.

30. Elizabeth Kenny "God Is My Doctor: Chapter I" *American Weekly* March 29 1944, 18. It was ghostwritten by RKO publicity agent Dan Mainwaring.

31. Elizabeth Kenny "God Is My Doctor: Chapter II" *American Weekly* April 2 1944, 18; Elizabeth Kenny "God Is My Doctor: Chapter III" *American Weekly* April 9 1944, 17; Elizabeth Kenny "God Is My Doctor: Chapter II" *American Weekly* April 2 1944, 19.

32. Alice Marble *Sister Elizabeth Kenny: Wonder Women of History as Told by Alice Marble* (New York: Wonder Women Publishing Co., Spring 1944). Thanks to Bert Hansen for sending me a copy of this comic book.

33. "[Script] BO'C Interview, WHAS—Louisville, Ky. 2-29-44; 4:40–4.45 PM," Public Relations, MOD-K.

34. *The Story of the Kenny Method* (New York: National Foundation for Infantile Paralysis, 1944), 4–8; see also Norine Foley "March of Dimes O.K.'s Sister Kenny Methods" *Los Angeles Examiner* March 24 1944; "Statement on Kenny Method By O'Connor" *Minneapolis Star-Journal* March 16 1944; Basil O'Connor "The Story of the Kenny Method" *Archives of Physical Therapy* (April 1944) 25: 231–234.

35. "The National Foundation and Sister Kenny's Work" February 8 1944, Public Relations, MOD-K; and see *The Story of the Kenny Method*, 4–6; John Lavan to My Dear Mrs. Miller, September 1 1944, Morris Fishbein Collection, vol. 77, Folder 8, Joseph Regenstein Library, University of Chicago; The National Foundation for Infantile Paralysis *Annual Report 1943* (New York: National Foundation for Infantile Paralysis, 1943), 46; "Sister Kenny's Work" *Hartford Courant* February 9 1944; Basil O'Connor "The Story of the Kenny Method" *Archives of Physical Therapy* (April 1944) 25: 231–234; Howard W. Blakeslee [science editor, AP] "Whispering Campaign" [enclosed in] Blakeslee to Dear Mr. O'Connor, February 21 1944, Public Relations, MOD-K; [Script] WPTF-"Fighting Infantile Paralysis," Raleigh, N.C. March 11 [1944]–7:30–8:00 PM, Public Relations, MOD-K; "Statement on Kenny Method By O'Connor" *Minneapolis Star-Journal* March 16 1944.

36. "Sister Kenny's Work" *Hartford Courant* February 9 1944.

37. "Sister Kenny's Work" *Hartford Courant* February 9 1944; [Script] WPTF-"Fighting Infantile Paralysis," Raleigh, N.C. March 11 [1944]–7:30–8:00 PM, Public Relations, MOD-K; *The Story of the Kenny Method*, 10.

38. "Paralysis Method Held Over[-]praised" *New York Times* April 11 1944.

39. [Script] WPTF- "Fighting Infantile Paralysis," Raleigh, N.C. March 11 [1944]–7:30–8:00 PM, Public Relations, MOD-K.

40. *The Story of the Kenny Method*, 5, 10; [Script] WPTF-"Fighting Infantile Paralysis," Raleigh, N.C. March 11 [1944]–7:30–8:00 PM, Public Relations, MOD-K; "The National Foundation and Sister Kenny's Work" February 8 1944, Public Relations, MOD-K.

41. PJAC to DWG Memorandum, March 8 1944, Public Relations, MOD-K.

42. *The Story of the Kenny Method*, 11.

43. Eddie Cantor to Dear Basil, March 20 1944, Public Relations, MOD-K. Cantor's "Show Business" was one of the top movies of 1944.

44. Mary [Pickford] to Dear Basil [O'Connor] March 11 1944, Public Relations, MOD-K. Pickford's work with the NFIP is not mentioned in Scott Eyman *Mary Pickford: America's Sweetheart* (New York: Donald I. Fine, 1990).

45. Peter J. A. Cusack to Dear Mary [Pickford] March 18 1944, Public Relations, MOD-K.

46. W. C. Higginbotham to Dear Sir, February 23 1944, Public Relations, MOD-K.

47. L. A. Karns, [secretary to W. A. Harriman] to Dear Mr. O'Connor, March 7 1944, Public Relations, MOD-K; Henry Ford to Dear Mr. Higginbotham, March 7 1944, Public Relations, MOD-K; James F. Bell to Dear Mr. O'Connor, March 2 1944, Public Relations, MOD-K; Peter J. A. Cusack to My Dear Mr. Clayton, March 7 1944, Public Relations, MOD-K; W. L. Clayton to Dear Mr. Higginbotham, March 6 1944, Public Relations, MOD-K.

48. F. B. Adams to Dear Mr. Higginbotham, March 13 1944, Public Relations, MOD-K.

49. Jack Alexander "Minneapolis-St Paul" *Saturday Evening Post* (April 3 1948), 23.

50. James F. Bell to My Dear Mr. O'Connor, March 8 1944, Public Relations, MOD-K.

51. Ibid.

52. O'Connor did however agree to accept Bell's letter of resignation from the NFIP board after Bell argued that there was a conflict of interest with his position as University of Minnesota regent; James F. Bell to My Dear Mr. O'Connor, July 22 1944, Public Relations, MOD-K; O'Connor to Bell, July 27 1944, Public Relations, MOD-K.

53. Basil O'Connor to My Dear Mr. Michaels, February 15 1944, Public Relations, MOD-K.

54. National Research Council, Division of Medical Sciences, "Report of Special Committee to Review Request Submitted by Elizabeth Kenny Institute, Inc. to National Foundation for Infantile Paralysis, Inc.," November 8 1944, Public Relations, MOD-K, 16 hereafter "Report of Special Committee."

55. Arthur D. Reynolds to My Dear Mr. O'Connor, November 22 1944, Public Relations, MOD-K.

56. "Statement By Marvin L. Kline Mayor of Minneapolis" [c.1943] MHS; see also Al Woodruff "Kline Opens Defense From Witness Chair" *Minneapolis Star* January 27 1961.

57. "Kline, Humphrey Step up Drive at Meeting" *Minneapolis Star-Journal* June 3 1943. For the debate around who deserved credit for promoting Kenny's work see F. J. Kottke, letter to editor, "Sister Kenny and the Kline Administration" [Minneapolis unnamed newspaper] June 19 [1943], Box 19, Sister Kenny Institute 1938–1946, Myers Papers, UMN-ASC; Editor's response to F. J. Kottke, letter to editor, "Sister Kenny and the Kline Administration" [Minneapolis unnamed newspaper] June 19 [1943], Box 19, Sister Kenny Institute 1938–1946, Myers Papers, UMN-ASC.

58. Ben Phillips "Kline Tells How City Won Kenny Institute" *Minneapolis Daily Times* June 3 1943; "Kline, Humphrey Step up Drive at Meeting" *Minneapolis Star-Journal* June 3 1943; Harry S. Sherwood "Kenny Report Awaited By Doctors" *Baltimore Evening Sun* October 31 1944.

59. Kenny "Data Concerning Introduction of Kenny Concept and Method of Treatment of Infantile Paralysis into the United States of America" [April 1944] Board of Directors, MHS-K.

60. Memorandum Re Conference On Kenny Program, February 10 1944, Am. 15.8, Folder 23, [accessed in 1992 before recent re-cataloging], UMN-ASC.

61. Harold S. Diehl "Summary of the Relationship of the Medical School of the University of Minnesota to the work of Sister Elizabeth Kenny," May 1944, Public Relations, MOD-K; "Sister Kenny's Work" *Hartford Courant* February 9 1944; "O'Connor Denies Foundation Break with Sister Kenny" *Hartford Courant* February 6 1944; "University Willing To Aid Sister Kenny" *New York Times* February 5 1944.

62. GBD [George Darling] "Preliminary Thoughts for a Tentative Draft: Special Committee for Investigation of Kenny Institute Request," [September 1944] Review Committee, 1944, NAS, 2; hereafter September Draft.

63. "Kenny Work Is Defended" *Minneapolis Star-Journal* [June] 1944, Poliomyelitis (Reprints, 1955–1964), MHS-K; "Institute Leader Comments" *New York Times* June 16 1944; September Draft, 2–3. See also John F. Pohl to Dear Mr. O'Connor, March 8 1943, Box 4, Basil O'Connor Papers, Manuscripts and Special Collections, New York State Archives, Albany; James S. Pooler "Kenny Complaint Based on Money" *Detroit Free Press* March 31 1945.

64. Miland E. Knapp "Observations on Infantile Paralysis: Its Symptoms and Treatment" *Journal-Lancet* (May 1944) 64: 164–168.

65. Harold S. Diehl to Dear Don [Gudakunst], August 3 1944, [attached with] O. H. Perry Pepper to Dear Doctor Winternitz, November 10 1944, Review Committee, 1944, NAS; "Kenny Method Again" *New York Times* September 10 1944; "Kenny Treatment Results" *Science News Letter* (September 16 1944) 46: 183.

66. Kenny "Data Concerning Introduction of Kenny Concept" [April 1944], Evidence, Reports 1943–1952, MHS-K.

67. Kenny to Dear Dr. Diehl, May 8 1944, Dr. Harold S. Diehl, 1941–1944, MHS-K.

68. "A.M.A. Meeting" *Time* (June 26 1944) 43: 50.

69. "Doctors Criticize Kenny Publicity" *New York Times* June 15 1944. The committee had also sent questionnaires to 900 orthopedic surgeons but did not include this information for "no definite conclusions could be drawn from the reports they submitted," a vague explanation suggesting that very vehement conclusions may well have been made but not in ways that could be easily integrated; Ralph K. Ghormley, Edward L. Compere, James A. Dickson, Robert V. Funsten, J. Albert Key, H. R. McCarroll and Herman C. Schumm "Evaluation of the Kenny Treatment of Infantile Paralysis" *JAMA* (June 17 1944) 125: 466.

70. J. Albert Key "Reasons Why the Orthodox Is Better than the Kenny Treatment of Poliomyelitis" *Surgery, Gynecology and Obstetrics* (October 1943) 77: 389–396; Key "The Kenny Versus the Orthodox Treatment of Anterior Poliomyelitis" *Surgery* (July 1943) 14: 20–31. See also H. R. McCarroll "The Role of Physical Therapy in the Early Treatment of Poliomyelitis" *JAMA* (October 17 1942) 120: 517–519; Lois Maddox Miller "Sister Kenny vs. The Medical Old Guard" *Reader's Digest* (November 1944) 45: 41.

71. Robert V. Funston [Report] in "Reports on Meeting of Committee to Investigate the Kenny Method of Treatment, Sunday and Monday, November 22 and 23, 1942, Minneapolis, Minnesota," Dr. R.K. Ghormley, 1943, MHS-K; "Doctor Favors New Paralysis Treatment" *Washington Post* August 24 1942; Robert V. Funsten "The Influence of the Sister Kenny Publicity on the Treatment of Poliomyelitis" *Virginia Medical Monthly* (October 1945) 72: 403–406. Robert Vivian Funsten (1892–1949) was the chair of the Department of Orthopedic Surgery at the University of Virginia (1932–1949); with Carmelita Calderwood he wrote *Orthopedic Nursing* (St Louis: C. V. Mosby, 1943).

72. Ghormley et al. "Evaluation of the Kenny Treatment of Infantile Paralysis," 467.

73. Ghormley et al. "Evaluation of the Kenny Treatment of Infantile Paralysis," 468.

74. See Key in Miller "Sister Kenny vs. The Medical Old Guard," 41. Key was said to be quoting an "Australian critic"; Funsten "The Influence of the Sister Kenny Publicity," 404. See a reference to a "Cynical Taunt by an Australian Medico Many Years Ago," Albert Deutsch "The Truth About Sister Kenny" *American Mercury* (November 1944) 59: 610.

75. Ghormley et al. "Evaluation of the Kenny Treatment of Infantile Paralysis," 466–468.

76. Ghormley et al. "Evaluation of the Kenny Treatment of Infantile Paralysis," 467–469.

77. Ghormley et al. "Evaluation of the Kenny Treatment of Infantile Paralysis," 469. This point was reiterated in the media; see "Doctors Criticize Kenny Publicity" *New York Times* June 15 1944.

78. Ghormley et al. "Evaluation of the Kenny Treatment of Infantile Paralysis," 468–469.

79. Deutsch "The Truth About Sister Kenny," 613. Polio historian Tony Gould claimed that the AMA report was "retribution" by the specialists; Gould *Summer Plague*, 105.

80. Albert Deutsch "Why Not a Scientific Test Of Kenny Polio Treatment?" *PM* June 20 1944.

81. "Paralysis Method Held Overpraised" *New York Times* August 11 1944; "Sister Kenny Treatment Hit by 7 Doctors" *Chicago Daily Tribune* June 16 1944.

82. Basil O'Connor to Peter J.A. Cusack, June 23 1944 [notice] *National Foundation News* (June 1944) 3: 1.

83. "O'Connor on Western Trip" *National Foundation News* (June 1944) 3: 1.

84. Editorial "Muscle Spasm in Poliomyelitis" *JAMA* (May 6 1944) 125: 35.

85. Fishbein "Facts About the Kenny Treatment" *Hygeia* (July 1944) 22: 573.

86. Thomas Parran to Miss Elizabeth Kenny [telegram], July 18 1944, Government—Misc., 1942–1951, MHS-K. Telegram in capital letters in original.

87. Howard Smith to Dear Sister Kenny, August 1 1944, Smith, Howard R., 1944, MHS-K.

88. Ibid.

89. See Michelle E. Osborn "Visscher, Maurice Bolks" *American National Biography Online* (February 2000), http://www.anb.org/articles/13/13-02004.html, accessed 1/16/2009. See also "$322,450 Grant to U. of M. Will Spur Kenny Program" *Minneapolis Star-Journal* June 21 1944; "New $320,000 Polio Grant Received by U" *Minneapolis Daily Times* June 21 1944.

90. Maurice B. Visscher to Dear Dr. Moldaver, June 5 1944, Minnesota Poliomyelitis Research Committee, Box 1, UMN-ASC.

91. A. B. Baker "The Central Nervous System in Poliomyelitis and Polio[-]encephalitis" *Journal-Lancet* (July 1944) 64: 224–233; Arthur I. Watkins "Electromyographic Studies in Poliomyelitis" *Journal-Lancet* (July 1944) 64: 233–236; Berry Campbell "The Physiology of the Spinal Cord with Relation to Poliomyelitis" *Journal-Lancet* (July 1944) 64: 236–239; Harland G. Wood "Metabolism of Nervous Tissue in Poliomyelitis" *Journal-Lancet* (July 1944) 64: 240–242; Ernest Gellhorn "The Effect of Muscle Pain on the Central Nervous System at the Spinal and Cortical Levels" *Journal-Lancet* (July 1944) 64: 243–245.

92. Editorial J. C. McKinley, Irvine McQuarrie, W. A. O'Brien, and M. B. Visscher "The Present Status of Poliomyelitis Management" *Journal-Lancet* (July 1944) 64: 249–250.

93. Lloyd [Ziegler] to Dear Chanley [McKinley], July 29 1944, Minnesota Poliomyelitis Research Committee, Box 1, UMN-ASC. See also H. M. Hines to Dear Dr. Visscher, July 31 1944, Minnesota Poliomyelitis Research Committee, Box 1, UMN-ASC; A. C. Icy to Dear Dr. Visscher, July 29 1944, Minnesota Poliomyelitis Research Committee, Box 1, UMN-ASC.

94. Thos. P. Bonner to Dear Madam, July 3 1944, Ray of Light Letters, 1944, MHS-K.

95. Otto E. Emrich to Dear Madame, June 27 1944, Ray of Light Letters, 1944, MHS-K.

96. H. A. Cosler to Dear Sister Kenny, June 23 1944, Ray of Light Letters, 1944, MHS-K.

97. [Reverend] F. E. Farrell [Minneapolis] to Dear Miss Kenny, January 9 1945, Churches, 1943–1946, MHS-K.

98. Harold S. Diehl, "Memorandum of Conference Concerning Future Plans for the Kenny Teaching Program of the Medical School" July 10 1944, Am. 15.8, Folder 16, [accessed in 1992 before recent re-cataloging], UMN-ASC

99. Roland Nicholson "Nurse Has Waged 33-Year Battle To Prove Ideas" *Washington Times-Herald* August 27 1944; "Medical, Govt. Experts Hosts At Dinner for Nurse Tonight" *Washington Times-Herald* September 1 1944; Dorothy Williams "D.C. Mission to Kenny Clinic Called 'Unnecessary Waste'" [Washington paper, c. August 1944], Supporting Data, Review Committee, 1944, NAS.

100. "Public Invited to Polio Forum Tomorrow Night at Statler" *Washington Times-Herald* September 1 1944.

101. "Notables View D.C. Premiere of Kenny Film" *Washington Times-Herald* October 23 1944.

102. J. E. Hulett, Jr. to Dear Sir [Peter Cusack] June 28 1944, Public Relations, MOD-K. Hulett wanted to do a study of the "sociological aspects" of Kenny's campaign "to gain professional and lay approval of her 'conception' of infantile paralysis." He assured Cusack that he would not be "making a judgment regarding the scientific validity of the 'Kenny method.'"

103. Howard Smith to Dear Sister Kenny, July 26 1944, Smith, Howard R., 1944, MHS-K.

104. Elizabeth Kenny to the President NFIP [telegram] July 8, 1944, Dr. Wallace H. Cole, 1940–1947, MHS-K; Elizabeth Kenny to My Dear Dr. Cole, July 11 1944, Dr. Wallace H. Cole, 1940–1947, MHS-K.

105. Elizabeth Kenny to Ladies and Gentlemen, [July 1944], Am. 15.8, Folder 23, [accessed in 1992 before recent re-cataloging] UMN-ASC

106. Lewis C. Mills "Sister Kenny Gives Answer to AMA in Dramatic Exhibition" *Minneapolis Star-Journal* June 20 1944.

107. "Notables View D.C. Premiere of Kenny Film" *Washington Times-Herald* October [23] 1944.

108. Elizabeth Kenny to Ladies and Gentlemen, [July 1944]; Albert Deutsch "Sister Kenny Again Engaged In Battle With Medicos" *PM* February 6 1944, 9; "Surgeons 'Severely Criticize' Claims Made for Her 'System'"—She Calls Their Statements 'Most Criminal Thing'" *New York Times* June 16 1944.

109. Edward L. Compere to Dear Miss Kenny, July 10 1944, Edward L. Compere, 1942–1945, MHS-K.

110. Elizabeth Kenny to Dear Dr. Compere, July 12 1944, Edward L. Compere, 1942–1945, MHS-K.

111. Edward L. Compere to Mr. E. E. Burr, February 28 1945, Edward Compere, 1942–1945, MHS-K.

112. Edward L. Compere ed. *The 1950 Year Book of Orthopedics and Traumatic Surgery* (Chicago: Year Book Publishers, 1951).

113. Charles J. Frankel and Robert V. Funsten "Use of Neostigmine (Prostigmine) in Subacute Poliomyelitis" *Southern Medical Journal* (June 1946) 39: 482–483; see also Funsten "The Influence of the Sister Kenny Publicity," 404–405; Charles J. Frankel "The Treatment of Acute and Subacute Anterior Poliomyelitis" *Virginia Medical Monthly* (September 1944) 71: 451–452.

114. Marvin L Kline to Dear Mr. O'Connor, July 18 1944, [attached with] O. H. Perry Pepper to Dear Doctor Winternitz, November 10 1944, Review Committee, 1944, NAS; "Yearly Program for Kenny Institute" [proposal enclosed in] Marvin L Kline to Dear Mr. O'Connor, July 18 1944, Public Relations, MOD-K; Marvin L Kline, Henry W. Haverstock, and John F. Pohl to Dear Mr. O'Connor, July 28 1944, Public Relations, MOD-K.

115. Harold S. Diehl to Dear Don [Gudakunst], August 3 1944, [attached with] O. H. Perry Pepper to Dear Doctor Winternitz, November 10 1944, Review Committee, 1944, NAS.

116. O'Connor to Diehl, May 18 1943, Dr. Harold S. Diehl, 1941–1944, MHS-K; Diehl to Dear Mrs. Miller, August 19 1944, Morris Fishbein Collection, vol. 77, Folder 8, Joseph Regenstein Library, University of Chicago.

117. "Kenny Methods Placed At Top" *Minneapolis Morning Tribune* [June 1944], Minnesota Poliomyelitis Research Committee, Box 2, UMN-ASC.

118. Mary Pohl, interview with Naomi Rogers, August 21 2003, Tallahassee, Florida. Pohl's awareness of gender discrimination in medicine had first been raised, according to his daughter, when he applied to the University of Minnesota's medical school under his childhood name "Florian Pohl" and was rejected because the medical school thought he was a woman.

119. Gould *Summer Plague*, 96–98; John F. Pohl "The Kenny Treatment of Anterior Poliomyelitis (Infantile Paralysis): Report of First Cases Treated in America" *JAMA* (1942) 118: 1428–1433.

120. Kenny to Dear Dr. Diehl, February 16 1942, Dr. Harold S. Diehl, 1941–1944, MHS-K; Kenny to Dear Mr. O'Connor, February 19 1942, Basil O'Connor, 1940–1942, MHS-K.

121. Editorial "The Kenny Treatment for Poliomyelitis" *Archives of Physical Therapy* (June 1942) 23: 364–367; [Cohn third interview with] John Pohl and Betty Pohl, October 9 1953, Cohn Papers, MHS-K.

122. "Sister Kenny Treatment Hit by 7 Doctors" *Chicago Daily Tribune* June 16 1944; "Institute Leader Comments" *New York Times* June 16 1944; "Kenny Methods Placed At Top" *Minneapolis Morning Tribune* [June 1944] Minnesota Poliomyelitis Research Committee, Box 2, UMN-ASC.

123. Harry S. Sherwood "Kenny Report Awaited By Doctors" *Baltimore Evening Sun* October 31 1944. See also Harry M. Marks *The Progress of Experiment: Science and Therapeutic Reform in the United States, 1900–1990* (New York: Cambridge University Press, 1997), 98–113; George B. Darling "How the National Research Council Streamlined Medical Research for War" in Morris Fishbein ed. *Doctors at War* (New York: E.P. Dutton & Company, 1945), 363–398.

124. Since 1940 the NFIP had provided a grant of $70,000 for an indefinite period of time to the NRC for fellowships in virus research and in orthopedic surgery; *Annual Report: For the Year Ended May 31 1945* (New York: National Foundation for Infantile Paralysis, 1945), 35.

125. O. H. Perry Pepper to Dear Darling, September 1 1944, Review Committee, 1944, NAS; O. H. Perry Pepper to Dear Mr. Bell, September 11 1944, Review Committee, 1944, NAS.

126. See Digby E. Baltzell *Philadelphia Gentlemen: The Making of a National Upper Class* (Chicago: Quadrangle Books, 1971); O. H. Perry Pepper *Old Doc* (Philadelphia: J. B. Lippincott Company, 1957).

127. Lewis H. Weed to My Dear Doctor [Ross] Harrison, August 16 1944, Review Committee, 1944, NAS; and see George B. Darling to Dear Mr. Kline, September 13 1944, Review Committee, 1944, NAS.

128. George B. Darling to Dear Mr. Kline, September 13 1944, Review Committee, 1944, NAS.

129. Pepper to Dear Doctor Darling, September 15 1944, Review Committee, 1944, NAS.

130. Kenny to Gentlemen, September 25 1944, Review Committee, 1944, NAS.

131. "Itinerary," Review Committee, 1944, NAS; Diehl to Dear Doctor Darling, September 8 1944, Review Committee, 1944, NAS. The 5 members who traveled to Minnesota were Bard, Darling, Pepper, Piersol, and Winternitz.

132. September Draft, 1–2, 5, 17; "Report of Special Committee," 2.

133. "Report of Special Committee," 4, 7. There were 3 small laboratories used for tissue pathology and chemical and hematological analysis, but no space "for any added activity and certainly not for any research."

134. "Report of Special Committee," 2–3; see also September Draft, 2.

135. "Report of Special Committee," 9; September Draft, 9, 19.

136. "Report of Special Committee," 4–6. The September Draft termed this group "home physicians," 5.

137. September Draft, 2, 5, 17.

138. "Report of Special Committee," 11–13, 16; September Draft, 17.

139. "Report of Special Committee," 16–17.

140. "Report of Special Committee," 14, 17–18.

141. "Report of Special Committee," 18–20.

142. Fred Fadell arranged for the Institute's board to invite Australian Prime Minister John Curtin and President Roosevelt, but both invitations were declined; Fred E. Fadell to Board of Directors, Memo, May 19 1944, Board of Directors undated and 1944–1945, MHS-K; Margaret Webber to Dear Honorable Sir [Prime Minister John Curtain], July 23 1944, Series A461, Item FA 347/1/7, AA-ACT; Marvin L. Kline to President, [1944], FDR-OF- 1930, Infantile Paralysis 1943–1945, Box 2, FDR Papers.

143. "Kenny Film Shown to 700" *Minneapolis Star-Journal* October 13 1944; "Kenny Drive Group Picked to Direct Pleas to Businesses" *Minneapolis Star-Journal* November 17 1944; "Speakers Ready for Kenny Drive" *Minneapolis Morning Tribune* November 5 1944; "Sister Kenny Returns From East as Big Drive Opens" *Minneapolis Star-Journal* November 15 1944; "Notables View D.C. Premiere of Kenny Film" *Washington Times-Herald* October 23 1944.

144. Lois Maddox Miller "Sister Kenny Wins Her Fight" *Reader's Digest* (1942) 41: 27–28

145. Miller "Sister Kenny Wins Her Fight," 27–28; see also notes taken by Naomi Rogers during the viewing of *The Kenny Concept of Infantile Paralysis,* Wilson Collection; "Fighter Ray Robinson Supports Crusade on Infantile Paralysis" *New York Amsterdam News* January 23 1943; on Lulu Boswell see "Typovision" *Chicago Defender* November 7 1942. On a group of "colored and white" children at the Institute see "Sister Kenny's 'Graduating Class'" *Atlanta Daily World* January 6 1944; "No Color Line Here as Children Are Cured of Polio" *Afro-American* January 15 1944.

146. "Progress Shown in Treatment On Infantile Paralysis In Tenn." *Atlanta Daily World* August 13 1943.

147. "Polio Patient" *Chicago Defender* September 30 1944; Dr U. G. Dailey "Until The Doctor Comes" *Chicago Defender* July 22 1944. See also "Sister Kenny's 'Graduating Class'" *Atlanta Daily World* January 6 1944.

148. "Fighter Ray Robinson Supports Crusade on Infantile Paralysis" *New York Amsterdam News* January 23 1943.

149. Kenny with Ostenso *And They Shall Walk,* 25–28. She wrote that "the aborigines of Australia are not the insensate animals that many ethnologists would make them out to be! They may be dirty, they may be lazy, but they are capable of displaying a heroism on occasion that would put many a white man to shame."

150. "Polio Committee Advocates Report on Method" *Los Angeles Evening Herald* October 14 1943; "Skin As A Paralysis Clue" *New York Times* October 16 1943.

151. "Sister Kenny Returns From East as Big Drive Opens" *Minneapolis Star-Journal* November 15 1944.

152. "Negroes To Join In Kenny Drive" *Minneapolis Star-Journal* November 10 1944; "Twin City Observer Committee for Kenny Institute" *Twin City Observer* November 10 1944; [editorial] "The Kenny Campaign" *Twin City Observer* November 10 1944. See also "Gold That Buys Health, Can Never Be Ill-Spent: Give to the Kenny Campaign" *Twin City Observer* November 17 1944; "Rev. Moore to Head the Sister Kenny Drive in St. Paul" *Twin City Observer* November 24 1944; "Sister Kenny Drive Extended" *Twin City Observer* November 24 1944; "Many Organizations Respond To Kenny Drive for Funds: St. Paul 'Kenny' Day Planned" *Twin City Observer* December 15 1944; "Elizabeth Kenny Mass Meeting At St. James Church" *Twin City Observer* December 22 1944. On the *Twin City Observer* as targeting "an older, more genteel readership" among African Americans and its "continued obsession with respectability" see Jennifer Delton "Labor, Politics, and African American Identity in Minneapolis, 1930–1950" *Minnesota History* (Winter 2001–2002) 57: 430.

153. "Successful 'Kenny' Mass Meeting Held at St. James Church in St. Paul" *Twin City Observer* December 29 1944.

154. "National Kenny Campaign Ready" *Minneapolis Morning Tribune* November 12 1944; "Hundreds Aid Kenny Drive" *Minneapolis Star-Journal* November 20 1944; "Kenny Gifts Coming In" *Minneapolis Star-Journal* November 14 1944; "Kenny Drive Sports Gift Total $4,792" *Minneapolis Morning Tribune* November 29 1944; "Bowlers Back Sister Kenny"

Minneapolis Morning Tribune November 21 1944; "Trade Dinner Will Boost Kenny Fund" *Minneapolis Star-Journal* November 1 1944.

155. "Jury Lays Gambling in Kline's Lap" *Minneapolis Star-Journal* November 3 1944; "National Drive for Kenny Funds Will Open Here" [Minneapolis newspaper] November 10 1944, Minnesota Polio myelitis Research Committee, Box 2, UMN-ASC.

156. "Liquor Dealers Aid Kenny Fund" *Minneapolis Morning Tribune* November 21 1944.

157. Miller "Sister Kenny vs. The Medical Old Guard," 38–43. The 5 were General Hospital, Wilmington, New York Orthopedic Dispensary and Hospital, Children's Hospital of Winnipeg, James Whitcomb Riley Hospital, Indiana University School of Medicine, and Willard Parker Hospital, New York.

158. Miller "Sister Kenny vs. The Medical Old Guard," 38–43.

159. Deutsch "The Truth About Sister Kenny," 610–615.

160. Ibid.

161. "Civic Leaders Vote Sister Kenny No. 1 Minnesotan of 1944" *Minneapolis Star-Journal* December 29 1944; "Audience of 7,100 Greets SJT [*Star-Journal and Morning Tribune*] Writers and Editors" *Minneapolis Morning Tribune* January 30 1945.

162. "$350,000 Given in Kenny Fund Drive" *Minneapolis Sunday Tribune* March 25 1945.

163. "O'Connor in Nationwide Broadcast, Opens 1945 Fund-Raising Appeal" *National Foundation News* (January 1945) 4: 9; National Foundation for Infantile Paralysis *The Miracle of Hickory* (New York: NFIP, 1945); Alice E. Sink *The Grit Behind the Miracle* (Lanham, MD: University Press of America, 1998); C. Hughes "The Miracle of Hickory" *Coronet* (February 1945) 17: 3–7.

164. "Report on Poliomyelitis Studies Made at Minneapolis General Hospital: Miland Knapp, John Moe, A. V. Stoesser, and J. S. Michael to Dear Doctor Harrington, October 12 1944" *Journal-Lancet* (January 1945) 65: 30–31.

165. Kenny to Mr. President, Ladies and Gentleman, January 15 1945, Board of Directors, undated and 1944–1945, MHS-K; and see Kenny to Dear Dr. Harrington, February 19 1945, Dr. F. E. Harrington, 1943–1946, MHS-K.

166. Kenny to Dear Mr. Moise, February 16 1945, *The American Weekly*, 1943–1945, MHS-K; John F. Pohl to Dear Mr. Kline, February 5 1945, [accessed in 1992 before recent re-cataloging], UMN-ASC.

167. John F. Pohl "The Kenny Concept and Treatment of Infantile Paralysis: Report of Five Year Study of Cases Treated and Supervised by Miss Elizabeth Kenny in America" *Journal-Lancet* (August 1945) 65: 265–271. See also J. A. Myers "Poliomyelitis (Infantile Paralysis) in Minnesota Including the Elizabeth Kenny Episode," Box 19, Sister Kenny Institute 1938–1946, Myers Papers, UMN-ASC 38–40.

168. DWG to SLJ [Memorandum] Notes on Questions Frequently Asked and Answers, January 2 1945, Public Relations, MOD-K.

169. Don W. Gudakunst "It's a Fifty-Fifty Chance" *Parents Magazine* (July 1944) 19: 32, 48, 50; and see Don W. Gudakunst and Marion O. Lerrigo "Minimizing Fear of Infantile Paralysis" *Understanding the Child* (June 1944) 13: 22.

170. Ephraim Fischoff and Don W. Gudakunst "The Fight Against Infantile Paralysis Continues" *American Journal of Nursing* (June 1944) 44: 533–546.

171. Gudakunst to Dear Sir [Kline], February 5 1945, Public Relations, MOD-K.

172. O'Connor [in] "Basil O'Connor Interview, Monday, Nov. 15 [19]44 10:05 to 10:15 KMOX The Voice of St. Louis," Public Relations, MOD-K.

173. Roosevelt to Dear Basil, December 1 1944, in "President's Birthday Fund" *Archives of Physical Therapy* (December 1944) 25: 743.

174. Peter J. A. Cusack to Dear Sir [Kline], March 16 1945, Mr. Marvin L. Kline, 1942–1959, MHS-K. See also "Rejected by Trustees 3-15-45" Application No CE CTAE, Public Relations, MOD-K.

175. PJAC to DWG Memorandum: Re Letter of January 7 1945, January 16 1945, Public Relations, MOD-K.

176. "Sister Kenny to Leave U.S." *Minneapolis Star-Journal* March 20 1945; Roland Nicholson "Parents of Ousted Child Tell How Sister Kenny Aided Boy" *Washington Times-Herald* March 28 1945.

177. "Sister Kenny Delays Plans to Leave City" *Minneapolis Morning Tribune* March 21 1945.

178. Elizabeth Kenny *Infantile Paralysis and Cerebral Diplegia: Methods Used for the Restoration of Function* (Sydney: Angus and Robertson, 1937). See also her comment to Australia reporters that her first textbook would be for "all kinds of paralysis"; "Queensland Nurse's Generous Action! Sister Kenny's Treatment for Paralysis a Gift for the Sick Poor" *Australian Women's Weekly* February 23 1935.

179. F. H. Mills "Treatment of Spastic Paralysis" *British Medical Journal* (August 25 1937) 2: 414–417; see also "The Treatment of Paralysis at the Elizabeth Kenny Clinic Royal North Shore Hospital of Sydney" *Medical Journal of Australia* (November 13 1937) 2: 888–894.

180. Kenny with Ostenso *And They Shall Walk*, 70–73.

181. "Yearly Program for Kenny Institute" [1944] [enclosed with] Marvin L Kline to Dear Mr. O'Connor, July 18 1944, [attached with] O. H. Perry Pepper to Dear Doctor Winternitz, November 10 1944, Review Committee, 1944, NAS.

182. Many children were cared for by relatives or placed in institutions for the feebleminded; Winthrop M. Phelps "Recent Significant Trends in the Care of Cerebral Palsy" *Southern Medical Journal* (February 1946) 39: 132–138; see also Editorial "The Problem of Cerebral Palsy" *JAMA* (October 25 1947) 135 [abstract] in *Physiotherapy Review* (1948) 28: 39.

183. Phelps "Recent Significant Trends in the Care of Cerebral Palsy," 132–138; see also "Medicine: Help for Spastics" *Time* (August 5, 1946) 48: 57; Howard J. Schaubel "Prostigmine as an Adjunct in the Treatment of Spastic Cerebral Palsy" *Physiotherapy Review* (1944) 24: 236–237.

184. "Birth-Spoiled Babies" *Time* (May 30 1932) 19: 45–46; "Tightrope Doctor" *Time* (February 17 1941) 37: 65; Earl R. Carlson *Born That Way* (New York: John Day Co., 1941).

185. "Kenny OKs Probe by Congress" *Minneapolis Morning Tribune* March 22 1945.

186. "Parents Win Return Of Spastic Children To Kenny Institute" *Minneapolis Star-Journal* March 21 1945; "Sister Kenny Delays Plans to Leave City" *Minneapolis Morning Tribune* March 21 1945; "Parents Win Return Of Spastic Children To Kenny Institute" *Minneapolis Star-Journal* March 21 1945; "Back In Kenny Institute" *Minneapolis Daily Times* March 22 1945.

187. "Kenny Resignation Refused by Board" *Minneapolis Morning Tribune* [March 1945]; Roland Nicholson "Parents of Ousted Child Tell How Sister Kenny Aided Boy" *Washington Times-Herald* March 28 1945. See also "Spastics Go Back to Kenny Care" *Minneapolis Star-Journal* March 21 1945; Myers "Poliomyelitis (Infantile Paralysis) in Minnesota Including the Elizabeth Kenny Episode," 36–37.

188. "Back In Kenny Institute" *Minneapolis Daily Times* March 22 1945; Roland Nicholson "Parents of Ousted Child Tell How Sister Kenny Aided Boy" *Washington Times-Herald* March 28 1945; "Sister Kenny Delays Plans to Leave City" *Minneapolis Morning Tribune* March 21 1945.

189. "Kenny OKs Probe by Congress'" *Minneapolis Morning Tribune* March 22 1945.

190. Clara Stoll to Dear Sister Kenny, April 2 1945, Congressional Investigation, Letters of Support, April–May 1945, MHS-K.

191. Deacon to Williams, March 10 1945, Minutes, Board of Directors 1938–1955, Children's Hospital of Winnipeg MG 10B33, Box 7, Province Archives, Manitoba.

192. Kenny to My Dear Mrs. Klock [Chicago], April 10 1945, Requests for Treatment 1942–1945, MHS-K.

193. "Sister Kenny Fights On" *Time* (April 2 1945) 45: 14; see also "O'Toole Invited By Sister Kenny to Visit Clinic" *Washington Times-Herald* March 30 1945; J. Earle Moser "Sister Kenny Hearing Asked" *Washington Times-Herald* April 11 1945.

194. Robert Conly "Only One in 1,500 Opposes Kenny Inquiry by Congress" *Washington Times-Herald* March 27 1945; "Sister Kenny OKs Probe by Congress" *Minneapolis Morning Tribune* March 22 1945.

195. Donald L. O'Toole to Dear Mr. President, March 26 1945, Public Relations, MOD-K; "Asks President's Aid" *New York Times* March 28 1945. See also Nat Fine "Probe Plea Declared Bid to Expose F.D.R. Patronage" *Minneapolis Morning Tribune* [March 1945], Public Relations, MOD-K; E. B. Cunningham and S. W. Whidden to President Franklin D. Roosevelt [telegram], March 28 1945, Public Relations, MOD-K; J. Earle Moser "Langer Seeks U.S. Supported Kenny Clinic" *Washington Times-Herald* March 29 1945; "Langer Asks 20 Million For Paralysis Clinic" *Washington Post* March 29 1945.

196. Nat Fine "Probe Plea Declared Bid to Expose F.D.R. Patronage" *Minneapolis Morning Tribune* March 1945, Public Relations, MOD-K.

197. "O'Toole Invited By Sister Kenny to Visit Clinic" *Washington Times-Herald* March 30 1945.

198. Kenny to My Dear Mrs. Fisher, March 28 1945 [accessed 1992 before re-cataloging] UMN-ASC; "Sister Kenny's Protest Taken to Roosevelt" *Chicago Daily Tribune* March 28 1945; Kenny to My Dear Mrs. Holman, March 26 1945, Case Files-Misc.: A-K, 1943–1946, MHS-K.

199. "Sister Kenny Would Air Row With O'Connor" *Washington Times-Herald* March 25 1945; Morris [Fishbein] to My Dear Basil, March 30 1945, Public Relations, MOD-K; Chicago Nurses Committee "We Urge You Now To Write or Wire Your Congressman…" [notice] March 27 1945 [enclosed with] Morris [Fishbein] to My Dear Basil, March 30 1945, Public Relations, MOD-K. See also Kenny to Dear Mr. President, Ladies and Gentlemen [of Board of Directors], [January 1945], Board of Directors, undated and 1944–1945, MHS-K.

200. "Fishbein Denies Kenny Polio Bias" *Los Angeles Times* March 24 1945.

201. Peter A. J. Cusack to Basil Waters, [telegram] March 24 1945, Public Relations, MOD-K; Basil L. Walters to Dear Mr. Cusack, March 28 1945, Public Relations, MOD-K. Pooler was one of 5 *Free Press* reporters who received the Pulitzer Prize for reporting in 1932, for an account of the American Legion parade in Detroit; "Best Reporting" *Time* (June 6 1932) 19: 28.

202. James S. Pooler "Fishbein Denies Unfairness Was Shown Sister Kenny" *Detroit Free Press* April 2 1945; Fishbein "Physiologic Nonsense and Poliomyelitis" *JAMA* (January 22 1944) 124: 236.

203. "Sister Kenny Fights On" *Time* (April 2 1945) 45: 56.

204. Kenny to Dear Sir [James Pooler], April 10 1945, Michigan-Newspapers, 1945, MHS-K; James S. Pooler to Dear Sister Kenny, [April 1945], Michigan-Newspapers, 1945, MHS-K. 945.

205. "Kenny Hearing Set for Tuesday" *Washington Times-Herald* April 12 1945; J. Earle Moser "Sister Kenny Hearing Asked" *Washington Times-Herald* April 11 1945.

206. "Sister Kenny Rebuffed" *New York Daily News* May 4 1945; "O'Toole to Talk On Kenny Case" *Washington Times-Herald* May 7 1945; "No Hearing for Sister Kenny" *New York Times* May 5 1945; "House Rules Group Agrees Not to Hear Sister Kenny" *Washington Post* May 5 1945.

207. J. Earle Moser "Sister Kenny May Appear On F.D.R. Memorial Talk" *Washington Times-Herald* May 11 1945.

208. "Decision Today On Hearing Plan For Sister Kenny" *Washington Times-Herald* May 4 1945.

209. Edward J. Noble to Dear Sister Kenny, April 25 1945, Blue Network, 1942–1943, MHS-K; see also "WTCN Radioscript: Sister Elizabeth Kenny, Fri. Apr. 13. 1945," Speeches (Radio) 1942–1945, MHS-K.

210. William Lawler [Illinois General Assembly] to Dear Nick [Keller], April 11 1945, Nick Keller, MHS-K; "Sister Kenny Visits Chicago" *Minneapolis Sunday Tribune* April 29 1945.

211. "Sister Kenny Tells Illinois About 'Organized Boycott'" [unnamed paper, maybe *Times-Herald*, May 1945], Kenny Institute, Box 10, Hubert. H. Humphrey Papers, MHS; "Kenny Method Boycotted, Nurse Tells Legislature" *Chicago Daily News* May 1 1945; Kenny "At the onset..." [May 1945 speech to Illinois legislature] Nick Keller, 1945, MHS-K.

212. "Experts Oppose Kenny Methods" *Brisbane Courier Mail* June 16 1944; see also [Elizabeth Kenny] "Elizabeth Kenny Institute (Physicians Class) March 19, 1945," Ray J. Lerschen, [Shorthand Reporter, Minneapolis], Kenny Collection, Box 1, Fryer Library; "Back to the Bush She Loves" *Australian* May 20 1945, Box 2, Folder 7, OM 65-17, Chuter Papers, Oxley-SLQ.

213. Frank E. Harrington, Stephen H. Baxter, and John F. Pohl [medical committee, Kenny Institute] to Honourable [sic] Sir [Sir Owen Dixon, Australian Legation], August 9 1944, Box 1, OM 65-11, Chuter Papers, Oxley-SLQ.

214. Later exposés detailed what were only rumors at the height of his career: his drinking, his temper, his violent disciplining of his 4 sons, and his neglect of his first wife Dixie (who died of cancer in 1952); see, for example, Charles Thompson *Bing: The Authorized Biography* (New York: David McKay Company Inc., 1975); Jib Fowles *Starstruck: Celebrity Performers and the American Public* (Washington: Smithsonian Institution Press, 1992).

215. "Bing Crosby Will Head Kenny Institute's Drive" *Chicago Daily Tribune* July 25 1945.

216. Smith *Patenting the Sun*, 64–87.

217. "American Salutes President's Birthday" *National Foundation News* (January 1945) 4: 11.

218. On anti-Catholicism continuing into the postwar era see Paul Blanshard *American Freedom and Catholic Power* (Boston: Beacon Press, [1949] 1958), 59–61, 90–91; Philip Jenkins *The Last Acceptable Prejudice* (New York: Oxford University Press, 2003).

219. Joe Savage to Dear Jim [James Bryan], November 8 1946, Public Relations, MOD-K; see also [Cohn interview with] Morris Fishbein, November 16 1953, Cohn Papers, MHS-K.

220. [cartoon] "5,000,000 Elizabeth Kenny Institute Campaign" *Los Angeles Herald-Examiner* November 20 1945.

221. See, for example, Lawrence J. Linck to Dear Mrs. Morey, November 30 1945, Public Relations, MOD-K; Minutes of November 14 1945 meeting of Hennepin County for Elizabeth Kenny Foundation Appeal, Box 10, Kenny Institute, Humphrey Papers, MHS; "S.F. Sets Tomorrow as Sister Kenny Fund Day" *San Francisco Examiner* December 7 1945.

222. Bing [Crosby] to Dear Mr. Parkin [form letter], December 4 1945, Public Relations, MOD-K.

223. William C. Bowen [Executive Assistant to the President] to Dear Mr. Comer, October 29 1945, Public Relations, MOD-K; Harry Brundidge "The Sister Kenny Controversy" *Cosmopolitan* (October 1945) 119: 56. On the support of Crosby by newspaper man Rocky Parks of Chicago "on loan" from the Hearst corporation as a field officer, see [Report] California Intelligence Bureau, November 30 1945, Public Relations, MOD-K.

224. Brundidge "The Sister Kenny Controversy," 56, 58, 131–132; James S. Pooler "Cripple Discards Crutches, Walks" *Detroit Free Press* March 29 1945.

225. Honorary County Chairman [Sister Elizabeth Kenny Foundation Infantile Paralysis Drive] to Dear Sir [form letter], December 4 1945, Public Relations, MOD-K. On therapists

who could "only be trained" at the Kenny Institute; Bing to Dear Mr. Parkin [form letter], December 4 1945, Public Relations, MOD-K; see also R. Kenneth Kerr [Ohio State Chairman KF] to Dear Friend, December [1945], Public Relations, MOD-K.

226. Michael F. Comer [Bloomfield, New Jersey] to Mr. O'Connor, October 18 1945, Public Relations, MOD-K.

227. Dorothy Ducas "Points in Kenny Article, Cosmopolitan, October 1945" October 25 1945, Public Relations, MOD-K. On the NRC report as "entirely independent of the National Foundation" see O'Connor to Dear Roy [Naftzger], September 7 1945, MOD-K.

228. Statement by Dr. Don W. Gudakunst, October 10 1945, Public Relations, MOD-K.

229. James P. Jennings to Dear Mr. [Walker] Wear, December 8 1945, Public Relations, MOD-K.

230. Frank E. McDonnell [Montana] to Mr. Stone Memorandum Re: Kenny, November 13 1945, Public Relations, MOD-K.

231. Hubert Humphrey, Fletcher Bowron, and Joseph J. Kelly to Dear Fellow Mayor, November 27 1945, Box 10, Kenny Institute, Humphrey Papers, MHS.

232. Mr. Wear to Mr. La Porte [Memorandum], November 20 1945, Public Relations, MOD-K; Chester LaRoche to Dear Marvin [Kline], December 3 1945, Clara and Chester LaRoche, 1945–1948, MHS-K.

233. Mr. Wear to Mr. La Porte Memorandum Re Elizabeth Kenny Campaign (Arizona), November 28 1945, Public Relations, MOD-K.

234. Dan Marovich [San Francisco] to Mr. D. Walker Wear Memorandum Re [Kenny Campaign], November 28 1945, Public Relations, MOD-K.

235. Roy E. Naftzger to Dear Basil, August 22 1945, MOD-K.

236. Mr. Stone to Mr. Wear Memorandum Re Scotts Bluff County, Nebraska, August 17 1945, Public Relations, MOD-K.

237. Harriet Pittman to Dear Mr. Wear, November 26 1945, Public Relations, MOD-K.

238. Arthur D. Reynolds to My Dear Mr. O'Connor, November 22 1944, Public Relations, MOD-K; see also Maurice B. Visscher to Dear Dr. McCarroll, October 19 1945, Minnesota Poliomyelitis Research Committee, Box 1, UMN-ASC.

239. Portland Better Business Bureau Inc. "Report: Sister Elizabeth Foundation, Inc." November 13 1945, Public Relations, MOD-K. The final goal was intended to be 5 million dollars; Dan Marovich [San Francisco] to Mr. D. Walker Wear Memorandum Re [Kenny Campaign], November 28 1945, Public Relations, MOD-K.

240. Dan Marovich to Dear Mr. O'Connor, August 16 1945, Public Relations, MOD-K; and see Dan Marovich [San Francisco] to Mr. D. Walker Wear Memorandum Re [Kenny Campaign], November 28 1945, Public Relations, MOD-K.

241. Roy E. Naftzger to Dear Basil, August 22 1945, MOD-K.

242. Robert G. McIntosh to Gentlemen [NFIP], November 26 1945, Public Relations, MOD-K. Harris was city editor of the Cincinnati Times Star.

243. John McGovern [Minnesota state KF chair] to Dear Sister Kenny, March 6 1946, [accessed in 1992 before re-cataloging], UMN-ASC.

244. Honorary County Chairman [Sister Elizabeth Kenny Foundation Infantile Paralysis Drive] to Dear Sir [form letter], December 4 1945, Public Relations, MOD-K.

245. Thompson Bing: The Authorized Biography, 114; Fowles Starstruck: Celebrity Performers and the American Public, 146; Donald Shepherd and Robert F. Slatzer Bing Crosby: The Hollow Man (New York: St. Martin's, 1981), 188–192.

246. Britton Budd to Dear Mr. O'Connor, September 20 1945, Public Relations, MOD-K.

247. Abner E. Larned to Dear Mr. MacRae, August 22 1945, Public Relations, MOD-K; Frank E. McDonnell [Montana] to Mr. Stone Memorandum Re: Kenny, November 13 1945, Public Relations, MOD-K.

248. Warren T. Kingsbury to Warren D. Coss Memorandum Re: Sister Kenny Campaign, December 4 1945, Public Relations, MOD-K.

249. John B. Middleton to Mr. George H. La Porte Memorandum, November 29 1945, Public Relations, MOD-K.

250. Robert H. MacRae to Dear Mr. Larned, August 19 1945, Public Relations, MOD-K.

251. "Just Between Us" *National Foundation News* (March 1943) 2: 21 ["those polio kiddies in the Greer Garson Metro-Goldwyn-Mayer trailer"]; see also "O'Connor in Nationwide Broadcast, Opens 1945 Fund-Raising Appeal" *National Foundation News* (January 1945) 4: 9; "Movie Preview" *National Foundation News* (January 1945) 4: 10.

252. Franklin D. Roosevelt to My Dear Mr. O'Donnell [Dallas] February 4 1943, FDR-P PF-4885, (1939–1945), Comm. Celeb. Pres. Birthday 1943, FDR Papers; Karl Hoblitzelle [Dallas] to Dear Jesse [Jones], January 19 1943, FDR-PPF-4885, (1939–1945), Comm. Celeb. Pres. Birthday 1943, FDR Papers.

253. Mr. La Porte to Dr. Gudakunst Memorandum Re Sister Kenny Camp[aign], July 26 1945, Public Relations, MOD-K.

254. Daniel W. De Hayas to Mr. D. Walker Wear Memorandum Re Sister Kenny Drive, October 12 1945, Public Relations, MOD-K.

255. "Foundation Tells Of Aid to Sister Kenny Treatment" *Motion Picture Herald* November 10 1945.

256. George La Porte to Dear Miss McGinn, January 4 1946, Public Relations, MOD-K; see also "S.F. Sets Tomorrow as Sister Kenny Fund Day" *San Francisco Examiner* December 7 1945.

257. George La Porte to C. C. Gaule Memorandum Your memo of August 27th, August 28 1945, Public Relations, MOD-K; Dan Marovich to Dear Joe [Schenck], August 2 1945, Public Relations, MOD-K.

258. [Bing Crosby to] Hulda McGinn [secretary of Board of Governors, California Theaters and Affiliated Industries, Inc.], November 21 1945, Public Relations, MOD-K.

259. J. David Larson to D. Walker Wear Memorandum Re Kenny Fund Raising—Bing Crosby, August 13 1945, Public Relations, MOD-K.

260. Dan Marovich to Dear Joe [Schenck], August 2 1945, Public Relations, MOD-K.

261. "Crosby Names 60 Aides for Kenny Drive" *Baltimore American* October 14 1945.

262. John B. Middleton to Mr. George H. La Porte Memorandum November 29 1945, Public Relations, MOD-K.

263. John B. Middleton to Mr. George H. La Porte [Memorandum] Re: Kenny Drive, November 21 1945, Public Relations, MOD-K; A. Harry Moore to Dear Friend, November 21 1945, Public Relations, MOD-K.

264. Arthur Potterton, the Jersey City chapter's treasurer and a "life-long friend" of Moore's, agreed to ask him if he knew that the Kenny drive "was being handled by a professional fund-raising concern" and to give him a confidential letter by Don Gudakunst; Major Nicholas Bernard to Public Relations Department Memorandum [Re: Kenny Campaign], October 18 1945, Public Relations, MOD-K.

265. Major Nicholas Bernard to Public Relations Department Memorandum [Re: Kenny Campaign], October 18 1945, Public Relations, MOD-K.

266. Charles K. Barton to My Dear Mr. [Grannell E.] Knox, November 24 1945, Public Relations, MOD-K.

267. NFIP "Program" [script] January 18 1945, FDR-PPF-4885, Comm. Celeb. Pres. Birthday 1945, (1944–1945), FDR Papers.

268. "Will Organize Polio Emergency Volunteers" *National Foundation News* (June 1945) 4: 29–30.

269. John B. Middleton to Mr. George H. La Porte Memorandum, November 29 1945, Public Relations, MOD-K. Roebling said she had taken on the position out of "personal respect" for the former Governor Harry Moore who was actively campaigning for the KF.

270. James P. Jennings to Dear Mr. [Walker] Wear, December 8 1945, Public Relations, MOD-K.

271. R.W. Gregory to Dear Mr. Joyce, October 25 1945, Public Relations, MOD-K.

272. Kenny "Results of Evidence Presented at the Medical Conference held in Minneapolis December 3rd to 6th [1945]," Public Relations, MOD-K; see also Kenny "I must thank you for your presence here today…" [December 1945], Marvin L. Kline 1942–1959, MHS-K; Kenny to Dear Mr. President [Kline], December 13 1945, Marvin L. Kline 1942–1959, MHS-K.

273. Kenny to My Dear Mr. O'Connor [form letter], January 18 1946, Public Relations, MOD-K.

274. [List of participants] "Conference On Poliomyelitis, December 3, 4, & 5 1945, Minneapolis, Minnesota," Record Group 29, vol. 201, file 311-P11-15, National Archive Centre, Ottawa; Savage to O'Connor Memorandum, January 19 1946, Public Relations, MOD-K. O'Connor referred to "Letter #1 by Gudakunst."

275. Kenny *Physical Medicine: The Science of Dermo-Neuro-Muscular Therapy as Applied to Infantile Paralysis* (Minneapolis: Bruce Publishing Company, 1946).

276. D. Paul Reed to Dear Member, October 11 1946, Kenny Foundation Fund Drive 1946, MHS-K.

277. [Report] California Intelligence Bureau, November 30 1945, Public Relations, MOD-K; D. Paul Reed to Dear Member, October 11 1946, Kenny Foundation Fund Drive 1946, MHS-K; see also George La Porte to Dear Doctor Robinson [Pittsburgh], November 26 1946, Public Relations, MOD-K.

278. "Kate Smith Heads Kenny Fund Drive" [*Minneapolis Morning Tribune*] [July 1946] Scrapbook 1945–1952, Henry Papers, MHS-K; "Kate Smith to Head Polio Drive" *New York Times* August 8 1946. On Kate Smith as embodying "cardinal American virtues" see Robert K. Merton *Mass Persuasion: The Social Psychology of a War Bond Drive* (New York: Harper and Brothers, 1946), 76, 83.

279. See Heather Green Wooten *The Polio Years in Texas: Battling a Terrifying Unknown* (College Station: Texas A&M University Press, 2009), 92–93; David M. Oshinksy *Polio: An American Story* (New York: Oxford University Press, 2005), 60.

280. "Physical Therapy Scholarship News" *National Foundation News* 4 (May 1945) 25–26; Gudakunst [Memorandum] Re: Kenny Institute, November 30 1945, Public Relations, MOD-K; Howard A. Rusk and Eugene J. Taylor *New Hope for the Handicapped: The Rehabilitation of the Disabled from Bed to Job* (New York: Harper & Brothers, 1946, 1949), 163–164; Roland H. Berg *The Challenge of Polio: The Crusade Against Infantile Paralysis* (New York: Dial Press, 1946), 156. Note also that two-thirds of the 24 illustrations of *Polio and its Problems* were devoted to images of patients working with physical therapists; Roland H. Berg *Polio and Its Problems* (Philadelphia: J.B. Lippincott, 1948), op. 84–op. 85.

281. "Dear Mr.____" September 19 1946, Public Relations, MOD-K.

282. "The Epidemic of 1946 (as of August 1, 1946) As detailed by Dr. Van Riper at Press Conference, 120 Bwy, NY 5, NY," Public Relations, MOD-K.

283. George La Porte to Dear Miss McGinn, January 4 1946, Public Relations, MOD-K.

284. Joe Savage to Dear Jim [James Bryan], November 8 1946, Public Relations, MOD-K; see also PJAC to DG et al Memorandum March 20 1944, Public Relations, MOD-K.

285. NFIP "In Daily Battle" [1947], MOD. By 1947 NFIP films included *When Polio Strikes, New Horizon, and Accent on Use.*

286. Oshinksy *Polio*, 86–89.

287. Berg *The Challenge of Polio*, 159–164, 169–170.

288. Anon. [review] *"The Challenge of Polio*, by Roland H. Berg" *New Republic* (September 23 1946) 115: 357.

289. H. M. Weaver "Why Chapters Cannot Sponsor Research" [speech given at] Hotel Roosevelt, April 1–5 1946, Public Historical Organizations, MOD. See also Hart Van Riper to Dear Dr. Lewin, May 16 1946, Public Relations, Lewin Files, MOD; George La Porte to Dear Miss McGinn, January 4 1946, Public Relations, MOD-K; *The Chapter's Role in Serving Infantile Paralysis Patients* (New York: National Foundation for Infantile Paralysis, publication #56, revised June 1948).

290. Chester La Roche to Dear Mr. O'Connor, September 3 1946, Clara and Chester La Roche, 1945–1948, MHS-K.

291. Francis P. L. Cronin to Dear Miss Keeler, January 20 1947, Public Relations, MOD-K.

292. Allen W. Fincke to Dear Mr. O'Connor, September 15 1947, Public Relations, MOD-K.

293. O'Connor to My dear Mr. Fincke, October 8 1947, Public Relations, MOD-K.

294. O'Connor in "Basil O'Connor Interview Monday, Nov 15 [19]44 10:05 to 10:15 KMOX "The Voice of St. Louis," Public Relations, MOD-K.

295. Gudakunst quoted in Richard Carter *Breakthrough: The Saga of Jonas Salk* (New York: Trident Press, 1966), 26.

296. Francis Reardon [chairman, Delaware Campaign Committee NFIP] to Dear Mr. Ward, January 22 1946, [enclosed in] Judson D. Ryon to Dear Sister Kenny, February 4 1946, Judson D. Ryon, MHS-K.

FURTHER READING

On medical populism see Kenny Ausubel *When Healing Becomes a Crime* (Rochester, VT: Healing Arts Press, 2000); Alan Brinkley *Voices of Protest: Huey Long, Father Coughlin, and the Great Depression* (New York: Knopf, 1982); David Cantor "Cancer, Quackery and the Vernacular Meaning of Hope in 1950s America" *Journal of the History of Medicine and Allied Sciences* (2006) 61: 324–368; Robert D. Johnston ed. *The Politics of Healing: Histories of Alternative Medicine in Twentieth-Century North America* (New York: Routledge, 2004); Robert D. Johnston *The Radical Middle Class: Populist Democracy and the Question of Capitalism in Progressive Era Portland, Oregon* (Princeton: Princeton University Press, 2003); Eric S. Juhnke *Quacks and Crusaders: The Fabulous Careers of John Brinkley, Norman Baker, and Harry Hoxsey* (Lawrence: University Press of Kansas, 2002); George Wolfskill and John A. Hudson *All But the People: Franklin D. Roosevelt and His Critics 1933–1939* (London: Macmillan, 1969).

On medicine, racism, and antisemitism see Gert H. Brieger "Getting Into Medical School in the Good Old Days: Good for Whom?" *Annals of Internal Medicine* (1993) 119: 1138–1143;

Edward C. Halperin "The Jewish Problem in Medical Education, 1920–1955" *Journal of the History of Medicine and Allied Sciences* (2001) 56: 140–167; Kenneth M. Ludmerer *Time to Heal: American Medical Education from the Turn of the Century to the Era of Managed Care* (New York: Oxford University Press, 1999); Dan A. Oren *Joining the Club: A History of Jews and Yale* (New Haven: Yale University Press, 1985).

On polio, medical care, and race see W. Michael Byrd and Linda A. Clayton *An American Health Dilemma, V. 2: Race, Medicine, and Health Care in the United States 1900–2000* (New York: Routledge, 2002); James P. Comer *Maggie's American Dream: The Life and Times of a Black Family* (New York: New American Library, 1988); Vanessa Northington Gamble *Making a Place for Ourselves: The Black Hospital Movement, 1920–1945* (New York: Oxford University Press, 1995); James H. Jones *Bad Blood: The Tuskegee Syphilis Experiment* (London: Free Press, 1981); Stephen E. Mawdsley " 'Dancing on Eggs': Charles H. Bynum, Racial Politics, and the National Foundation for Infantile Paralysis, 1938–1954" *Bulletin of the History of Medicine* (2010) 84: 217–247; Dorothy Roberts *Killing the Black Body: Race, Reproduction, and the Meaning of Liberty* (New York: Pantheon, 1997); Naomi Rogers "Race and the Politics of Polio: Warm Springs, Tuskegee and the March of Dimes" *American Journal of Public Health* (2007) 97: 2–13.

On Fishbein and medical politics see Edward D. Berkovitz and Wendy Wolff *Group Health Association: A Portrait of a Health Maintenance Organization* (Philadelphia: Temple University Press, 1988); James G. Burrow *AMA: Voice of American Medicine* (Baltimore: Johns Hopkins University Press, 1963); Frank D. Campion *The A.M.A. and U.S. Health Policy since 1940* (Chicago: Chicago Review Press, 1984); Jonathan Engel *Doctors and Reformers: Discussion and Debate over Health Policy 1925–1950* (Charleston: University of South Carolina Press, 2002): Elizabeth Fee and Theodore Brown eds. *Making Medical History: The Life and Times of Henry E. Sigerist* (Baltimore: Johns Hopkins University Press, 1997); Daniel S. Hirschfield *The Lost Reform: The Campaign for Compulsory Health Insurance in the United States from 1932 to 1943* (Cambridge: Harvard University Press, 1970); Elton Rayack *Professional Power and American Medicine: The Economics of the American Medical Association* (Cleveland: World Publishing Co., 1967); Patricia Spain Ward *"United States versus American Medical Association et al.:* The Medical Anti-Trust Case of 1938–1943" *American Studies* (1989) 30: 123–153;.

On Crosby, movies and anti-Catholicism see Paul Blanshard *American Freedom and Catholic Power* (Boston: Beacon Press, [1949] 1958); Bing Crosby as told to Pete Martin *Call Me Lucky* (New York: Simon & Schuster, 1953); Jib Fowles *Starstruck: Celebrity Performers and the American Public* (Washington: Smithsonian Institution Press, 1992); Philip Jenkins *The Last Acceptable Prejudice* (New York: Oxford University Press, 2003); Les Keyser and Barbara Keyser *Hollywood and the Catholic Church: The Images of Roman Catholicism in American Movies* (Chicago: Loyola University Press, 1984); Ruth Prigozy and Walter Raubicheck eds. *Going My Way: Bing Crosby and America Culture* (Rochester: University of Rochester Press, 2007); Donald Shepherd and Robert F. Slatzer *Bing Crosby: The Hollow Man* (New York: St. Martin's Press, 1981); Charles Thompson *Bing: The Authorized Biography* (New York: David McKay Company Inc., 1975); Frank Walsh *Sin and Censorship: The Catholic Church and the Motion Picture Industry* (New Haven: Yale University Press, 1996).

6

Celluloid

⌒⌒————————————————————————————————————

ALL HER LIFE, Kenny loved movies. While running her clinic in Brisbane in the 1930s she had regularly "popped out" for an afternoon show at the local Regents Theater, and in Minneapolis she sought escape from the tensions of her work in the cinema's fantasy and anonymity.[1] But she also saw film as a valuable means of persuasion. When she first came to the United States she brought with her a silent film showing the transformation in her Australian patients, some of whom had been profoundly disabled for many years.[2] After only a year in Minnesota she produced another silent film about "the treatment carried out at Minneapolis and its results" and warned Basil O'Connor that if he refused to see it "I will understand the Foundation is not interested in my work and I am wasting my time in [the] U.S.A."[3] Her early films were of poor quality, jerky, and hard to see, and despite her warning to O'Connor she wanted to remain in Minneapolis and improve them. She began to discuss making a sound film with National Foundation for Infantile Paralysis (NFIP) secretary Peter Cusack, editor of the *National Foundation News*, although they both agreed that for "satisfactory" accuracy they needed to wait until the next polio epidemic.[4] In 1942 she showed her "moving pictures" at the American Physiotherapy Association's annual meeting in June, the biennial nursing conference in July, and during the visit of the American Medical Association (AMA) orthopedic committee in November.[5]

While these short films were clearly intended to demonstrate the efficacy of her methods to medical professionals, Kenny considered them accessible to lay audiences as well. In 1943, after she had been awarded the 1942 Humanitarian Award by the Variety Clubs, she noticed that other recipients of the award had a film showing their work. She therefore offered Variety officials one of her short silent films, and was gratified when a senior Variety official screened the picture and reported that "it is very good."[6] Members of the women's auxiliary of the Los Angeles Children's Hospital heard Kenny had a film "showing you treating children afflicted with Infantile Paralysis" and asked for a copy to show their volunteers.[7] Michigan physician Ethel Calhoun asked for a loan of one of her films to help her "spread the 'gospel' in Michigan," suggesting the film would convert viewers into Kenny supporters.[8]

FILM AND MEDICAL AUTHORITY

By the 1940s, medical films played a critical role in American medicine. They were regularly screened at medical societies and health department meetings, and functioned as entertainment, pedagogy, and on occasion as research. Philanthropies such as the National Tuberculosis Association and the American Social Hygiene Association used films as educational and fundraising tools. Even before the NFIP was established, polio films were widely used, including ones on treatment during acute, paralytic, and postparalytic phases, orthopedic operations, a virological study of the "experimental production of infantile paralysis," and a study of polio's epidemiology.[9] The NFIP made short films a prominent part of its March of Dimes campaigns and as early as 1938 the head of the NFIP's committee on the treatment of after-effects proposed buying films to be part of a polio library to be housed in either the Surgeon General's Library or the library of the New York Academy of Medicine.[10]

In the 1910s and 1920s many physicians had seen medical films as "undignified and even unethical."[11] Many early films, one commentator recalled, "were made as hobbies to show a particular method of operation" and were not of good quality. Indeed surgeons often had to leave the making of the film to a cameraman who knew little or nothing about what he was filming.[12] Films also contradicted the pedagogic philosophy at the heart of professional medical training: that clinical skills should be gained on the job through seeing and touching individual patients.

Still, teachers sought out films to show medical students. Especially popular were those produced by Brooklyn surgeon Jacob Sarnoff, whose films included dissections, medical anomalies, general and plastic surgery, rehabilitation, and anatomy.[13] By the 1930s films were used in most medical schools and projection equipment became a crucial part of medical education. The AMA reviewed these films and set up a film loan library.[14] During the war the Army and Navy used films to teach surgery and other medical procedures. This experience created great enthusiasm for, as one physician later noted, "what soldier has not been taught complicated techniques by film and don't they know it."[15]

In fields like pediatrics and physical medicine, where diagnosis and therapy involved the visible physical manipulation of the body, films were particularly successful. During the 1930s the AMA's Council on Physical Therapy (a group of physician specialists) developed a series of films to remind hospital administrators and medical staff of "the importance of physical therapy as an adjunct to the practice of medicine and surgery."[16] At the 1937 AMA annual meeting an exhibit by the American Physiotherapy Association on physical therapy and polio home care included the Kendalls' 1 hour, 5-reel film on the "Examination, Protection, and Treatment of Convalescent Poliomyelitis Cases."[17]

At the annual meetings of medical societies screenings of technical films, usually announcing a new technique and demonstrating its validity and utility, were so popular that they were "clogging the aisles with visitors and interfering with the demonstration of exhibits." In response the AMA arranged for several cinemas to be set up next to the scientific exhibits.[18] At the AMA's annual meeting in 1942 there were 4 theaters adjacent to the exhibits where technical films were shown continuously.[19] The widespread use of commercial medical films designed by pharmaceutical companies, food producers, and other manufacturers led some professional societies to try to ensure that films shown in their scientific exhibits were serious contributions to medical science and not propaganda or advertisement. In January 1943, for example, the New Orleans Graduate Medical Assembly sent participants a printed form that had to be filled out if they were planning to show a film. Speakers were warned that "all movie films, except those previously approved by organized medical societies, must be previewed and approved by the Scientific Exhibits Committee before being shown . . . No exhibits will be accepted which are in any way commercialized."[20]

KENNY AND THE POWER OF FILM

For Kenny film was a powerful and transformative medium, opening eyes and changing minds. Not only could it demonstrate the achievements of her method, but, in her eyes, a technical film was a form of scientific proof, a kind of virtual witnessing equivalent to the experiential persuasion conveyed by in-person demonstrations. In her 1943 autobiography she described an incident in Australia in which she had confronted the physical therapist and doctor who were in charge of a child she had been treating. The doctor was impressed with the "satisfactory" changes in his patient, but the physical therapist was more skeptical. Kenny invited her "to see a moving picture which would give her a complete history of the case. She refused to see the picture, began to weep bitterly, and left the clinic."[21] Here, Kenny felt, was an example of the power of film as clinical evidence, so overwhelming that, without even having been seen, it had stripped a professional of her rational equilibrium.

Film could also bear witness to the damage done by orthodox treatment. John Pohl had shown her a technical film showing patients he had treated during his postgraduate orthopedic training in England and Germany in the 1930s. After he had worked with Kenny and changed his view of polio's therapy and prognosis, Pohl sometimes showed these films as examples "of the unhappy results that had followed the neglect of these symptoms" that Kenny had pointed out to him.[22] It was the same film but presented from a very different point of view.

With her love of films, it is hardly surprising that Kenny was more than receptive to suggestions that her life story might have wider cinematic possibilities. From the time she had arrived in America she had crafted her life's story: a courageous nurse healing children and battling resistant doctors. Versions of this story were retold on radio shows and in magazines, beginning with the 1941 *Reader's Digest* article. Public response hinted at its cinematic potential, and Kenny, who was finishing her first autobiography, was certainly open to the idea.

HOLLYWOOD CALLS

Kenny's direct connection with Hollywood began when Mary Eunice McCarthy, a B-movie screenwriter, read "Sister Kenny vs. Infantile Paralysis" in *Reader's Digest*. McCarthy had worked on comedies such as *Slightly Married* (1932), *Woman Unafraid* (1934), and *Theodora Goes Wild* (1936). She had also been one of the script writers for the controversial medical horror film *Life Returns* (1935). With an eye for a good story, McCarthy took the train from Los Angeles to Minneapolis in early 1942 and sought out Kenny. The 2 women delighted in their shared Irish Catholic background. But it was the possibility that Kenny's story could rival those of other Hollywood scientist-heroes seen in films such as *The Story of Louis Pasteur* (1936) and *Dr. Ehrlich's Magic Bullet* (1940) that most excited both of them. "One can say, without fear of contradiction," McCarthy declared in the screen proposal she sent to studio executives a few months later, "that the persecution [Kenny] endured makes the lives of Pasteur and Dr. E[h]rlich sound like Sunday School picnics."[23]

Although McCarthy depicted Kenny as a reluctant subject who forced McCarthy to "pry the dramatic story of her life out of her," Kenny was neither reluctant nor naïve.[24] By August 1942 Kenny, worried that "a motion picture could be made without my consent," was careful to make sure that the material in her almost completed autobiography would be protected for "I will hold the copyright."[25] Some years later Martha Ostenso discovered that even before she began working with Kenny as coauthor on the autobiography, Kenny had sold the film rights for her manuscript for $50,000.[26] It was clear that Kenny intended to be in charge of the making of her story. She confidently told a friend in Brisbane that "the film story of my life is now in process of preparation," and assured an Australian reporter that Hollywood would film her story.[27] But she eventually found that although she retained the rights to the film's technical aspects she was unable to control the movie's scripts or its presentation of herself and her life.

McCarthy quickly claimed Kenny as an intimate friend, calling her "my beloved Elizabeth," and telling her about her love life.[28] McCarthy understood how Hollywood worked and recognized her own limited power: to make a movie she had to gain the interest of a studio and a star.[29] Her film proposal interested United Artists and then RKO, and she was able to present both the proposal and Kenny herself to Rosalind Russell, a movie star who had raised money for the League of Crippled Children.[30]

The star of comedies such as *His Girl Friday* (1940), Russell was becoming tired of being typecast as a comic career woman and saw the role of Sister Kenny as a way to boost her career.[31] She had received an Academy Award nomination for the comedy *My Sister Eileen* (1942), but felt she needed a leading dramatic role to win an Oscar.[32]

Russell expressed interest in McCarthy's project and welcomed Kenny to Hollywood. Like McCarthy and Kenny, Russell was a Catholic with a sardonic sense of humor; she had once dubbed her local Beverly Hills church "Our Lady of the Cadillacs." She supposedly hounded RKO's new head of production Charles Koerner, who would say "Oh, please, Rosalind, not that story about the nurse," but he finally agreed to "take a chance if you star" and if she would do 2 other films for RKO.[33] Russell recalled the difficulties of attracting a producer, a director, and cast members who "all shrugged me aside." As she remembered it, Kenny "solved this last problem for me. I had her at my home to meet the director and reluctant cast members, and from then on it was smooth sailing."[34]

When Russell first met Kenny she was struck by her dowdy appearance. She looked, Russell thought, "like a[n] M4 tank" with a black dress, a big hat, and a suitcase with a leather strap around it that didn't match. Russell bought her some fashionable clothes and took her to cocktail parties and other Hollywood events.[35] Russell was also worried about Kenny's naivety. (In the early days, Russell noted, Kenny "would talk to anyone.")[36] Russell feared that an association between a movie star and a nurse might threaten Kenny's professional reputation. And indeed there were occasions when she noticed that physicians showed little respect for Kenny. At one California hospital, Russell recalled, after Kenny was shown a patient she turned to the doctor saying, "that's not nice, that's not nice." The child did not have polio but another form of paralysis, and the hospital staff had been trying to trick her. Caught out, the physician in charge "turned red."[37]

Kenny enthusiastically embraced the culture of Hollywood. She and Mary Kenny, who accompanied her on her frequent visits, were fascinated by the stars, the gossip, the fashion; they were, in Mary's words, "two film-struck Aussies."[38] In July 1942, after conferring with screenwriters and conducting clinics in Los Angeles, Kenny flew to Minneapolis wearing white orchids, a gift from Russell.[39] She became a celebrity guest, ready to speak to groups, visit local hospitals, and be introduced to admiring potential donors. During one visit to Los Angeles Kenny and Mary were photographed with Cary Grant who, a friend kidded Kenny, seemed to be "more interested in Mary than you."[40] By December 1942, at the dedication of her new Institute, Kenny was already boasting to NFIP officials about a Hollywood film of her life as she accepted flowers from McCarthy and Russell and a "very beautiful garland of red roses" from RKO Studios.[41]

Kenny made much of Russell's character, praising her as "not only a fine person, but a fine actress." In a slightly joking way she pointed to Russell's Catholicism in comparison to the typical immorality of Hollywood stars, telling reporters that she approved of Russell "because she hasn't been divorced, for one thing."[42] Russell, in turn, was impressed with Kenny's work, and her faith in Kenny's healing powers truly solidified when Kenny identified a "spastic" leg muscle in Russell's 10-month-old son Lance. Kenny admitted the boy to the Institute under a false name, and he recovered after 2 months.[43] When the film was finally shot, Russell sought to protect Kenny from the less attractive mechanics of movie production. She insisted that the makeup and prosthetics that she used to make her look like Kenny—including "things on my legs to make them fatter"—had to be removed when Kenny came to visit the set.[44]

But Kenny's frequent appearance at Hollywood events also had a down side. Her growing celebrity status threatened to contradict her efforts to gain respect as a medical innovator. A true scientific discoverer was supposed to be suspicious of Hollywood's glamorous, scandal-ridden culture. She began to remind journalists of the distance between herself and others who sought personal fame and wealth. Hers was a life, she claimed, of courage and sacrifice, befitting a great humanitarian. In a confusing characterization, a reporter for the *Los Angeles Examiner* praised "her lack of pretentiousness" as "beguiling," but also noted that when Kenny was asked to pose for a close-up "she tilted her nose in the air at an angle all her own and told the astonished camera-man, 'This is my Hollywood profile; I always save it for best!' "[45]

A scientific hero was also unworldly in matters of money. Kenny frequently told reporters she received no salary and devoted her life to patient care; and her autobiography, as one commentator noted, offered a "highly romantic and dramatic picture of a lowly life of sacrifice."[46] In McCarthy's sentimentalized screen proposal, Kenny had never received "a single cent for all the magnificent work she was doing. Moreover, she had beggared herself through the years by donating her own money for the care of countless children."[47] While reporters commented on the large payment Kenny had received from RKO for the rights to her autobiography, they usually added that it had been all donated to her Institute, or, in one account, put in trust for her 17 nephews who were all in the Australian air force.[48] But the argument that Kenny did not care for wealth or its trappings was contradicted by her frequent sojourns at the Waldorf-Astoria and other fancy hotels. Such benefits, of course, could be explained away as expressions of gratitude from the friends and families of her patients.[49] Those who knew Kenny well, though, remained skeptical about her claims of sacrifice. When her former Brisbane secretary saw her dressed in a stylish black dress with pearls and white diamonds, talking about how she had "never charged a fee," she was contemptuous. "That lying old bugger," the secretary commented to one of Kenny's Brisbane allies, "did you see all those pearls and all those diamonds?"[50]

MAKING THE MOVIE

Kenny had hoped that with the proper guidance, the Hollywood film would simultaneously entertain and educate the public about the Kenny method. "This picture will have the rare combination of wit and pathos," Kenny wrote McCarthy, "and also a message of healing which has not yet been combined in anything in the film world that I know of."[51] Her contract specified that she would supervise all the technical parts of the movie and she believed that its portrayal of her method would be accurate enough to guide parents of paralyzed children "in case of emergency."[52] But to her disappointment the movie took on a life of its own. Like her autobiography, it dramatized her life's story from her earliest days in Australia to her arrival in the United States, but it also fit carefully into what studio executives felt would make a commercial product and skirted the politically sensitive chapters about her efforts to convert American doctors. The final script presented a romanticized depiction of Kenny's life and work, and a message of hope at a time when Americans lived under the specter of epidemic polio.

The movie Sister Kenny took 4 years to make. Like all Hollywood films, it did not spring full-grown from the head of a single screenwriter, producer, or studio executive. Its construction was a process of negotiation. RKO did not consider this property especially valuable: crippled children and a middle-aged nurse did not sound like the stuff of a Hollywood hit. Although polio was not a socially unacceptable disease like syphilis, putting the disabled on screen could make a film seem too close to an RKO horror film or a medical teaching film.[53] RKO executives complained to McCarthy that there were "entirely too many scenes...dealing with the Kenny method," and other advisors told her that "it would be nothing but a dull and rather clinical portrayal of hospitals, etc."[54]

Portraying a nurse-clinician as a scientific discoverer was awkward. It was not easy to translate the firmly masculinized image of Louis Pasteur and Thomas Edison into a woman's life. The story of discovery was almost always popularized as a man's achievement. MGM's successful drama Madame Curie (1943) was a rare exception and showed that as long as the discovery could be combined with a love story, scientific research could be claimed on occasion as a woman's sphere. But Kenny's story went even further. Kenny was surrounded not by laboratory equipment, but by patients and technicians in long veils. She didn't even look like a scientist; she looked like a nurse.

Russell's interest in the project also seemed to wane as the development of the script limped on, and her time was taken up by other movie commitments. In early 1944 she also took a lengthy break to recuperate after the birth of her son.[55] Gossip columnist Hedda Hopper, a powerful force in Hollywood, chided her for neglecting a project that "may save thousands of little children from being crippled for life."[56] The "collapse" of the movie became part of a wider public sense of conspiracy: that somehow the NFIP and the AMA were scheming to defeat Kenny in Hollywood as well.[57] Kenny expressed her frustration privately, telling McCarthy that "every father's and mother's heart in America shall be saddened when they know that some frivolous picture has superseded the one with a great message."[58] But she had underestimated the power of Hollywood rumor and was horrified when some of her remarks appeared in the California press. Fearing that they might cause both RKO and Russell to back away from the project, she sent a telegram to Hopper defending Russell, arguing that Hopper had been "very much misinformed with regard to Rosalind Russell's attitude toward the picture." Russell, Kenny wrote, "has promoted my work ten times more than [any] other individual in America," and the text of her telegram was repeated in print.[59]

The project also had trouble attracting a good director. Dudley Nichols, a respected screenwriter who was interested in directing, was RKO's final choice. Nichols had worked with John Ford on *The Informer* (RKO 1935)—for which he had won an Academy Award—and *Stagecoach* (United Artists 1939). He had also written popular comedies like *Bringing up Baby* (RKO 1938) and was working with Bing Crosby on *The Bells of St Mary's* (RKO 1945). Nichols' involvement in the movie was another conversion story: a skeptical Hollywood professional committed only after visiting the Institute and seeing Kenny at work. French director Jean Renoir recalled that he traveled to Minneapolis with Nichols and watched a meeting of Kenny and many doctors as "questions were rained on her, and she answered them with great spirit." She ended her demonstration by showing photographs of the limbs of a boy projected on a screen and asking her audience if it would be possible for him to be cured. After everyone had replied that it was impossible, the door opened and a hefty young man appeared, saying he had been the sick boy and was now a truck driver.[60] In a less publicized, more pragmatic bargain, Nichols agreed to direct and produce *Sister Kenny* if Russell would star in his next big project, a screen version of Eugene O'Neill's "Mourning Becomes Electra."[61] Nichols was credited in the film as producer, director, and as one of its screenwriters.[62] Although he later praised her distinctive clinical insights as the sign of an "isolated genius," Nichols disliked seeing Kenny on his set and paid little attention to her suggestions about the script.[63]

DESIGNING THE SCRIPT

As Nichols took over, he discarded McCarthy's original scripts, and RKO brought in Milton L. Gunzburg, a more experienced screenwriter.[64] He and McCarthy began to try to design a story of a woman in white whose life, while focused on healing crippled children, also included love and romance.

McCarthy's original proposal had framed the story as "a stirring saga of a fighter who battled against odds... [with] complete unselfishness." Gunzburg disagreed, telling her, "Baby, *this is a love story*! Rich, full and warm!"[65] Kenny's autobiography had spent only a few pages on the story of Dan, a local farmer, but McCarthy's and Gunzburg's scripts made a romance between Kenny and a local rancher (named Dan, then Larry, and then

Kevin) more central. "Personally, I think there is too much Dan Cunningham and, I may also say, rapturous kissing which is not Elizabeth Kenny," Kenny complained after reading one draft.[66]

But the love interest stayed, and Kenny's attitude to the film's emphasis on a love story vacillated between a proper disdain and a willingness to be seen as a woman with a passionate, romantic past. She told a friend in Brisbane that Hollywood studios were not interested in making a movie without "a love affair."[67] On one of her rare visits to the RKO set, they were filming the scene where the rancher surprises her character in the pantry and then a plate drops from behind the pantry door. Kenny, supposedly shocked, said "I wasn't that kind of a girl."[68] When an Australian friend asked her about that scene with the remark "Gee, Sister, that must have been a beaut clinch," Kenny replied that she was "very annoyed with the film people for putting it in."[69] On the other hand, during the final shooting in November 1945, Kenny sent the director a copy of a cable she had received from the lawyers of a man who had just died, with a message for her: "Here in the silent hills you loved so well I wait for thee."[70] Russell was convinced that Kenny had had a secret romantic life. McCarthy, on the other hand, told a reporter after Kenny's death that Kenny had said to her, "Oh, I never wanted to bother with any man."[71] Kenny's resistance to the portrayal of the love story may have also reflected her abhorrence of rumors that Mary Kenny was her illegitimate daughter. During the filming of Sister Kenny she asked Charles Chuter to send copies of Mary's birth certificate and adoption papers to counter this rumor.[72]

McCarthy's and Gunzburg's depiction of Kenny drew on both the feisty independent professional woman typical of 1930s Hollywood films that had made Katharine Hepburn and Rosalind Russell famous, and presaged the harsher stories of women in later films such as Mildred Pierce (1945). Although both knew Mary Kenny as Kenny's ward and one of her most accomplished technicians, neither McCarthy nor Gunzburg considered adding her character to the script. The writers tempered Kenny's fierce devotion to her cause with a sympathetic femininity. In McCarthy's original proposal Kenny, forced by a medical emergency to break a date with her fiancé, rides her horse "still wearing her evening gown with its beautiful long white satin train."[73] In typical Hollywood fashion Kenny's character is forced to choose between professional success and personal happiness. Throughout the film her fiancé returns, eager to marry her, only to be put off as Kenny copes with one epidemic after another. Finally, although he protests "I'm not going to let you throw yourself away on this work any longer," she chooses helping the world's children over having her own.

The scriptwriters were aware that the story's drama needed to be balanced with moments of humor, a point John Pohl also made in 1944 after reading a version of the script.[74] Gunzburg had considered depicting Kenny as an Australian naïf, urging McCarthy to consider that "the mere thought of Kenny in Manhattan offers comedy situations...hamburgers, automats."[75] Pohl suggested dramatizing Kenny's initial work at the Minneapolis General Hospital "showing you trying to demonstrate patients upon the stairway landing between two elevators...with the elevator unloading laundry, food carts, etc. and nurses and interns coming and going up and down stairs through your demonstration." Pohl also proposed adding an episode whereby Kenny loses the special hat she has bought to meet the Queen of England out of a train window in Australia, and then finds it later on the head of an Aboriginal woman.[76] In a later version of the script,

Queensland doctors mistakenly test Kevin for evidence of polio while he protests "Miss Kenny knows there's nothing wrong with me."[77] None of these episodes was used in the film, but there is a gentle comedy around a busy doctor mistaking Kevin for a patient he has no time to examine.

Questions about Kenny's nursing qualifications, the screenwriters recognized, were also being raised and, unusual for a nurse's autobiography, *And They Shall Walk* had said little about her training.[78] The writers sought to resolve this issue unambiguously. The film opened with Kenny arriving home in her new nurse's cap and cape after graduating from an unnamed school. She continues to wear a version of a white nurse's uniform, when she is an army nurse and then in her practice afterward. To reinforce the idea that officials regarded her as a reputable professional, the film also suggests that Kenny was supported and sanctioned by the government. Kenny is shown receiving a letter from members of the London City Council who "want you in England," and later has a request from the Australian government that sends a government plane.

But the film writers did not want to portray Kenny as too professional. Early- and mid-twentieth century nursing leaders promoted nursing to the public as an altruistic vocation rather than a career offering professional satisfaction. Thus, her physician-mentor tells her "you're a born nurse" and is frustrated when she turns down his offer of a hospital position to work as a bush nurse. In the film local rural families give her a black horse in gratitude for her 3 years of work with them because "you won't take a penny for what you've done."

A Hollywood nurse was usually a clever supportive assistant whose innocent insight aids the more brilliant male scientist or doctor. The most successful part of the screenwriters' efforts to balance Kenny as a nurse and humane crusader were showing her in relation to dismissive physicians. She never strays far from the path of the good nurse, is soft-spoken with patients, and defiant but not disrespectful with doctors. When she is faced with her first patient with polio, for example, her professionalism is shown by her ability to ignore the girl's constant crying and not do anything until she hears back from her physician-mentor by telegram. As she develops her own theory of polio and begins presenting it to disbelieving doctors, she is sometimes clearly frustrated by their rudeness, but she is never openly angry.

Unlike Kenny's experience in Australia and America the film showed no adult patients or male therapists. The gender relations in the film are stark: all the nurses and technicians are women, all the doctors are men, and all the patients are children. During the 1930s a few films (*The White Angel*, Warner Brothers, 1936 and *Nurse Edith Cavell*, RKO, 1939) had gone beyond the "nurse-handmaiden" approach, but not many. During the war, stoic and courageous nurses were becoming familiar characters, central to movies such as *Cry 'Havoc'* (MGM, 1943) and *So Proudly We Hail* (Paramount, 1943). Perhaps these movies and the recent success of MGM's *Madame Curie* (1943) explained RKO's willingness to stretch the conventions of commercial film storytelling and allow Kenny to be portrayed both as a healing nurse and a scientific innovator, challenging physicians to accept her concept of the disease. Both movies ended with a cautious feminist message: women scientists can achieve great things, but at a great cost.[79]

And then the screen writers had to deal with the question of how to depict the medical establishment. Gunzburg had at first wanted to dramatize an episode from Kenny's autobiography in which a medical antagonist steals her manuscript and tries to publish it under his own name. To balance this picture of a bad doctor, Gunzburg was willing to portray Kenny as angry, explaining to McCarthy: "in justice to the medical profession, as well as to the humanization of Kenny, we have established that her temper was responsible for some of the misunderstandings and prejudices against her."[80] But the plagiarist did not appear in the film and neither did the anger.

In the film the dichotomy between medical right and wrong is exemplified by the 2 central male physicians. Aeneas McDonnell, Kenny's mentor and the "good" doctor, is the rural general practitioner and a man of the people. He has an old-fashioned unpretentious office, the final script suggested, unlike his medical opponent's office that "is large and very modern, full of scientific paraphernalia and new books."[81] In the words of one reviewer, he "speaks with a fine, thick Scotch burr and looks on Miss Russell as the greatest thing in medicine since Pasteur."[82] The "bad" doctor and Kenny's main antagonist is contemptuous Brisbane orthopedic specialist Dr. Brack. He is presented as elitist, rational, and inflexible. In the film's most memorable scene, based on an episode in Kenny's autobiography, Kenny confronts Brack while he is lecturing on the virtues of splinting to a group of nurses and doctors seated in a Brisbane hospital amphitheater. Kenny, simmering with frustration, interrupts him, asking why he refuses to meet with her and why he has colluded with the city health authorities to close her clinic. Brack invites her to speak to his audience. Although he tells Kenny that "as open-minded men of science we do not reject ideas without examination," he dismisses her, saying her words "are not scientific terms." Kenny replies that "the words I use describe the things I see." When Brack asks her why doctors do not see them, she says "because you've got a book in front of your eyes" and turns to Brack's audience to remind them that "medical ideas change: your fathers bled their patients." Throughout the scene a patient lies at the center, fully encased in splints, and when Brack warns Kenny not to debate "in front of the patient," Kenny retorts "it's his life, not yours or mine."

In another scene, the 2 doctors debate Kenny's work by arguing about the evidence of books versus bodies. "Are we to take her word or Sir Robert Jenkins?" Brack asks McDonnell, who retorts "you only recognize a fact when it's printed in a book." Brack berates McDonnell for encouraging "a nurse to contradict the greatest medical authorities in the world." McDonnell replies "If she'd been a doctor, she'd have followed the orthodox treatment. She wouldn't have done the things she did, she wouldn't have dared." In the final script Gunzburg suggested that Brack ask McDonnell "do you often get these mad ideas about fake cures brought in by untrained people?"[83] But in the film Brack does not say that Kenny is "untrained." In one of the film's few references to Kenny's claim that she had identified a new disease, Brack comments: "If her ideas were correct she'd have discovered not a new treatment, but an entirely new disease." McDonnell replies, "Well, I don't mind her discovering a new disease so long as she can cure it."[84] To explain his refusal to try her methods, Brack declares dramatically that "I will not experiment with the lives of children! . . . Guinea pigs, yes—children no." His ethical qualms are presented seriously, and McDonnell says later with reluctant admiration: "He's a brilliant man, he's absolutely sincere. In his mind he's defending the rights of children."

Near the end of the film Brack attacks Kenny, saying that "instead of aiding physicians you have the arrogance to try to teach [them] . . . in the opinion of many doctors you are no longer a nurse." Kenny's self-sacrifice and nursely behavior, shown by many examples before this, is intended to refute any such accusation, and she responds with quiet defiance, "I have given up too much to wear this nurse's uniform."

The film's ending reinforces the idea of Kenny's sacrifice. As the AMA committee's critical report plays over the loudspeaker of a lecture room Kenny bravely continues to give a lecture to orthopedic surgeons. She returns to her office at the Institute, lonely and unhappy, having learned of McDonnell's death and now another medical committee's rejection. As she walks to the Institute's front gates a flock of happy children (former patients) come running to greet her singing "Happy Birthday." They are all healthy children walking without crutches or wheelchairs, but it is a poignant scene, hardly a sign of uplifting success.[85]

Pohl felt that the scene showed that "the happiness and well bodies of children are of more importance than rebuffs from the medical profession," but he did "not like to see Sister Kenny as a bitterly disappointed woman without a future."[86] Kenny agreed—this was not the ending she had imagined. She urged Nichols to use a scene based on one he himself had witnessed at the Institute where "doctors stood on chairs and tables to watch me correct a deformity." The film, she suggested, could offer "a grand climax" such as when an orthopedic surgeon told the group of physicians that "the deformity had been corrected and function restored and said 'Gentlemen, that is the answer to the accusations.'"[87]

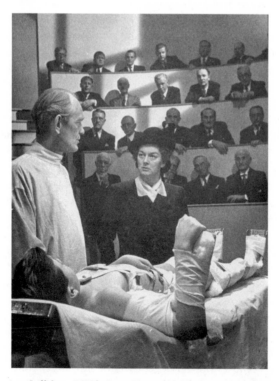

FIGURE 6.1 Still from RKO's *Sister Kenny* (1946) showing Philip Merivale as orthopedist Dr. Brack debating with Rosalind Russell as Kenny in a Brisbane amphitheatre. Courtesy of Time & Life Pictures/Getty Images.

In August 1946, after Kenny learned that the ending remained the same, she sent a telegram to RKO protesting that as it conveyed "a message of defeat," RKO should "not release the picture" without a more positive ending, "otherwise it would not be my life."[88] By this time, however, the upcoming Kenny Foundation (KF) fundraising campaign was using footage of the film and claiming (inaccurately) that all the child actors except for Doreen McCann were "cured patients from the Kenny Institute."[89] More importantly, Kenny had staked her professional career on it. It was not easy to admit that she had lost creative control. A day later she sent another telegram presenting her change of heart as the result of speaking to calmer heads. Both Russell and Valerie Harvey, one of her technicians who was working as an advisor on the Hollywood set, Kenny explained, had disagreed with her assessment. She was "willing to take their verdict [that]... the ending of the film was satisfactory."[90]

The KF campaign and Kenny's own extensive fundraising also made her earlier harsh depiction of elite women seem inappropriate. McCarthy and Gunzburg had planned to dramatize one of the few class conflicts in Kenny's autobiography through the figure of Lady Latham, described by McCarthy as a parody of a female British aristocrat with "three chins, a lorgnette and a nose perpetually pointed upward in disapproval." [91] In one script version McCarthy made Latham a trustee of the Toowoomba Nurses Home, where Kenny is finishing her training. "Elizabeth Kenny may be a good nurse, but she must be taught to keep her place," Latham announces; her off-duty clothes are "too frivolous" and "beyond her station in life." "No good Australian has any patience with that 'station in life' nonsense," young Kenny retorts. "We nurses resent people who give money to hospitals just for their own personal glory and amusement. Laymen should consider it a privilege to give such checks, but, after giving them, they should go away quickly and permit experts to run the affairs of the sick."[92] Gunzburg at first liked this character, adding "this was not to be the first nor the last society woman to become peeved when Kenny refused to permit them to bask in the sunshine of her career at [the] expense of her treatment."[93] But as wealthy women like Latham loomed larger in Kenny's fundraising, the character was dropped. One of the few references to the financing of medical care comes when Kenny learns that a donation from Kevin was paying for 10 beds at the Toowoomba Hospital.

Kenny's claim to have contributed to polio science was also avoided. The film offers a safely domesticated story of scientific discovery. Kenny's understanding of polio comes from her heart and from her clinical experience. Kenny succeeds in healing a paralyzed child because she does not understand polio and is thus free from the constraints of any orthodox medical knowledge. Her hands, her knowledge of sick bodies, and her ability to use tools of the domestic environment such as strips of blanket and hot water build on her "natural" understanding of healing. In McCarthy's words, she succeeds "using nothing but her shrewd eyes and her common sense, plus her great knowledge of the muscular system."[94] In the bush cabin where she meets her first patient, she directs the girl's parents to tear up blankets, pour boiling water over them, and twist them so that every drop comes out. After treating the pain and spasm she and the parents realize that the girl's legs still cannot move. The mother cries, but Kenny in cape and long-sleeved white uniform keeps her emotions under control. She tells the child she is "going to have to teach them [her legs] how to walk." She gently moves a leg and, when she notices a tendon react, she tells the child calmly "your leg just told me something."

The film makers, perhaps pressured by RKO, stayed away from the direct portrayal of groups of "deformed" children. In the film Kenny and her mentor examine a textbook by "Sir Robert Jenkins," which is identified as Brack's "bible," and note the similarities between its images and some of the patients she has recently treated. One of the scripts proposed a close-up of a plate from the Jenkins book "showing us a typical posture in the acute stage," but the film does not show any such images.[95] In fact, other than a scene of a ward of children in splints and braces, there are very few groups of severely disabled children. In the final script this ward was described as "full of horribly crippled children, in wheel-chairs, braces, walking cages, etc." but the camera avoids any close ups and there are no wheelchairs or walking cages.[96] Brack doubts Kenny's evidence that her method works and dismisses her first healed patient, saying "this child never had infantile paralysis... the symptoms were not accurately observed." He suggests that Kenny "stick to nursing and not meddle with orthopedic medicine. It's a complicated subject which is difficult enough for those who have spent a lifetime studying it." Meanwhile, the film lingers on Dorrie, one of Kenny's patients (child actor Doreen McCann), turning cartwheels while Brack's own patient David, a small boy in braces and crutches, whom Brack proudly shows as an example of orthodox success, watches morosely. This image is interpreted with horror by Kenny who ends the scene saying quietly "I will never forget David."

By 1945 Kenny had constructed a story of her life that downplayed the role that the NFIP had played in her career. She reminded Nichols that O'Connor was not responsible for the introduction of her work to America; rather, that a group of Australian doctors had arranged for her to arrive "as an official visitor... with a definite statement that I had made a brilliant contribution to medicine." In fact, O'Connor "told me to go home."[97] Russell believed that the movie script had been sent to the NFIP for approval, but O'Connor later assured a reporter that he had stayed away from "the movie." While Fishbein's role as a movie censor has been well documented for other scripts, his role here is unknown.[98] In any case, although Kenny's 1943 autobiography had dwelt for some chapters on her struggles to convert American physicians, the filmmakers avoided mentioning either O'Connor or the NFIP and depicted very few of Kenny's experiences in the United States, omissions that must have seemed strange to American audiences when the movie came out in 1946.

Despite these omissions and the script's many additions to Kenny's history, the film was promoted as a "true" story. RKO publicity claimed that Russell's depiction of Kenny herself was accurate. The studio told reporters that Russell was doing an intensive course in the Kenny method, and had "the nurse's magic hand motions down pat."[99] Mary Kenny recalled that Russell, a great mimic, was able to copy Kenny's own accent perfectly. But after Kenny protested that she did not "sound like that," Russell used a bland English accent instead.[100] The movie's appearance of cinematic documentary was reinforced by old-fashioned clothes and backdrops. A newspaper reported that the Toowoomba hospital, where a member of the merchant marine had been treated during the war, was being copied by the same man, who was now a set dresser at RKO.[101]

Convinced that accuracy was important, Kenny warned Nichols that the script had a "few little things that will annoy Australians exceedingly." A story about a bull added to dramatize the founding of the Sylvia stretcher would lead to "a lot of criticism" and "give the whole picture a phony atmosphere." Her clinic in Brisbane also had not been in "an old dilapidated building" but one that was "wonderfully renovated and beautifully

equipped."[102] Chuter was asked to assess scripts for their accuracy and in 1945 the managing director of RKO in Sydney thanked him for cooperating "in the research that we have
been required to carry out by our Studio in the interests of authenticity."[103] Chuter also
dispelled what he considered to be misapprehensions about Kenny's main antagonist.
To some who had seen the script, Brack suggested orthopedist Harold Crawford, whom
Kenny had named in her autobiography. But Chuter was sure that Brack was meant to
be Sir Raphael Cilento. "No one will waste any sympathy on this person," Chuter assured
an RKO official; "he has been Sister Kenny's most implacable enemy, and really deserves
all opprobrium which can be heaped upon him."[104] Two years later, Chuter was able to
use his authority to counter protests about the content of the film. In 1947, just before
the film's premiere in Australia, Queensland's state censor threatened to cut a dramatic
scene between Kenny and Brack, claiming it was not "authentic." Chuter prevented this,
arguing: "This scene is, in my opinion, the great scene in the picture. It focuses and crys-
tallizes the issue fought over many years and in many Countries. The brave nurse forces
her way into the teaching citadel and fights out the issue. Dr. Brack portrays the concept
[and] attitude of traditional medicine admirably and accurately."[105]

In promotions for the film RKO was able to highlight the danger of polio, the hope
of Kenny's work as a cure, and the allure of romance. A full page advertisement in *Life*
featured Kenny, Dorrie, and her parents inside a bush cabin, while the text referred to
the darker side of polio: "it might strike in far away Toowoomba—or hit next door."[106] In
a letter from Rosalind Russell to Kenny ally James Henry that was intended to be published in the local paper, she described the previews of the film to "bobbysoxers" in San
Francisco, shipyard workers in Oakland, "high type[s]" in Burlingame, Mexicans in Indio,
and a mixed group in downtown Los Angeles. Every group, she said, "pull for Kenny like
mad ... [and are] ONLY interested in the polio part of the story. That amazed us so that the
love story will be cut quite a bit. It still runs through the picture, but the polio part of the
story predominates and you can hear a pin drop during the medical portion of the film."[107]

But it was the love story that appeared in most advertisements. Another advertisement in *Life* feted "the drama of a desirable woman who turned her back on all that *most*
women hold dear—love, family, home—to write in glorious deeds one of the most thrilling chapters in all human history."[108] In one poster Russell stood in a bridal gown (never
shown in the film) under the heading "The wedding gown that waited" with the caption
"Tucked away in a cedar chest for half a lifetime by a courageous nurse who wanted desper-
ately to wear it ... but wanted even more to help children walk again."[109] An advertisement
in *Colliers* referred to "one of the greatest love stories ever screened."[110] In another poster
Russell faced Brack with the words "She won FAME ... but lost LOVE!"[111] For a Hollywood
woman to succeed in the world of medical science she had to sacrifice everything else.

One casualty of the filmmaking process was Kenny's friendship with McCarthy. As
McCarthy's original scripts were discarded, she began to worry that she would lose credit
for her work. But when she tried to have Kenny defend her, she found that Kenny was
no longer her champion. Friends later speculated that the end of their friendship was the
result of Kenny's discovering that McCarthy was a lesbian. But Kenny already knew this
and had even offered advice to McCarthy over a break-up.[112] In fact the break was caused
by Kenny's assessment of movie politics. As she learned that the studio did not like
McCarthy's scripts, she distanced herself from the writer. While Kenny recognized that
for McCarthy receiving screen credit "would mean a lot for her future financial status," in

her view the script was based partly on McCarthy's first script and partly on Kenny's own autobiography with "a dash of *The Kenny Concept* book."[113] "Mary rather amuses me with her protestations of a great friendship," Kenny commented to Nichols, yet "the first time anything occurs to interfere with what she considers her financial position the friendship takes a very secondary position." Mary had "many good qualities," Kenny added, but she needed to "cultivate them and try to obliterate her bitterness and mischief making propensities."[114] McCarthy sent Kenny and her Minneapolis friend James Henry an angry telegram, threatening to spread scandal about Russell, but Kenny "threw it in the waste basket."[115] After Nichols agreed to give McCarthy screen credit as co-writer in August 1944, Kenny urged her to "forget that the picture ever existed." Kenny thanked her for her friendship, but declared that she had "no time to waste on Hollywood jealousies," and added "for the sake of my own peace of mind which affects my work, I respectfully request that all further associations and bickering shall cease."[116]

THE TECHNICAL FILM

In 1944, as the Hollywood machinery slowly ground on, Kenny decided to replace her short silent films with a longer sound film to be produced by Ray-Bell Films, a St. Paul production company. She financed *The Kenny Concept of the Disease Infantile Paralysis* by selling some of her property in Queensland, and with donations from local businessmen and Rosalind Russell.[117] At one dinner, Russell later recalled, Kenny was going "on & on" about what the Hollywood movie had to include. Frederick Brisson finally said Kenny must realize his wife could not make an "honest" picture but an "entertaining and commercial" picture. If Kenny wanted to make a documentary film, she needed to recognize that was not what Hollywood did. That, Russell claimed later, was "how I happened to pay for the [technical] film."[118]

Initially, Kenny saw this film as a supplement to the Hollywood movie. It would "contain material the lay people would not understand or appreciate."[119] But the Hollywood movie was taking years longer to make than she had anticipated, so the technical film had to stand on its own. The film was part of Kenny's effort to control the meaning and significance of her work. It was intended to dramatize her theory of polio, using the camera to point to what the viewer should be seeing while her voice as narrator told the viewer what the scene meant.

Her allies in Minneapolis assumed that it would be a teaching film but Kenny initially resisted this, saying she did not "expect to include anything about treatment in the film." Instead it was intended to provide evidence "to the world of science" so that scientists could explore her ideas "further," a task that seemed even more urgent after the critical AMA report in June 1944.[120] But she soon recognized that if the film were to "explain to the Orthopedists of the world how to keep the body straight when affected by this disease," it would need to have a teaching component. She therefore produced 2 reels: *The Kenny Concept of the Disease Infantile Paralysis* and *Second Phase of the Kenny Treatment*. The second reel provided practical information about the making and applying of hot packs and demonstrated specific muscle exercises that would help "to stimulate the muscles from their focal point," but she usually showed both under the title *The Kenny Concept*.[121] Kenny noted that the film was the result of a direct request from medical officers of the Army and Navy, who had come to the Mayo Clinic for postgradu-ate study in physical medicine and had traveled to Minneapolis to attend a course at the Institute. They had told her, Kenny claimed, that "it was impossible for them to absorb (as they explained it) one or both of my presentations in the short space of one week, and advised me to make a documentary film explaining the revolutionary concept and presenting result[s] of my clinical research."[122] This gave her film, produced during the war, the approval of both physicians and the military.

In September 1944, during the NRC committee visit, Kenny invited the committee to see an early version of this new film.[123] In their subsequent report the NRC committee members praised the film as "persuasive and interesting, especially with regard to results accomplished by muscle reeducation." But they criticized its style as "spectacular and definitely of a propaganda nature" and found fault with its use of unscientific-sounding statements such as "the muscle is host to the virus."[124] Nonetheless, the committee recog-nized the potential power of Kenny's film for both medical and lay audiences and urged the NFIP to make a "series of teaching films for the professions on the care of individuals with poliomyelitis, including the Kenny method."[125] NFIP officials did not initially fol-low this recommendation and continued to rely on films produced by other professional groups. Then in 1945 the NFIP produced *Your Fight Against Infantile Paralysis* for the pub-lic and later *Accent on Use* for physical therapists.[126]

In October 1944 Kenny organized what she called a "world premiere" for a Twin Cities audience of local physicians, clergy, members of social and civic organizations, and medi-cal and science university faculty. The audience, estimated at 700, gave Kenny a standing ovation, and she was presented with several gifts of flowers during a reception in the the-ater's lounge. To reporters unable to attend, Institute board member Henry Haverstock described the film's "graphic scenes" and its story of "the progress of patients from the time they entered the Institute as cripples to the day they were released as normal, active individuals." Although it was "technical in nature," Haverstock believed "the film never-theless carries a powerful emotional appeal."[127] Kenny then took her film on a tour that included Washington, D.C. and several towns in Illinois and Ontario.[128]

THE KENNY CONCEPT

Kenny was convinced that the power of her film was its first reel, which would enable doctors and other professionals to hear her explain how and why her techniques worked, and thereby recognize the truth of her concept of the disease. "Many statements have been made concerning this work," she warned, "by those who have preferred to view it from afar."[129] Thus, in an early scene, *The Kenny Concept* brought the viewer directly into the wards of the Institute to watch a "well trained" Kenny technician in a white gown and mask who was "familiar with the newer knowledge of the classification and typing of the muscular system" treat a patient with hot packs.[130] She was also proud of her film's narra-tive arc. It showed patients whose "severe pain is overcome in three days," and then after their "deformities" were "combated" the full function of their muscles was "restored" in 2 months. The patients then waved "goodbye to all treatment and hospitalization and walk out," after a period of treatment that "prior to my visit to the United States" would not even have begun.[131]

The Kenny Concept was structured around 2 sites: patients at the Institute—before, during, and after therapy—and Kenny in her office, seated at a desk like a kind of senior stateswoman, reading from her lectures to explain what the viewer had seen and why it was important. Despite the film's portrayal of Kenny as Institute director, Kenny reminded her audience that as a nurse she had not breached professional conventions, for all of her patients were examined in the presence of "medical men" who were members of the AMA.[132]

The patients (but not the therapists shown on screen) were named and personalized: Patsy, Allen, Robert, Rosemary, Colleen, Bobby, Vernon, Jack, Wally, and Virgil. And, viewers were assured, they were all real people, not actors.[133] It is not quite clear how Kenny distinguished between acting and demonstrating, for she later sent each patient $50 for their participation in the film. "I am always only too happy to help you in any way in your lectures and clinics by being there if you need me," one recipient replied, "because some doctors really do have to be shown."[134]

Kenny was usually careful not to identify the patients with a surname, but she did boast to a group of university officials that after meeting a young man called Jack MacArthur and finding out that he was related to General Douglas MacArthur, "I felt it absolutely incumbent upon me to try do something for him." In her film MacArthur's body was used to dramatize the harmful effects of orthodox polio care. He is first seen lying on a table while Kenny explains that "this patient did not receive treatment by the newer science." To show "the devastating effect of peripheral involvement" (the term she used to imply viral infection in places outside the brain and spinal cord) MacArthur, flanked by Kenny and a nurse in white, tries to sit up. Then he is shown as completely recovered after 2 months of treatment for "peripheral damage."[135]

Kenny saw this transformation as testimony not only to her method but also to her theory. She believed that the patients in the film, like her other patients at the Institute and around the country, were "clinical proof" demonstrating "that the concept of this disease infantile paralysis presented by me as the result of my research is correct."[136] For Kenny the film provided visual confirmation of her ideas, democratically available to anyone who watched the film. "Dr. Fishbein and anyone else may see living proof of the value of the newer science of dermo-neuro-muscular therapy introduced by me for the newer concept discovered by me," she told one reporter. "This proof can be produced anywhere at any time in the documentary films."[137] To bring home the lessons of the film she wrote *A Brief Description of the Film Presenting The Kenny Concept*, a pamphlet intended to be handed out to audiences, reiterating that the film provided "indisputable evidence directly contradicting the theories upon which all previous treatment had been based."[138] As further evidence of a serious engagement with medical science, the film reproduced photographs of patients featured in Robert Lovett's *Treatment of Infantile Paralysis* in order to show the poor results of orthodox care.

Kenny's theory that the polio virus attacked muscles more often than the nervous system was difficult to prove by showing only the body's clinical appearance. The American public was used to seeing cinematic dramatizations of germs as well as men in white coats and test tubes in laboratories. *The Kenny Concept* used bodies to talk about the polio virus. As the camera focuses onto Virgil's back, the narrator explains that "the virus evidently found a host in the spinal muscles alienating the abdominals."[139] (It was this kind of statement that had annoyed the NRC committee visitors.) But it was difficult to demonstrate that what the viewer saw was actually the picture of a virus in the muscles.

Alienation was also difficult to demonstrate. In the case of Colleen, Kenny's voice explains, "the quads are stretched and the hamstrings are stimulated in order to bring about subconscious contraction and preserve the pattern of movement in the cerebrum." But while stretching and stimulating could be shown on film, the other comments were simply words, as was the narrator's statement, "We are now ready to overcome condition of alienation of the quadriceps...by relaxing and contracting, the subconscious mind is reached, then it is necessary to get the brain power back to the point of attachment."[140] Such phrases and terms made sense only to a fully trained Kenny technician or perhaps to a professional who had attended one of Kenny's courses. For most audiences, these were serious-sounding words indicating the wisdom and skills of a polio expert, but neither they nor the images that accompanied them explained or proved the validity of Kenny's concepts.

In Kenny's staged lecture in the film she compares the comments of her medical critics to the evidence her audience has just seen. She quotes O'Connor admitting in August 1944 that the results of NFIP-funded researchers "had been negative." She tries to denigrate orthodox treatment without demonizing its practitioners, saying "in this film you have seen fettered muscles crippling their victims even with the best and most conscientious treatment."[141] But her pamphlet attacked polio care more harshly, warning of the dangers of any modification of the Kenny method: "all investigators, whether antagonist or kindly disposed, have admitted that deformities have been eliminated in all patients receiving the unadulterated Kenny treatment."[142]

Kenny was most convincing when she appeared as the active clinician giving a patient special muscle exercises, saying "Don't think of anything, don't think of anything at all, don't think I am doing anything with you. Now think with me, relax that, let your brain power extend to here. I am taking it back, don't you try to take it back, I am taking it for you." Then she shifts from clinician to teacher and theorist as she turns to the audience explaining "it will take some little time to correct the mistake [of] non-treatment of in-coordination." To reiterate the economic as well as physiologic necessity of functionality she features Wally, a patient who after 16 months of orthodox treatment could not sit up or feed himself, but is shown transformed after 16 months of Kenny treatment. Kenny, dressed in a white suit with a corsage, stands proudly besides Wally, now a young aspiring businessman in a suit, one hand casually in his pocket.[143]

Still, Kenny continued to believe that her film constituted proof of her theories. Her "documentary film," she proudly announced during a fundraising event, presented "indisputable evidence and proof of my clinical findings. I have forgotten the weary 34 years of loneliness, humiliation and sacrifice in the joyouse [sic] consciousness that as a result of the knowledge gained by me through research, your child will walk again and play again— perhaps you yourself may again enjoy a happy normal life."[144]

Most viewers who disliked the film said nothing to Kenny. But on occasion sympathetic doctors did try to help her turn her film into a medium that might convince a scientific audience. James Perkins, the head of the Division of Communicable Diseases of New York State's health department, had attended Kenny's course in Minneapolis in June 1942, and continued to be interested in her work. In May 1945, after watching a copy of *The Kenny Concept* with other officials in the health department's screening room,

Perkins wrote to Kenny to explain why he believed its use of dramatic cinematic conventions made it untrustworthy as a medical film.[145]

The strength of the film, Perkins assured Kenny, involved "those portions showing you at work at the bedside [which] make clear, as no amount of printed matter can, your mastery of muscle anatomy and physiology, as well as your understanding of the mental factors involved." But there were certain aspects of the film that he believed would "hinder your cause rather than help it so far as the medical profession is concerned." Two elements had left him and other physicians in his department with "mixed emotions": the testimonials quoted in the film and the "direct comparison of your cases with horrible examples of deformities resulting from treatment by the orthodox method."[146]

The testimonial, Perkins warned, was the strategy of choice for defenders of alternative medicine. The sincerity and social standing of these defenders did not give their words any greater credibility. At a recent hearing on the licensing of chiropractors in New York's state legislature, for example, the "most glowing and yet worthless testimonials were presented by such individuals as a retired brigadier general, an Army nurse, a Rabbi, a Catholic priest, and a Metropolitan opera star." These men and women were "absolutely sincere," but their conclusions were "completely erroneous." This technique, further, was likely to raise professional hackles. Physicians "are so well aware, through bitter experience, of the utter worthlessness of testimonials, that I think there is almost an automatic reaction *against* the device or method being advocated when testimonials are used."[147]

Worse than the use of testimonials, Perkins argued, was Kenny's comparison of patients treated by her methods and patients treated with orthodox therapies. Not only did such scenes humiliate the unfortunate, but physicians found no scientific validity in this kind of comparison for, as "each group represents selected cases," it did not prove "the superiority of your method." Perkins tried to think of a way that her film could appropriately compare patients, and suggested that a comparison of cases could be valid "*if your cases and the orthodox cases represented strictly alternate cases meeting rigid diagnostic criteria upon admission to a given hospital,*" and then showing "final results in a consecutive series of cases admitted to a hospital and treated by you, *with no omissions made in the series.*" And perhaps at the beginning of this reel there should be "a certification by the chief of staff of the hospital that each case met certain (specified) criteria of diagnosis, and that every case meeting such criteria has been included in the series."

Perkins regretted that "a carefully controlled study was not conducted on the value of your method when you first came to the United States." But it was "too late now" for polio's clinical care had altered so profoundly that he doubted whether anyone "will be willing to treat the alternate cases in such a study rigidly in the manner practiced so widely prior to your coming here." "Although I know some of the above remarks will not be to your liking," he concluded, "they have been written in a friendly and constructive manner."[148]

"Constructive, or even destructive criticism, is always helpful," Kenny replied, noting that Perkins's criticisms of her film were the only ones "recorded up to date." She defended her use of testimonials in the film as extracts from "the scientific reports of duly qualified medical practitioners" rather than from lay people. Nor was she willing to accept the idea that the film showed selectivity bias. The patients had been

chosen objectively, for they had been "examined in the presence of a group of medical men with Dr. Melvin Henderson as Chairman, and evidence was taken from the
doctor who supervised both groups. These cases were selected owing to their similar-
ity."[149] Kenny-trained professionals at the Institute had checked other patients who
had been treated by orthodox methods and released "as complete recoveries" 3 years
later, and found "there wasn't one normal child amongst the whole forty cases." But
patients treated with the Kenny method—"the same type of cases and treated under
the supervision of the same medical man and presented to other medical men"—
were, the physicians all agreed, "normal—as a matter of fact, better than normal
children. This can be understood when you take in the findings of science." In her
mind a clinical trial would be torture rather than science. She would reject any "controlled study of a method of treatment that would condemn children to suffer pain
from two to four months [when]... as you saw in the film this pain can be reduced to
a few days."[150]

Perkins started to answer Kenny's reply "paragraph by paragraph, but thought better
of the idea," remarking sadly "I thought I probably would get about the sort of answer
which I did." He hoped that she would still heed his advice with regard to her film for
he believed it would "definitely help your cause and, personally, I think your cause is
worth helping." "Your difficulties arise principally from your complete lack of conception of what is known as the scientific method," he concluded in frustration, "but that is
simply that, and I doubt there is anything anybody can do about it."[151] Perkins was quite
right, Kenny agreed, that she found it "very difficult to conceive just what is a truly scientific method." Not only had the AMA orthopedic committee, for example, "religiously"
avoided studying the Kenny method at the Institute during their investigation, but after
their report one of the committee members published a paper in the *Journal of Pediatrics*
that referred to symptoms such as muscle spasm and painful muscles with "contractures
and deformities," which were all based on a concept that was "exactly the opposite of
the concept he and his colleagues wrote the paper about." Further, instead of the purported ideal of scientific objectivity, the AMA report had been full of personal attacks
that undermined her personally and hindered the expansion of her work. When these
"untruthful" statements were then "distributed throughout the world... the rest of the
world has to suffer."[152] Perkins did not answer this second letter and remained eager to
use the film.[153]

The Kenny Concept was also reviewed quietly by the NFIP. After seeing the film in
Minneapolis a local NFIP official told the New York headquarters that Kenny had quoted
a letter by O'Connor "in which he recognized the value of her treatment" but that Kenny
was "liberal with her cracks when speaking of the medical profession generally." In his
estimation the film was too long and, despite its useful practical depiction of therapies,
used too many technical terms to suit a lay audience. Overall, it appeared to be simply a
propaganda vehicle centered around a single person: her voice "predominated the whole
picture," and she "was the center of all demonstrations."[154] When the NFIP's New York
office got its own copy, the NFIP's research director agreed with this assessment and
pointed out further that the film used several illustrations from Lovett's 1917 textbook
to show the contrast between his patients and Kenny's, yet "some of these illustrations
were actually used by Dr. Lovett to indicate the deformities resulting from lack of any
treatment."[155]

THE FILM IN EUROPE

The European war ended in May 1945, and a month later Kenny took *The Kenny Concept* to England where she met up with Mary. It was a horrific time for Mary who had traveled to London to meet her fiancé, Flight Lieutenant Peter Sinclair Jennings, a New Zealand pilot whom she had met in 1943. When Mary arrived she was told his plane had been shot down and that he was missing. It took many months until it was clear that he was dead. Kenny and Mary were guests of one of the physical therapists from Carshalton. Kenny kept Mary busy to try to distract her, knowing "she will be pretty lost and very sad."[156]

News of the AMA report, Kenny discovered, had reached Europe. Undaunted, she convinced Philippe Bauwens, head of the physical medicine department at St. Thomas's Hospital, to allow her to present her film to members of the British Association of Physical Medicine, a group Bauwens had founded a year before. Kenny showed the film, she boasted later, to "a very appreciative and respectful audience" at the Royal Society of Medicine in London chaired by "Lord Horder, the King's Physician."[157] According to Kenny, an enthusiastic Australian army physician declared that "all Doctors in Australia should see this film." He had used his watch to time Kenny on screen correcting a pelvic obliquity. It took her, he said, 7 minutes, yet "orthodoxy could not do this in seven years or seventy-seven years."[158]

In the *British Journal of Physical Medicine* a different picture emerged. According to this journal, before Kenny's film was shown, Horder warned the audience that "owing to the controversy which had surrounded her unorthodox concept of the disease" both the British Association of Physical Medicine and the Royal Society of Medicine disclaimed all responsibility for any views expressed in the film. Bauwens then explained that Kenny's clinical observations had led her to emphasize "the treatment of some peripheral disturbances which the medical profession held to be entirely secondary to the involvement of the central nervous system." Her new terminology as well as her methods, he admitted, "from the orthodox point of view, appeared to be irrational, if not futile." Yet, he assured his peers, Kenny did recognize the existence of cord lesions and her film "studiously avoided" most neuropathological topics. Bauwens, who had already seen the film, warned that it "embodied many of the worst features of a 'Hollywood Movie'" and regretted its "exaggerated sentimentality" and "offensive sensationalism." These defects were regrettable "since [they]...constituted an abuse of the very medium best capable of illustrating those points to which Miss Kenny [sought]...to draw attention." Bauwens especially disliked the film's final portrayal of orthodox-treated patients shown side by side with patients treated by Kenny's method, a depiction that put "the orthodox method...in a very unfavorable light" and was both "reprehensible" and "misleading."[159]

The physical medicine physicians in the audience seemed to have shared Bauwens' limited enthusiasm. Harold Balme, a respected specialist who had written on the clinical care of pain, told the *Lancet* that he had found the film "interesting and suggestive." Like Bauwens, Balme found some virtues in Kenny's work. He especially liked her emphasis on the value of very early treatment, the importance of focusing attention on painful and spastic muscles instead of inert ones, and her critique of immobilization. For him her skills in relieving pain and securing relaxed muscles were aspects of modern rehabilitative methods that could be used to treat other serious injuries such as fractures. But Balme drew a clear distinction between Kenny's methods and her theories. He saw her pathological claims as a "farrago of nonsense" that he felt ruined the film's value for any medical audience. Notions that the polio virus appeared in the skin and muscles, or that immobile muscles were "alienated," or that the chief factor in restoring mobility was educating a patient's mind in "the pattern of movement" were all signs of "jargon . . . reminiscent of a certain type of 'osteopath pathology.'"[160]

Despite his own qualms, Bauwens, like Perkins, was convinced that the film could be remade to attract rather than repel medical audiences. He urged Kenny to make her film less sensational and to highlight "those points which you have observed and which are of great interest to the Medical Profession."[161] Bauwens' suggestions were expounded in greater detail by Brian Stanford, a London physician who was becoming known as an expert in directing medical films. Stanford argued that Kenny's film was too long and that "the phraseology" used in her commentary was too obscure for her audiences "to draw a coherent argument." He urged her to shorten it to appeal to a medical audience that would not want to "assemble . . . for much longer than forty minutes." Many physicians, he added, might "come in a critical, and sometimes even an antagonist, frame of mind, therefore the material must be presented in the clearest and most concise manner possible." Stanford offered to help edit the film, and suggested he travel to the Institute to do this. The Institute's board of directors agreed to pay his expenses and an honorarium. Unfortunately Stanford found postwar international travel restrictions too difficult and was unable to come to Minneapolis.[162]

In August 1945, after the London presentation Kenny traveled to Belgium where she and 2 of her technicians visited the Neurological Institute in Brussels, which had been converted into makeshift wards during that summer's polio epidemic.[163] Leon Laruelle, the director of the Brussels center, was not happy to see Kenny. He told her, she recalled, that "there were several other centers in Belgium that no doubt would appreciate a visit," a comment that Kenny understood as "a polite way of letting me know he personally did not desire to waste too much time."[164] But Laruelle did agree to have her accompany him and other members of his staff on rounds where Kenny pointed out "in one patient after another. . .the condition in the periphery that was preventing recovery." Laruelle allowed Kenny's technicians to treat a few of the patients, including a woman whose paralyzed face was so stiff that she was unable to sleep. After these demonstrations a number of the doctors asked her to see their patients, and she was invited to show her film first to "a select few" and then "to a large audience."[165] With her typical brashness along with her medical connections, Kenny may have seemed, in war-torn Belgium, to be the personification of the American crusader, free from the trauma and deprivation of war. Certainly the analogy drawn by a local physician suggested this when he commented that her film showed "indisputable evidence of a greater knowledge of the disease. As a matter of fact you have produced an 'atomic' bomb."[166]

After seeing the film and its effect on his colleagues Laruelle, Kenny reported happily to Bauwens, became "very cooperative." He told Kenny that both her film and her work with patients had shown him "conditions he had no idea existed." Laruelle did not, Kenny noted, "complain about anything in the film but told me it was like a great interesting book which he could read many times."[167] Kenny seemed to have heard this remark as an unambiguous compliment, but perhaps Bauwens heard something else as well, a hint that Laruelle found the film a messy, complex piece of evidence with the clinical results more intriguing than the interpretation. In any case, Laruelle and Kenny began to discuss the idea of sending a group of doctors, nurses, and physical therapists from Belgium for training at the Minneapolis Institute.[168] When Kenny returned to Minneapolis, she left behind 2 copies of her film: one with Mary in London and the other at the Brussels center.[169]

BATTLES AT HOME

Kenny arrived home to find herself besieged by reporters who had just read the August 1945 issue of the *Journal-Lancet*, the local medical journal edited by University of Minnesota physiologist Maurice Visscher and tuberculosis expert Jay Arthur Myers.[170] The journal had published a glowing report by John Pohl of 5 years of work with 364 patients treated at the Institute. Pohl described his staff's increasing enthusiasm and concluded that "continuing observation has served to increase this enthusiasm and to prove the great merit of the Kenny methods."[171] In the same issue, however, an editorial by Visscher and Myers disagreed forcefully. Visscher and Myers highlighted Pohl's statistics showing that 22 percent of Kenny's patients had died or had "extensive residual paralysis." This, they pointed out, was "an account slightly different from that which one reads in the newspapers." Thus, Pohl had "unwittingly perhaps, performed a real service to humanity in exposing these figures to public view." Most of all, they disliked Pohl's enthusiastic promotion of Kenny's ideas and accused Pohl and other Kenny proponents of deliberately misleading the public and the wider medical community. "The 'Kenny concept' has been built up to fictitious importance largely by salesmanship and wishful thinking," they argued, and "it would not be worth refuting were it not for the international publicity which has been given to the view." They hoped that "someday the public will be wise enough and sufficiently informed to refuse to be misled by unsound theories." "Science is the search for truth," they concluded dramatically, and "it is a misfortune when anything is permitted to confuse that search."[172] "'U' Medics Clash Over Success of Kenny Concept" said the local papers, and in a confusing mélange noted that Pohl's results were "far superior to those obtained by any previously known method," but that, as Visscher and Myers had noted, 22 percent of Pohl's patients had died or remained "extensively paralyzed."[173]

Kenny had long boasted that almost all Minnesota physicians supported her work, so the editorial was a blow to her pride and to the Institute's reputation. Deciding that this was an opportunity to target the University of Minnesota and demand an "apology" from Visscher and Meyer's superiors, she called for a special hearing before the University of Minnesota's Regents. At the hearing she made much of her recent European experiences, pointing out that her technical film had been shown at the Royal Society of Medicine "by invitation" and that "Lord Horder, King's Physician [had] presided." Angry with Visscher and Myers's remark that her work should not have had international publicity, she assured the Regents that the doctors of England and Europe "were big enough to allow me to present my clinical findings." She also recognized the attack on herself as a theorist. Visscher and Myers "admit the treatment is all right . . . [but] I shouldn't say anything about a concept [yet] . . . without explaining the symptoms it is impossible to explain the treatment." Science, she agreed, was a search for truth yet "these gentlemen apparently object to being shaken out of a rut and refuse to accept the truth if that truth takes them out of this rut."[174] The Regents thanked her and expressed their interest in her work, but were careful to avoid any mention of an apology.[175]

In Australia, as polio outbreaks became more frequent during 1945, Kenny's film gained a small audience, although mainly in Queensland. Charles Chuter, the Brisbane civil servant who had remained her friend and ally since the 1930s, became the film's Australian agent, promoter, and interpreter. Chuter considered donating the film to the Queensland government, but he knew the dangers of bureaucracy, and in order not to "risk the film being relegated by the State Health Department to the 'mud of oblivion'" he decided to show it first to "representative" audiences and provide short introductions himself.[176]

Chuter struggled to find occasions for physicians to see Kenny's film. Most of Kenny's clinics had closed during the war, and Sir Raphael Cilento, her longstanding enemy, was still head of the Queensland's state health department.[177] Australian physicians were well aware of the 1944 AMA report, and Chuter had heard that many were now saying "the Kenny bubble has burst in America."[178] Reflecting this widespread antagonism, University of Queensland pathologist James Duhig, a former member of the Queensland Royal Commission, refused to see the film. He had become one of Kenny's most vocal antagonists. He described her textbook to the Brisbane Sunday Telegraph as "drivel" and argued that American doctors who were Kenny supporters were "of much poorer scientific and professional standing than those who reject her claims to novelty, originality, or superiority."[179] Duhig then informed Chuter that "in view of the highly condemnatory reports of her ideas and methods, particularly in the manipulation of statistics, I would remain extremely sceptical even if I saw the film."[180] Charles Thelander, who had chaired the Commission, also refused to see the film, telling Chuter "he would not believe a word Kenny had to say."[181] Chuter was able to convince a few other former members of the Commission to attend a screening, along with the head of the Brisbane branch of Australia's medical society, who later assured Chuter he was sure that his colleagues would want to see the film although, he admitted, "there is strong opposition."[182]

The reception from other professionals was more mixed. At a screening before residents, physical therapists, and nurses at the Brisbane Hospital, Chuter reported, "there was unanimous agreement that the picture had been wonderfully produced; the nurses were favourably impressed; the physical therapy staff still prejudiced; resident medical staff, silent."[183] Physicians at the University of Queensland's medical school agreed that "the film was well presented," Chuter informed Kenny, "and that it established that you had got 'something'" but they also identified "exaggeration."[184]

Lay viewers, in contrast, were markedly enthusiastic. Local officials in Brisbane were so impressed that they passed a resolution "demanding the Kenny treatment for this State." Members of the Irish Association turned out in numbers, "notwithstanding that the night was stormy and wet," and a friendly audience of around a hundred members of the National Council of Women urged Chuter to exhibit the film more widely.[185] The film raised Chuter's own reputation as an expert on Kenny's work. A Brisbane assemblyman asked him to help a 15-year-old boy paralyzed by polio who was not, the parents believed, getting the proper treatment at the Brisbane General Hospital. In a response that suggested that Chuter saw the film as both a technical guide and propaganda vehicle, he organized a special screening for the parents and invited 5 members of Parliament and "a substantial number of other people."[186] Chuter became more convinced than ever that the film illuminated what he had long suspected: a division between thoughtful members of the public and prejudiced Australian professionals. "Lay audiences have been fascinated," he reflected, while most doctors "have been shocked into silence . . . [and] some of them are floundering in an endeavour [sic] to find defects."[187]

These responses to *The Kenny Concept* reminded Kenny that most Australian physicians, whom she had largely been able to ignore during her early years in Minnesota, were not impressed by her American success. Like Chuter, she saw her film illuminate a chasm between lay Australians and medical professionals. She had intended the film to end professional bickering, public ignorance, and the tyranny of distance. It needed, she felt, only viewers of good will and honorable character who would believe in what they saw. Why was it not reaching physicians? Were their prejudices stronger than their eyes? Or was there something in the design of the film that marked it as not scientific enough?

REEDITING THE FILM

Kenny's technical film became her great hope, a way of simultaneously demonstrating and confirming her ideas. However, it carried many of the same failings as her textbooks and lectures: it juxtaposed sentimentalized language and dramatic vignettes with scientific terms, giving it a tone and style far from the typical medical films of the day.

Kenny at first refused to acknowledge these failings. But supporters such as Perkins, Bauwens, and Stanford convinced her that the etiquette of cinematic science required less talk of pain and emotion. By mid-1945 Kenny had come to acknowledge that she had to edit her film to bring it closer to the universal language of science.

She cut the film in half and found several doctors to translate the soundtrack into German, Dutch, Spanish, Russian, French, and Italian.[188] It was the first time she had ever responded positively to even mild criticism from anyone outside her immediate circle. She was beginning to feel that this film, remade with its narration in a number of languages and then sent all over the world, could stand as her legacy and as the concrete example of her contribution, satisfying enough to allow her to return to Australia and claim that she had achieved what she had set out to do in 1940. The new film could become a kind of global ambassador, and, she hoped, "draw attention to the indisputable presence of the disturbance in the peripheral structures and in this way perhaps scientific research may find out the reason for these disturbances."[189]

Bauwens's advice to take out the film's "sensational" elements and his warnings against its "Hollywood" features spoke directly to the dangers of personality politics in science, which Kenny had exacerbated by accompanying her film during 1944 and early 1945. She now became more willing to separate herself from the promotion and explication of her work. Leaving the original version of the film in England and Belgium, and preparing the new version in various languages to be sent around the world without her—all were significant steps in breaking the link between Kenny herself and the Kenny method.

Bauwens was glad to hear that Kenny was preparing a shortened edition of the film and asked to look over the new version with a colleague to make "an abstract of the portions which I consider of the highest clinical importance." The film, he believed, should be made available for distribution to any medical society or association "which might want the loan of it." To achieve this he had put the film in the catalogue of the Scientific Films Association.[190] Delighted, Kenny used Bauwens's letter to confirm her claims that eminent physicians had recognized the authority of her work through her film. Her technical film, which presented "indisputable evidence," she informed O'Connor, was now accepted by a British expert who had presented it to the "Scientific Film Association of Great Britain."[191] To the *Chicago Herald-American* Kenny noted that her film been adopted as a "great scientific document" by the "Royal Medical Society of England" and would be "made available to every medical society and university in the land." British physicians, she assured Chicago supporters, had initially been skeptical before seeing the film. They had told her "we in England had been led to believe the Kenny treatment was evolved from some fantastic theory of infantile paralysis, but your film proved your treatment is based on definite clinical findings."[192]

UPHEAVAL

Other events served to make Kenny even more dependent on the success of her film. In London, grieving for the death of her fiancé, Mary met Stuart McCracken, an Australian soldier who had been a German prisoner of war. They became engaged, and Mary left for Australia to marry and raise a family. Her move to Brisbane, according to her American friends, helped her free herself from Kenny's tight control.[193] Kenny had not wanted to have Mary leave, recognizing the emotional and physical sustenance Mary offered. Stuart, who years later became a fervent guardian of Kenny's legacy, recalled the money Kenny had offered him not to marry Mary so she could help Kenny "carry on her work."[194] Although Kenny wished them "life-long" happiness she missed Mary terribly and felt bereft without her help.[195] And there was further upheaval. Margaret Opdahl, her secretary since 1942, left the Institute for a new position at the Red Cross. Kenny had recognized Opdahl's "ability to maintain harmonious relations [and]...trusted her with my most intimate and private affairs."[196] She was never able to replace her with anyone as reliable and loyal.

Local political alliances altered as well. Hubert Humphrey, the city's new mayor, was, NFIP officials noted with delight, "not in sympathy with the Kenny Institute being run as a project of the Board of Public Welfare."[197] Still, although most of the Institute's board members were Republicans, Democrat Humphrey found it politically expedient to work enthusiastically for the annual Institute fundraising campaigns. Kenny's sense that only a small group of people were loyal to her—and that physicians in the city hospital and at the University of Minnesota were not—intensified. "I may be a little selfish," she wrote to Marvin Kline after the results of the 1945 mayoralty election in which he had run and lost were announced, "but to be candid, I think now that you are relieved of your parochial responsibilities your sympathetic heart and your sound judgment will have more opportunity to reach out to wider horizons and help to bring joy and comfort and security to a greater number."[198] Kline remained on the Institute's board as its senior executive, but, as the NRC committee had feared, he began to see the burgeoning Kenny movement as an opportunity to make as well as to raise money.

Kenny's own sense of mortality exacerbated her dependence on the film. Not only did it have to stand for concrete and unambiguous achievement, it had to portray an Institute without politics where, she recognized, she would not always be in charge. She took her film to the Mayo Clinic and showed it to Melvin Henderson and his colleagues, trying to ensure regional loyalties.[199] She continued to feel that the situation in the United States was "chaotic" but that her efforts were starting to come to fruition. When she had finished editing and translating the film she wrote to President Truman that fall, "I [will] have fulfilled my obligation to my own country and presented my clinical findings by documentary film to research institutions where clinical presentation and scientific research can be instituted side by side."[200] "This is the crown of my life['s] work," she wrote to Chuter the same week, "I am sure when the scientists of the world see the indisputable evidence presented in the film, research will bring the conquest of the disease centuries nearer."[201]

INITIAL REACTIONS TO *THE KENNY CONCEPT*

Kenny was delighted by the public response to her film. She loved the ovations and the postscreening receptions where she was treated as a celebrity.[202] She was eager to hear the reactions of particular viewers, asking a Hearst newspaper executive whether "your Chief has seen the Documentary film and what were his reactions to it?" "Mr. Hearst had viewed the documentary film," the official replied, "and thought it most impressive. He asked me to express his appreciation to you."[203]

Kenny was especially interested in her film's impact on professional audiences. She was not surprised when Morris Fishbein told the Institute's public relations director that, as "the editor of a scientific magazine," he was interested only in "controlled scientific evidence regarding the results of methods submitted by people capable of evaluating the results" and was therefore "not interested in Sister Kenny's film."[204] Fishbein's reaction— refusing to look—suggested the film might indeed have the power to sway its observers, a power she had frequently found in her own clinical demonstrations. One Iowa physician assured her that "Waterloo physicians were greatly impressed by the documentary film . . . Too bad there are so many 'die hards' but Pasteur had the same trouble in putting over his germ theory."[205]

John Pohl liked the film but he felt its main strength was to help allies who wished to understand further details of Kenny's work.[206] Kenny technicians, similarly, tended to use the film to inform students who had already "grasped the concept." They found that students who were finishing their training were able "to get so much more from it."[207]

From the beginning, Kenny challenged critics to see her film and retain their skepticism. In early 1945 she urged the members of the AMA committee to return to Minneapolis to see her film because "they would find it most instructive, and I am sure that many of the opinions expressed in their report would in all honor be contradicted."[208] When physicians from the Minneapolis General Hospital published a report that was critical of Kenny's concept in the state medical journal and stated that there was no proof that muscles had "direct virus involvement," Kenny retorted that "if all of these gentlemen had kept themselves abreast of the results of research and had waited to see the documentary film" none of those comments "would ever have been written."[209]

For some lay viewers the film's impact was tremendous and positive. A North Dakota woman who saw the film after hearing Kenny lecture told her that "what you have done in the field of medical science seems to me like a great sermon, which I wish the world might hear." Watching the film, she had "received a spiritual vision": just as patients with polio were "crippled [so] ... our spirits are imprisoned in braces and splints and corsets [for] ... we use only a small fraction of the spiritual life which is rightfully ours."[210] Clara Russell La Roche, Rosalind Russell's sister, showed the film to potential donors in New York City, and, according to her husband, the occasion spurred the founding of the New York KF chapter.[211]

While Kenny continued to see *The Kenny Concept* as appropriate for both professional and lay audiences, she also produced a 12-minute film *The Value of a Life*, designed specifically "for the lay person."[212] Institute officials found this film particularly useful to show to families and potential donors, but Kenny continued to show *The Kenny Concept* to members of the public as well as medical professionals who visited the Institute. [213]

THE SILVER SCREEN

In 1946 Kenny was caught up in the excitement of the Hollywood movie's premiere and promotion. She flew to New York to attend the movie's premiere in Time Square, and spoke at a gathering of New York's social elite at the Waldorf-Astoria, where she was presented with a large book of photographs commemorating the movie. "Wish you were here to go with me," she wrote to Mary; "I have a new green evening frock to wear as I am not quite sure what these bally Americans will do to me at such a premiere."[214]

According to the *Minneapolis Star-Journal*, traffic in Times Square was "a mad mix up" as more than 20,000 people "jammed in for a close look at arriving celebrities," along with extra squads of policemen. Kenny arrived escorted by Russell's husband Frederick Brisson. She told the crowd "it is a pleasure to see you here and I know you will see a fine film ... It has been gratifying to be able to do something for your country, that has done so much for mine." The crowd broke through the barriers and jostled the platform on which Kenny stood, "nearly throwing her off balance."[215] The northwest premiere the next month in Minneapolis rivaled the New York premiere "in color and fanfare," as a crowd of over a thousand milled outside the RKO-Orpheum theater to watch local and regional celebrities enter.[216]

Advertised as "one of the world's great stories of love, sacrifice and conflict," the film was clearly made to capitalize on public curiosity about a controversial and popular figure, and on the celebrity attraction of Rosalind Russell.[217] Although *Sister Kenny* did not do well at the box office, audiences and many film critics liked it. In November 1946 the National Screen Council, comprised of local civic film committees, gave it that month's Blue Ribbon Award for family entertainment, even though the film's average gross was lower than that of the council's usual award choices.[218] Russell's performance was widely praised, and few were surprised when she received a Golden Globe award for best dramatic actress and an Academy Award nomination.[219] The Oscar for Best Actress, however, went to Olivia de Haviland in *To Each His Own*.

The movie's message was harder to assess. Howard Barnes of the *New York Tribune* called it "a fascinating documentation of a ceaseless and stirring medical struggle."[220] The

Pittsburgh Sun Telegraph considered it "a sympathetic and indignant photoplay" with "a depth of feeling and sincerity that occasionally takes on a documentary tinge."[221]

As sentimental as any March of Dimes preview, *Sister Kenny* drew its appeal from dramatizing the fear of ignoring the value of the Kenny method. On this occasion it offered the American public a heroic "woman in white" who provided alternative, perhaps even antiorthodox, solutions to puzzles the American medical establishment could not solve. The film's image of scientific discovery—the outsider versus the conservative professional establishment—was, leaders of organized medicine realized, one that fit all too well with the public's distrust of what it considered the overblown claims of America's medical elite. Members of the audience would leave the cinema convinced they had the right to choose between experts to care for a child paralyzed with polio. This was, of course, an option they had always had, but one that was now recognized by Hollywood's powerful silver screen. Kenny's critics feared the movie would sway a public already eager to embrace a miracle worker.

James Hulett, Jr., a young sociologist at the University of Illinois, decided that the movie provided the perfect research subject to follow "the conflict between scientific medicine and the Kenny group as it affects the attitudes of the public." He wrote to the NFIP's national office to ask for "a reliable statement on the question whether the Kenny therapy represents anything new or 'revolutionary' that was unknown before Kenny 'discovered' it." "My purposes in studying the Kenny movement are strictly objective," he assured NFIP officials.[222]

The NFIP had always paid close attention to movies about polio. In 1944 it had advised its Minneapolis chapter not to sponsor the film *They Shall Have Faith* (later renamed *Forever Yours*), produced by the B-studio Monogram. It was the story of a doctor's daughter paralyzed by polio who defies her father's old-fashioned splinting methods and is healed by the experimental treatment of Army surgeon Tex O'Connor. The NFIP headquarters concluded that polio was hardly central to the plot, which was "the usual Hollywood romance," but suggested the chapter not sponsor the film, for "the picture will do no damage but is the type of thing which we should have no part of."[223] RKO's *Sister Kenny* was different. Not only was polio central to the plot, but there was also an explicit discussion of medical orthodoxy, and the doctors who disagreed with Kenny's ideas were the ones leaving children deformed.[224] Further, Kenny had made the film her personal triumph. After talking with his staff, who noted that Hulett had written an "outstanding article on 'The Kenny Cult,'" the head of NFIP's Public Relations suggested that Hulett contact Maurice Visscher, Harold Diehl, and other members of Minnesota's medical faculty who were "living as it were in the middle of the Kenny movement."[225] In the article Hulett published a few years later he saw the film's success as the result of a misguided popular beliefs.[226]

Some reviewers turned to physicians to try to balance the film's pro-Kenny stance. In the *New York Herald Tribune* Judith Klein noted the film's "distortion and omission of facts," a problem that "not only tends to shake public faith in the medical profession but also raises false hopes as to the universal effectiveness of treatment." She referred to Pohl's 1945 study of the numbers of Kenny patients who were left with extensive residual paralysis and she also quoted NFIP medical director Hart Van Riper. While Van Riper praised Kenny's "brilliant results in treatment" and credited her with the demise of the orthodox use of plaster casts, he made it clear that praising Kenny as a clinician did not mean accepting her theories of polio. "If Miss Kenny had remained on the clinical side—instead of invading the laboratory field of the physician—the great schism between her and the medical profession would not have occurred." The movie, he feared, might revive the feuding between doctors and Kenny. "Let's not worry about cause," Van Riper told Klein and her readers, "but concentrate on the treatment...there is no known cure for poliomyelitis." After all, he concluded, "doctors cure very few people. The Lord cures them. Doctors just help Him along."[227]

The disjunction between clinical ability and scientific understanding was picked up by other reviewers as well. Kenny "will never forsake her theory [that polio is]...essentially a disease of certain muscles," Archer Winsten reflected in the New York Post. But physicians base their theories on "much more penetrating research into the nature of the causative virus [and]...point to actual nerve destruction." Thus, doctors may "grant her good therapeutic innovations" but they "consider her scientifically ignorant."[228] "A little knowledge is a dangerous thing when it touches the field of medicine," agreed Florence Fisher Parry of the Pittsburgh Press. The movie, she believed, "misrepresents the medical profession in a manner shocking to those who hold it in high regard." Parry quoted Nebraska orthopedist H. Winnett Orr who questioned even Kenny's clinical methods. He argued that the promotion of Kenny's treatment had been a cruel fraud that had led to the spending of millions of dollars "in a campaign which has had only a minor effect upon the care of a few patients." In Orr's view the polio epidemics of the past few years had abundantly demonstrated that splints, braces, and surgical care were "necessary in order to put these patients on their feet, to restore them to usefulness in society, and to make them independent of the care of families, relatives, and institutions."[229]

Life featured the film as its movie of the week, calling Kenny "the most publicly controversial figure in the medical world today" with "a host of utterly devoted followers and a host of strongly skeptical medical opponents." Life recognized that "many medical men will utter howls of protest against it—and not without reason—for Sister Kenny is frank propaganda for the Kenny treatment and, by inference, against other methods employed by most doctors." The magazine included 2 pages of stills from the movie and a full-page photograph of Russell as Kenny in Brack's auditorium with the caption "Sister Kenny Glares at a Doctor Who Thinks She is a Quack."[230] But the same issue also contained a short review by New York pediatrician Philip Stimson entitled "A Doctor Comments on 'Sister Kenny.'" In a stunning reversal, Stimson, who had been a strong Kenny supporter since the early 1940s, now argued that "millions of people will be stirred by the movie and believe all its implications." He warned it was not true that all acute patients treated by Kenny recover completely and rapidly or that "all but a few orthopedists are opposed to Sister Kenny and have nothing to do with her treatment." He praised the Kenny method but noted many similarities between Kenny and orthopedists, arguing that the best treatment of polio involves the services of many experts.[231] Stimson had recently been featured in the National Foundation News as the director of a new unit providing specialized polio training for doctors, nurses, and other professionals at New York's Knickerbocker Hospital.[232]

Life also provided a separate story about Kenny herself, describing her as 59 and "undaunted." Even though the KF was now a large and growing institution and Kenny was a local celebrity, success had not "made her any less determined or cantankerous." "She is still caustic toward all critics" and regards the AMA and the NFIP "as woefully far from the true faith." The story included a photograph of Kenny and a girl patient who was standing for the first time and another photograph of Kenny with Russell and an RKO executive.[233]

In October 1946 Ed Sullivan came out on Kenny's side in his syndicated column "Little Old New York." "Basil O'Connor's richly-endowed National Foundation won't let Sister Kenny have the money," he told readers, even though the NFIP had formally endorsed her work. He warned that "the future of tens of thousands of polio victims is being jeopardized by temperament and false pride" and suggested that "Basil O'Connor, custodian of $20,000,000 of public contributions, should render an accounting of this curious situation." As for the difference in quality of care between ordinary therapists and Kenny-trained therapists, Sullivan quoted Kenny saying "it is as if a Boy Scout's knowledge of first aid were opposed to the knowledge of a specialist."[234] This immediately became a national story. The editor of *New York Medicine* responded by calling Sullivan "a romantic partisan" and Kenny "tragically egotistical."[235] "If I'm a 'romantic partisan' of Sister Kenny," Sullivan retorted in print, then Kenny's allies such as Robert Bingham and the late Don Gudakunst were "in the upper brackets of romanticism." As for the accusations of egotism, "the parents of a child afflicted with infantile paralysis don't care whether the healer is an egotist—all they want is to see that child walk again." Sullivan framed this as a public interest story, arguing that "the public, which volunteers the money gladly to fight this cruel disease" had "a financial stake" in any meeting between NFIP and KF leaders. He also doubted the good faith of many physicians. "Somewhere along the line, deliberately or accidentally, the medical profession apparently tossed the Kenny method overboard, [and] turned instead to a modification of her method which perhaps relieved them from acknowledging that all along they had been in error."[236]

Marvin Kline thanked Sullivan for his "clear exposition of the facts," noting "the tremendous reader interest in your column and the enormous circulation of your newspaper."[237] In the *New York Post* Archer Winsten praised Sullivan's "great-hearted attempt to reconcile Nurse Kenny and the medical profession," and suggested that O'Connor "invent a diversion by which all faces are saved."[238]

In private notes NFIP officials were delighted with the *New York Medicine* editorial, which they described as carefully thought out and "logical."[239] In public the NFIP issued a 13-page statement on "The Kenny Question" to clear up "a slight confusion in the public mind as to the present status of the Kenny method of treatment [raised by] ... the recent film depicting the life of the Australian nurse, Elizabeth Kenny." Doctors had accepted her method and most now practiced a modified version. Moreover, NFIP funds were available for any polio treatment prescribed by a doctor, including at the Kenny Institute. It was Kenny's concept of the disease that doctors rejected. "True scientists," the statement read, "are willing to follow any clue, any lead that seems to promise new discoveries. They merely are unwilling to disbelieve the evidence of many competent investigations and reports already made, though less publicized than the Kenny concept among laymen."[240] Thus, the NFIP portrayed the film as a sign of Kenny's inappropriate use of publicity to try to persuade patients and doctors to employ a technique only a quack would resort to.

Theater managers, uneasy about the film's antidoctor tone, were advised by their trade journals "to draw attention to the performance of Rosalind Russell and to the name of Sister Kenny ... [and] to avoid the controversial aspect of the Sister Kenny vs. the medical profession fight."[241] Some exhibitors, Dudley Nichols told Kenny, were "reluctant to run the film because they fear it lacks popularity and therefore will not bring them in a profit."[242] An official from RKO drafted a letter to be written on KF letterhead and signed by Kenny, which presented her as altruistic and fully committed to the movie and its makers. Thus, she had "no financial stake" in the movie; she had "personally approved and endorsed the story that Mr. Dudley Nichols wrote and produced and directed"; and she hoped the film would "help to light up the darknesses [sic] of ignorance... [and] save lives before it is too late."[243]

Many medical societies delighted in the controversy and reprinted the film's critical reviews as a way of attacking both Kenny and also journalists who preferred fantastical drama to the less exciting, scientifically proven truth. "We would suggest a few movies, books, and magazine articles portraying the heartaches, the emotional catastrophes which every reputable physician encounters as counsellor in the ultimate facing of the bitter truth by those whose hopes have been falsely aroused," wrote the editor of the *Westchester Medical Bulletin*. Referring implicitly to the Hearst papers' support of both Kenny and the antivivisectionists, the editor continued, "Let those who have in their control the tremendously powerful media for moulding the thinking of the masses through press, radio and motion picture screen realize and live up to their great educational responsibility!"[244] The reviewer in the nursing journal *The Lamp* praised this "sincere story of devotion to a cause" but protested that objections by physicians "to novel ideas on treatment devised by unqualified persons [were]... often soundly rooted." As "Sister Kenny's idea has been thoroughly examined and as thoroughly rejected by the main body of opinion" it would have better if RKO "had chosen a subject that doctors should have examined, but have not."[245]

Most of the film's critics tended to portray the public as a passive audience, easily swayed by this populist attack not only on polio orthodoxy but medical orthodoxy.[246] Eileen Creelman of the *New York Sun* warned that the film might "keep people from accepting the standard methods," for "whether 'Sister Kenny' will do harm or good is not for the layman to decide."[247] After *Time* made a list of the film's "most outstanding distortions," Pohl protested that the magazine's "Cinema section" was not "the proper place in which to pass upon the relative merits of a highly scientific medical subject."[248]

The film's sanctification of Kenny also disturbed critics. Exaggerating the heroism of a central figure was, of course, a standard part of the Hollywood bio-pic.[249] However, the idea of producing a film about a *living* person whose "noble accomplishments"—unlike the work of Marie Curie and Louis Pasteur––had not yet "been established in history... had social and moral perils," warned Bosley Crowther, the leading film reviewer for the *New York Times*, comments that were quoted extensively in an editorial on "Sister Kenny: Problem Child of Medicine" in *New York Medicine*.[250]

Both the film's sanctification of Kenny and its harsh dichotomy between medical right and wrong were at the heart of film critic John McCarten's review in the *New Yorker*. "The business of treating Miss Kenny's clinics with the kind of reverence that suggests the miracles of Lourdes is obviously dangerous," he argued. "There is in this picture no hint that Miss Kenny is fallible. Her patients, one and all, are represented as being completely cured, whereas the patients of physicians unwilling to subscribe *in toto* to her ideas are uniformly revealed to be hopelessly warped and twisted." McCarten found the film not only boring but exaggerated and not medically sound. Unlike other reviewers he was not impressed with Russell's acting, which he described as "a series of grimaces that grow more and more arch as 'Sister Kenny' moves glumly along."[251]

THE PUBLIC RESPONDS

After the RKO movie was distributed letters poured into the Kenny Institute. The vast majority of these writers saw the film as the true story of a great figure who could heal the crippled and who understood polio better than doctors. The film had clearly convinced many Americans that Kenny was a polio expert and probably also a miracle worker. Writers variously interpreted her work as Hollywood legend, as medical resource, and sometimes as generalizable to other disabling diseases such as multiple sclerosis or osteomyelitis.

Just as NFIP officials had feared, writers appealed to Kenny as healer and medical consultant. Paralyzed 49 years earlier, Ray Pospisil of Miami, Florida, saw Kenny's work as a medical resource, explaining, "I saw the moving picture of you treating the infinitile [sic] paralysis with hot packs that gave me a new idea how to treat my paralysis." He asked her to "please send me the book so I can get well."[252] Kenny was a preferable alternative to a doctor, partly for her skills and partly for her empathy for the suffering, as shown by her personal sacrifices on the silver screen.

Some felt the film confirmed their doubts not just of an individual doctor but the whole orthodox profession. With a daughter who was always in pain from osteomyelitis, Mrs. H. P. Schoening of Allegan, Michigan, was "so happy that you have told the truth about so many doctors and how many people have been cripple[d] for life from Polio, through so many doctors." It had taken 9 doctors to diagnose her daughter's illness and "the doctors even went so far as to tell us it was a mental condition."[253] Leon Colton of Milwaukee admitted that "I do not go to shows very often, and do not care much for them but this one I stayed awake." He had no doubt that he and Kenny agreed on the flaws of organized medicine. "I have know[n] for some time that Doctors of today could not live under the present system, if everybody were well. So it is the duty of a Dr. *not* to make you well, and not to kill you, but to prolong your life as long as posble [sic], so as to give the Dr. a meal ticket...I am for you and with you in this work 100 percent & wish you much luck & success."[254]

Responding to the film's unsympathetic portrayal of Brack, many saw Kenny's method as a promising alternative to orthopedic surgery. Alda Cononna of River Edge, New Jersey, who had been paralyzed by polio since 1939, had become interested in the Kenny method since seeing the movie. Her doctor had urged her to have an operation, but she first wanted to try the Kenny treatment and to have Kenny's "personal advice about it."[255] Others like Helen E. Sente of Hastings on Hudson, New York, had had a number of operations, "and would still go throu[gh] more if there was ever the slightest hope of getting rid of one brace." Paralyzed by polio during the 1916 epidemic, Sente thought "the picture of your life...was to[o] wonderful for words...You certainly have given a lot to humanity." She was also willing to be part of any scientific research. "I know it is asking a lot after all these years, but I do believe in mericals [sic] and am will[ing] to be a 'human guinea pig' if I may use that expression...I've had a lot of disappointments in my life, so please don't hesitate to give me your honest opinion."[256]

Some viewers saw the movie as implying clinical options for cerebral palsy patients as well. Mrs. Don Lariscy of Savannah had taken her 7-year-old daughter who had been "injured at birth" to "several Medical Doctors, Specialists in Polio Cases and to Chiropractors" who had all told her that "there is not anything that can be done." "At present I am massaging her with Coco-Butter and have had her in a Walker since last September." Mrs. Lariscy ran a beauty shop to care for her 2 children. "After seeing the wonders you have obtained for other children I do have some hope."[257] But Kenny and her staff had put aside their previous efforts to extend her work to cerebral palsy patients, and her secretary replied that the Kenny method was intended primarily for the treatment of polio in the acute stage. Kenny had worked "with spastics in Australia but while in the United States all her work has been with infantile paralysis."[258]

Kenny's experiences depicted in the movie made many writers sure that she would have special empathy as well as knowledge, as this heart-wrenching yet unsentimental letter suggests. Arthur, the son of Mrs. Mary Cavallaro of Brooklyn, had been paralyzed by polio in 1944. He spent 4 months in the St. Charles Hospital and was then sent home and told to use therapy daily to stretch his foot. His mother took him to another doctor who suggested "a stretching with instruments and his leg in a cast for 6 weeks," but "our doctor" disagreed, warning that his foot might deform and then require an operation. "Last night I saw your picture," Cavallaro told Kenny, "and after seeing what you gave up to help the children, I knew I had to write to you." She had thought her son accepted his brace, but "last week I heard him cry for the first time because he can't go skating. I hear that cry in my head day and night and it[']s almost driving me crazy." She believed Kenny could advise her on what medical option to follow: "if you tell me it's all right to do that, I'll do it because I have a lot of faith in you. Because to me, you are like a God." Her friends, she added, told her she was crazy and that "you wouldn't help me or see my son, but I feel different[ly] . . . after seeing your picture and reading about your work you've done with children with braces and corsets, I think you can make my son well." In a combination of a bargain and a plea, she promised, "Sister Kenny, if you do this, so help me God, I'll do anything in my power to help you in any way. I'll even help your fight against those Doctors who still don't believe in you . . . He's the only child I have and everytime I watch him walk a nail go[es] through my heart deeper and deeper."[259]

DEFENSIVE KENNY

Kenny's own reaction to the film was intense and defensive. She was appalled that *Life* had published the Stimson article, even though it was juxtaposed with the magazine's fulsome review of the film as its movie of the week.

Kenny was already frustrated with the publicity surrounding the Knickerbocker unit.[260] She especially disliked the NFIP's announcement that Knickerbocker had been the site of a 6-week NFIP-funded course to teach the Kenny method. Such an announcement, she warned Stimson, was "pure exploitation and a delusion as far as the students and public are concerned," for the clinic was staffed by therapists with a few months experience, "just enough time to give them an idea of the value of the work [but] . . . not enough time to let them know what were the symptoms and conditions present for which the work was really evolved."[261]

Stimson's *Life* article left her furious. In the angry tone she often used when converts recanted, she told reporters that "Dr. Stimson knew nothing about the early treatment except what I taught him, and there's still quite a bit he doesn't know."[262] Distressed, Stimson wrote asking for a public apology for this "belittling of my professional qualifications."[263]

But by this time Kenny had learned that the NFIP was sending out reprints of Stimson's comments in *Life* to chapter officials and other NFIP supporters.[264] Instead of apologizing Kenny grandly reiterated the reasons she felt so embattled: "May I be pardoned if I say that the National Foundation for Infantile Paralysis and certain members of the American Medical Association have shown a very poor spirit of gratitude for these priceless gifts and have remained cruelly silent...[when] inaccurate and untruthful statements have been published in medical journals." Nor did she accept Stimson's mild criticism of the impact of the movie. "You are entirely in the wrong if you think that any presentation in the entertainment picture can do harm," Kenny told him privately. Showing "a mother what to do for a child in agony [was]...of world wide importance."[265]

Sister Kenny, she began to assure wealthy allies, would have "a tremendous influence on the minds of the medical men of the world" and in Rochester physicians from the Mayo Clinic had already "flocked to see the picture."[266] The Hollywood film had become part of her work to be defended as strongly as her clinics, textbooks, or technicians.

Over the next months Kenny became stiffer and more suspicious, partly in response to the continuing criticism and partly as she tried to hide her age. Although reporters saw a lighthearted side of her in social occasions they found her unwilling to show any lightness in discussing her ideas; on those "she displays a solid, granite-like fanaticism [speaking with]...a stilted, formal quality that sounds almost like what is known in the patent medicine and carnival world as a 'pitch.'"[267] Adopting the attire of Hollywood celebrities, Kenny began to wear even larger corsages and decorative jewelry, and ordered stylish clothes from stores like Lane Bryant that specialized in large sizes. She began a life of fundraising rather than clinical care, and, like Basil O'Connor, she openly sought out a life of luxury. The KF provided her with "a big car," although she supposedly insisted on riding with the chauffeur. When she was in New York, she went to nightclubs like the Copa or the Stork Club where performers and club owners would come and talk to her, and she was disappointed if there was not a crowd around. With her house paid for by the city of Minneapolis, a regular allowance from the Exchange Club, and additional funds from the Institute's board, Kenny became a lady bountiful. She always carried "a big pocketbook with a big load of dough in it," a KF official recalled, and would take $50 or $60 and give it to some poor patient who needed it.[268]

Stimson remained a well-regarded polio expert. His growing distance from Kenny led him closer to the NFIP. He began to describe Kenny as "the best physiotherapy technician" he knew who "would get a lot further" if she limited her activities to clinical care.[269] At a meeting of the American College of Physicians in 1947 he declared, in a dramatic turnaround, that the "so-called Kenny treatment" had been described in a pamphlet published by New York health authorities in 1928, a reference to Boston therapist Wilhemine Wright's work.[270] Kenny later protested that she asked Stimson "to produce this health pamphlet describing my treatment in the year 1928" and that he was unable to do so.[271] Stimson realized that Kenny would always see any recanting convert as an enemy; she had no middle ground. He remained fascinated by her, however, and began to compile private letters, unpublished reports, and newspaper clippings into a scrapbook that he later called "Sister Elizabeth Kenny and Her Treatment of Acute Poliomyelitis in The United States as Experienced and Taught by Philip M. Stimson, M.D."[272]

JOURNEYING

At the Institute, Visscher and Myers continued their quiet campaign against Kenny. In December 1946, while Kenny was away, 2 respected physicians, Abraham Fryberg, a Queensland bureaucrat who had known Kenny for some years, and Brisbane orthopedic surgeon Thomas Stubbs Brown visited the Institute. They had been sent to America and Britain under the auspices of the Queensland government to investigate medical and rehabilitative care for polio, industrial hygiene, and tuberculosis.[273] Based on a visit to the Kenny wards at Carshalton in Surrey as well as the Institute in Minneapolis and other American hospitals, they concluded that polio treatment in the United States was "in a phase of change." Physicians were "uncertain" about therapeutic procedures: "old principles have been discarded and in their place treatments have been formulated which have a clinical rather than a scientific basis." They praised Kenny's work and clinical innovations, but her concepts, they concluded, were "not proven."[274]

By February 1947 Myers had received not only a copy of the Fryberg–Stubbs Brown report but additional reports from Australia suggesting that Kenny had never been a registered nurse. "I wonder," he wrote to Visscher, "if we have not had among us a worse imposter than we had realized." He was keeping "all of this material about Elizabeth Kenny in a special file so it will be available to you or anyone else who wishes to use it."[275] "She isn't quite on the level!" his friend Visscher agreed.[276]

Kenny was disappointed at the Fryberg–Stubbs Brown report. She had already visited Australia during the spring of 1946, her first opportunity since 1941. The visit was disappointing in many ways: her beloved Mary was now married and engrossed in domestic life; the report of the AMA committee had reinforced a wider dislike of her methods among Australian physicians; and even her Labor Party allies in the Queensland government had unhelpfully passed her request for an inquiry to the state's new Medical Research Council.[277] She showed her technical film in several places, but it was not well received. She sent a protesting report to Queensland Premier Ned Hanlon, and made sure Brisbane reporters heard her side of the story.[278]

Back in Minneapolis Kenny found that she had begun to be pushed to the side. She was now called Honorary Director at the Institute, although she retained a place on the KF board of directors.[279] Still she returned to Australia in October 1947, determined to be present for the Brisbane premiere of her Hollywood movie. She had already heard that the film had "not gone too well" in Melbourne or Sydney, the result, Chuter believed, of "medical threats."[280]

In Brisbane Kenny was featured in Hoyts Regent advertisements as the "famous Australian, whose dramatic and adventurous career is the subject of this outstanding picture." But despite Kenny's appearance at the Brisbane opening and generally positive reviews in the press, Sister Kenny did not do well in Brisbane either.[281] This may partly have been the result of a campaign of critical comments by the Brisbane Telegraph, which had mocked the idea that Australian physicians were "selfish, narrow-minded men, who refuse to accept or listen to new medical discoveries or treatments." The paper also quoted a local "cynic" who suggested the movie be retitled "Saint Elizabeth Kenny."[282] Members of Brisbane's medical elite, especially pathologist James Duhig who had long disliked Kenny, promised that when the movie was shown, they would provide pamphlets attacking Kenny's treatment to theatre audiences.[283]

Where the movie did find a delighted audience was in Toowoomba. Flashes of train carriages with words "Queensland Railways" and old-time railway stations caused "gasps of surprise from picture[-]goers who are so seldom treated to a sight of their own institutions on the screen," noted the *Toowoomba Chronicle*. The audience also enjoyed comparing the actors to the people they knew well: the actor who played McDonnell "had the physical and facial characteristics of Dr. McDonnell to a degree that made the identification easy" but his "rather strong Irish-Scottish tone" did not resemble " the thinner tone of the well-known Toowoomba medico." The actor playing Chuter, though, was "excellently drawn, bearing a reasonable likeness for those who know Mr. Chuter." Some of the actors "had traces of the American accent" but the *Chronicle* felt that "in all, much of the Australianism of the language was achieved."[284]

Aware of growing antagonism in Australia and even at her own Institute Kenny had become convinced that only in Europe would she find serious medical supporters. She traveled widely in 1947, visiting England, Ireland, France, Belgium, Sweden, Russia, Norway, Germany, Denmark, Switzerland, Spain, Italy, and Holland. She met with orthopedic surgeons, pediatricians, public health officials, and some ministers of health, assuring her audiences that the American physicians who "knew the least about my work during these last five years were the only ones to...supply reports in the medical journals." In Madrid she was met at the airport by doctors carrying a large bouquet; "it was very cheering to me to receive this floral tribute from a world famous Institute while I was yet able to smell them."[285] This was a joke she would repeat often, but its reference to her mortality made the humor rather black.

NOTES

1. Mary Kenny McCracken, interviews with Naomi Rogers, November 1993, Caloundra, Queensland, Australia.

2. Kenny "Paper Read at the Northwestern Pediatric Conference, Nov. 14, 1940, Saint Paul University Club," Kendall Collection; Kenny with Ostenso *And They Shall Walk*, 106–107, 111.

3. Kenny to O'Connor, September 12 1941, Basil O'Connor, 1940–1942, MHS-K; Kenny to Dear Mr. O'Connor, September 5 1941, Public Relations, MOD-K; Kenny to Dear Dr. Fishbein, October 5 1941, Public Relations, MOD-K.

4. Kenny to Dear Mr. Cusack, November 11 1942, Public Relations, MOD-K.

5. Kenny to Dear Miss [Catherine] Worthingham, June 24 1942, American Physiotherapy Assoc., 1941–1942, MHS-K; Catherine Worthingham to Dear Miss Kenny, July 20 1942, American Physiotherapy Assoc., 1941–1942, MHS-K; "The Biennial" *American Journal of Nursing* (July 1942) 42: 754–762; J. Albert Key [Report] in "Reports on Meeting of Committee to Investigate the Kenny Method of Treatment, Sunday and Monday, November 22 and 23, 1942, Minneapolis, Minnesota," Dr. R. K. Ghormley, 1943, MHS-K. Key was shown a movie at the General Hospital "from which I could draw no conclusions as to the relative value of the Kenny and the orthodox treatment."

6. Secretary to Sister Elizabeth Kenny to Dear Mr. Harris, July 16 1943, John H. Harris, 1942–1944, 1952, MHS-K; Secretary to Sister Elizabeth Kenny to Dear Mr. Harris, November 1 1943, John H. Harris, 1942–1944, 1952, MHS-K; John H. Harris to Dear Sister Kenny, December 16 1943, John H. Harris, 1942–1944, 1952, MHS-K.

7. Mrs. Sydney Sanner and Mrs. George Leslie Smith [Kate Crutcher Works of the Children's Hospital, Los Angeles] to Dear Sister Kenny, July 17 1943, Los Angeles-Misc., 1942–1951, MHS-K.

8. Ethel Calhoun to Dear Sister, November 24 1943, Ethel Calhoun, MHS-K.

9. [Philip Lewin] "Report of the Proceedings of the Committee on Treatment of After Effects," December 1 1938, Public Relations, Historical Organization, MOD. In the early 1940s the NFIP produced a one-reel sound motion picture on epidemiology and treatment of polio that was available to chapters; D. B. Armstrong and John Lentz "Credit Lines: A Selective Digest of Diversified Health Interests: Jottings" *American Journal of Public Health* (January 1942) 32: 94.

10. [Lewin] "Report of the Proceedings of the Committee on Treatment of After Effects," December 1 1938.

11. Howard A. Rusk "Motion Pictures Changing Form of Medical Education" *New York Times* November 7 1948.

12. Thomas G. Hull "Bureau of Exhibits" in Morris Fishbein *A History of the American Medical Association 1847–1947* (Philadelphia: W.B. Saunders Co., 1947), 1055; Brian Stanford "The Evolution of the Medical Film in Britain" *Canadian Medical Association Journal* (October 1947) 57: 385.

13. See "[Obituary] Sarnoff, Jacob" *JAMA* (1961) 178: 345.

14. Rusk "Motion Pictures Changing Form of Medical Education."

15. Hull "Bureau of Exhibits," 1056–1057; Stanford "The Evolution of the Medical Film in Britain," 386. For examples of some Navy films including *Morning Care, Bathing the Bed Patient, Beds and Appliances, Evening Care, Taking Blood Pressure, Postoperative Care,* and *Temperature, Pulse, Respiration* see "Sound Films: Nursing Procedures" *American Journal of Nursing* (September 1944) 44: 917–918.

16. "Films on Physical Therapy" *Physiotherapy Review* (1938) 18: 318. On the movies shown by the AMA's Council on Physical Therapy, including *Massage, Occupational Therapy, and Underwater Therapy* see Medical Motion Pictures *JAMA* (September 4 1943) 123: 43–44.

17. "Report of the Executive Committee [of the American Physiotherapy Association]" *Physiotherapy Review* (July–August 1937) 17: 152; Lucie P. Lawrence "Florence Kendall: What a Wonderful Journey" *PT Magazine of Physical Therapy* (May 2000) 8: 41.

18. Hull "Bureau of Exhibits," 1047.

19. "The Program of the Sections, American Medical Association, Ninety-Third Annual Session, Atlantic City, June 8–12, 1942: The Scientific Exhibit" *JAMA* (May 2 1942) 119: 60.

20. Max M. Green to Dear Sister Kenny, January 27 1943, Louisiana 1943–1944, MHS-K; [form "If you desire to have a Scientific Exhibit…"] [enclosed in] Max M. Green to Dear Sister Kenny, January 27 1943, Louisiana 1943–1944, MHS-K.

21. Kenny with Ostenso *And They Shall Walk*, 128. See also Kenny's offer to the Townsville city council of a film of her work; "Sister Kenny: City Council Motion" *Townsville Daily Bulletin* May 17 1935.

22. Kenny with Ostenso *And They Shall Work*, 245.

23. Mary McCarthy "'Sister Kenny' Outline," [1942], Paul Kohner Inc., Hollywood, Sister Kenny Collection, Margaret Herrick Library Special Collections, Academy of Motion Picture Arts and Sciences, Beverly Hills, 13. Mary Eunice McCarthy was no relation to the novelist and critic Mary Therese McCarthy. For a longer version of this section see Rogers "American Medicine and the Politics of Filmmaking: *Sister Kenny* (RKO, 1946)" in Leslie J. Reagan, Nancy

Tomes, and Paula A. Treichler eds. *Medicine's Moving Pictures: Medicine, Health, and Bodies in American Film and Television* (Rochester: University of Rochester Press, 2008), 199–238.

24. McCarthy "Outline," 2–3.

25. Kenny to McCarthy, August 26 1942, Mary McCarthy, 1942–1944, MHS-K; Kenny to Dear Dr. Diehl, September 16 1942, Dr. Harold S. Diehl, 1941–1944, MHS-K.

26. Martha Ostenso quoted in George Grim "Entertainers? Brainerd's Got Dandies" *Minneapolis Sunday Tribune* April 17 1950, 1, 5.

27. Kenny to Chuter, April 15, 1943, OM 65-17, Box 2, Folder 8, Chuter Papers, Oxley-SLQ; John B. Davies "Sister Kenny Triumphs in America" *Australian Women's Weekly* (March 6 1943) 10: 9.

28. Mary McCarthy to My Beloved Elizabeth, February 7 1944, Mary McCarthy, 1942–1944, MHS-K; Mary McCarthy to Sister Dear, February 25 1944, Mary McCarthy, 1942–1944, MHS-K.

29. On Russell's assessment of McCarthy as "a terrific saleswoman; full of Irish palaver" see [Cohn first interview with] Rosalind Russell, August 18 1953, Cohn Papers, MHS-K.

30. [Cohn first interview with] Rosalind Russell, August 18 1953; see also "Screen News Here And In Hollywood" *New York Times* July 24 1942; "Screen News Here And In Hollywood" *New York Times* September 5 1942.

31. By 1955 she had starred in 19 career-woman movies; Richard G. Hubler "The Perils of Rosalind Russell" *Saturday Evening Post* (October 1 1955) 228: 78. As Russell commented in 1953, "the plot was always the same, and I used to even get the same desk in each picture"; "The Comic Spirit" *Time* (March 30 1953) 61: 40.

32. Russell in Roy Newquist *Showcase, A Candid Cross Section of the Show World by the People Who Make It Show Business* (New York: William Morrow & Company, 1966), 396.

33. "The Comic Spirit," 42–44; [Cohn first interview with] Rosalind Russell, August 18 1953; Lowell E. Redelings "The Hollywood Scene" *Citizen News* September 26 1946; and see Rosalind Russell and Chris Chase *Life Is a Banquet* (New York: Random House, 1977), 143–147; Rosalind Russell "The Role I Liked Best…" *Saturday Evening Post* (August 2 1955) 228: 104. On the RKO studio reaction "What, a story about cripples and a nurse? No!" see Nicholas Yanni *Rosalind Russell* (New York: Pyramid, 1975), 86. She was married to Danish-born agent Frederick Brisson.

34. Russell "The Role I Liked Best," 104; see also "The Comic Spirit," 44; Redelings "The Hollywood Scene"; Russell and Chase *Banquet*, 145–146, 154.

35. "Famed Paralysis Nurse Here to Discuss Film" *Los Angeles Times* July 14 1942; Hedda Hopper "Star Nurses An Enthusiasm!" *Washington Post* July 27 1942; [Cohn first interview with] Rosalind Russell, August 18 1953; [Cohn interview with] Rosalind Russell, April 20 1955, Cohn Papers, MHS-K. See also "The Comic Spirit," 44; Russell and Chase *Banquet*, 143–144.

36. [Cohn first interview with] Rosalind Russell, August 18 1953.

37. Ibid.

38. McCracken, interviews with Rogers, November 1993.

39. "Famed Paralysis Nurse Here to Discuss Film" *Los Angeles Times* July 14 1942; Hedda Hopper "Star Nurses An Enthusiasm!" *Washington Post* July 27 1942.

40. Chuter to Dear Sister Kenny, June 29 1943, Wilson Collection.

41. Kenny to McCarthy, August 26 1942; PJAC [Peter Cusack] to BOC [Basil O'Connor], December 8 1942, Public Relations, MOD-K; Kenny to McCarthy, December 21 1942, Mary McCarthy, 1942–1944, MHS-K. See also "Rosalind Russell" in Mike Steen *Hollywood Speaks: An Oral History* (New York: G.P. Putnam's Sons, 1974), 82; Cohn *Sister Kenny*, 167–169.

42. Hedda Hopper "Star Nurses An Enthusiasm!" *Washington Post* July 27 1942; McCarthy to My Beloved Elizabeth, October 21 1943, Mary McCarthy, 1942–1944, MHS-K; Kenny to McCarthy, August 26 1942 Cohn *Sister Kenny*, 167–169; Russell and Chase *Banquet*, 12. For Kenny's divorce comment see E. B. Radcliffe "Show Mirror" *Enquirer* [1946], Public Relations, MOD-K.

43. On the Lance story, see McCracken, interviews with Rogers, November 1993; and see Kenny to Dear Mr. Henry, November 22 1949, Henry Papers, MHS-K; [Cohn first interview with] Rosalind Russell, August 18 1953; [Cohn interview with] Rosalind Russell, April 20 1955; Cohn *Sister Kenny*, 192–193. The story is not mentioned in Russell's autobiography, *Life Is a Banquet*.

44. [Cohn interview with] Rosalind Russell, April 20 1955.

45. Margaret Buell Wilder "Noted Nurse Gives Hope To Stricken" *Los Angeles Examiner* [1943], Clippings, MHS-K.

46. J. B. Hulett, Jr. "The Kenny Healing Cult: Preliminary Analysis of Leadership and Patterns of Interaction" *American Sociological Review* (1945) 10: 365.

47. McCarthy "Outline," 16.

48. Cohn *Sister Kenny*, 203–204. In "Angel of Mercy" *New York Times* November 21 1946 the amount was $100,000.

49. "Famed Paralysis Nurse Here to Discuss Film" *Los Angeles Times* July 14 1942.

50. Aubrey Pye, interview by Douglas Gordon and Ralph Doherty, November 8 1980, [transcript of sound recording], Fryer Library.

51. Kenny to McCarthy, August 26 1942.

52. Kenny "Data Concerning Introduction of Kenny Concept and Method of Treatment of Infantile Paralysis into the United States of America" [April 1944], Board of Directors, MHS-K; Kenny to Dear Dr. Diehl, September 16 1942, Dr. Harold S. Diehl, 1941–1944, MHS-K.

53. RKO had, for example, produced *The Hunchback of Notre Dame* (1939) and *I Walked With a Zombie* (1943).

54. McCarthy to Sister Dear, February 25 1944.

55. Mary McCarthy to My Beloved Elizabeth, February 7 1944; Russell in Newquist *Showcase*, 396.

56. Hedda Hopper "Looking at Hollywood" *Los Angeles Times* September 22 1944; Louella O. Parsons "'Roz' Russell Seriously Ill" *Los Angeles Examiner* September 24 1944; Russell and Chase *Banquet*, 146–147.

57. Hedda Hopper "Fans Object to Cancellation of Film About Sister Kenny" *Sioux Falls (S.D.) Argus-Leader* February 26 1944, Clippings 1944, MHS-K; James F. Bell to My Dear Mr. O'Connor, March 8 1944, Public Relations, MOD-K; Editorial "Heard and Read" *The A-V* (November 1946) 54: 152. On Russell, Hopper, and Kenny see Bernard F. Dick *Forever Mame: The Life of Rosalind Russell* (Jackson: University Press of Mississippi, 2006), 103–104.

58. Kenny to Dear Mary [McCarthy], February 17 1944, Mary McCarthy, 1942–1944, MHS-K; see also Mary to Sister Dear, February 25 1944.

59. Kenny to Hedda Hopper, [telegram] September 23 1944, RKO-Misc., 1942–1948, MHS-K; and see Louella O. Parsons "In Hollywood: Sister Kenny Protests Blaming of Rosalind Russell for Polio Film Delay" *Los Angeles Examiner* September 27 1944.

60. Jean Renoir *My Life and My Films* transl. Norman Denny (London: Collins, 1974), 220–221. See also Redelings "The Hollywood Scene"; Erskine Johnson "Hollywood Diary" *Los Angeles Daily News* September 12 1946; "Russell" in Steen *Hollywood Speaks*, 83; Russell and Chase *Banquet*, 145. Russell recalled that Nichols and Renoir had gone to Minneapolis and

returned enthusiastic, and then bought McCarthy off; [Cohn first interview with] Rosalind Russell, August 18 1953. Nichols recalled that RKO executive Charles Koerner had "begged" him to take it, and that he had later gone to Russell's house where he met Kenny and was "terribly impressed"; [Cohn interview with] Dudley Nichols, [c.1955], Cohn Papers, MHS-K.

61. "The Comic Spirit," 44.

62. The other credited screenwriters were Alexander Knox and Mary McCarthy. Most of the featured cast were respected studio actors, without Russell's star reputation. Alexander Knox, a Canadian character actor who played Anneas McDonnell, had been nominated for an Oscar for best actor for his role as Woodrow Wilson in *Wilson* (1944). Kevin Connors was played by Dean Jagger who had roles in *Woman Trap* (1936) and *Revolt of the Zombies* (1936), and as the central character in *Brigham Young* (1940). Kenny's mother was played by Beulah Bondi, a well-known character actor who had played Arrowsmith's mother-in-law in *Arrowsmith* (1931), another mother in *Mr. Smith Goes to Washington* (1939), and Jimmy Stewart's mother in *It's a Wonderful Life* (1946), and had been nominated for 2 best supporting actress Oscars in the 1930s [*The Gorgeous Hussy* (1936) and *Of Human Hearts* (1939)].

63. Dudley Nichols to Dear Mr. Cohn, November 1 [1954], Cohn Papers, MHS-K; [Cohn interview with] Rosalind Russell, April 20 1955.

64. Milton L. Gunzburg (circa 1910–1991) was the founder and president of Natural Vision 3-D Corporation. He was not credited in the film.

65. McCarthy "Outline," 3; Milton Gunzburg to McCarthy, [1942] in Kenny Collection, Margaret Herrick Library.

66. Kenny to McCarthy, September 1 1943, Mary McCarthy, 1942–1944, MHS-K.

67. [Cohn interview with] Mrs. Mary McCrae, April [n.d.] 1953, Cohn Papers, MHS-K.

68. McCracken interviews with Rogers, November 1993; see also Cohn *Sister Kenny*, 195.

69. "Sister Kenny" [Sydney] *People Magazine* June 20 1951, 7.

70. Kenny to Dear Mr. Nichols, November 9 1945, [enclosed cable to] Kenny, November 2 1945, [copy in] Cohn Papers, MHS-K.

71. [Cohn interview with] Rosalind Russell, April 20 1955; [Cohn interview with] Mary McCarthy, April 4 1953, Cohn Papers, MHS-K.

72. [Cohn interview with] Mary and Stuart McCracken, [El Monte] April 15 1955, Cohn Papers, MHS-K; Chuter to Dear Sister Kenny, September 6 1945.

73. McCarthy "Outline," 7.

74. John F. Pohl and Betty Pohl to Dear Sister Kenny, August 17 1944, Cohn Papers, MHS-K.

75. Milton Gunzburg "'Sister Kenny:' Rough Outline of Fictionized Fact" [1943], Kenny Collection, Margaret Herrick Library, 82. See also Gunzburg's suggestions that the appearance of paralyzed children be "done for laughs" so that the audience is not "wincing" with the tragedy of children becoming ill, "Rough Outline," 12.

76. Pohl and Pohl to Kenny, August 17 1944.

77. [Milton Gunzburg] "Final Script: Sister Kenny" October 27 1945, Kenny Collection, Margaret Herrick Library.

78. Kenny with Ostenso *And They Shall Walk*, 18–19. Kenny vaguely mentioned working in a "private hospital" for 3 years and winning "my certificate."

79. Curie, born in 1867, a generation before Kenny, was certainly the best-known woman scientist of the early and mid-twentieth century. In 1921 Curie had traveled to the United States, been greeted by President Warren Harding, and been widely feted. She died in 1934 at 67.

80. Gunzburg "Rough Outline," 36. Gunzburg also proposed that an angry father or grand-father threaten Brack with a gun and that Kenny save his life, "Rough Outline," 57.

81. [Gunzburg] "Final Script."

82. John McCarten "Experiment Perilous" *New Yorker* September 28 1946; see also RKO Studios "Call Bureau Cast Service" June 10 1946, Clipping File, Kenny Collection, Margaret Herrick Library.

83. [Gunzburg] "Final Script."

84. Ibid.

85. On the "somewhat hollow victory of Sister Kenny, who receives the acclaim of the children and families helped by her therapeutic methods but remains a figure on the margin of the medical profession," see Jacqueline Foertsch *Bracing Accounts: The Literature and Culture of Polio in Postwar America* (Madison: Fairleigh Dickinson University Press, 2008), 170–181.

86. Pohl and Pohl to Kenny, August 17 1944.

87. Kenny to Dear Mr. Nichols, August 12 1944, Cohn Papers, MHS-K; Kenny to Dear Mr. Nichols, September 18 1944, Cohn Papers, MHS-K.

88. Kenny to RKO Studios, August 2 1946, RKO-Misc., 1942–1948, MHS-K.

89. On the movie "jam-packed with crippled kids" with all but 6-year-old Doreen McCann "actual Institute patients" see anon. *Liberty* October 12 1946; and see Kenny to Edward Donahoe, October 4 1945, RKO-Misc., 1942–1948, MHS-K; Eddie Donahoe to Sister Kenny, October 12 1945, RKO-Misc., 1942–1948, MHS-K. Donahoe told Kenny that in most of the scenes "the little boy, David Martinson, appears. His affliction is spinal abifida [sic], and I don't know whether you would want to use him or not."

90. Kenny to RKO Studios, August 2 1946; Kenny to Manager, RKO Studio, August 3 1946, RKO-Misc., 1942–1948, MHS-K.

91. McCarthy "Kenny" [Script 1943], Kenny Collection, Margaret Herrick Library, 24. This battle would have made sense only if Kenny's background had been portrayed as working-class or lower middle-class. In the film her background is left ambiguous, but in other script versions McCarthy had tried to distance Kenny from nurses' typical class origins by making her family middle class. "When Elizabeth announced to her startled family that she wished to become a nurse, they objected heatedly. They were in quite comfortable financial circumstances, and were horrified that their daughter should set out to take a job of any kind," McCarthy "Outline," 5; on the Kenny family home as large and comfortable with many verandas and a beautiful garden, see McCarthy "Kenny," 2.

92. McCarthy "Kenny," 24–29. On Latham see Kenny and Ostenso *And They Shall Walk*, 127–129. Kenny supposedly said that what she "hated most" was to "go to teas with a lot of fat, overdressed, overbejewelled [sic] women who've never done one honest day's work in their lives"; Cohn *Sister Kenny*, 168.

93. Gunzburg " Rough Outline," 51.

94. McCarthy "Outline," 7.

95. [Gunzburg] "Final Script."

96. Ibid.

97. Kenny to Dear Mr. Nichols, August 12 1944.

98. [Cohn interview with] Rosalind Russell, April 20 1955; [Cohn interview with] Basil O'Connor, June 20 1955, Cohn Papers, MHS-K.

99. Anon. *Liberty* October 12 1946.

100. McCracken interviews with Rogers, November 1993. Guards had to be stationed to give warning when Kenny appeared on the set, for Russell "between takes, could not resist

throwing out her chest in a burlesque of the woman she admired"; Louis Berg "A Tomboy Grows Up" *Los Angeles Times* February 22 1948.

101. "War Veteran Expert on Set Authenticity" *Hartford Courant* December 9 1945.

102. Kenny to Dear Mr. Nichols, September 18 1944.

103. Ralph R. Doyle [managing director of RKO Radio Pictures in Sydney] to Dear Mr. Chuter, October 24 1945, OM 65-17, Box 3, Folder 12, Chuter Papers, Oxley-SLQ; see also Chuter to Dear Sir, September 15 1944, Box 3, Folder 19, OM 65-17, Chuter Papers, Oxley-SLQ. Nichols told the Sydney distributor to assure Chuter that "the whole script will be handled with the utmost dignity and in the pursuit of truth." Nichols admitted that some "surface details" were "inexact" but this was "only because we want to grasp more fully the spirit of truth"; Dudley Nichols to Dear Mr. Doyle, October 29 1945, OM 65-17, Box 3, Folder 12, Chuter Papers, Oxley-SLQ.

104. Chuter to Mr. Schneider [RKO Pictures, Brisbane] Memorandum: Re Script of Picture "Sister Kenny" October 23 1945, OM 65-17, Box 3, Folder 12, Chuter Papers, Oxley-SLQ.

105. Chuter to Dear Duncan [McInnes, Secretary, Toowoomba Hospitals Board], January 9 1947, Box 1, Folder 1, OM 65-17, Chuter Papers, Oxley-SLQ; Chuter to D. Schneider [RKO Pictures, Brisbane], October 15 [1947], Box 1, Folder 1, OM 65-17, Chuter Papers, Oxley-SLQ; Chuter to George Bayer [manager of Brisbane's Regent Theatre], October 30 [1947], Box 1, Folder 1, OM 65-17, Chuter Papers, Oxley-SLQ; Chuter to Kenny, October 15 [1947], Box 1, Folder 1, OM 65-17, Chuter Papers, Oxley-SLQ. Kenny attended the film's premiere in Brisbane, and also showed her technical films; on "the deep silence, and intense interest with which the films were followed" see Miss I. Martin to Dear Madam [Sister Kenny], November 6, 1947, Wilson Collection.

106. "RKO presents Sister Kenny" [advertisement] *Life* (September 16 1946) 21: 17.

107. Cedric Adams "In This Corner" *Minneapolis Star-Journal* July 5 1946.

108. "RKO presents Sister Kenny" [advertisement] *Life* (September 16 1946) 21: 17.

109. "The Wedding Gown that Waited" [advertisement] *Woman's Home Companion* [1946] 81, author's possession.

110. "RKO Presents Sister Kenny" [advertisement] *Colliers* (September 28 1946) 118: 31.

111. Poster in author's possession; for other posters see Victor Cohn "Sister Kenny's Fierce Fight for Better Polio Care" *Smithsonian Magazine* (November 1981) 12: 196; and see Hulett "Net Effect of a Commercial Motion Picture," 267.

112. [Cohn interview with] Dudley Nichols, [circa 1955], Cohn Papers, MHS-K; [Cohn interview with] Mary and Stuart McCracken, April 14 1953, Cohn Papers, MHS-K. The McCrackens told Cohn that Kenny and McCarthy had broken up after McCarthy was drinking and it became obvious that Elizabeth Dickinson and she were lesbians; Kenny was shocked and did not want to have her working on the picture. But compare: McCarthy had confided in Kenny about a nasty breakup with her girlfriend, and later wrote delightedly to tell Kenny about a new friend, saying "I'm deeply fond of her and I know you would approve of her utterly;" Mary McCarthy to My Beloved Elizabeth, February 7 1944; Mary McCarthy to Sister Dear, February 25 1944.

113. Kenny to Dear Mr. Nichols, August 12 1944; Kenny to Dear Mary [McCarthy], August 28 1944, Cohn Papers, MHS-K; Kenny to Dear Mary [McCarthy], August 12 1944, Cohn Papers, MHS-K; [Cohn first interview with] Rosalind Russell, August 18 1953; see also Alexander *Maverick*, 158–159.

114. Kenny to Dear Mr. Nichols, August 18 1944, Cohn Papers, MHS-K; Kenny to Dear Mr. Nichols, September 18 1944.

115. Kenny to Dear Mary [McCarthy], August 12 1944.

116. Ibid.

117. "Kenny Film to Be Shown Here Tonight" *Washington Times-Herald* October 22 1944; Cohn *Sister Kenny*, 193.

118. [Cohn interview with] Rosalind Russell, April 20 1955.

119. Kenny to Dear Mr. Bell, May 4 1944, James Ford Bell 1942–1946, MHS-K.

120. Harold S. Diehl "Memorandum of Conference Concerning the Future Teaching of Sister Kenny's Work and the Relation of the Medical School to the Kenny Institute and the Kenny Foundation" July 18 1944, [accessed in 1992 before recent re-cataloging], Am. 15.8, Folder 16, UMN-ASC; Kenny in [Minutes] Adjourned Meeting, Elizabeth Kenny Corporation, August 8 1944, Board of Directors, undated and 1944–1945, MHS-K.

121. Kenny to Ladies and Gentlemen, [July 1944], [accessed in 1992 before recent re-cataloging], Am. 15.8, Folder 23, UMN-ASC; [Script enclosed with] C. A. Abbott [sales manager, Ray-Bell Films] to Dear Sister Kenny, July 28 1944, Ray-Bell Films, 1944–1945, MHS-K; Kenny to Dear Dr. Boines, April 5 1945, Dr. George J. Boines, 1941–1946, MHS-K.

122. Kenny to Honorable Sir [President Truman], October 12 1945, Board of Directors, MHS-K; and see Kenny to Lionel Moise, [March 1944] [Statement], *The American Weekly*, 1943–1945, MHS-K; Kenny "Data Concerning Introduction of Kenny Concept."

123. Kenny to Gentlemen, September 25 1944, Committee to Review Request of Elizabeth Kenny Institute to National Foundation for Infantile Paralysis: General, Medical Sciences, 1944, National Academy of Sciences, Washington D.C. (hereafter Review 1944, NAS).

124. National Research Council, Division of Medical Sciences, "Report of Special Committee to Review Request Submitted by Elizabeth Kenny Institute, Inc. to National Foundation for Infantile Paralysis, Inc.," November 8 1944, Public Relations, MOD-K, 17–18.

125. "Recommendations Suggested by GBD as a Basis of Discussion," Review 1944, NAS.

126. "Sound Motion Picture on Infantile Paralysis Ready for Distribution" *National Foundation News* (June 1945) 4: 32; "Physical Therapy Film" *Archives of Physical Medicine* (September 1946) 27: 580.

127. "Kenny Film Shown to 700" *Minneapolis Star-Journal* October 13 1944; Diehl to Dear Sister Kenny, October 5 1944, Dr. Harold S. Diehl, 1941–1944, MHS-K; "Kenny Film to Be Shown Here Tonight" *Washington Times-Herald*, October 22 1944.

128. "Kenny Film Shown to 700" *Minneapolis Star-Journal* October 13 1944; "Sister Kenny Returns From East as Big Drive Opens" *Minneapolis Star-Journal* November 15 1944.

129. Kenny *A Brief Description of the Film Presenting The Kenny Concept* [pamphlet, 1945] [accessed in 1992 before recent re-cataloging], Am. 15.8, Folder 25, UMN-ASC, 9.

130. Kenny *A Brief Description of the Film Presenting The Kenny Concept*, 12; Notes taken by Naomi Rogers during the viewing of *The Kenny Concept of Infantile Paralysis*, Wilson Collection.

131. Kenny to Dear Sir [James Pooler], April 10 1945, Michigan-Newspapers, 1945, MHS-K.

132. Notes taken by Rogers of *The Kenny Concept of Infantile Paralysis*.

133. Kenny *A Brief Description of the Film Presenting The Kenny Concept*, 5; see also notes taken by Rogers of *The Kenny Concept of Infantile Paralysis*.

134. Jean Anderson to Dear Sister Kenny, September 10 1944, Case Files—Misc., A-K, 1943–1946, MHS-K.

135. Proceedings Before the Board of Regents, University of Minnesota, Minneapolis, Minnesota. In the matter of Sister Elizabeth Kenny, Elizabeth Kenny Institute, Inc., 18th and Chicago Avenue, Minneapolis, Minnesota, October 10 1945, University of Minnesota—Board

of Regents, 1945–1946, MHS-K; [Script enclosed with] C. A. Abbott [sales manager, Ray-Bell Films] to Dear Sister Kenny, July 28 1944, Ray-Bell Films, 1944–1945, MHS-K. For an example of a still from the film with caption see Sister Elizabeth Kenny *My Battle and Victory: History of the Discovery of Poliomyelitis as a Systemic Disease* (London: Robert Hale Limited, 1955), opposite 48.

136. Kenny to Dear Mr. President, Ladies and Gentlemen [of Board of Directors], [January 1945], Board of Directors, undated and 1944–1945, MHS-K.

137. Kenny to Dear Sir [James Pooler] April 10 1945.

138. Kenny *A Brief Description of the Film Presenting The Kenny Concept*, 5.

139. Notes taken by Rogers of *The Kenny Concept of Infantile Paralysis*.

140. Ibid.

141. Ibid.

142. Kenny *A Brief Description of the Film Presenting The Kenny Concept*, 7.

143. Notes taken by Rogers of *The Kenny Concept of Infantile Paralysis*; for a still of Wally see Kenny *My Battle and Victory*, opposite 65.

144. Kenny "This Is Elizabeth Kenny Speaking" [opening speech of campaign for Kenny Foundation, c.1945], [accessed in 1992 before recent re-cataloging], UMN-ASC.

145. Perkins was Harold Diehl's brother-in-law; see "Biographic Sketch of Harold Diehl," James E. Perkins, March 4 1958, Diehl, 1932–1959, Box 9, Myers Papers, UMN-ASC.

146. James E. Perkins to Dear Miss Kenny, May 15 1945, Dr. James E. Perkins, 1944–1945, MHS-K.

147. Ibid.

148. Ibid.

149. Kenny to Dear Dr. Perkins, May 23 1945, Dr. James E. Perkins, 1944–1945, MHS-K.

150. Ibid.

151. Perkins to Kenny, June 4 1945, Dr. James E. Perkins, 1944–1945, MHS-K.

152. Kenny to Dear Dr. Perkins, June 6 1945, Dr. James E. Perkins, 1944–1945, MHS-K.

153. "Doctors See Film of Kenny Cure" *New York Journal-American* [October 31 1945], Clippings, MHS-K.

154. Kent H. Powers to Dear Mr. Stone, October 13 1944, Public Relations, MOD-K.

155. JLL to CK Memorandum re Miss Kenny's Film, December 11 1944, Public Relations, MOD-K.

156. Kenny to Dear Sir [Captain L. W. White, New Zealand Air Mission], April 23 1945, Personal Correspondence and Related Papers, 1942–1951, MHS-K; Kenny to My Dear Dr. Boines, April 23 1945, Dr. George J. Boines, 1941–1946, MHS-K; [Cohn notes, after interview with] Mary and Stuart McCracken, May 19 1955, Cohn Papers, MHS-K; Alexander *Maverick*, 164, 167–169.

157. Kenny to President and Members of the Board of Directors [Institute], September 10 1945, Public Relations, MOD-K; Kenny to Honorable Sir [President Truman], October 12 1945.

158. Kenny to President and Members of the Board of Directors [Institute], September 10 1945; Kenny to Dear Doctor Bauwens, August 31 1945, Dr. Philip[pe] Bauwens, 1945–1947, MHS-K. Bauwens was a major figure in British and European physical medicine, and later was one of the founders, along with Frank Krusen, of the International Federation of Physician Medicine and Rehabilitation. A specialist in electrotherapy and clinical electromyography, he made these fields professionally respectable by bringing together the disparate physicians

working with electricity and other physical modalities into a formal organization in the 1930s, which became the British Association of Physical Medicine in 1944.

159. "Report of the Meeting of the British Association of Physical Medicine on the 'Kenny Treatment'" *British Journal of Physical Medicine* (1945) [reprinted in] *Archives of Physical Medicine* (September 1946) 27: 579–580.

160. Harold Balme, letter to editor, "The Kenney [sic] Treatment" *Lancet* (August 11 1945) 2: 186.

161. Bauwens to Dear Sister Kenny, July 31 1945, Minnesota-Hospitals, Sister Kenny Institute, 1944–1961, Judd Papers, MHS.

162. Brian Stanford to Dear Sir [Marvin Kline], September 27 1945, England—Misc., 1942, 1950, MHS-K; Marvin L. Kline to Dear Doctor Stanford, September 10 1945, England—Misc., 1942, 1950, MHS-K. See also Stanford "The Evolution of the Medical Film in Britain," 385–387.

163. Widely respected and with family connections in Belgium, Bauwens may have suggested to Kenny that she contact Leon Laruelle at the Neurological Institute in Brussels; F. S. Cooksey "Philippe Bauwens, F.R.C.P." *Rheumatology and Rehabilitation* (May 1942) 13: 49–50. According to Kenny, it was Baron Waha de Baillonville, the Belgian representative of the Red Cross in Britain, who arranged for Kenny to visit Brussels; Kenny to President and Members of the Board of Directors [Institute], September 10 1945.

164. Kenny to President and Members of the Board of Directors [Institute], September 10 1945.

165. Kenny to Dear Doctor Bauwens, August 31 1945; Kenny to President and Members of the Board of Directors [Institute], September 10 1945; Kenny to Gentlemen [Board of Regents, University of Minnesota], September 20 1945, University of Minnesota—Board of Regents, 1945–1946, MHS-K.

166. Kenny to Dear Doctor Bauwens, August 31 1945.

167. Kenny to Dear Doctor Bauwens [September 1945], Dr. Philip[pe] Bauwens, 1945–1947, MHS-K; Kenny to Dear Doctor Bauwens, August 31 1945. Laruelle had produced medical films himself in the 1930s on paraplegia, encephalitis, and other neurological conditions.

168. Kenny to Dear Doctor Bauwens, August 31 1945; Kenny to Dear Doctor Bauwens [September 1945].

169. Marvin L. Kline to Dear Doctor Bauwens, September 10 1945, Dr. Philip[pe] Bauwens, 1945–1947, MHS-K.

170. Kenny to My Dear Dean Diehl, September 22 1945, University of Minnesota—Board of Regents, 1945–1946, MHS-K.

171. John F. Pohl "The Kenny Concept and Treatment of Infantile Paralysis: Report of Five Year Study of Cases Treated and Supervised by Miss Elizabeth Kenny in America" *Journal-Lancet* (August 1945) 65: 265–271.

172. Maurice B. Visscher and Jay A. Myers [Editorial] "Sister Kenny Five Years After" *Journal-Lancet* (August 1945) 65: 309–310.

173. "'U' Medics Clash Over Success of Kenny Concept" [Minneapolis newspaper] August 23 1945, Minnesota Poliomyelitis Research Committee, Box 1, UMN-ASC.

174. Kenny to Gentlemen [Board of Regents, University of Minnesota], September 20 1945; Proceedings Before the Board of Regents, University of Minnesota, Minneapolis, Minnesota: In the matter of Sister Elizabeth Kenny, Elizabeth Kenny Institute, Inc., 18th and Chicago Avenue, Minneapolis, Minnesota, October 10 1945, University of Minnesota—Board of Regents, 1945–1946, MHS-K.

175. J. A. Myers "Poliomyelitis (Infantile Paralysis) in Minnesota Including the Elizabeth Kenny Episode" Box 19, Sister Kenny Institute 1938–1946, Myers Papers, UMN-ASC, 42.

176. Chuter to Dear Sister Kenny, May 22 1945, Box 3, Folder 12, OM 65-17, Oxley-SLQ.

177. Chuter to Dear Sister Kenny, October 29 1945, Box 3, Folder 12, OM 65-17, Chuter Papers, Oxley-SLQ; Chuter to Dear Sister Kenny, May 22 1945; [Chuter] to Dear Sister Kenny, September 27 1945, Box 3, Folder 12, OM 65-17, Chuter Papers, Oxley-SLQ; Chuter to Dear Sister Kenny, November 22 1944, Wilson Collection.

178. [Chuter] to Dear Mr. Editor, June 17 1945, Box 3, Folder 12, OM 65-17, Chuter Papers, Oxley-SLQ.

179. "Professor Attacks Sister Kenny" *Brisbane Sunday Telegraph* April 15 1945.

180. J. V. Duhig to Dear Mr. Chuter, August 5 1945, Box 3, Folder 13, OM 65-17, Chuter Papers, Oxley-SLQ.

181. [Chuter] to Dear Professor Wilkinson, August 21 1945, Box 3, Folder 12, OM 65-17, Chuter Papers, Oxley-SLQ; [Chuter] to Dear Sister Kenny, September 27 1945.

182. [Chuter] to Dear Professor Wilkinson, August 21 1945ary of Queensland; [Chuter] to Dear Sister Kenny, September 27 1945; Chuter to Dear Sister Kenny, September 6 1945.

183. [Chuter] to Dear Sister Kenny, October 5 1945, Box 3, Folder 12, OM 65-17, Chuter Papers, Oxley-SLQ.

184. [Chuter] to Dear Sister Kenny, December 20 1945, Box 3, Folder 12, OM 65-17, Chuter Papers, Oxley-SLQ.

185. [Chuter] to Dear Sister Kenny, September 27 1945; Chuter to Dear Sister Kenny, September 6 1945; Chuter to Dear Sister Kenny, October 29 1945; Chuter] to Dear Sister Kenny, October 5 1945.

186. [Chuter] to Dear Sister Kenny, September 27 1945.

187. Ibid.

188. Kenny to Dear Dr. Bauwens, October 26 1945, Dr. Philip[pe] Bauwens, 1945–1947, MHS-K; Kenny to My Dear Dr. Bauwens, December 20 1945, Dr. Philip[pe] Bauwens, 1945–1947, MHS-K. For a reference to the film in 8 different languages (French, Spanish. German, Italian, Czech, Russian, Greek and English) see "Move on Kenny Training Centre For Australia" *Toowoomba Chronicle* October 25 1951.

189. Kenny to My Dear Dr. Bauwens, February 9 1946, Dr. Philip[pe] Bauwens, 1945–1947, MHS-K.

190. Bauwens to Dear Miss Kenny, November 5 1945, Minnesota-Hospitals, Sister Kenny Institute, 1944–1961, Judd Papers, MHS; Bauwens to Dear Miss Kenny, January 15 1946, Minnesota-Hospitals, Sister Kenny Institute, 1944–1961, Judd Papers, MHS.

191. Kenny to Basil O'Connor, December 26 1946, James A. Crabtree, MHS-K. She also claimed that the Royal College of Surgeons and Physicians of Australia had "also placed this film in their library."

192. "Sister Kenny Wins Fight for Recognition" *Chicago Herald-American* February 3 1946.

193. [Cohn second interview with] Valerie Harvey, August 27 1953, Cohn Papers, MHS-K; see also [Cohn interview with] Rosalind Russell, April 20 1955; [Cohn notes, after interview with] Mary and Stuart McCracken, May 19 1955, Cohn Papers, MHS-K.

194. [Cohn interview with] Stuart McCracken, April 14 1953, Cohn Papers, MHS-K.

195. Kenny to Dear Mary [Kenny], [November 1945], Mary Stewart Kenny, 1942–1947, MHS-K.

196. Kenny to Dear Margaret [Opdahl], August 10 1945, Kenny Collection, Fryer Library; Marvin Teeter to My Dear Sister Kenny, May 10 1945, Red Cross 1942–1945, 1950, MHS-K; Kenny to Dear Miss Fraser, May 15 1945, Red Cross 1942–1945, 1950, MHS-K.

197. DWG to BO'C Memorandum: Re: Miss Kenny, July 13 1945, Public Relations, MOD-K; see also [Cohn interview with] Frank Krusen, March 24 1953, Cohn Papers, MHS-K.

198. Kenny to Dear Friend [Marvin Kline], June 13 1945, Mr. Marvin L. Kline, 1942–1959, MHS-K.

199. Secretary to Sister Elizabeth Kenny to Dear Doctor Henderson, October 6 1945, Dr. Melvin Henderson, 1942–1948, MHS-K.

200. Kenny to Honorable Sir [President Truman], October 12 1945.

201. Kenny to My Dear Mr. Chuter, October 17 1945, Box 3, Folder 12, OM 65-17, Chuter Papers, Oxley-SLQ.

202. Kenny to Dear Rosalind [Russell], October 13 1944, Cohn Papers, MHS-K.

203. Kenny to My Dear Mr. Moise, April 24 1945, *The American Weekly*, 1943–1945, MHS-K; Lionel C. Moise to Dear Sister Kenny, May 25 1945, *The American Weekly*, 1943–1945, MHS-K.

204. Nathan E. Jacobs to Dear Sister Kenny, April 9 1945, Bozell and Jacobs, 1944–1945, MHS-K.

205. Eugene Smith to Dear Sister Kenny, August 29 1946, Ray-Bell Films, 1944–1948, MHS-K.

206. F.E. Harrington and John F. Pohl to Dear Mr. Chuter, April 26 1945, Box 3, Folder 12, OM 65-17, Chuter Papers, Oxley-SLQ.

207. Nora Housden to Dear Sister Kenny, December 9 1948, Belgium—Nora Housden, 1948–1950, MHS-K.

208. Kenny to Dr. Edward L. Compere, February 12, 1945, Edward L. Compere, 1942–1945, MHS-K.

209. Kenny to Mr. President, Ladies and Gentlemen [of Board of Directors], February 14 1945, Board of Directors, undated and 1944–1945, MHS-K.

210. Ruth McMahon to My Dear Sister Kenny, September 25 1950, General Correspondence–M, MHS-K.

211. "Sister Kenny Seeks an Institute Here To Care for Infantile Paralysis Victims" *New York Times* November 11 1944; Chester LaRoche to Dear Marvin [Kline], December 3 1945, Clara and Chester LaRoche, 1945–1948, MHS-K.

212. Kenny's description "for the lay person" is from Kenny to Dennis Rigan, February 27 1948, Michigan-Misc., 1942–1951, MHS-K; see also notes taken by Naomi Rogers during the viewing of *The Value of a Life*, Wilson Collection.

213. Kenny to Mrs. A. D. Cohen, November 14 1945, Kenneth Kerr and Dolly Cohen, Ohio Fund Drive, 1945–1946, MHS-K.

214. Kenny to My Dear Mary and Stuart [McCracken], September 24 1946, Mary Stewart Kenny, 1942–1947, MHS-K.

215. Robert Murphy "20,000 Break Lines to See Sister Kenny" *Minneapolis Star-Journal* [c. September 1946], Scrapbook 1945–1952, 1956, Henry Papers, MHS.

216. "'Sister Kenny' Premiere Complete With Stars and Bright Lights" [Minneapolis newspaper, unnamed] [October 1946], Scrapbook 1945–1952, 1956, Henry Papers, MHS; "At 'Sister Kenny' Premier" [Minneapolis newspaper, unnamed] [October 1946], Scrapbook 1945–1952, 1956, Henry Papers, MHS.

217. "The Wedding Gown That Waited" [advertisement], *Woman's Home Companion* [1946] 81, copy in author's possession.

218. Velma West Sykes "'Sister Kenny' Is Voted the Winner of November Blue Ribbon Award" *Boxoffice* (December 14 1946) 50: 20.

219. "From the New York PM" *Minneapolis Morning Tribune* October 5 1946; Louella O. Parsons "In Hollywood: Sister Kenny Triumph for Rosalind Russell" *Los Angeles Examiner*, October 11 1946; "Movie of the Week: 'Sister Kenny'" *Life* (September 16 1946) 21: 77.

220. See Howard Barnes, *New York Tribune* [1946] in Clipping File, Kenny Collection, Margaret Herrick Library.

221. Karl Krug "'Sister Kenny' Good" *Pittsburgh Sun Telegraph* [November] 1946, Public Relations, MOD-K.

222. Hulett to Gentlemen [National Foundation], August 22 1946, Public Relations, MOD-K; see also J. E. Hulett, Jr. "Estimating the Net Effect of a Commercial Motion Picture Upon the Trend of Local Public Opinion" *American Sociological Review* (April 1949) 14: 263–275. Note that Hulett had already contacted Peter Cusack about doing a study of the "sociological aspects" of Kenny's campaign; J. E. Hulett, Jr. to Dear Sir [Peter Cusack], June 28 1944, Public Relations, MOD-K; see also J.E. Hulett, Jr. "The Kenny Healing Cult: Preliminary Analysis of Leadership and Patterns of Interaction," *American Sociological Review* (June 1945) 10: 364–372.

223. Cusack to Naftzger, November 22 1944, Public Relations, MOD-K; Peter J. A. Cusack to Frank H. Higgins, [telegram], January 10 1945, Public Relations, MOD-K; Phillip K. Scheuer "New Picture Poignant" *Los Angeles Times* December 12 1944.

224. Unlike later movies such as *Sunrise at Campobello* (Warner Brothers, 1960) and *Interrupted Melody* (MGM, 1955), this film "calls constant attention to the name of polio and its specific clinical manifestations"; Foertsch *Bracing Accounts*, 170–181.

225. [Handwritten note, no signature] "This man wrote..." Public Relations, MOD-K; George La Porte to Dear Professor Hullett [sic], September 23 1946, Public Relations, MOD-K.

226. Hulett, Jr. "Estimating the Net Effect of a Commercial Motion Picture," 263–275.

227. Judith Klein "'Sister Kenny' Film Seen Raising False Hopes" *[New York] Herald Tribune* October 6 1946.

228. Archer Winsten "Movie Talk: Movie House Murals as Clean As Pictures Shown on Screen" *New York Post* November 1 1946.

229. Florence Fisher Parry "I Dare Say: Difference Between Therapy and Cure" *Pittsburgh Press* November 13 1946.

230. "Movie of the Week: 'Sister Kenny'" *Life* (September 16 1946) 21: 77–78, 80.

231. "A Doctor Comments on 'Sister Kenny'" *Life* (September 16 1946) 21: 77–82.

232. "New Polio Center Set Up in N.Y." *National Foundation News* (September–October 1945) 4: 41–42.

233. "At 59 Sister Kenny Is Undaunted" *Life* (September 16 1946) 21: 82.

234. Ed Sullivan "Little Old New York: I've Got News for You" *New York Daily News* October 17 1946; "Little Old New York: The Passing Show" *New York Daily News* October 31 1946.

235. Editorial "Sister Kenny: Problem Child of Medicine" *New York Medicine* (November 20 1946) 2: 413–414.

236. Ed Sullivan "Little Old New York: I Have News for You" *New York Daily News* December 5 1946; Sullivan "Little Old New York: The Passing Show" *New York Daily News* October 31 1946; see also Cohn *Sister Kenny*, 207.

237. Marvin Kline to Dear Mr. Sullivan, December 6 1946, Ed Sullivan, 1946–1947, MHS-K.

238. Winsten "Movie Talk: Movie House Murals as Clean As Pictures Shown on Screen."

239. Joe Savage to Dear Jim [James Bryan], November 8 1946, Public Relations, MOD-K.

240. "The National Foundation for Infantile Paralysis Discusses the Kenny Question" [January 1947], Public Relations, MOD-K. On "fears that Rosalyn [sic] Russell's motion picture might injure us" John B. Middleton [Regional Director] "Memorandum: Re: Statement on Kenny Drive Activities 1946" to George La Porte, June 26 1946, Public Relations, MOD-K.

241. "Sister Kenny" *[New York] Motion Picture Daily* July 16 1946.

242. Dudley Nichols to Dear Sister, April 15 1947, RKO-Misc., 1942–1948, MHS-K. On Russell's recollections that "RKO had a hard time drumming up much enthusiasm among exhibitors" see Russell and Chase *Banquet*, 145–146.

243. Paul Hollister to Dear Perry [Lieber], April 8 1947, RKO-Misc., 1942–1948, MHS-K; [draft of letter to be signed by Kenny] [enclosed in] Paul Hollister to Dear Perry [Lieber], April 8 1947, RKO-Misc., 1942–1948, MHS-K.

244. Editorial "Experiment Perilous" *Westchester Medical Bulletin* (November 1946) 14: 25–26, [copy in] Public Relations, MOD-K.

245. "The Sister Kenny Film" *The Lamp* (February 1947) 4: 14, Wilson Collection.

246. "A great many uniformed people will be badly confused by this film, which is presumably intended to spread confidence and light"; Bosley Crowther "Sizing 'Sister Kenny" *New York Times* October 6 1946. See also "vitally interested families may take its one-sided message too deeply to heart. They should be wanted that the picture's natural enthusiasm of the biography renders it somewhat misleading as present-day scientific gospel"; Winsten "Movie Talk: Movie House Murals as Clean As Pictures Shown on Screen."

247. Eileen Creelman *New York Sun* [1946] in Clipping File, Kenny Collection, Margaret Herrick Library.

248. *Time* review [September 30 1946], reprinted in *Minneapolis Morning Tribune* October 3 1946; John Pohl to Dear Sir [*Time*] [1946], [accessed in 1992 before recent re-cataloging], UMN-ASC.

249. At the end of a review of "Madame Curie" the *New Yorker* film critic did ask plaintively whether "someday" a film would "be made about a scientist who was not scoffed at by the authorities...who did not have to surmount insurmountable obstacles to reach his goal...who lolled in luxury, [and] knocked off an invention or two when he felt like it"; David Lardner "Popular Science" *New Yorker* (December 18 1943), 19: 53–54.

250. Crowther "Sizing 'Sister Kenny'"; Editorial "Sister Kenny: Problem Child of Medicine," 413–414; see also Crowther's comments on the "eulogistic and romantic treatment" of growing numbers of "living biography" Hollywood films; Crowther "Living Biographies, Hollywood Style," *New York Times* January 20 1946.

251. John McCarten "Experiment Perilous" *New Yorker* (September 28 1946) 22: 91–93. The title of the review was a reference to the 1944 RKO thriller of the same name.

252. Ray Pospisil [Miami Florida] to Sister Kenny, February 14 1947, General Correspondence, February 11–28 1947, MHS-K.

253. Mrs. H. P. Schoening [Allegan, Michigan] to Sister Kenny, December 26 1946, General Correspondence, February 1–10 1947, MHS-K.

254. Leon A. Colton [Milwaukee] to Sister Kenny, January 19 1947, General Correspondence, February 1–10 1947, MHS-K.

255. Alda Erma Cononna [River Edge, New Jersey] to Sister Kenny, December 29 1946, General Correspondence, February 1–10 1947, MHS-K.

256. Helen E. Sente [Hastings on Hudson, New York] to Sister Kenny, January 30 1947, General Correspondence, February 1–10 1947, MHS-K.

257. Mrs. Don D. Lariscy to My Dear Sister Kenny, May 15 1947, General Correspondence, June 1947, MHS-K.

258. Secretary to Sister Elizabeth Kenny to My Dear Mrs. Lariscy, June 6 1947, General Correspondence, June 1947, MHS-K.

259. Mrs. Mary Cavallaro [Brooklyn] to Sister Kenny, January 16 1947, General Correspondence, March 15–31 1947, MHS-K.

260. [Lewin] "Preamble to the Proposal for the Establishment of a Polio Unit at Michael Reese Hospital" [1946], Public Relations, Lewin, MOD; Kenny to My Dear Mr. O'Connor [form letter], January 18 1946 [1947], Public Relations, MOD-K.

261. Kenny to Dear Doctor Stimson, October 8 1945, Public Relations, MOD-K.

262. "New Controversy Forecast as Result of Kenny Movie" *Minneapolis Morning Tribune* September 13 1946.

263. Stimson to Kenny, September 19 1946, in Stimson, [Scrapbook] "Sister Elizabeth Kenny and Her Treatment of Acute Poliomyelitis in The United States as Experienced and Taught by Philip M. Stimson, M.D." [1969], Rare Book and Manuscript Collection, New York Academy of Medicine, New York City.

264. Excerpts from minutes of the staff meeting [Public Relations], September 10 1946, Public Relations, MOD-K. "If you have not already seen it, I would like to call your attention to the statement by Dr. Philip Stimson in Life Magazine for September 16, relative to the Sister Kenny movie"; "Dear Mr.____" September 19 1946, Public Relations, MOD-K.

265. Kenny to Philip M. Stimson, October 2 1946, in Stimson [Scrapbook].

266. Kenny to Dear Mr. Hearn, December 2 1946, Richard J. Hearn 1946, MHS-K.

267. E. B. Radcliffe "Show Mirror" *Enquirer* [1946], Public Relations, MOD-K.

268. [Cohn interview with] Al Baum and Mrs. Baum, June 14 1955, Cohn Papers, MHS-K.

269. Philip Stimson in "Conferences on Therapy: Treatment of Poliomyelitis" *New York State Journal of Medicine* (April 1 1945) 45: 1–6.

270. Hazel Macdonald "Doctors, Discuss Polio, Sister Kenny" [unnamed newspaper] May 2 1947, Clippings 1945–1947, MHS-K; see also "Conferences on Therapy: Treatment of Poliomyelitis" *New York State Journal of Medicine* (April 1 1945) 45: 3.

271. Kenny, Report to Board of Directors of the Sister Elizabeth Kenny Foundation; Kenny to Mr. President, Mrs. Webber and Gentlemen, May 24 1948, Board of Directors, MHS-K.

272. Stimson, [Scrapbook].

273. Minister for Health and Home Affairs to Dear Mr. Pike [Agent General for Queensland, London] July 23 1946, Home Secretary's Office, Special Batches, Kenny Clinics, 1941–1949, A/31753, QSA; [Cohn interview with] Abe Fryberg, [c. 1953], Cohn Papers, MHS-K; "Doctors For U.S. To See Kenny Style" *Brisbane Courier-Mail* May 22 1946.

274. "Report on Concepts and Treatment of Poliomyelitis by Thomas Victor Stubbs Brown, M.B., B.S., F.R.C.S. Ed., Senior Orthopaedic Surgeon, Brisbane Hospital and Abraham Fryberg, M.B., D.P.H., D.T.M., Deputy Director-General of Health and Medical Services, Brisbane, 6th December, 1946," OM 65-7, 2/5, Chuter Papers, Oxley-SLQ.

275. J. A. Myers to Dear Maurice [Visscher], March 31 1947, Box 19, Folder 1, Myers Papers, UMN-ASC; Myers to Dear Dr. Visscher, June 13 1946, Box 1, Minnesota Poliomyelitis Research Committee Collection, UMN-ASC.

276. [handwritten] Maurice [Visscher] to Myers, n.d., on Myers to Dear Maurice, March 31 1947, Box 19, Folder 1, Myers Papers, UMN-ASC.

277. [Chuter] to Dear Abe [Fryberg] December 24 [19]46, Wilson Collection; Kenny to Dear Doctor Diehl, February 7 1946, Dr. Harold S. Diehl, 1941–1944 [sic], MHS-K; Chuter to Dear

Mr. Kelly, May 27 1946, Box 3, Folder 12, OM 65-17, Chuter Papers, Oxley-SLQ. Mary Kenny was married in May 1946.

278. H. J. Summers "Sister Kenny Says It's Goodbye This Time" *Brisbane Courier Mail* November 18 1947; "Sister Kenny Scorns 'Modern' Polio Methods" *Brisbane Courier Mail* November 11 1947.

279. "Sister Kenny to End U.S. Work, Aide Says," *New York Times* February 14 1947; "Says Sister Kenny Retires Friday" *Philadelphia Evening Bulletin* February 13 1947.

280. Chuter to Dear Sister Kenny, August 19 1947, Box 1, Folder 6, OM 65-17, Chuter Papers, Oxley-SLQ; Chuter to Dear Sister Kenny, April 21 1947, Box 1, Folder 1, OM 65-17, Chuter Papers, Oxley-SLQ.

281. Hoyts Regent [advertisement] "Sister Kenny" *Brisbane Telegraph* October 16 1947. See also [advertisement] "Sister Kenny" [unnamed Brisbane newspaper] December 31 1947, OM 65-17, Box 3, Folder 19, Chuter Papers, Oxley-SLQ.

282. Lon Jones "Bitter Storm Likely Over Kenny Film" *Brisbane Telegraph* November 21 1945; "Kenny Film Hits At Doctors Here" *Brisbane Telegraph* July 12 1946.

283. "Will Attack Kenny Film" *Brisbane Sunday Mail* December 9 1945; "Sister Kenny Prepares For Her Hardest Battle" *Brisbane Telegraph* September 25 1947; "Sister Kenny" *[Sydney] People Magazine* June 20 1951, 6–7.

284. "Sister Kenny: Life Story in Film" *Toowoomba Chronicle* [October] 1947, Box 3, Folder 19, OM 65-17, Chuter Papers, Oxley-SLQ.

285. Kenny "My First Experience with the Disease...[Report of European Trip 1947]" [1947], Biographical Data, MHS-K.

FURTHER READING

On the history of medicine and film see Bruce Babbington "'To Catch a Star on Your Fingertips': Diagnosing the Medical Biopic from *The Story of Louis Pasteur* to *Freud*" in Graeme Harper and Andrew Moor eds. *Signs of Life: Medicine and Cinema* (London: Wallflower, 2005), 120–131; Timothy M. Boon *Films of Fact: A History of Science in Documentary Films and Television* (London: Wallflower Press, 2008); David Cantor "Uncertain Enthusiasm: The American Cancer Society, Public Education, and the Problems of the Movie, 1921–1960" *Bulletin of the History of Medicine* (2007) 81: 39–69; T. Hugh Crawford "Glowing Dishes: Radium, Marie Curie, and Hollywood" *Biography* (2000) 23: 71–89; George F. Custen *Bio/Pics: How Hollywood Constructed Public History* (New Brunswick: Rutgers University Press, 1992); Peter E. Dans *Doctors in the Movies: Boil the Water and Just Say Ahh* (Bloomington, IL: Medi-Ed Press, 2000); Thomas Doherty *Projections of War: Hollywood, American Culture and World War II* (New York: Columbia University Press, 1993); Marianne Fedunkiw "Malaria Films: Motion Pictures as a Public Health Tool" *American Journal of Public Health* (2003) 93: 1046–1057; Lester D. Friedman ed. *Cultural Sutures: Medicine and Media* (Durham: Duke University Press, 2004); Bert Hansen *Picturing Medical Progress from Pasteur to Polio: A History of Mass Media Images and Popular Attitudes in America* (New Brunswick: Rutgers University Press, 2009); Graeme Harper and Andrew Moor eds. *Signs of Life: Cinema and Medicine* (London: Wallflower Press, 2005); Philip A. Kalisch and Beatrice J. Kalisch "The Image of the Nurse in Motion Pictures" *American Journal of Nursing* (1982) 82: 605–611; Anne Karpf *Doctoring the Media: The Reporting of Health and Medicine* (London: Routledge, 1988); Susan E. Lederer *Frankenstein: Penetrating the Secrets of Nature* (New Brunswick: Rutgers University Press, 2002); Susan E. Lederer "Repellent Subjects: Hollywood Censorship and Surgical Images in the 1930s" *Literature and Medicine* (1998) 17: 91–113; Susan E. Lederer and John Parascandola "Screening Syphilis: Dr. Ehrlich's Magic Bullet Meets the Public Health Service" *Journal of the History of Medicine and Allied Sciences* (1998) 53: 345–370; Susan E. Lederer and Naomi Rogers "Media" in Roger Cooter and John Pickstone eds. *Medicine in the Twentieth Century* (London: Harwood, 2000), 487–502; Gregg Mitman "Cinematic Nature: Hollywood Technology, Popular Culture, and the American Museum of Natural History" *Isis* (1993) 84: 637–661; Martin F. Norden *The Cinema of Isolation: A History of Physical Disability in the Movies* (New Brunswick: Rutgers University Press, 1994); Kristin Ostherr *Cinematic Prophylaxis: Globalization and Contagion in the Discourse of World Health* (Durham: Duke University Press, 2005); John Parascandola *Sex, Sin, and Science: A History of Syphilis in America* (Westport, CT: Praeger, 2008); Martin S. Pernick *The Black Stork: Eugenics and the Death of 'Defective' Babies in American Medicine and Motion Pictures since 1915* (New York: Oxford University Press, 1996); Leslie J. Reagan, Nancy Tomes, and Paula A. Treichler eds. *Medicine's Moving Pictures: Medicine, Health, and Bodies in American Film and Television* (Rochester: University of Rochester Press, 2007); Miriam Posner "Depth Perception: Filmmaking and Narrative in American Medicine" Ph.D. dissertation in Film Studies and American Studies, Yale University, 2011; Naomi Rogers "'Sister Kenny'" *Isis* (1993) 84: 772–774; Eric Schaefer *"Bold! Daring! Shocking! True!:" A History of Exploitation Films, 1919–1959* (Durham: Duke University Press, 1999); David Serlin ed. *Imaging Illness: Public Health and Visual Culture* (Minneapolis: University of Minnesota Press, 2010); Kay Sloan *The Loud Silents: Origins of the Social Problem Film* (Urbana: University of Illinois Press, 1988); Christopher R. Smit and Anthony Enns eds. *Screening Disability: Essays on Cinema and Disability* (Lanham, MD: University Press of America, 2001); Ken Smith *Mental Hygiene: Classroom Films, 1945–1970* (New York: Blast Books, 1999).

PART THREE

7

Kenny Goes to Washington

IN MAY 1948 Kenny went to Washington to speak as an expert witness before the House Committee on Interstate and Foreign Commerce investigating whether and how the government should fund medical research. Wearing a corsage, a circle pin, strands of pearls, and a plumed hat, the white haired nurse praised a proposed Medical Research Foundation that would study polio as well as cancer and other "degenerative diseases." "Mobilization of forces and pooling of knowledge concerning this disease are imperative," Kenny told the committee. As the cameras clicked in a room packed with Congressmen and their aides, Kenny admitted that friends had advised her "not to interfere in any way with American politics" but she was nonetheless certain that the federal government should support medical research and "should undertake to see that every avenue is explored to wipe out this disease."[1]

Kenny was invited to testify as a healer and medical celebrity, but most of all she was welcomed as a medical populist. Her presence transformed the Washington hearings into a platform to attack organized medicine, especially the policies of the nation's largest polio philanthropy, the National Foundation for Infantile Paralysis (NFIP). The NFIP, Kenny complained, used its power as a polio monopoly to deny her scientific respect. NFIP officials were organizing an international conference on polio to be held in July, but Kenny had heard that "my appearance at this meeting would mean that they would have to close the door."[2] A new government research agency run by unbiased officials could, she was sure, challenge the NFIP's power and, in this era of global tensions, demonstrate to other nations America's commitment to providing children with the best polio care based on the most modern knowledge of the disease.

Many members of the House committee agreed that the NFIP was an elitist medical monopoly, "a sort of medical closed shop, run for the benefit of certain doctors and certain politicians, perhaps more than for the benefit of the patients," as a Republican Congressman from Missouri noted.[3] Although Roosevelt's death in April 1945 had left the NFIP without a political patron in the White House, Basil O'Connor, Roosevelt's former friend and advisor, had strong ties to America's social and scientific elite, especially the conservative leadership of the American Medical Association (AMA) through his friendship with Morris Fishbein. Fishbein's antipathy to alternative medicine and any government incursion into traditional medicine was reflected in the NFIP as well. Over the previous decade the NFIP had come to play a significant if somewhat hidden role in shaping American medical politics. O'Connor had moved the professional weight of the NFIP behind some of the more conservative forces in medicine, including the provivisection National Society for Medical Research and Fishbein's campaign against government health insurance. The NFIP was growing away from its early Democratic affiliations and closer to the Republican Party, the political affiliation of most American physicians in the 1940s and 1950s.

Scientific research and health care were crucial elements of national politics between 1945 and 1950. The experience of World War II had reinforced the notion that a government agency could effectively direct research priorities and that such research, based on widely shared goals, would provide concrete solutions. The American public, already impressed with the scientific achievements made during the war—penicillin, radar, the atomic bomb—saw research as having the potential to improve the world and everyday lives. World War II, as historian Victoria Harden described it, "enhanced public belief that scientific research offered an endless frontier on which a happier, healthier life could be built."[4] Not surprisingly, many witnesses at congressional hearings framed the debate on research policy within a broader project by liberal Truman Democrats to centralize and restructure American health care.

The federal government was becoming a major player in shaping the confusing quilt of medical research programs in peacetime. The Cold War now provided a new urgency for Congress to take a more active role in funding research. Against this cultural attitude and opponents like Kenny the NFIP had to defend its control of polio research funding in terms of democratic, responsive, health care management and to convince Congress and the public that private philanthropies should retain a respected place in the unsettled world of health policy.

Kenny came to Washington in the midst of a raucous debate over the National Science Foundation (NSF). In August 1947, President Truman had vetoed an NSF bill giving scientists significant control, explaining he was not willing to "vest the determination of vital national policies...in a group of individuals who would essentially be private citizens...[and] would be divorced from control by the people to an extent that implies... the state's lack of faith in the democratic process."[5] Immersed in postwar politics, the NSF bill became a powerful symbol of the changing relationship between government and the research community. Scientists feared rigid government bureaucrats; federal officials distrusted ivory-tower researchers; politicians wanted research that would lead to innovative technologies as dramatic as penicillin and the atomic bomb; and the public sought a fair, democratic, and representative science research policy. Privately Truman told science advisor Vannevar Bush that a science foundation run by a board of scientists outside government would become "simply a log-rolling affair to make grants to things that its members were interested in."[6]

The story of the battle between Kenny and the NFIP allows us a new, rather unexpected look at the ways medical populism shaped postwar science policy. Populism in medicine is difficult to analyze and even harder to categorize. The version of medical populism, spurred by Kenny and her allies, challenged orthodox medicine's claims to authority, yet demanded access to medical science so that the people's health could be protected through scientific research. What Kenny and her allies promoted was a vision of populist science that idealized science and its products but attacked representatives of professional authority. A focus on such critics of medical orthodoxy thus complicates the accepted picture of postwar America as the era of organized medicine's Golden Age, when public respect for medical science was unrivaled and doctors in film and radio were always the good guys.[7]

The stream of populism that Kenny drew on was composed of elements from both the left and the right. These dissidents were against the medical establishment; they feared elitism and corporate conspiracy but idealized the tools and products of science. The people's health was threatened, according to Kenny and her supporters, by narrow-minded medical professionals unwilling to consider ideas promoted by anyone outside elite medical institutions. Yet truth could be gained not only by the work of mainstream scientists but also when scientific tools became resources available to all.

The struggle between Kenny and the NFIP that played out publicly at the 1948 hearings was part of a wider battle over the direction of research policy, especially over whether Congress should mandate lay representatives on the boards of its new research agencies to provide alternative views to the scientific and medical establishment. Kenny's testimony in Washington blasting medical elitism and parochial, inaccurate science exemplified the debate among politicians, philanthropic officials, the public, and even a few scientists in postwar America over the relationship between research and democracy.

POPULISM AND THE GOLDEN AGE OF AMERICAN MEDICINE

Leaders of organized medicine tended to lump all medical populists together as quacks and cultists, and fought them with the help of state legislatures, the courts, and the media. To fight back, populists spoke of medical freedom—sometimes as an antigovernmental ideology, and sometimes as a resource to battle elitist professionals. Across American history medical populists have simultaneously pushed away and reached for government resources in their efforts to challenge medical trusts. Discoverers of anticancer tonics and rejuvenating operations, naturopaths, chiropractors, and others on the margins of the medical profession developed a populist ideology that drew on the public sympathy for outsiders fighting elitism. When these struggles entered the political arena they tended to find allies among right-wing politicians. Kenny was a newcomer to American politics but her claim that as an outsider she deserved scientific respectability and needed to be defended against Big Medicine and Big Science (as represented by the AMA and the NFIP) had deep political resonance.

Despite a lingering faith in the Thomas Edison-type lone inventor, the prospect of massive government investment into medical research grabbed the public imagination. But there was no consensus on how the government would ensure that its resources would be provided to researchers who would make the most important medical breakthroughs.

At the time of the Congressional hearings, most medical research remained diffuse and unregulated, relying on donations from large and small private organizations, often known as foundations, which were frequently single-disease charities that also paid for patient care.[8] After the war this patchwork system of research funding seemed old fashioned and inefficient, but what model should replace it was less clear.

Elite scientists argued that research funding should be based on a "best science" model, but politicians in postwar America recognized the competing popular appeal for a "geographic" model, a kind of science democracy in which government money was distributed state by state, available not just for privileged academic researchers but for ordinary investigators. In what historian Harry Marks has called the "highly pluralist postwar system of medical research" Congress divided over whether the development of such research should be left in the hands of universities, private research institutes, and philanthropies or should be overseen by a government agency.[9]

As the NSF bill was reintroduced in 1948 a provocative study in *Science* reinforced Truman's sense that scientists could not be relied on to put the public's interest ahead of loyalty to their own institution or discipline. The study, quoted during the NSF Congressional hearings, found that almost 75 percent of the research funds distributed by scientists on the advisory boards of 10 private philanthropies—including the NFIP—went to researchers based at elite, Northeastern universities. Thus, it concluded, "our top scientists are no more able to provide equitable distribution of funds at their disposal than are the politicians they have so castigated."[10] Although Fishbein pointed out to O'Connor privately that the NFIP "comes off very well in comparison with other similar agencies," the *Science* study was a blow to the idea of objective peer review, and useful for those who argued that geographic distribution of research funds would be just as meritorious as any other system.[11]

An early test of whether the country was ready to apply populist-defined democratic principles to scientific research came in 1945 when Harry Hoxsey, accompanied by 3 Congressmen, traveled to Washington, D.C. to ask the National Cancer Institute for a federal investigation of his anticancer powder. Hoxsey was the founder of his own National Cancer Research Institute in Taylorsville, Illinois.[12] The Institute turned down this request, but North Dakota Senator William Langer, a distinctive Plains populist who mistrusted big government, Communists, and Jews took up Hoxsey's cause. Langer championed Kenny's cause as well. In 1944 Langer had introduced a Senate resolution proposing $10,000,000 for an Infantile Paralysis Control Board to be chaired by the Surgeon General and composed of Kenny herself and a "leading medical man" from each of the 48 states and Washington, D.C. "to investigate and study the origin, causes, and means of control of infantile paralysis."[13] The resolution did not pass but Langer continued to try to have the government support Kenny's work. In 1945 he suggested that the federal government establish a national polio clinic run by a board made up not of physicians but of "persons who have had infantile paralysis and have been treated for such disease in accordance with the methods discovered and practiced by Sister Elizabeth Kenny." He also proposed federal funding for a polio research program to foster the national adoption of Kenny's method.[14]

Hoxsey and others demanded a populist version of medical research, and hoped that the federal government would respond with respectful attention and perhaps funding. This nascent research populism fit awkwardly with a growing anticommunist, antiintellectual populist movement that feared the liberal Eastern establishment and its decadent bureaucracy. Members of the public, enthusiastic about government-sponsored research as an antidote to elitism, hoped that federal oversight would temper the power of elite scientists and physicians.

In the postwar years many Americans saw the NFIP, a lay-run disease-oriented charity, as old-fashioned and out of touch with modern epidemiological and structural changes in American life. The NFIP's distinctive style—especially its extensive resources and access to celebrities—was under attack. During the late 1940s, reinforced by public attention to the shift from infectious to chronic diseases, Americans began to see disease philanthropies as often inefficient and led by directors who were "aristocratic, aloof, and egotistical." Social scientists pointed out that without proper yardsticks to measure the organizations' effectiveness, many programs were duplicated.[15] The solution seemed to be single, federated fund drives such as Community Chest and Red Feather campaigns that were seen as more efficient and more effective.[16] In 1947 when Henry Ford II became the new head of the Ford Motor Company he began to organize a United Health and Welfare Fund with the cooperation of the AFL and the CIO.[17]

Polio epidemics were still as frightening as ever, but there was now a sense that perhaps too many resources were being used to fight a disease that affected a relatively small number of people compared to the funds being spent on research into diseases such as heart disease and cancer, which, as one science writer noted in 1946, "are the chief killers in America."[18] In 1947, when medical historian Richard Shryock wrote a brief history of medical research in America, he made almost no reference to the NFIP, a striking omission. In a footnote Shryock did compare the amount of money spent on research of serious health problems such as heart disease (17 cents per death) to polio (over 500 dollars) to show that "standard research expenditures are seriously unbalanced."[19]

Across the country communities began to set up United Fund agencies in response to "the nuisance of multiple fund raising appeals."[20] A widely read expose by Selskar Gunn and Philip Platt, financed by the Rockefeller Foundation, of 569 charities (or as they called them "voluntary agencies") and 143 official agencies out of the approximately 20,000 nonprofit health agencies in the United States found that many had no centralized organization, poor leadership, and, despite vast expenditures, did not meet community health needs. In their opinion, most services performed by individual health agencies should be combined, especially fundraising activities.[21] Reviewers praised the study's "valid and objective analysis" that had pointed out "the emotional, sentimentalized, and frequently misdirected efforts of expensively planned and disproportionately financed programs [and]...the waste, inefficiency, duplications of service, and actual selfishness inherent in unco-ordinated planning."[22] They also noted the tremendous disparity between the resources of the NFIP ($12 million in 1944) compared to other agencies like the American Heart Association (only $100,000 the same year).[23]

KENNY AS POPULIST EXPERT

Kenny's path from unknown nurse in the Australian bush to medical celebrity had become a familiar tale by the late 1940s, retold in family magazines, her autobiography, and the 1946 movie *Sister Kenny*. She embraced her celebrity status, and liked to talk to reporters and be photographed. But she did not like to be contradicted and increasingly sought out occasions in which she was surrounded by friends and supporters. "The best seats in every theatre are at her disposal; the Police recognize her and stop the traffic; and altogether I felt on my visit with her that I was with Royalty," one Australian visitor gushed.[24]

Despite her claims of political naiveté Kenny demonstrated a keen understanding of the nation's medical politics. She had long argued that American patients with polio needed more than improved therapy. They needed to be protected from practice by professionals who understood polio only in orthodox ways. In her technical film, which she showed the Congressional committee, the narrator highlighted her concept the polio, praising the "newer science" based on the "advanced concept."[25] Kenny had also hoped that her Institute in Minneapolis would become a research facility like New York's Rockefeller Institute. But she and her supporters had come to realize that no scientist was going to base himself at the Institute to do research to demonstrate the veracity of her theories.[26] When, despite its deep pockets, the NFIP had rejected the Institute's formal request for research funding, Kenny's sense that scientific research was organized by an elite group that funded themselves and their friends was confirmed. "Universities interested in studying poliomyelitis," John Pohl had noted bitterly to KF executive director Marvin Kline, "are already under the thumb of the National Foundation through the issuance of financial grants." Like Kenny, Pohl disassociated himself from the NFIP. His daughter Mary who was treated for a mild case of polio in 1946 recalled that, unlike most of her friends' families, her parents did not contribute to March of Dimes campaigns and "never had anything to do with the March of Dimes."[27] Even though in 1948 talk of a vaccine was only talk, Kenny assured the Congressional committee that no vaccine would be possible until the scientific community accepted her concept of the disease.[28]

Throughout her life Kenny tried to balance her role as a medical celebrity (having cocktails with Rosalind Russell and her Hollywood friends), as the people's healer (attacking medical elitism and rescuing patients from disabilities and from unnecessary orthopedic operations), and as a scientific innovator directing a research and teaching institute. These somewhat contradictory elements of her public persona had come to serve her well. In a 1947 poll of the 10 most admired living people in the world, Eleanor Roosevelt (sixth) and Sister Kenny (ninth) were the only women to make the list.[29]

Being a populist expert, though, was tricky. Kenny yearned to be welcomed as a scientific discoverer, invited to speak at conferences, have her work quoted in medical journals, and see her concepts become the basis for scientific investigation. At the hearings she repeated a promise she had made to her Australian medical mentor Aeneas McDonnell "that I would keep with the duly qualified medical practitioner until he saw the light [for]... I know that if I did veer out a little from the straight and narrow path, that the duly qualified medical practitioners would have nothing to do with me."[30] But she directed an Institute named after herself and promoted a method and theory that carried her name. It made her sound uncomfortably like a patent medicine hawker. Her use of publicity—her many speeches, her technical film, her interviews with local and national reporters—was as extensive as the NFIP's but lacked the patina of the latter's elite medical connections.

By the time she appeared before Congress there were 3 new Kenny centers: in Buffalo, Jersey City, and Centralia, Illinois. In Buffalo Kenny's work had been promoted by Marvin Israel, a pediatrician whose teenage son had recovered from polio after being treated by his father based on advice from John Pohl. In May 1948, after Israel's death, a wide movement encompassing local Jewish, Catholic, and Protestant religious groups, as well as the local Variety Club, established a Kenny clinic in Buffalo and made fundraising for it a civic cause.[31] In Centralia, a small railroad and coal mining town in southern Illinois, parents had been frustrated during a 1946 epidemic by a lack of facilities that had left their paralyzed children "all night in motor cars, unattended and uncared [for]."[32] Kenny and Marvin Kline attended the dedication ceremony for Centralia's new Kenny clinic in August 1947. The ceremony included benedictions by a priest and a Baptist minister, followed by speeches from the town's mayor, the head of the local medical society, the state's health commissioner, officers of the clinic's advisory committee, and a representative of the International Union of Operating Engineers.[33] The Jersey City clinic, opened in April 1948, was featured in *Newsweek* as "Sister Kenny's New Center." It took up 2 floors of the Jersey City Medical Center, a facility that had been expanded in the 1930s by the city's powerful mayor Frank Hague with New Deal funding. The clinic's medical director was orthopedic surgeon Marvin (Mal) Stevens, a former navy officer who had been part of the first American unit to enter Nagasaki after it had been bombed. Stevens had gone to Minneapolis in 1947 to study with Pohl at the urging of his friend New York advertising executive and KF promoter Chester LaRoche.[34]

While these 3 clinics were a source of great pride for Kenny, who traveled frequently to be part of their fundraising activities, she disliked the local tensions that surrounded them. There were bitter fights in Buffalo over whether an NFIP-funded ambulance would carry paralyzed children to the Kenny clinic; and officials at the Illinois crippled children's division threatened to refuse to recognize the Centralia clinic since its medical staff had no permanent consulting pediatrician or orthopedic surgeon. Only the Jersey City clinic, supported by Frank Hague's nephew Mayor Frank Eggers, had political and financial stability.[35]

By the late 1940s, although O'Connor was still a powerful force in American philanthropy, Fishbein's influence was waning. His caustic rejection of any kind of prepaid group practice (even organized by physicians themselves) had alienated patients as well as many doctors trying to give the public alternatives to the attractive government health insurance proposals being debated in Congress and supported by governors such as California's Earl Warren. After the war, Fishbein and the AMA initiated a fierce campaign against Truman's health insurance plan and anyone who supported it. In 1947 Truman's Justice Department began a second antitrust investigation of the AMA.[36]

Even before Congress decided to support a new National Science Foundation it had begun to enlarge what became the National Institutes of Health (NIH). Proposals to expand the NIH were enthusiastically received by a number of disease-oriented philanthropies, including the American Cancer Society and the American Heart Association, but not the NFIP. Liberal reformers testifying in congressional hearings during the 1940s castigated Fishbein's AMA policies and welcomed an expansive role for government in health care and scientific research. Left-wing physicians groups such as the Physicians Forum (founded in 1941) voiced these populist arguments as did other progressive organizations such as the Progressive Citizens of America and the American Veterans Committee. A physician representing the latter during Congressional hearings in 1947 assailed *JAMA* as a journal that "damns other points of view without presenting them," creating a "shockingly prejudiced" medical profession, and urged that government health agencies be "placed in the hands of administrators responsible to the public, and not in the control of a private doctors' association."[37] Although the intense anticommunism of the Cold War later isolated and defeated these groups, such moments were, nonetheless, signs of instability in the power and prestige of organized medicine.

The state of polio science, moreover, weakened the NFIP's claim to stand proudly embodying America's polio expertise without the need for any government oversight. Its promoters praised its breadth of research pursued in universities, medical schools, and hospitals organized in an efficient and democratic way. With more than 2,700 county chapters run by around 30,000 volunteers, the NFIP's polio program, officials assured Congress, was "the greatest research campaign ever carried out against a single disease by the voluntary effort of a free people."[38] Yet scientists funded for a decade, critics pointed out, had not found a cure; perhaps the government could do it better. Even respected members of the AMA began to express their frustration with the NFIP's stagnant research program. A Pittsburgh surgeon, outraged that *JAMA* would not publish an article on the efficacy of curare, complained to Fishbein: "How can the A.M.A. justify the refusal to publish this article when they and the National Foundation, despite the millions of dollars collected, have to date little or nothing to offer the profession, patients, or the public?"[39] The association between the AMA leadership and the NFIP had worked well in the interwar years, but with such postwar critiques the benefits were unraveling. With its movement away from the Democratic Party, some of the NFIP's former allies were no longer falling in line. In a rare comment on polio fundraising Eleanor Roosevelt in one of her "My Day" columns noted that a neighbor had told her "that a considerable organization is being formed to promote Sister Kenny clinics." "Her treatment should certainly be known in every hospital in the county," the former First Lady wrote, adding with an edge directed at both Kenny and the NFIP, "she has not found a cure any more than have the people to whom research grants are made by the National Foundation."[40]

KENNY IN WASHINGTON

By the time she came to Washington in 1948 Kenny was struggling to establish her legacy. Medical texts and public health bulletins on polio rejected splinting in favor of hot packs and muscle training but they often left out Kenny herself. Physicians mixed elements of her method with their own therapies and called this the "modern treatment."

Not only was the Kenny method no longer new, but the drama of its promise to heal, and its stark comparison to harmful previous therapies, was waning. The vision of a healing nurse could not trump the public's fascination with the scientist in a white coat, the drama of the laboratory, and the magical products possible from research. By the late 1940s NFIP posters featured not only a walking child but also a scientist holding a test tube. The prominent University of Cincinnati virologist Albert Sabin told the local medical society in 1948 that "the Kenny treatment is a waste of energy, effort and money. It fills the hospitals with extra nurses and creates an unnecessary bedlam." The money spent on such techniques, he argued, "could be better used for rehabilitation of the few crippled by the disease and for further research." Its widespread use was "part of a wave of hysteria," Sabin concluded, quoting the now familiar line that "what is good about the Kenny treatment is not new. What is new about it is not good."[41]

Kenny's claims to a theoretical discovery that would alter polio science were increasingly easy to dismiss as the overwrought words of a nurse with good clinical skills who had gone too far. Her results were impressive, but the methods were messy, labor-intensive, and expensive. Not surprisingly, many physicians began to search for other therapies that were more under medical control.

RESEARCH, PUBLIC RELATIONS, AND THE NFIP

NFIP officials recognized that public support for science populism threatened their organization. They were therefore eager to use the 1948 hearings to contest the claim that their refusal to fund Kenny's Institute proved that they were using public funds in an undemocratic way. The NFIP had consistently sought to defend itself by emphasizing that it was both democratic and meritocratic, in fact "the *people's* Foundation," as O'Connor had assured one donor during the polio wars.[42] It had also long claimed for itself the role of director and perhaps even instigator of research. During the polio wars NFIP officials had contrasted medical research conducted before its founding—"faltering, unorganized and without coordination"—to research progress afterward.[43] In 1948 the foundation boasted of ten years of promising research in its new pamphlet *A Decade of Doing* and bragged about a new understanding of the mechanism of immunization after Johns Hopkins researchers described experiments showing that polio antibodies in the central nervous tissue of a monkey injected with the live virus could protect the animal from developing paralysis. This research suggested that such antibodies might offer resistance to the "crippling after-effects of this disease" in humans.[44]

The 1948 hearings gave the NFIP a chance to speak as the nation's expert on polio and explain the danger of too much government interference in medical and scientific affairs. Of course, the NFIP did not want to portray itself as unreasonably antagonistic to all government funding. NFIP officials thoughtfully pointed to the "crying need" for research in other fields such as multiple sclerosis and cerebral palsy.[45] Research funding, one official admitted frankly to Congress, was a crucial part of the NFIP's public fundraising and was the "interest and hope" of the thousands of men and women who "work at the grass-roots level." If the NFIP's research program were "taken over by the Government...we believe our greatest appeal for public support will be removed."[46] NFIP representatives were strongly opposed to the idea of a special polio commission within the proposed NSF or any other government agency, warning that "such a step might jeopardize a voluntary program which is achieving important gains."[47]

O'Connor had a longstanding belief in free-market medicine, research, and philanthropy, and he had always been opposed to federated fundraising. With the power of the NFIP behind him he defended medical charities. Charity-directed medical research was, he claimed, the "American way." The nation's great philanthropic agencies were "a peculiarly American type" supported "by funds derived from the mass of the people [and]...led by individuals who join together for the common good...without any thought of emolument in terms either of money or privilege." Any change would threaten the entire system of philanthropy, for the strength of these agencies was "their voluntary and independent nature." Without naming Gunn and Platt's study O'Connor decried their proposal for setting up "a central group with a permanent directorate which all agencies would join."

Each agency would then be compelled to accept the dictums of this directorate about when to seek funds and how to distribute them. This would lead to a loss of humanity in philanthropy and would be part of a wider, more dangerous form of totalitarianism in society at large. American charities required "integrity and independence" to ensure their continued work in "aiding and assisting the less fortunate so that they may participate in and enjoy our standard of life."[48]

Fishbein made similar arguments when he praised America's system of voluntarism in the organization of both philanthropy and medical care. The NFIP's research program, he told a group of polio experts at Warm Springs, was "as fine a program of research...as any developed by any agency in the world in relation to any other disease." Attacking the NFIP, he argued, was like attacking America's fee-for-service medical system. People sometimes said, Fishbein remarked sarcastically, that health charities were not systematic or democratic. But they were "in accord with the democratic traditions of the United States"; rather than being communistic or socialistic, they were "an inspired effort arising out of the hearts and souls of a free people." In defending both the NFIP and America's current fee-for-service health system Fishbein added his own interpretation of attacks on government-directed research agencies. President Truman, Fishbein claimed, had vetoed an earlier version of the NSF bill because he could see that "the research developed with freedom and private initiative gave the better results." As for the argument that there was too much money being collected for "one disease that afflicts so few people," Fishbein dared his audience to "place a child with T.B. above one with infantile paralysis, or one with heart disease above one with infantile paralysis." The NFIP's attitude to polio should be "a model to be emulated in relationship to other diseases."[49] Prompted by an NFIP suggestion, Fishbein then wrote a *JAMA* editorial on medical research urging Congress to "omit any and all special commissions for specific diseases" from the current NSF bill.[50]

Fears that government-funded research could lead to socialized medicine was most starkly laid out before the House committee by Basil's brother John O'Connor, a former New York Democratic congressman who was now an NFIP official. Even if the proposed NSF would be only a "government research bureau" collecting data, John O'Connor argued, "we believe [it] is the proverbial camel getting its nose under the tent and from that time on you have the whole animal, and the whole carcass, right in the center of the ring. You have got the government taking care of the personal disease of our people, a completely totalitarian idea that never was intended in America." He asked the Congressmen to imagine their own families threatened by polio. In 1947, his son, who had just graduated from Harvard Medical School, had become a victim, and the father explained, "I did not want then, and I do not want now any Government representative whether he is a scientist or a doctor, treating me or my people under such circumstances. I want to get the best private treatment. And this proposed research by the Government is bound to develop by the Government taking over completely."[51]

KENNY IN CONGRESS

As a witness at the Congressional hearings Kenny sought to benefit from the complicated medical politics of the times. She enjoyed the effusive, over-the-top language common in Congress and was able to tell her story in terms that fit well with the current congressional climate. Republicans, who had gained control of the House and Senate in 1946, found that supporting Kenny—an underdog battling a medical trust—made good politics and good press.[52] Minnesota Republican Congressman Joseph O'Hara described relations among Sister Kenny, the NFIP, and some of the doctors as a "civil war."[53] New Jersey Republican Charles Wolverton, chair of the House committee, was especially concerned, and, reiterating many of Kenny's own arguments, pointedly questioned NFIP officials about their refusal to fund her work.[54] According to *The Washington Times-Herald*, Wolverton gave the NFIP "a severe tongue lashing," warning that its refusal to support Kenny was "inconceivable" and that the NFIP had clearly "given her the run-around" when she offered to design an exhibit for the upcoming conference.[55] "In all my experience on this committee," Wolverton told Kenny on her second day at the hearings, "you have had more photographers interested in taking your picture than any witness we have ever had before the committee." "I am afraid I do not make a very pretty one," Kenny replied with unconvincing modesty.[56] In fact, according to one commentator, the hearings

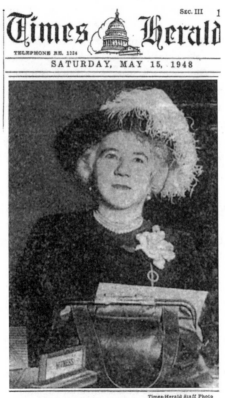

Times-Herald Staff Photo

Sister Kenny Takes the Stand

Sister Elizabeth Kenny is shown as she testified yesterday before a House interstate commerce committee hearing on legislation to set up a national foundation for research on cancer and other degenerative diseases.

FIGURE 7.1 A proud and dignified Kenny was a witness at a Congressional committee hearing in 1948; "Sister Kenny Takes the Stand" *Washington Times-Herald* May 15, 1948.

had the aspect of a trial whose defendants were O'Connor and Roosevelt. Although the late President's name was not mentioned, the critical questioning leveled at NFIP spokesmen and the relish with which Republican members listened to Kenny's attacks on an organization founded by Roosevelt, heightened the feeling that both the former president and his New Deal were under attack.[57]

Kenny made her work a symbol of medical populism. She sought to draw in her congressional audience by demonstrating her trust in the abilities of lay observers to judge evidence put before their own eyes. She showed her technical film at the hearings, noting that she had shown it the previous summer in Europe. This "documentary evidence," she said in introducing the film, could be rejected only through neglect, ignorance, or prejudice. Kenny then recommended that the film be shown to all state health departments and that pamphlets be printed and distributed to inform every family about the Kenny concept.[58]

Kenny was aware that the State Department was sending out invitations for the NFIP conference to some 60 countries. Pressing her claim to be included, she spoke in terms of the new global health politics (the first assembly of the World Health Organization would be meeting in Geneva that summer), reminding the committee of her visits to both Western and Eastern Europe.[59] Thus, she argued, her participation in the NFIP's conference would give the federal government an opportunity to present to "governments of all countries... [a] link in the golden chain of friendship." Turning this argument into a threat, she warned that friends could become enemies. While the gift of her knowledge might "cement the much desired friendships," if it were withheld it was possible that "a bitterness will enter the hearts of the people when the truth finally becomes known." And the NFIP was at fault. Its refusal to allow her to participate in the upcoming conference was "perpetrating a grave injustice on the people of this country by assuming this attitude which, to me, is not American."[60] Many Congressmen caught the implications of the politics of medical openness. If the NFIP's International Conference could carry "governmental implication... to the people of this country and other countries," Massachusetts Republican John Heselton reflected, the committee should "inquire as to what further consideration has been given to the [Kenny] Institute's request, and as to whether or not... there has been a run-around or a pigeon holing of this very reasonable request to participate in developing all the facts."[61]

KENNY AND JUNGEBLUT

One of the most provocative moments in the case against the NFIP was the appearance at the hearings of a pro-Kenny scientist. Claus Washington Jungeblut, a bacteriologist at Columbia University, had been working as a polio researcher for the previous 2 decades, and had been funded by the Milbank Committee, the Rockefeller Foundation, and the Birthday Ball Commission.[62] Kenny had met him in January 1948 along with other Columbia scientists when she had shown her film at the medical school. She had immediately begun to claim him as an ally.[63]

Born in Minnesota but brought up in Switzerland, Jungeblut had received a medical degree in 1921 from the University of Berne and worked as a bacteriology assistant at Berne's public health institute and later at the Robert Koch Institute in Berlin. Fluent in German and English—which he spoke with a Swiss-German accent—he had been hired as an assistant professor of bacteriology at Stanford in 1927 and after 2 years moved to Columbia University to study polio. In the early 1930s William Park and his colleagues had established the failure of polio convalescent serum to protect children from polio, an insight followed by the disastrous testing of a polio vaccine that Park had helped to develop. These events convinced Jungeblut that polio was not like other infectious diseases and that its etiology was more complicated. He proposed that as patients' previous exposures to the polio virus did not explain the patterns of paralysis, there must be additional "poliocidal substances"—perhaps in vitamins or hormones—that would explain why some children developed paralysis and others did not.[64] Jungeblut became a full professor in 1937. His work was praised by the Queensland Royal Commission and 35 of his articles were cited in the NFIP's collection *Infantile Paralysis: A Symposium Delivered at Vanderbilt University April, 1941.*[65]

Impressed by Kenny's clinical results Jungeblut saw in her a new funding source and hoped to gain respect as a KF-funded scientist standing apart from the NFIP. But he did not want to go too far. During her testimony, for example, Kenny had mentioned her plan to set up a rival international polio conference and scientific council and boasted that "several outstanding scientists" were willing to be part of this council.[66] But Jungeblut had already told Kenny privately that he was not willing to be part of any such council and that he thought a separate conference was a bad idea, fearing that few of his fellow scientists would be willing to proclaim such "open rebellion against the National Foundation." "The course I have chosen for myself—not without considerable mental anguish—is to continue my experimental work," he told her, "and hope that with further diffusion of knowledge the objective facts will eventually be accepted."[67]

The NFIP had refused to fund his work, he explained at the hearings, because he worked with mice rather than primates. His research, in other words, was out of the mainstream compared to other virologists favored by the NFIP's science advisors. Nor was he the only scientist in this position. There were, he claimed, "a considerable number of people who have either refused to go with the regimentation of research by the National Foundation, or otherwise have been pushed out by them." He believed that a government agency would be more likely to be fair and disinterested than the NFIP "monopoly" or at least that such an agency could be organized with "devices that make this sort of thing impossible."[68] Kenny had similarly declared that non-NFIP-funded research was crucial for progress in polio science. "Despite the millions of dollars that have been spent on research and investigation," she argued, "the findings that have been of greatest value to humanity concerning this disease" had been the result of work by Jungeblut, virologist Julian Sanz Ibanez at the Cajal Institute in Madrid, and herself, none of them "grantees of the National Foundation."[69]

The characterization by Jungeblut and Kenny of a dangerously autocratic NFIP swayed some members of the House committee. "Too often the medical profession is too orthodox, and unwilling to recognize the individual who is traveling along a path that is different from what is recognized by orthodox medicine," Wolverton told Jungeblut sympathetically, "yet . . . so many of our great inventions have come about in a most unexpected way . . . through the vision or the thought of some individual who was thinking differently than others thought."[70] Although Jungeblut had not referred to Kenny's lack of medical training, a few Congressmen did—not to criticize but to show their explicit support of medical populism. Minnesota Republican Joseph O'Hara pointed out that a person's lack of professional training should not necessarily undermine his or her scientific respectability: "[O]ftentimes the layman contributes something in the way of science to something in the way of relief that too often we might be inclined to be a little jealous of it or overlook it."[71] In his understanding of scientific progress every contribution should be valued, irrespective of physicians' unreasonable envy.

Hart Van Riper was the NFIP's most articulate defender at the hearings. He briefly criticized Jungeblut's science – noting that "we are not going to solve the mystery of polio by working with mice" - but addressed the bulk of his testimony to Kenny's assertions. The gist of his attack was that Kenny was unfit to participate in the upcoming conference or in any serious scientific meeting, and that she had no legitimate claim to scientific insight. While he noted that the NFIP had "not argued about the quality of her treatment," Van Riper claimed that her work was not particularly new and was widely practiced under a variety of names throughout the country. He also identified what he considered 2 glaring weaknesses in Kenny's claims to scientific respectability: her reluctance to abide by the conservative etiquette of the scientific establishment—exemplified by her speaking so brashly to the press of her "contribution"—and her inability to recognize the kinds of evidence professionals regarded as authoritative. "Miss Kenny is not a physician," physician Van Riper explained, and "has made statements that certain things do not exist which, in the laboratory animal we can reproduce." Further, he added, "unfortunately Miss Kenny feels that unless you accept her concept of the cause you cannot accept her treatment."[72] In short, she refused to separate her technical work—as healer and therapist—from her theoretical insights; she was not content to be lauded only as a nurse.

Although Kenny spoke often of her desire to obtain scientific confirmation of her theories through clinical and laboratory studies, she had always relied heavily on personal testimonials as evidence. These she described as "reports of unbiased medical men and the findings of science."[73] This kind of strategy did not impress the NFIP. In letters between conference organizer Stanley Henwood and Marvin Kline that formed part of Kenny's Congressional evidence, Henwood dismissed any proposed submission that would be merely "a restatement of Sister Kenny's contribution to the field of poliomyelitis" and requested instead "some concrete scientific evidence and not merely statements that are based on personal opinion." He suggested that "actual scientific evidence" be submitted in manuscript form showing "the presentation of a sufficient number of case reports covering all of the patients treated with the end results as compared with cases in the same area treated by other methods."[74] In vain did Kline protest that the KF did not intend to provide a restatement but "to present scientific evidence confirming the contribution of Sister Elizabeth Kenny [through]... the medium of visual education in six different languages" (that is, by showing her film *The Kenny Concept*). Kenny also quoted Henwood's additional disapproving comment that her request to show a film was one of many from "several large institutions and personalities throughout the world who felt that their story should be told."[75]

Kline along with Kenny and members of the KF Board recognized that nothing would convince the conference organizers to allow Kenny to participate and concluded that the reason was NFIP prejudice and elitism. "Owing to the many stumbling blocks presented we would assume that it is your intention to maintain your original attitude in considering scientific exhibits from the [NFIP]... grantees only," Kline told Henwood.[76]

Kenny knew that her work appealed to antivivisectionists and to other antiorthodox critics. But in public she no longer acknowledged such alliances, and her friends noticed that when first meeting a physician she wanted to know "what kind of doctor is he?"[77] At the 1948 hearings she made much of her commitment to professional orthodoxy. While Van Riper pointedly called Kenny "Miss" instead of "Sister," he carefully did not call her a quack. His reluctance to attack Kenny this way reflected her national popularity, her shrewd use of the press, and the fact that, in the 1940s and 1950s, antivivisectionists remained a potent political force in some states.

Charles Wolverton heard the testimony by Kenny and Jungeblut with great sympathy. Wolverton had been a member of Congress since 1927, and chaired the House Interstate and Foreign Commerce committee during the 80th and 81st Congresses. He supported the distinctive kind of research populism Kenny was promoting, and had told Surgeon General Leonard Scheele at the hearings that he was very strongly convinced that much knowledge necessary for "the proper functioning of research and research foundations is not reposed in doctors, with all due respect to doctors... much can be gained by the presence on these councils of lay members."[78] To Kenny, Wolverton expressed his committee's "very great appreciation for your attendance here today." He praised her film and her marvelous work, and said he was impressed by "the disdain you apparently have for any financial reward." His committee was "anxious... to assist you in the great work you are doing," he assured her, for "you are doing a great service for humanity [and]... are entitled to the respect and the support of all who are in [a] position to give it to you."[79]

As a New Jersey representative, Wolverton made much of Kenny's newly established clinic in Jersey City. He held up the front page of Camden's *Courier Post* showing a picture of Kenny at the Jersey City center with a patient who hailed from a town "about three miles from my home." He paid tribute to Irish-Catholic Democratic boss Frank Hague who had, Wolverton admitted, "not always been spoken of in the highest terms." Yet Hague's support of the Jersey City center "will stand as a monument for as long as he should live, and will remain long after he has gone." Hague's recognition of the importance of Kenny's treatment by making it "a part of his Medical Center" was a gesture Wolverton wished more local officials would emulate in their own communities and thus "make possible the teaching of this new concept that Sister Kenny has developed with such wonderful results."[80]

NSF DEFEAT

Despite the appearances of Kenny and Jungeblut and the support of many Republicans on the committee, the version of the NSF bill they were debating was defeated. In June 1948 only weeks after Kenny's appearance in Washington the NSF bill passed the Senate but was held up in the House Rules Committee long enough to miss being put on the House calendar so it could not be voted on before Congress adjourned.[81] Truman was beginning his presidential campaign, and the bill floundered over the issue of governance and over the highly charged inclusion of disease commissions. While the American Cancer Society and the American Heart Association welcomed federal funding of "cure-oriented research" through a government agency, the NFIP rejected any agency that included a special commission on polio. Behind the scenes, the NFIP made sure that any version of the NSF bill that included polio research would fail, assuring Congress that such a provision was part of a "'Communistic' un-American... scheme."[82]

With the unexpected election of Truman in November 1948 the politicization of organized medicine intensified. For the first time the AMA established an office in Washington,
D.C. and a new Council on Medical Service and Public Relations, whose job was to lobby
both politicians and physicians. The transformation of relations among universities,
business, and the government in scientific research begun during the war continued, but
Truman's national health insurance plan was firmly and effectively defeated by some of
the most sophisticated activist AMA-directed campaigns the nation had ever seen.[83]

It was not until 1950 after the Democrats regained control of Congress that Truman
finally signed a watered-down version of the NSF bill. The President appointed its director, but the director shared power with a board made up of academic and industrial scientists. And there was no polio commission. By this time the funding of medical research
was clearly shifting from private to government organizations, and the NIH's emerging empire expanded with the new National Institute of Mental Health, National Heart
Institute, and National Institute of Dental Research.[84]

Kenny was unable to muster enough support to establish a government research
agency that targeted polio, much less one that supported her distinctive theory of the
disease, and the NFIP was able to make sure that no National Polio Institute was ever
established. The 1948 hearings nonetheless brought populism into the politics of science
research, and the new Institutes were overseen by councils that included a few lay community representatives. In June 1948, despite AMA protests that "it may be questioned
whether a leader in the field of public affairs will be particularly equipped to make very
much of a contribution to the promotion of [that] kind of research," the surgeon general
appointed wealthy lobbyist Mary Lasker, wife of advertising executive Albert Lasker, as
the first lay member of the National Heart Institute's advisory council. Lasker had already
rejuvenated the American Cancer Society and had lobbied for laymen to serve on the
Heart Institute's advisory council.[85] Naturopath critics wondered sardonically whether
she would be willing to attack "enterprises that [had] helped to make her husband rich
[such as]...the white flour industry, the alcohol industry, the soft drinks industry, and
other evil industries that spend billions yearly in advertising?"[86] Lasker's appointment
was a reminder that lay representation did not mean class or regional diversity; indeed,
"public" could easily be interpreted to mean "patron."

THE INTERNATIONAL CONFERENCE

On the defensive, the NFIP turned the First International Poliomyelitis Conference into a
public relations project. Held at New York's Waldorf-Astoria Hotel, amid banquets, films,
and poster exhibits, the conference program was filled with Kenny's work—although
mostly uncredited. The July 1948 conference had 10 sessions, 3 official languages, and
was attended by over a thousand representatives from around 40 countries.[87]

The conference provided an exciting opportunity to bring together American and
European researchers who had been kept apart by the war. Polio had only just become a
significant problem in Europe, and physicians were looking across the Atlantic for expertise.
Making polio research an international issue showed the American public as well as Congress
that NFIP policies went beyond parochial medical politics. Indeed, the word *international*
was a coded Cold War term, indicating American allegiances with other "free" nations.[88]

Kenny's appearance at the Congressional hearings had not gained her access to the international conference as a scientific participant. But she was able to attend as a reporter with a press card from the American Newspaper Guild.[89] While she could not formally participate during the sessions, she did attend press conferences amid the country's leading science writers where she stood out in her distinctive, elegant attire. *Newsweek* described her as a "majestic, white-haired woman in a long black frock, large plumed hat, and heavy ropes of pearls."[90] To the press corps Kenny complained frequently of her exclusion. She made sure her fellow reporters learned that she had not been invited as a scientific participant as a result of "the personal attitude and ambition of Mr. Basil O'Connor [who refused] . . . to recognize the merit of anything connected with polio treatment that cannot be identified in some way with his name."[91] Her sense of conspiracy was reflected in her private detective escort who accompanied her to these public events along with a man who she claimed was a reporter but, according to a pro-NFIP commentator, was in fact "her own personal press agent who tried to conceal his identity at the Conference."[92]

While Kenny's name was avoided by most of the speakers, her ideas were not. Many of the exhibits and technical films showed aspects of her treatment and featured some of the physical therapists she had trained, and, following Kenny's lead, speakers sought to link clinical signs to pathology.[93] Both spasm and pain were now recognized symptoms, although some presenters argued that spasm was rare, and others argued that its presence did not indicate a new pathology.[94] Virologist David Bodian of Johns Hopkins agreed that an "important component of muscle weakness in the acute stage may be a partial and temporary loss of function of some motor units." He believed that "the origin of muscle pain in poliomyelitis also requires further exploration" and referred vaguely to "the re-routing of neuron-chain discharge pathways from interrupted primary paths to secondary alternative paths."[95] Fritz Buchthal, a physiologist from Copenhagen, noted that "the occurrence of 'spasm'" had been "the subject of intensive discussions and controversies," although in his research spasm rarely occurred unless "passive therapies" were employed too vigorously.[96] During the discussion following Buchthal's paper, Lewis Pollock, a Chicago neurologist, declared dramatically that 11 neurologists assigned to Chicago's city hospitals had conducted around 9,000 examinations of individual muscles and could not find a single instance of spasm.[97] Oxford orthopedist W. Ritchie Russell, the author of a textbook on polio which Kenny had read in the 1930s, said firmly that patients must have "physiologic rest" for any "so-called spasm" could be a muscle's "response to stretch if nothing else, and perhaps a defense against pain."[98] While the cause of pain in polio, commemorators admitted, was still obscure, most continued to argue that the pathology of polio was without doubt based on affected nerve cells. Stanford pediatrician Harold Faber was sure that the polio virus was "strictly neurotropic."[99] Bodian—a neurobiologist and not a clinician—was one of the few who wondered out loud about "the possibility . . . that a peripheral disease may exist in the absence of central infection."[100]

Kenny did not pay much attention to this kind of debate. She was upset when someone asked a question about the cause of spinal deformities, which members of the panel on stage could not answer. Some of her physician allies asked her to explain this symptom, but when this request was sent to the session's moderator Robert Bennett he did not recognize her as an appropriate respondent.[101]

Kenny did respond dramatically after a session in which Herbert Seddon, a respected British orthopedist, criticized her method by name. Seddon may not have noticed that the

American participants were avoiding Kenny's name, or he may not have cared. Speaking as a specialist still reeling from the reorganization of the British health system and without the backing of a major polio philanthropy, he called on physicians to seek more economical treatments, arguing that the public "should get value for money." He was one of the few participants to discuss the cost of medical care openly. "Everyone agrees that the Kenny treatment is expensive," he said, quoting an estimate from Nicholas Ransohoff that Kenny treatment was around 5 times as expensive as orthodox care. According to the views of "dispassionate critics," Seddon declared, this expenditure was not justified. He was unsparing in his attacks on his own colleagues as well. "It is not sufficient to dismiss Miss Kenny's work as an expensive nine days' wonder; we must ask ourselves whether our own methods of treatment are altogether rational. Maybe we are, in fact, wasting money in prolonging treatment beyond the point when it is of the slightest use to the patient." He also noted what he called "curious inconsistencies" in current polio practice, urging his peers to "abandon the notion that denervated muscle is in a peculiarly delicate state [for] . . . it does not degenerate; it atrophies."[102] Physicians, Seddon argued during the discussion of his paper, needed better studies of recovery based on "carefully controlled clinical experiment[s]."[103] While he was uncomfortable with Ransohoff's promotion of curare, he did praise Ransohoff's arguments in favor of early ambulation compared to the "slavish enforcement of bed-rest that most of us had practised [sic]."[104]

Kenny then demanded a news conference with Seddon and Ransohoff. She had contested Seddon's views before, assuring her Australian critics that his claim in 1947 that spasm was rare in his own patients was because "Professor Seddon is viewing the disease from the orthodox point of view."[105] Now she and "a corps of assistants began feeding statements into a mimeograph machine and within a few hours she had a batch of handout[s] for other members of the press." Seddon and Ransohoff attended this press conference as did Fishbein. Wearing a royal purple dress and large garden-party hat, Kenny challenged Seddon's calculations and his critique. Kenny treatment at both the Minneapolis Institute and at the Jersey City center, she argued, cost between $9.12 and $12.50 a patient daily, while Ransohoff had previously told her that in his hospital such care cost $17 a day. In any case, the comparison was inappropriate, for it was comparing good care to poor care and therefore any discussion "was a waste of time." As for the "dispassionate critics"—who she guessed were the members of the 1944 AMA committee—she gave Seddon copies of a telegram showing their refusal to give out the names of the cities or hospitals they visited and one from Alfred Deacon noting that at the end of a 2-year period his Kenny-treated patients were "ten times better."[106]

Ransohoff refused to back down, and while Seddon responded politely, he also did not yield. He thanked her publicly "for methods which you have given me that are advantageous to my patients. You got rid of braces. But I do not agree with you on everything. I have to treat the very poor. And for them, when speaking on economic grounds, I cannot recommend the Kenny treatment on account of expense."[107] Kenny technician Amy Lindsey recalled later that Seddon came back into the meeting room after the reporters had left and shook Kenny's hand saying he admired her although they didn't agree on everything.[108] In contrast, Fishbein recalled that Seddon had said to him after this press conference "I think the old girl is potty."[109]

Reporters were split between admiring Kenny's bravado and finding her amusing and embarrassing. NFIP publicist Roland Berg reported in an internal note that when "Miss Kenny attempted to voice her pseudo-scientific facts . . . the press was not at all impressed and reported nothing of her claims."[110] But science journalist Albert Deutsch disagreed. In his article "Sister Kenny and the Foundation" he wrote that Kenny had "made a greater contribution to its treatment than any other personality of our generation" and for 30 years "had to fight the bigoted opposition of medical groups who were outraged by the notion that a nurse could teach them anything." Deutsch castigated NFIP officials who had deliberately ignored her and "apparently have allowed personal peeves and prejudices to get in the way of scientific duty and humanitarian consideration." Like "many great medical pioneers," he admitted, Kenny could be difficult and placed too high a value on her work, but she had "beyond all doubt, made a most valuable contribution to the understanding and treatment of polio." "Under no circumstances," he cautioned, "should personal feuding be allowed to stand between children fighting off the crippling after-effects of polio and the best possible means of helping them get well."[111]

In a deliberate rebuttal to the film Kenny had shown Congress 2 months earlier, University of Illinois's Division of Services for Crippled Children, funded by the NFIP, presented a new technical film called *Nursing Care of Poliomyelitis* at the international conference. It was 4 reels and in sound and color. Kenny's methods appeared throughout, without her name and once again in a modified version. Thus, the first reel, *The Acute Stage*, showed the use of footboards and hot packs (both Kenny hallmarks); the second reel, *Treatment of Spasm*, demonstrated details of administering hot packs as well as how to use baths as a substitute; the third reel dealt with the iron lung; and the fourth, on the convalescent stage, showed ways of applying splints "to prevent deformity" and various muscle tests. A *JAMA* reviewer thought the film was likely to be useful in training physicians, advanced medical students, nurses, and physical therapists, "who may not always appreciate how elaborate the procedure must be if the patient is to have the best possible care and [be] spared unnecessary suffering."[112] Humane polio care, this film suggested, could be obtained by mixing old and new methods, not by slavish adherence to a single program.

AFTER THE HEARINGS

By December 1948 2 main changes in polio treatment, research, and funding were in place. The first was a new organizational structure for the KF. Donald Dayton, a Minneapolis businessman whose son had been paralyzed by polio and treated by Kenny, now headed its Board, and pediatrician Edgar Huenkens directed the Institute. The second change occurred far from Minnesota with the organization of a Citizen's Polio Research League, a lay group inspired by the Congressional hearings, based in California's San Fernando Valley.

In Minnesota Huenkens, who had come to local prominence as the head of the state's polio commission during the 1946 epidemic, reorganized the Institute's medical staff, appointing Miland Knapp, who was already in charge of polio technicians at the University hospital, as head of a new physical medicine unit with authority over the Institute's technicians. Huenkens was eager to reestablish relations with the University of Minnesota and with the NFIP, but he recognized the delicate balance between maintaining Kenny's trust and working with those she considered her enemies. "I firmly believe in the value of her treatment," he declared in the formal announcement of his new position, and "we hope to do away with the antagonism that exists between Sister Kenny and the medical profession, which has caused both to be misunderstood by the public." Once these misunderstandings were resolved he believed that "physicians will be able to judge the Kenny method objectively," and he invited every doctor to the Institute "to observe for themselves the treatment and its results."[113] In a statement reported in local Minneapolis papers Kenny declared, "I quite agree with the procedures of members of the medical profession for their caution in not embracing new ideas that may from time to time be presented, including my own, until they are satisfied they are effective."[114] Huenkens had helped to craft this statement, and he boasted to Van Riper that "this is the most forward statement she has made yet and I got her to make it." The Institute under his direction was now successful in "getting the doctors to adopt her methods and ignore her."[115] Van Riper did feel that "for the moment that the Kenny situation in Minneapolis is under control," but he remained suspicious. Huenkens urged him to come out to the Institute, but Van Riper refused, adding he "would come out if I was sure I would not have to encounter her—the only way I can remain something of a gentleman is to avoid meeting her."[116]

In California, to Huenkens's chagrin, Kenny was fully in control of the Citizens Polio Research League. It had a number of vocal women members including its president Mrs. Sonja Betts, and Rosalind Russell agreed to be its "patroness."[117] The league began planning a Sister Kenny Hospital to be affiliated with the Southern chapter of the California KF. It also circulated petitions asking Congress to create a federal research foundation to study polio, implying that only government-directed research into polio could be unbiased.[118] The implications of this populist ideology were not lost on NFIP officials. In a private phone conversation, Van Riper told Huenkens that he was sure this new league was a kind of "Kenny Foundation No. 2," reflecting Kenny's resentment at the shifting power relations at the Institute and in the KF.[119]

The *San Fernando Sun* became the mouthpiece of the new California movement. It began to publish provocative letters claiming that Kenny had been prevented from presenting the results of her polio research at the Congressional hearings "because of pressure from the National Foundation for Infantile Paralysis, members of Congress and/or the medical profession." Herbert Avedon, the paper's editor, sent open letters to local politicians, the NFIP's national office, and Kenny herself arguing that "if any group, official, unofficial, charitable, social, medical or any other sort, actively works to prevent such information from being made known or even investigated, we believe the people ought to know."[120] Congressman Harry Sheppard, a Democrat representing northern Los Angeles, assured Avedon and his readers that the hearing had been courteous; the NFIP's executive director Joseph Savage wrote a careful and defensive reply; and Kenny sent an 8-page letter defending Congress and attacking the NFIP.[121] Kenny's argument that her work could not achieve its best results when it was modified was reiterated in a letter the *Sun* published from a patient who had been recently discharged from the Los Angeles County General Hospital and could now "only walk a little." Had he been given "the best treatment available," he wondered. He had been reading about the Citizens Polio Research League and also heard a discussion on the radio. "If what they say is true, then I may be crippled for the rest of my life merely because I was not treated by the Kenny method."[122]

In December 1948 Sonja Betts and other league representatives went to Jersey City to attend a 1-day conference. Seeking to reach over the head of the NFIP and the AMA by focusing on national organizations with clout over the nation's health and welfare institutions as well as scientific research, Kenny and her allies had invited representatives of the Federal Security Agency and the Public Health Service along with Bernard Baruch and

John D. Rockefeller. The league received "courteous replies" from Baruch and Rockefeller, regretting that they could not attend.[123] Representatives from the 2 federal agencies did attend along with a number of physicians and physical therapists.

Kenny loved this new forum. She urged the league to demand that findings of the research that had shown that polio was a disturbance in peripheral structures be published and made available to all American voters. This research, she promised, would "result in the rewriting of the medical books of today."[124] Foreign delegates, she told the Jersey City audience, had been "disappointed" at the way she was treated at the recent international conference. She quoted the sympathetic remarks of a Spanish participant that she had been "thwarted and frustrated while at the conference...unable to answer questions, [and] given no recognition." Thousands of American children and adults with polio, she warned, would "become needlessly deformed and crippled" because they were not being treated with her methods in its entirety. She showed Public Health Service and Federal Security Agency patients as evidence of the danger of such modified treatment. Every 6 months she had tried to present scientific reports on the Kenny concept to the NFIP in "a friendly conference with representatives of all bodies interested in this particular disease," but she had been consistently rejected. Along with a heated discussion of Roland Berg's recent book *Polio and Its Problems* Kenny quoted Alfred Deacon, who had said his patients treated with her methods were "ten times better." She also announced triumphantly that a new affiliation with the Mayo Clinic, the University of Minnesota, and the Institute was "now in the process of culmination."[125]

The Jersey City meeting was described by the *New York Times* and in a private note by an NFIP official who estimated that there were only 22 people in attendance, including Philip Stimson, Marvin Stevens, another 5 doctors, young women who were probably physical therapists, several press representatives, and a photographer. In the meeting's hostile environment, Stimson's mild protests that the NFIP had indeed authorized money to pay for Kenny and her technicians had been ignored.[126]

Neither Chester LaRoche nor Mal Stevens was comfortable with the Citizens Polio Research League or the heights to which it inspired Kenny. Such publicity, LaRoche warned Kenny, "hurts our efforts" as it seemed to emphasize "that the medical profession is not with us." "Let's not get people feeling that we are fighting," he urged her, but have everyone know "that the Kenny treatment is accepted all over the country."[127] Unrepentant, Kenny claimed she had been trying "to get known to the public that the doctors are with us" and the NFIP is "against us." As for any impact on the KF's campaign, "your drive shall be a failure until the truth is known."[128]

Stevens was even more disturbed than La Roche. He felt Kenny's speech, which had been widely reported, "spreads salt on old wounds and opens new ones." He told LaRoche that he doubted whether the Mayo Clinic "would condone this statement of affiliation." While it was true that the Mayo Clinic taught Kenny technicians as part of their regular physical therapy course, that was "a far cry from being a medical tie-up" with the Institute. Stevens agreed that Kenny's clinical observations "have been and are of great value," but noted that a number of people, including doctors, had warned him that she "should not be the spokesman on medical matters or on the foundation's plans for expansion unless she is so instructed to be by the medical board or the foundation."[129]

Learning of these remarks Kenny disagreed vehemently, replying that the *New York Times* version of her speech in Jersey City had given "great satisfaction to Doctor

Huenkens who especially asked me had I seen it." In a confusing effort to combat Stevens' metaphor she added that "if the truth rubs salt on old wounds and opens new ones, the more salty the old wound becomes and the more numerous the new ones become, the better for humanity." As for relations with the Mayo Clinic, she had received a letter from Melvin Henderson "congratulating me on the fact that a great burden had been removed from my shoulders and exhorting me to take life much easier." She did not, she protested, aspire to be a spokesman on medical matters other than on those that were "still unknown to the medical world to a great extent, such as my own contribution." In any case, she noted to LaRoche, Stevens was not proving himself a particularly good proponent of her work. He had ignored a suggestion by the head of New Jersey's Crippled Children's Association that "all doctors in the state should be presented with my findings." He had also excused himself from a meeting with a physician from the Children's Bureau who had come to visit Jersey City, and had ignored an offer by the New York Academy of Medicine to show her technical film.[130]

As Van Riper shrewdly recognized, even in her own Institute Kenny was being pushed to the side. Never easy to work with, she had lost much of her patience and tact without Mary Kenny's watchful eye. She pretended to a heroic humility, telling audiences in London "I am of no consequence...It is only my great gift—my work—which matters," but she was annoyed when her contribution to American medicine was called the Kenny method instead of "an entirely new concept of the disease."[131] Her suspicions of conspiracy also deepened after she returned from one of her European trips in 1947 and discovered that her technical film "had been cast aside" by Institute officials, a pamphlet she had prepared for parents during the 1946 epidemic had not been distributed, and her gray book *Physical Medicine* was not mentioned in any of the KF reference lists.[132] Worse, she learned in early 1948 that a script writer from Hollywood had been employed without her knowledge to write a script about her methods. All these were efforts, she warned, "to eliminate my name."[133]

Kenny believed correctly that these policies were the work of William O'Neil, the KF's new director of information services. O'Neil saw his role as reestablishing relations with local physicians and the medical school and ending "wild promotion schemes." He contacted Fishbein and got him to agree to publish a leading article by John Pohl on the early diagnosis of polio in *JAMA*.[134] He defended the Hollywood script project by arguing that "the public is anxious to know just what training is in back of a Kenny technician." Kenny relied on technical films but she wanted only her cinematic vision, which combined clinical evidence and theoretical explanation. The public, she told O'Neil, was "not anxious to know anything about the training [but was]...only interested in the end results of treatment."[135] Worried that O'Neil was making alliances with her own medical supporters she warned Pohl that O'Neil was boasting "about being able to twist you around his little finger."[136] She sent a series of annoyed letters to the KF board and finally called Kline from New York and said she was "not going to come back to Minneapolis as long as that man is there." O'Neil was fired in April 1948.[137]

Kenny continued to seek additional celebrity testimonials. She met President Truman's daughter Margaret who had expressed interest in the Citizen's League and asked her to become the League's "national patroness" (a request Truman gracefully ignored).[138] Kenny enthusiastically allied herself with William Fox, owner of the Fox theater chain, and his daughters Mona and Belle, who had become Kenny supporters.[139] She graciously accepted effusive praise from English suffragist Christabel Pankhurst who described her as "our modern Florence Nightingale as well as great medical pioneer." Pankhurst wanted to know Kenny's view of "the actual *cause* of Poliomyelitis" and described her own theory of "a poisonous element in pools and ponds."[140] Kenny did not respond.

In November 1948 the celebrity photographer Yousuf Karsh produced a new portrait of Kenny titled "Polio-Fighting Australian Nurse." It was published in the family magazine *Coronet* just in time for the 1948 KF campaign.[141] It was a full length black-and-white picture of Kenny, arms outstretched, wearing no jewelry or hat. She is dressed in black with a white cape around her shoulders. The light shines on her hands, her lined face, and her strong shoulders. It is a portrait of a woman who has struggled, but—bereft of laboratory instruments or patients—it is not a picture of a scientific researcher or even a clinician. In contrast, Karsh's later depiction of Jonas Salk placed him with a child patient and a syringe.[142]

Kenny's distinctive personality was widely used to explain why working with her was so difficult. *Newsweek* noted her "stubborn will and sharp tongue" and her "bitterly undiplomatic...dealings with American physicians" who had "resisted taking peremptory orders from a nurse with no formal medical training." "She has," the magazine continued, "'resigned,' flounced out of hospital wards and executives offices—and later reconsidered her resignation."[143] Albert Deutsch agreed that Kenny was "a strong-willed stubborn woman, given to exaggerating the importance of her work, just as her enemies tend to minimize it."[144] Van Riper said privately that at any meeting "called by her or her representatives...she will make her claims just as she always has in the past, and if intelligent questions are asked or if she is crossed in any way, you are subjected to humiliation and ridicule."[145] He repeated this argument to explain to donors why the NFIP refused to fund additional efforts to evaluate Kenny's work. "It is unlikely that any evaluation would satisfy Miss Kenny or her staunch supporters," he explained to one woman; "I think we must realize that nothing less than a complete and total surrender to Miss Kenny will ever satisfy her or anyone who supports her."[146] Around this time Kenny learned that O'Connor was describing her as an "Amazon," a term which both she and O'Connor found denigrating, implying inappropriate independence and defiance of gender norms.[147]

WHEN FOUNDATIONS FIGHT

Kenny's claim to scientific discovery did not sway the organizers of the First International Poliomyelitis Conference. But it certainly enhanced her celebrity status. A few months after the international conference, Gallup pollsters asked the American public: "What woman, living today in our part of the world that you have heard or read about do you admire the most?" The top 3 women listed were first Eleanor Roosevelt, then Madame Chiang Kai-shek, and third Sister Kenny.[148]

The NFIP's public image was buffeted by the polio wars and the Congressional hearings. Although O'Connor made a point of sending major donors social science research to confirm his argument that voluntary health agencies were vital to American democracy, doubts lingered. In private memos, John Rockefeller III's advisors argued that he should not support the NFIP as it was "well-heeled" and did not "disclose its financial situation to the public." The NFIP, they warned him, also "overdramatizes" its case and raises massive funds for a disease compared to "diseases of far greater importance in terms of their incidence and toll."[149] Virologist Thomas Rivers, a member of the NFIP's scientific advisory committee, told Rockefeller quietly that he agreed that "there are other fields of medicine that need your help more urgently."[150]

In *Consumer Reports* science journalist Harold Aaron agreed that the NFIP—"one of the world's richest and most powerful voluntary health organizations"—was misdirecting public resources to a single disease that was far less significant in the public's health than the NFIP's scare campaigns claimed. In 1948, for example, the NFIP had spent $17,0000,000, while Congress had given the Children's Bureau only $7,500,000 for the care of all types of disabled children. Yet according to statistics gathered by the Crippled Children bureaus at least as many children in 1948 were disabled by cerebral palsy as by polio (about 175,000 for each), and many had other neglected diseases with major disabling effects including diabetes (35,000), epilepsy (200,000), and rheumatic heart disease (500,000).[151] Progress in the treatment of polio was also harmed by fights between the KF and the NFIP, Aaron suggested, especially fights over "the controversial figure of Sister Elizabeth Kenny." The NFIP and the KF competed with each other "in the promotion of research methods of treatment, and provision of medical facilities." The battle was based on "fundamental differences of opinion as to proper treatment of a disease which stubbornly resists the development of vaccines for its prevention and drugs for its control." Parents of patients would "continue to suffer from the doubts raised in their minds by claims and counterclaims." In Aaron's assessment the NFIP had not given Kenny "an adequate opportunity to make further contributions" and had also denied her supporters any part of the "abundant harvest of the annual March of Dimes." Fights over "matters of prestige, antagonisms and jealousies, personal as well as professional," had, he believed, led the NFIP to withdraw its national support of Kenny's program and had widened the breach between the 2 groups.[152]

Aaron also pointed to conflicts between the NFIP's national office and its state and local chapters, almost 3,000 across the country. Too often chapters were run by lay citizens who might be excellent fundraisers but who often lacked other experience in health activities. "In the opinion of medical consultants," Aaron reported, the national officers of the NFIP did not "hold sufficient authority over the various state and local chapters to assure conformity to high medical standards."[153] The NFIP's national office had tried in vain to set up rules about paying only for treatment carried out at a facility recognized by a state's crippled children's commission. Although the Federal Security Agency directed these commissions and set federal guidelines, state politics always played a part in influencing those institutions deemed "appropriate." With 2,800 local chapters, O'Connor admitted to one potential donor, the NFIP "cannot expect perfection" in following national policy.[154]

Indeed, the KF was able to highlight and exploit idiosyncrasies of individual NFIP chapters. KF officers claimed that the NFIP did not pay for Kenny treatment, but that was only partly true. NFIP chapters usually paid for all polio treatment—whether "Kenny" or not—as long as it was approved by a physician. There were many anecdotes about bigoted local NFIP officials who pressured families to go to a doctor who did not use Kenny's methods: in Buffalo, a family was told by a local official that he would pay their unpaid balance only if they agreed to have a particular doctor examine their son; another family quoted an official who told the parents "how much good the March of Dimes was doing and that the Sister Kenny group was no good at all."[155] Making the distinction between care provided by Kenny technicians and general hospital care the KF argued that while the NFIP paid for hospitalization, it did not fund Kenny treatment of any patient. No patients with polio at the Jersey City clinic, according to the KF, had ever had their bill paid by the NFIP. As a result, the KF claimed, the new foundation was forced to divert funds earmarked for training Kenny technicians and research to absorb these hospitalization costs.[156] Other incidents demonstrated that chapters were interpreting NFIP propaganda for their own purposes. A woman from Manhattan Beach, California, spent 5 months as a patient in the Minneapolis Institute, but California NFIP officials refused to pay any part of the Institute's bill, telling her family "they didn't have any money to spend on 'experimental treatment.'"[157]

In Minneapolis the delicate balance between the Institute and the local NFIP chapter was constantly upset by national policies. In early 1949 the head of the Minneapolis chapter was taken aback to learn that the national office had informed Kline that it would no longer pay for patient care at the Institute. This ill-advised policy was, Minneapolis officials protested, clearly the result of not having consulted local officials. Altering this policy "would rupture the harmonious relationship" between the Institute and the NFIP and "would prejudice all Minnesotans against the National Foundation." Many local officials might then have to resign from the NFIP and its March of Dimes January campaign "would fall flat."[158] So tricky were public relations around this issue that University of Minnesota president J. L. Morrill expressed his regret and embarrassment at having to decline the opportunity to serve as a formal sponsor of the NFIP's state drive. If he did this, he explained to an NFIP official, "it would be very difficult for me thereafter to decline similar service and connection with the Kenny campaign," which for personal and professional reasons he would prefer not to do.[159]

Attacks on the NFIP were also voiced by the Citizen's League, working with the newly invigorated California KF chapters.[160] State politicians responded to this public pressure. California's Republican Governor Earl Warren served as the honorary chair of the KF's Northern chapter and proclaimed state Sister Kenny days, as did the mayor of San Francisco for that city. Judge Georgia Bullock, who had been appointed to the state's high court by a Republican governor in the 1930s, urged full support of the KF campaign.[161] According to Sonja Betts, head of the Citizen's League, NFIP officials "have blocked Sister Kenny at every turn, and with their money and power are exercising every strategy to prevent her from getting in on the West Coast." Betts planned to seek the aid of both Republican and Democratic California politicians for a Congressional resolution to increase funding to the Public Health Service and to earmark part of those funds to fight polio. "The National Foundation is strong and powerful, but it is time the people took the matter into their own hands and fight to get the Kenny treatment here if we are ever going to get any relief from the ravages of polio," Betts told reporters dramatically.[162]

FIGHTS IN CENTRALIA

Unlike the thriving center in Jersey City and the growing nucleus of supporters in California, the Kenny clinic in Centralia, Illinois, proved a disappointment. The clinic's first administrator resigned in early 1948, and, although the clinic's medical board appointed a successor, the Minneapolis KF board refused to approve him. The KF board claimed it was still waiting to receive formal approval of the clinic from the state's crippled children's division. The state agency hesitated to approve sending patients to the clinic, arguing that the clinic needed more permanent specialists, specifically a pediatrician and an orthopedist.[163] John Lucian Matthews, a labor leader on the Centralia clinic's board of directors, urged both Kenny and Kline to back the clinic's board in its efforts to maintain high standards. "Labor like the physicians in this area," Matthews told Kenny, "have a warm spot in their hearts for you."[164] Although Matthews and other directors urged her to visit the clinic, Kenny initially refused, saying that Kline would visit and assuring her supporters that she had "every confidence in his ability to meet the wishes of the medical profession [and to]...solve any difficulties which may have arisen."[165]

As the calls for help from Centralia continued, Kenny finally acted. She contacted Illinois Governor Dwight Green, warning that if the situation were not cleared up "it will be my painful duty to recall my Staff from the Centralia Clinic and place them in other Centers and in other States that are so eagerly awaiting the service now being given to the State of Illinois." The "repeated stumbling blocks" around the formal certification of the clinic by the state's crippled children's division had prevented the clinic from receiving the funds "donated for purposes of caring for the children afflicted by the disease," funds that were in the NFIP "coffers."[166] In August, 2 months after the 1948 Congressional hearings, Green arranged a meeting at his campaign headquarters attended by Kenny, the mayor of Centralia, clinic officials, and the director of the State Division of Services for Crippled Children. Green was in the midst of his campaign for his third term as Illinois's Republican governor, and he may have hoped the meeting would distract voters from the uproar over the mining accident in Centralia the year before in which 111 miners had died, one of the nation's worst mining disasters.[167] Before the meeting Kenny travelled to Centralia where she spoke to a crowd of an estimated 5,000 including hundreds of workers who had helped to renovate the clinic.[168]

At the meeting hosted by Green, physicians on the Crippled Children Division's advisory board noted that state officials could not "purchase medical care in an institution where only one method of treatment of crippled children is practiced."[169] The director of the Crippled Children Division reiterated his agency's policy: the clinic must have a board-certified pediatrician and orthopedist living and practicing in Centralia. The clinic's selection of a pediatrician from St. Louis and an orthopedic surgeon from Chicago did not meet these requirements for these physicians were not suitable for emergency care.[170] Centralia was a small coal-mining town without the medical facilities of nearby larger communities; its physicians were frustrated but not surprised when all the pediatricians they asked to serve at the clinic—in one estimate 50—turned them down.[171]

The Centralia community refused to accept this decision and believed that Kenny could alter the clinic's fate. In 1949 while Kenny was in Australia John Lucian Matthews, who had contracted polio in November 1948 and been treated at the Centralia clinic, flew to Toowoomba to see Kenny about keeping the clinic open.[172] Kenny's limited influence became clear when the clinic's new administrator announced that Kenny had ordered the clinic to remain open pending her return from Australia in early 1949. Kline contradicted this immediately, saying the KF would no longer back the clinic, as it was unable to "economically meet the foundation's medical standards," and he began to arrange for current Centralia patients to be treated at the Michael Reese Hospital in Chicago. He also said that the town of Centralia was too small and not close enough to a medical center, arguments that supporters pointed out could just as well have been made about Warm Springs.[173] Suddenly, however, a polio epidemic in June 1949 changed this story. The state department of public health agreed to fund the clinic—now called the "Centralia Polio Center"—along with assistance from the NFIP and the KF. But when the epidemic ended in September the center closed again and did not reopen.[174]

The Centralia center collapsed despite backing by a local medical society, grateful parents, and an enthusiastic community. Kenny alone had not been powerful enough to alter antagonistic bureaucrats backed by unhelpful prominent physicians, and the KF board in Minneapolis had not supported her. If she had another opportunity to open a new Kenny clinic she was determined to shore up all of these alliances from the outset.

THE HOPE OF GOVERNMENT POWER

The Congressional hearings in 1948 did not lead to the formation of a federal Polio Institute or convince Congress to support the idea of a federal Kenny clinic. Nonetheless, Kenny remained convinced that the regulatory power of government could help to promote her work and counter the influence of the NFIP. Both in America and especially on her trips to Europe Kenny focused more and more on a particular group of experts: public health officers. Hers was a vision of medical power based partly on her success in 1930s Queensland when she had the ear of bureaucrats within the state ministry of health, and also on her awareness of the power of federal and state officials within the expanding New Deal and Fair Deal administrations to control access to facilities for the care of disabled and infectious disease patients. Conscious of the tricky medical politics of her time, she carefully avoided speaking to European audiences about the organization of medical care, the status of nurses, or other health policy issues.[175] It is possible that she did not see that her visits to European hospitals and health departments bore the imprimatur of an appearance by an American dignitary, but it is likely that the respect she received stemmed from that perception. Her discussion of polio care, just as epidemics were becoming a growing health problem in Europe, attracted attention from both European physicians and the public.

In America, as Kenny recognized, medical populism had deep popular and political roots. A number of congressmen and members of the public shared her sense that laymen and women should play a role in directing medical policy (including scientific research) to ensure fairness and objectivity. In the 1940s and 1950s, the expansion of government investment in medicine and science provided a new platform for the articulation of populist critiques of professional elitism and monopoly, phrased in the Cold War language of democracy and freedom.

To be sure, Kenny, Congress, the AMA, and the NFIP all agreed that modern scientific research was the best way to fight polio. However, populists such as Kenny and her supporters demanded that science be linked to medical freedom, which in Kenny's case meant freeing her patients from braces and crutches and from the crippling effects of elitist orthodoxy. Populists wanted more than the freedom to chose the medical treatment they wanted; they also wanted some say over the kinds of research that would be funded. For Kenny twentieth-century science was a resource, not a threat, and she confidently demanded the right to the vocabulary and technology of the laboratory. Clinicians' access to the fruits of laboratory science, she warned, was blocked by the monopoly of the NFIP and the AMA. Only the government, responding to popular outrage, could ensure a true democracy of science. Kenny's demands for scientific respect and her self portrayal as an isolated outsider attracted a public suspicious of corporate elitism. Perhaps medical freedom could be ensured by government fiat, opening the doors of hospitals and laboratories so that the resources of medical science would be available to all.

The excitement of being a Congressional witness, surrounded by eager reporters, Congressmen, and members of the public was not matched by Kenny's personal experience. By the late 1940s Kenny was in a newly isolated position. In the years after the war most of her Australian technicians left the Institute. Mary Farquarson, Kenny's niece from Queensland, had replaced Mary Kenny as Kenny's assistant and companion in 1946. Unwilling to endure the restricted social life Mary Kenny had led, Farquarson married a local Minnesota businessman in 1949 and began to raise a family.[176] Bill Bell, Kenny's nephew and technician who had come from Australia to work with her in 1941, moved to New Zealand where, backed by the minister of health, he introduced Kenny's work in hospitals across the North Island, and began to work at a hospital in Wanganui designated for Kenny's work. Bell, who combined Kenny's "crusading zeal and optimism" with his own "persuasiveness and tact," later trained his sons to work as Kenny therapists.[177] Only Valerie Harvey, the former Brisbane nurse, remained in the United States, practicing at the Jersey City clinic. Harvey was convinced of the value of Kenny's work, but she had a gentler and more patient style, and many technicians considered her a better teacher than Kenny herself.[178]

Most disappointing for Kenny was the quiet retreat by her beloved ward Mary. Back in Brisbane Mary was not continuing to fight for the expansion of the Kenny method in Australia. Instead Kenny found that her ward was "very happily married" and "a very busy housewife." Mary was also no longer putting Kenny's needs ahead of her own. Thus, while Kenny was "very pleased" that Mary had a husband and a home, she complained throughout the late 1940s that she had written several letters and received no reply. "I get anxious when I don't hear from you," she admitted.[179] With so many members of her family and medical associates so far away Kenny leaned on her close Minneapolis friends like James Henry. But the Institute and the city no longer felt like home.

NOTES

1. Kenny, May 14 1948, *Hearings before the Committee on interstate and Foreign Commerce, House of Representatives, 80th Congress, Second Session on H.R. 977 [Cancer and Polio Research]...H.R. 3257 [Cancer Research Commission]...H.R. 3464 [Cure of Cancer, Heart Disease, Infantile Paralysis, and other diseases]...May 13, 14 and 19 1948* (Washington DC: Government Printing Office, 1948), 97, 114 hereafter *Hearings*; Gerald Gross "Sister Kenny Has Her Say Against Polio Foundation" *Washington Report on the Medical Sciences* (May 17 1948) 50: 1. Part of this chapter is a version of Rogers "Sister Kenny Goes to Washington: Polio, Populism and Medical Politics in Postwar America" in *The Politics of Healing: Histories of Alternative Medicine in Twentieth-Century North America* ed. Robert D. Johnston (New York: Routledge, 2004), 97–116.

2. Kenny to Mr. President, Mrs. Webber and Gentlemen, May 24 1948, Board of Directors, MHS-K.

3. Marion T. Bennett, *Hearings*, May 14 1948, 108. Bennett, a Republican Congressman from Missouri, was in the House 1943–1949.

4. Victoria A. Harden *Inventing the NIH: Federal Biomedical Research Policy, 1887–1937* (Baltimore: Johns Hopkins University Press, 1986), 181.

5. Quoted in Homer W. Smith "Present Status of National Science Foundation Legislation" *JAMA* (1948) 137: 18. The NSF bill of 1947, for example, had included special disease commissions to be directed by an eleven member board made up of 6 "eminent scientists" and 5 representatives of the general public; see Donald C. Swain "The Rise of a Research Empire: NIH, 1930–1960" *Science* 138 (1962) 1233–1237; Toby A. Appel *Shaping Biology: The National Science Foundation and American Biological Research, 1945–1975* (Baltimore: Johns Hopkins University Press, 2000), 34–35.

6. See J. Merton England *A Patron for Pure Science: The National Science Foundation's Formative Years, 1945–1957* (Washington DC: National Science Foundation, 1982), 85; Daniel J. Kevles *The Physicists: A History of a Scientific Community in Modern America* (New York: Knopf, 1977), 363.

7. John Burnham "American Medicine's Golden Age: What Happened to It?" *Science* (1982) 215: 1474–1479; and see also Allan M. Brandt and Martha Gardner "The Golden Age of Medicine?" in Roger Cooter and John Pickstone eds. *Medicine in the Twentieth Century* (London: Harwood, 2000), 21–37.

8. A study of all sources of American medical research funding during 1947 found 45% from industry, 28% from federal, state, and local governments and 13% from foundations; Smith "Present Status of National Science Foundation Legislation," 19.

9. Harry M. Marks "Cortisone, 1949: A Year in the Political Life of a Drug" *Bulletin of the History of Medicine* (1992) 66: 421.

10. Clarence A. Mills "Distribution of American Research Funds" *Science* (1948) 107: 127–130 [reprinted in] *Hearing before the Committee on Interstate and Foreign Commerce, House of Representative Eightieth Congress Second Session on H.R. 6007 and S. 2385 [on a National Science Foundation] June 1, 1948* (Washington: Government Printing Office, 1948), 138–142.

11. Morris Fishbein to My Dear Basil, February 23 1948, Public Relations, AMA, MOD.

12. James Harvey Young *The Medical Messiahs: A Social History of Health Quackery in Twentieth-Century America* (Princeton: Princeton University Press, 1967), 360–389; Eric S. Juhnke *Quacks and Crusaders: The Fabulous Careers of John Brinkley, Norma Baker and Harry Hoxsey* (Lawrence: University Press of Kansas, 2002), 76–86, 140–142.

13. Charles M. Barber "A Diamond in the Rough: William Langer Reexamined" *North Dakota History* (1998) 64: 2–18; Glenn H. Smith *Langer of North Dakota: A Study in Isolationism, 1940–1959* (New York: Garland Press, 1979); Agnes Geelan *The Dakota Maverick: The Political Life of William Langer, also Known as "Wild Bill" Langer* (Fargo: Geelan, 1975); Lawrence H. Larsen "William Langer: A Maverick in the Senate" *Wisconsin Magazine of History* (1961) 44: 189–198; Ted Kincaid "Senator Langer Sponsors Polio Study Measure" *Washington Times-Herald* September 1 1944; Amendment, S.J. Res. 147, 78th Congress, 2d Session, Children's Bureau Central File 1941–1944, Record Group 102, Infantile Paralysis 4-5-16-1, National Archives.

14. William Langer May 7 1945 *Congressional Record Appendix, 79th Congress* volume 91, part 2 (Washington: Government Printing Office, 1945), A2110; Langer "S. 800: A Bill to provide for the establishment of a National Infantile Paralysis Clinic," 79th Congress 1st Session, March 28 1945, Mayoralty Files 1945–1948, Box 10, Kenny Institute, Humphrey Papers, MHS; J. Earle Moser "Langer Seeks U.S. Supported Kenny Clinic" *Washington Times-Herald* March 29 1945; "$20,000,000 Fund to Foster Kenny Plan Proposed by Langer" *Washington Evening Star*, March 29 1945; see also David A. Horowitz *Beyond Left and Right: Insurgency and the Establishment* (Urbana: University of Illinois Press, 1997), 151–152.

15. Mrs. Eugene Meyer "Judgment Day for the Private Welfare Agent" *Public Opinion Quarterly* (1945) 9: 338–345.

16. Ralph M. Kramer *Voluntary Agencies in the Welfare State* (Berkeley: University of California Press, 1981), 114–115.

17. See Scott M. Cutlip *Fund Raising in the United States: Its Role in America's Philanthropy* (New Brunswick: Rutgers University Press, 1965); Kramer *Voluntary Agencies in the Welfare State*; Richard Carter *The Gentle Legions* (Garden City, NY: Doubleday, 1961).

18. David Dietz "Cost of Fighting Polio: Why March of Dimes Is Needed" *New York World Telegram* January 29 1946.

19. Richard H. Shryock, *American Medical Research: Past and Present* (New York: Commonwealth Fund, 1947), 165 n 20. These statistics were taken from a paper by Henry S. Simms read before the American Association for the Advancement of Science in September 1944.

20. Horace A. Brown "Organization of a Voluntary Health Agency" (thesis, Masters of Public Health, Yale University, 1953), 67–69; Bernhard J. Stern "[Review of] *Voluntary Health Agencies*" *American Sociological Review* (1946) 11: 757.

21. Selskar M. Gunn and Philip S. Platt *Voluntary Health Agencies: An Interpretive Study* (New York: Ronald Press Company, 1945). See also "Selskar Michael Gunn" *American Journal of Public Health* (1944) 34: 1096–1097; "Deaths: Philip S. Platt" *American Journal of Public Health* (1979) 69: 191.

22. Dora Goldstine "[Review of] *Voluntary Health Agencies*" *The Social Service Review* (1946) 20: 277; see also Carter *The Gentle Legions*, 257–260.

23. Edward G. Huber "Official and Non-Official Health Agencies" *Public Administration Review* (1946) 6: 189; Brown "Organization of a Voluntary Health Agency," 70. The NFIP raised $6.5 million in 1943, $12 million in 1944, and $19 million in both 1945 and 1946; while the American Cancer Society raised $4 million in 1945, and $10 million in 1946; Angela N.H. Creager *The Life of a Virus: Tobacco Mosaic Virus as an Experimental Model, 1930–1965* (Chicago: University of Chicago Press, 2002), 152.

24. Pearl Baldock (Mrs. R. G. Baldock) to Dear Mrs. Sterne, June 2 1949, General Correspondence-B, MHS-K; and see Mrs. R.G. Baldock to Sir [Prime Minister], October 6 1952, #707/9/A, Series A462, AA-ACT.

25. "My Report on Conferences with the Medical Profession in Fourteen Foreign Countries—Elizabeth Kenny" [reprinted in] *Hearings*, May 14 1948, 153; [film transcript in] Kenny, *Hearings*, May 19 1948, 198.

26. *New York Journal-American* March 22 1945, [abstract] Public Relations, MOD-K; "Sister Kenny Delays Plans to Leave City" *Minneapolis Morning Tribune* March 21 1945.

27. John F. Pohl to Marvin L. Kline, February 5 1945, [accessed in 1992 before recent re-cataloging], UMN-ASC; Mary Pohl, interview with Rogers, August 21 2003, Tallahassee, Florida.

28. Kenny, *Hearings*, May 14 1948, 116.

29. George H. Gallup *The Gallop Poll: Public Opinion 1935–1971* (New York: Random House, 1972), 1: 663.

30. Kenny, *Hearings*, May 19 1948, 103-4.

31. [Cohn interview with] William O'Neill, May 20 1955, Cohn Papers, MHS-K; "Sister Kenny Polio Center, First In East, to Open Here June 15" [unnamed newspaper] 1947, Public Relations, MOD-K; "Kenny Center Opens" *Buffalo Courier-Express Pictorial* May 16 1948; "A Higher Force Has Helped Her Work, Sister Kenny Says" *Buffalo Evening News* November 23 1948.

32. Kenny to Sir [Governor Dwight Green], June 4 1948, Dwight Green 1948, MHS-K.

33. Kenny to Mr. President, Mrs. Webber and Gentlemen, May 24 1948; Kenny to Sir [Governor Dwight Green], June 4 1948; "Dedication Ceremonies: Sister Elizabeth Kenny Clinic, Centralia, Illinois, Sunday, August 24, 1947," George W. Gould, 1946–1948, MHS-K; "Sister Kenny Clinic Dedicated In Illinois" *New York Times* August 25 1947.

34. "Paralysis Clinic For East" *New York Times* February 27 1948; "Medicine: Sister Kenny's New Center" *Newsweek* (March 15 1948) 31: 49; Kenny to Mr. President, Mrs. Webber and Gentlemen, May 24 1948; "Sister Kenny Asks [for] A Medical Inquiry" *New York Times* March 3 1948; "Sister Kenny Institute Opens" *New York Herald-Tribune* April 6 1948; [Cohn interview with] Al Baum and Mrs. Baum, June 14 1955, Cohn Papers, MHS-K; "Polio Cure Goal of Mal Stevens" *New York Times* September 4 1949.

35. "Kenny Unit Accepts Dimes Board Offer To Confer On Rift" *Buffalo Evening News* November 18 1949; "Sister Kenny Asks [for] A Medical Inquiry"; "Kenny Institute in Illinois Faces Closing" *Minneapolis Star* July 22 1948.

36. See Jonathan Engel *Doctors and Reformers: Discussion and Debate over Health Policy 1925–1950* (Charleston: University of South Carolina Press, 2002), 209, 295–296; on Fishbein and the AMA see Frank D. Campion *The AMA and U.S. Health Policy since 1940* (Chicago: Chicago Review Press, 1984), 118–130; Carl F. Ameringer "Organized Medicine on Trial: The Federal Trade Commission vs. the American Medical Association" *Journal of Policy History* (2000) 12: 445–472. The second investigation lasted until 1951. For Fishbein's version of events, see Morris Fishbein *Morris Fishbein, M.D.: An Autobiography* (New York: Doubleday, 1969), 208–223.

37. Dr. Allan M. Butler [Progressive Citizens of America], July 3 1947, *Hearings before a Subcommittee of the Committee on Labor and Public Welfare, United States Senate, Eightieth Congress, First Session, on S. 545 [NIH funding] and S. 1320 [National Health Program]... Part 2, June 25, 26, 27 and July 2 and 3, 1947),* (Washington, D.C.: Government Printing Office, 1947), 1002.

38. Joe W. Savage, *Hearings*, May 13 1948, 71.

39. William O'Neill Sherman [M.D., Pittsburgh] to Morris Fishbein, January 17, 1947, Public Relations, MOD-K. Nicholas Ransohoff's paper was submitted to *JAMA* for publication but was rejected by the AMA's Orthopedic Section.

40. Eleanor Roosevelt "My Day" September 4 1947, http://www.gwu.edu/~erpapers/myday/displaydoc.cfm?_y=1947&_f=md000749, accessed 12/11/2009.

41. Helen Waterhouse "Akron No Polio Nest, County Doctors Told" *Akron Beacon Journal* June 2 1948.

42. Basil O'Connor to My Dear Mr. Michaels, February 15 1944, Public Relations, MOD-K.

43. [Script] WPTF- "Fighting Infantile Paralysis," Raleigh, N.C. March 11 [1944]-7:30–8:00 PM, Public Relations, MOD-K. See also Roland H. Berg *Polio and Its Problems* (Philadelphia: J.B. Lippincott, 1948), 97–98. The appointment of anatomist Harry Weaver as director of research in 1946 further demonstrated the fund's belief in centralized and coordinated investigation; On Weaver see Richard Carter *Breakthrough: The Saga of Jonas Salk* (New York: Trident Press, 1966), 56–59. For comments that this direction of scientific research ran counter to "scientific tradition" and was "controversial," see Paul *A History*, 412–413.

44. The National Foundation for Infantile Paralysis *A Decade of Doing: The Story of the National Foundation For Infantile Paralysis, 1938–1948* (New York: National Foundation for Infantile Paralysis, 1948), 11.

45. Hart Van Riper, *Hearings*, May 13 1948, 79; Joe W. Savage, *Hearings*, May 13 1948, 71.

46. Joe W. Savage, *Hearings*, May 13 1938, 71.

47. Gerald Gross "Demurrer By O'Connor, Et Al" *Washington Report on the Medical Sciences* (May 17 1948) 50: 1.

48. Basil O'Connor "The American Way" June 7 1947, Public Relations, AMA, MOD. On O'Connor's longstanding campaign against federal giving see Oshinksy *Polio* 80–81; and O'Connor "Foreword" in Berg *Polio and Its Problems*, vii-viii.

49. "Address by Dr. Morris Fishbein, Editor of the Journal of the American Medical Association Given at a Dinner in the Ansley Hotel, Atlanta, Georgia on Wednesday, September 17, 1947 Marking the End of the Clinical Conference on Poliomyelitis Held at Georgia Warm Springs Foundation, September 15th Thru the 17th Commemorating the 20th Anniversary of its Founding," Public Relations, Fishbein, MOD.

50. Joe W. Savage to Morris A. Fishbein, February 25 1948, Public Relations, AMA, MOD; Fishbein to Savage, February 28 1948, Public Relations, AMA, MOD; Editorial, "Medical Research," *JAMA* (1948) 137: 465.

51. John O'Connor, *Hearings*, May 13 1948, 41, 49–50. New York Democrat John Joseph O'Connor (1885–1960) had been in the House 1923–1939.

52. Gross "Sister Kenny Has Her Say Against Polio Foundation," 1.

53. Joseph P. O'Hara during Van Riper's testimony, *Hearings*, May 13 1948, 81. Joseph Patrick O'Hara (1895–1975), a Minnesota Republican, was in the House 1941–59.

54. Wolverton, *Hearings*, May 14 1948, 107; Edwin D. Neff "Kenny Polio Fund Denial Is Denounced" *Washington Times-Herald*, May 15, 1948.

55. Neff "Kenny Polio Fund Denial Is Denounced."

56. Wolverton and Kenny, *Hearings*, May 14 1948, 101.

57. Gross "Sister Kenny Has Her Say Against Polio Foundation," 1.

58. Kenny, *Hearings*, May 19 1948, 193; Gerald Gross "Sister Kenny Shows Her Film To House Interstate Group" *Washington Report on the Medical Sciences* (May 24 1948) 51: 2.

59. Kenny, *Hearings*, May 14 1948, 103, 112; Neff "Kenny Polio Fund Denial Is Denounced"; Kenny to Mr. President, Mrs. Webber and Gentlemen, May 24 1948.

60. Kenny, *Hearings*, May 19 1948, 204; Kenny to Wolverton, May 26, 1948, reprinted in Kenny, *Hearings*, May 14 1948, 154. See also Gross "Sister Kenny Has Her Say Against Polio Foundation," 1.

61. John Heselton, *Hearings*, May 14 1948, 111. John Walter Heselton (1900–1962) was a Massachusetts Republican in the House 1945–1959.

62. Jungeblut "Vitamin C Therapy and Prophylaxis in Experimental Poliomyelitis" *Journal of Experimental Medicine* (1937) 65: 127–146; Jungeblut "Further Observations on Vitamin C Therapy in Experimental Poliomyelitis" *Journal of Experimental Medicine* (1937) 66: 459–477; Jungeblut and R.R. Feiner "Vitamin C Content of Monkey Tissues in Experimental Poliomyelitis" *Journal of Experimental Medicine* (1937) 66: 479–491; Jungeblut "A Further Contribution to Vitamin C Therapy in Experimental Poliomyelitis" *Journal of Experimental Medicine* (1939) 70:315–332. See also Paul de Kruif to Dear Doctor Jungeblut, February 19 1936, Box 1, Folder D, Jungeblut Papers, NLM; de Kruif to Dear Dr. Jungeblut, December 16 1938, Box 1, Folder D, Jungeblut Papers NLM.

63. Kenny to Mr. President, Mrs. Webber and Gentlemen, February 24 1948, Board of Directors, MHS-K.

64. Jungeblut "Vitamin C Therapy and Prophylaxis in Experimental Poliomyelitis," 141; Victor Cohn "Sister Kenny Wins New Medical Praise" *Minneapolis Morning Tribune* October 4 1949; "Polio Clues: Vitamin C" *Time* (September 18 1939) 34: 35–36; "Claus Jungeblut, Bacteriologist, 78" *New York Times* February 2 1976.

65. "Report of the Queensland Royal Commission on Modern Methods for the Treatment of Infantile Paralysis" *Medical Journal of Australia* (January 29 1938) 1: 195–198; National Foundation for Infantile Paralysis *Infantile Paralysis: A Symposium Delivered at Vanderbilt University April, 1941* (Baltimore: Waverly Press, 1941), 207–209.

66. Kenny, *Hearings*, May 19 1948, 202; Jungeblut to Kenny, February 24 1948, Dr. Claus W. Jungeblut, 1945–1950, MHS-K; Kenny to Jungeblut, February 16 1948, Dr. Claus W. Jungeblut, 1945–1950, MHS-K.

67. Kenny, *Hearings*, May 19 1948, 202; Jungeblut to Kenny, February 24 1948; Kenny to Jungeblut, February 16 1948.

68. Jungeblut, *Hearings*, May 13 1948, 67–69; Gerald Gross "'Monopoly' Charge Hurled" *Washington Report on the Medical Sciences* (May 17 1948) 50: 1.

69. Kenny to Dear Sir [Wolverton], June 9 1948, U.S. House of Representatives Committee on Interstate and Foreign Trade, MHS-K.

70. Wolverton in Jungeblut testimony, *Hearings*, May 13 1948, 68.

71. O'Hara in Van Riper testimony, *Hearings*, May 13 1948, 83.

72. Van Riper, *Hearings*, May 13 1948, 79–81.

73. Kenny quoted by William Langer May 7 1945, *Congressional Record Appendix, 79th Congress* volume 91, no. 2 (Washington: Government Printing Office, 1945), A2109.

74. Stanley Henwood to Marvin Kline, May 21 1948, [reprinted in] Kenny, *Hearings*, May 14 1948, 155.

75. Martin L. Kline to Dear Mr. Henwood, May 25 1948, [reprinted in] Kenny, *Hearings*, May 14 1948, 156; Henwood to Kline 1948, [reprinted in] Kenny, *Hearings*, May 14 1948, 105.

76. Kline to Henwood, May 25 1948.

77. [Cohn interview with] Al Baum and Mrs. Baum, June 14 1955, Cohn Papers, MHS-K; [Cohn first interview with] Rosalind Russell, August 18 1953, Cohn Papers, MHS-K.

78. Wolverton [during testimony of Dr. Leonard A. Scheele, Surgeon General], *Hearings*, May 13 1948, 22.

79. According to reporters, Wolverton gave the NFIP "a severe tongue lashing," warning that its refusal to support Kenny was "inconceivable" and that the NFIP had clearly "given her the run-around" when she offered to design an exhibit for the conference; Neff "Kenny Polio Fund Denial Is Denounced"; Wolverton, *Hearings*, May 14 1948, 118; Wolverton, remarks, *Hearings*, May 19 1948, [enclosed in] Kenny to Mr. President, Mrs. Webber and Gentlemen, February 24 1948; Gross "Sister Kenny Shows Her Film To House Interstate Group," 2.

80. Wolverton, *Hearings*, May 19 1948. Kenny had been the guest of honor at a luncheon hosted by Jersey City Mayor Frank Eggers who had promised the KF his full cooperation and recalled that his uncle, Frank Hague, had urged Kenny 7 years ago to have a clinic in the Medical Center; "Sister Kenny Asks [for] A Medical Inquiry" *New York Times* March 3 1948.

81. Appel *Shaping Biology*, 34–35; Kevles *The Physicists*, 324–366.

82. England *Patron for Pure Science*, 91; Marks "Cortisone," 429, 438 n.88.

83. Campion *The AMA and U.S. Health Policy*, 127–164.

84. Kevles *The Physicists*, 356–364; Appel *Shaping Biology*, 18–37; Gerald Gross "Clinical Research Center Nearing Contract Stage" *Washington Report on Medical Sciences* 57 (July 5 1948), 4, Washington Report File, MHS-K.

85. Dr. Edward L. Bortz [AMA president], *Hearings before the Committee on Interstate and Foreign Commerce, House of Representatives Eightieth Congress Second Session on H.R.*

5159, H.R. 3059, H.R. 3464, H.R. 3762, H.R. 5087 May 5 and 6, 1948 (Washington: United States Government Printing Office, 1948), 102; Steven P. Strickland *Politics, Science and Dread Disease: A Short History of United States Medical Research Policy* (Cambridge: Harvard University Press, 1972), 53; Roger L. Geiger *Research and Relevant Knowledge: American Research Universities Since World War II* (New York: Oxford University Press, 1993), 180–181.

86. [Herbert M. Shelton] "Women To the Rescue," *Dr Shelton's Hygienic Review* (July 1945) 6: 257–258.

87. Morris Fishbein "Introduction" in *Poliomyelitis: Papers and Discussions Presented at the First International Poliomyelitis Conference* (Philadelphia: J.B. Lippincott, 1949), vii; "Polio Conference Opens Here Today," *New York Times* July 12 1948; William I. Laurence "Older Age Groups Attacked by Polio" *New York Times* July 13 1948. This conference inaugurated a series of international polio meetings sponsored by the NFIP, held every 3 years until 1962, with Fishbein assisting with the publication of the proceedings.

88. These conferences, Yale epidemiologist John Paul later reflected, "set both the stage and the American standard for a global type of representation that had not existed before, and was especially welcome [by researchers] in the immediate post-World War II period." But, he added, the conferences were "conducted in a lavish manner, and it was obvious that they could not have been put on without the unique financial backing of the NFIP." This "spectacle of medical science being closely allied to fund-raising and fund-spending techniques," Paul believed, resulting in "the raising of eyebrows" among both American and European scientists; Paul *A History*, 320–323. Paul compared these conferences to meetings held by the WHO Expert Committee on Poliomyelitis which began in 1952 and "in the eyes of the world had a truly authoritative ring," 323.

89. "Sister Kenny Joins Guild" *New York Times* July 10 1948.

90. "News: Sister Kenny" *Newsweek* (July 26 1948) 32: 53.

91. Harold Aaron "Polio: A Story of Conflicting Personalities, Promotional Methods and Treatments for a Crippling Disease," *Consumer Reports* (February 1949) 14: 80. See also Kenny's report of a foreign doctor about the recent conference that "when weighed in the balance, [it] left the scales empty for the National Foundation...and with gold for Sister Kenny;" Kenny to Dear Mr. LaRoche, November 8 1948, Clara and Chester LaRoche, 1945–1948, MHS-K. On "The Incomprehensible Tabu" cited by Kenny see "Polio Foundation Fights Her Method, Sister Kenny Says" [*Freeport NY] Leader* October 21 1948.

92. Roland Berg to Roy Naftzger [chairman, executive committee of the Los Angeles County Chapter], November 23 1948, Public Relations, MOD-K.

93. "First International Poliomyelitis Conference" *Physical Therapy Review* (September-October 1948) 28: 252–253.

94. Irvine McQuarrie "The Evolution of Signs and Symptoms in Poliomyelitis" in *First International Poliomyelitis Conference*, 57, 59.

95. David Bodian "Poliomyelitis: Pathologic Anatomy" in *First International Poliomyelitis Conference*, 81, 83, 81.

96. Fritz Buchthal "Some Aspects of the Pathologic Physiology of Poliomyelitis" in *First International Poliomyelitis Conference*, 85, 88.

97. Pollock [in Discussion of Fritz Buchthal] "Some Aspects of the Pathologic Physiology of Poliomyelitis" in *First International Poliomyelitis Conference*, 99.

98. Russell [in Discussion of Fritz Buchthal] "Some Aspects of the Pathologic Physiology of Poliomyelitis" in *First International Poliomyelitis Conference*, 96–97, 104.

99. Faber [in Discussion of Fritz Buchthal] "Some Aspects of the Pathologic Physiology of Poliomyelitis" in *First International Poliomyelitis Conference*, 97.

100. Bodian [in Discussion of Fritz Buchthal] "Some Aspects of the Pathologic Physiology of Poliomyelitis" in *First International Poliomyelitis Conference*, 99.

101. Kenny "This Report Was Presented to The Honorable The Premier of the State of Queensland E.M. Hanlon, M.L.A. and to Doctors Pye, Nye, Lee, Arden, Wilkinson, and Fryberg of the City of Brisbane, Queensland, Australia Concerning the disease Poliomyelitis [1950]," Kenny Collection, Box 1, Fryer Library, 11.

102. Herbert J. Seddon "Economic Aspects of the Management of Poliomyelitis" in *First International Poliomyelitis Conference*, 35–36; Laurence "Older Age Groups Attacked By Polio"; Nicholas S. Ransohoff "Intocostin in the Treatment of Acute Anterior Poliomyelitis" *New York State Medical Journal* (1947) 47: 151–153.

103. Seddon [in "Discussion" of Herbert J. Seddon] "Economic Aspects of the Management of Poliomyelitis" in *First International Poliomyelitis Conference*, 53.

104. Seddon [in Discussion], "Great Britain: Orthopaedic Section of the Royal Society of Medicine" *Journal of Bone and Joint Surgery* (May 1948) 30: 386–388.

105. H.J. Seddon "The Early Treatment of Poliomyelitis" *British Medical Journal* (August 30 1947) 2: 319–321; Kenny "For the Information of: Dr. Aubrey Pye, Dr. Felix Arden, Dr. Jarvis Nye, Dr. Alan Lee, Dr. Abraham Fryberg, Professor Wilkinson" November 10 1947, Kenny Collection, Fryer Library; Kenny "For the Information of the Staff of the Royal North Shore Hospital, St. Leonards, Sydney" [1947] [enclosed in] Kenny to Sir [Hanlon] November 11 1947, Wilson Collection.

106. Laurence "Older Age Groups Attacked by Polio"; "Paralysis Trend Found to Adults And Teen-Agers" *New York Herald-Tribune* July 13 1948; "News: Sister Kenny," 53; Kenny [Report] July 19 1948, First International Poliomyelitis Conference, 1948, MHS-K; "Polio Treatment Costs Defended by Sister Kenny" *Los Angeles Times* July 13 1948. For the claim that the cost of the Kenny method was at least 10 times as great as therapy used several years ago see Joseph G. Molner "The Kenny Method" [paper presented at] Post-Graduate Course in Physical Medicine and Rehabilitation, University of Texas, Medical Branch, Galveston, March 7 1946, Public Relations, MOD-K; "Medicine: Sister Kenny's New Center," 49.

107. Laurence "Older Age Groups Attacked by Polio."

108. [Cohn interview with] Amy Lindsey, May 19 1955, Cohn Papers, MHS-K

109. [Cohn interview with] Morris Fishbein, November 16 1953, Cohn Papers, MHS-K; and see Fishbein *An Autobiography*, 233.

110. Roland Berg to Roy Naftzger, November 23 1948, Public Relations, MOD-K.

111. Albert Deutsch "Sister Kenny and the Foundation" *New York Star* July 14 1948.

112. "Illinois: Film on Poliomyelitis" *JAMA* (1948) 137: 1325; "Medical Motion Pictures" *JAMA* (1948) 138: 111.

113. "New Kenny Institute Setup Announced" *Minneapolis Star* December 6 1948; "The Kenny Institute" *Minnesota Medicine* (December 1948) 31: 1349.

114. "New Kenny Institute Setup Announced."

115. [Transcript] "Telephone Conversation between Dr. Van Riper and Dr. Huenkens, Medical Director, Kenny Institute, Minneapolis—Dec. 8, 1948," Public Relations, MOD-K.

116. [Transcript] "Telephone Conversation between Dr. Van Riper and Dr. Huenkens"; Van Riper to Dear Mr. [Charles B.] Sweatt, January 25 1949, Public Relations, MOD-K.

117. "Citizens Form Polio Research League, to Ask Congress to Institute New Project" *San Fernando Sun* [1948], Clippings 1948, MHS-K; "Anti-Kenny Stand Hit By League" *Glendale*

News-Press August 4 1949; "Sister Kenny Hospital Plans Mapped; L.A. to Hail Polio Foe" *Los Angeles Examiner* October 23 1949; [editorial] "The Polio Controversy", *San Fernando Sun* October 28 1948; "Polio Conference Set" *New York Times* December 9 1948; [Transcript] "Telephone Conversation between Dr. Van Riper and Dr. Huenkens."

118. "Citizens Form Polio Research League"; "Group Launches Federal Polio Research Drive" [newspaper name missing], September 30 1948, Public Relations, MOD-K.

119. Citizen's Polio Research League Petition, Public Relations, MOD-K; [Transcript] "Telephone Conversation between Dr. Van Riper and Dr. Huenkens." We know little about this group, although it may well be part of the wider postwar conservative movement in southern California; see Kurt Schuparra *Triumph of the Right: The Rise of the California Conservative Movement 1945–1966* (Armonk, N.Y.: M. E. Sharpe, 1998).

120. Herbert Avedon to My Dear Sister Kenny, "A Third Open Letter," *San Fernando Sun*, October 14 1948; Herbert Avedon to My Dear Mr. Sheppard, "An Open Letter," *San Fernando Sun*, October 14 1948; Herbert Avedon to My Dear Mr. O'Connor, "Another Open Letter," *San Fernando Sun*, October 14 1948.

121. Herbert Avedon to Sister Kenny, October 29 1948, General Correspondence, July–December 1948, MHS-K; Harry R. Sheppard to Herbert Avedon, October 21, 1948, *San Fernando Sun*; "Sister Kenny Answers Sun Open Letter," *San Fernando Sun*, October 28 1948.

122. Barbaralu Sanderson to My Dear Mr. O'Connor, *San Fernando Sun,* December 2 1948.

123. "Polio Conference Set"; Sonja Betts to Dear Miss Truman, December 2 1948, General Correspondence-T, MHS-K.

124. "Citizens Form Polio Research League."

125. "Sister Kenny Gives Counsel On Polio" *New York Times* December 17 1948; Mildred Freeston to R. A. Burcaw, December 16 1948, Memorandum on Citizens Polio Research League Conference, Jersey City, December 16 1948, Public Relations, MOD-K.

126. "Sister Kenny Gives Counsel On Polio"; Freeston to Burcaw, December 16 1948.

127. Chester LaRoche to Dear Sister, October 28 1948, Clara and Chester LaRoche, 1945–1948, MHS-K.

128. Kenny to Dear Mr. LaRoche, November 8 1948, Clara and Chester La Roche, 1945–1948, MHS-K.

129. Marvin Stevens to Dear Chet [LaRoche], December 20 1948, Clara and Chester La Roche, 1945–1948, MHS-K.

130. Kenny to Dear Mr. LaRoche, December 27 1948, Clara and Chester La Roche, 1945–1948, MHS-K. Note that in June 1948 a subcommittee of the Committee on Medical Education of the New York Academy of Medicine viewed the Kenny film and after consulting with its sections on Pediatrics and Orthopedic Surgery decided not to request showing the film at its next general meeting; Mahlon Ashford to Dear Sister Kenny, January 21 1949, General Correspondence-A, MHS-K.

131. John Ralph "My Struggle By Sister Kenny" [Britain] *Sunday Graphic* May 11 1947, OM 65-17, Box 1, Folder 4, Chuter Papers, Oxley-SLQ; Kenny to Mr. President, Mrs. Webber and Gentlemen, May 24 1948.

132. Kenny to Dear Sir [Haverstock as secretary of KF], September 2 1947, Henry W. Haverstock, 1942–1951, MHS-K; Kenny to Mr. President, Mrs. Webber and Gentlemen, February 24 1948.

133. Kenny to Mr. President, Mrs. Webber and Gentlemen, February 24 1948; Kenny to Dear Sir [Haverstock as secretary of KF], September 2 1947.

134. [Cohn interview with] William O'Neil, May 20 1955; John F. Pohl "Early Diagnosis of Poliomyelitis" *JAMA* (July 26 1947) 134: 1059–1061.

135. Kenny to Dear Sir [Haverstock as secretary of KF] September 2 1947.

136. Kenny to Dear Dr. Pohl, September 20 1947, [accessed in 1992 before recent re-cataloging], UMN-ASC.

137. [Cohn interview with] William O'Neill, May 20 1955.

138. Kenny to Dear Miss Truman, January 6 1949, General Correspondence-T, MHS-K; Sonja Betts to Dear Miss Truman, December 2 1948.

139. "Kenny Picture Shown" *New York Times* July 1 1948; [Advertisement] "To the Publishers, Editors, Columnists and Reporters of Metropolitan Area Newspapers, Leaders of Parent-Teacher, Civic, Fraternal, Trade Union, Business, Women's and Public Service Organizations, Men and Women in All Branches of Public Life, the Medical and Nursing Professions" [unnamed New York newspaper 1948], Public Relations, MOD-K; "Kenny Polio Therapy Film Shown" *New York World-Telegram* [1948] Public Relations, MOD-K; "Asks Unity on Kenny Method" [unnamed New York newspaper] [1948], Public Relations, MOD-K; "Change Arrival Time For Sister Kenny's Visit to Centralia" *Centralia Sentinel* September 24 1951.

140. Christabel Pankhurst to Dear Sister Kenny, January 15 1948, Rosalind Russell (Brisson) 1947–1952, MHS-K.

141. "18,000 Begin Kenny Drive" [with Karsh photograph and caption "Sister Elizabeth Kenny, Polio-Fighting Australian Nurse"] *Minneapolis Sunday Tribune* November 7 1948; Doris B. Medsger to Dear Sister Kenny, October 26 1948, General Correspondence, July-December 1948, MHS-K; Yousuf Karsh "Women of Achievement" *Coronet* (November 1948) 25. This portrait is not mentioned in Maria Tippett *The Life of Yousuf Karsh* (New Haven: Yale University Press, 2007).

142. Mary Kenny McCracken said later that the cape was Karsh's own; McCracken, interviews with Rogers, November 1992.

143. "Medicine: Sister Kenny's New Center," 49.

144. Deutsch quoted in Aaron "Polio: A Story of Conflicting Personalities," 80.

145. [Transcript] "Telephone Conversation between Dr. Van Riper and Dr. Huenkens."

146. Hart Van Riper to Dear Mrs. Karlsteen, January 5 1950, Public Relations, MOD-K.

147. McCracken, interviews with Rogers, November 1992; See also "the Amazonian figure of the gray-haired, steely-eyed, strong-jawed Elizabeth Kenny;" Albert Deutsch, "The Truth About Sister Kenny," *American Mercury* (November 1944) 59: 610.

148. Gallup, *Gallup Poll*, 1: 775. The poll was done on December 26 1948.

149. Dana S. Creel to Isabel Robertson Memorandum Re: National Infantile Paralysis Foundation, December 11 1950, Record Group III-2K, OMR, Series Medical Interest, Box 14-171A, Folder 115, Rockefeller Archive Center, Tarrytown.

150. Thomas M. Rivers to Dear Mr. Rockefeller, December 7 1950, Record Group III-2K, OMR, Series Medical Interest, Box 14-171A, Folder 115, Rockefeller Archive Center, Tarrytown.

151. Aaron "Polio: A Story of Conflicting Personalities," 78.

152. Aaron "Polio: A Story of Conflicting Personalities," 78–81.

153. Aaron "Polio: A Story of Conflicting Personalities," 79.

154. Basil O'Connor to Dear Mr. Rockefeller, February 21 1951, Record Group III-2K, OMR, Series Medical Interest, Box 14-171A, Folder 115, Rockefeller Archive Center.

155. "Polio Foundation Leader Denies Pfeifer Charges" *Buffalo Courier-Express* October 14 1949; "'Dimes' Accounting Is Asked; Kenny's Unit's Charges Denied" *Buffalo Evening News*

October 14 1949, Public Relations, MOD-K; "Dimes Drive Has Failed To Aid Kenny Center, Foundation Says" *Buffalo Evening News* October [n.d.] 1949, Public Relations, MOD-K.

156. "Sister Kenny Foundation Scores March of Dimes Head" [unidentified newspaper 1949], Public Relations, MOD-K.

157. Inez Mattson to Dear Mrs. White, October 10 1948, Public Relations, MOD-K.

158. C. W. Plattes [chair of NFIP Hennepin County Chapter] to Dear Mr. Savage, October 5 1949, Public Relations, MOD-K.

159. J.L. Morrill to Dear Mr. [Charles Bolles] Rogers, November 15 1946, Presidents Papers, Box 119, UMN-ASC.

160. "Mapping Campaign" [photograph of Kenny, Sonja Betts and Mrs. J. Harold Dexter planning a West Coast Kenny Hospital] *Los Angeles Examiner* October 23 1949; "Sister Kenny Hospital Plans Mapped; L.A. to Hail Polio Foe" *Los Angeles Examiner* October 23 1949.

161. George D. Roberts "Activities of the Northern California Chapter," November 4 1949, San Francisco-Misc., MHS-K; Kenny "Concerning the Extension of My Work in the State of California" [1949]; "Judge Bullock Commends Sister Kenny Fund Drive" *Los Angeles Times* June 5 1950.

162. "Anti-Kenny Stand Hit By League"; "Gird for Total War on Polio" *Herald Express* July 28 1949. Betts identified Representative Republican Carl Hinshaw, Republican William Knowland and conservative Democrat Sheridan Downey.

163. Herbert J. Levine to Marvin H. Kline [telegram], [January 1948] Centralia, Illinois, MHS-K; H.D. Gillette to Sister Kenny [telegram], February 20 1948, Centralia, Illinois, MHS-K; Harley Queen to Marvin Kline [telegram], February 21 1948, Centralia 1948, MHS-K; Marvin Kline to Dr. Herbert J. Levine [telegram], [1948] Centralia 1948, MHS-K; Kline to Dr. H. Logan [president, Medical Board, Salem IL] et al [telegram], [1948] Centralia, 1948, MHS-K.

164. John L. Matthews to Sister Kenny [telegram], February 21 1948, Centralia, Illinois, MHS-K; John L. Matthews to Marvin H. Kline, February 21 1948, Centralia, Illinois, MHS-K.

165. Kenny to John L. Matthews [telegram], February 23 1948, Centralia, 1948, MHS-K; Kenny to Harley Queen [telegram], February 23 1948 Centralia, 1948, MHS-K; Kenny to Julius Kissel [telegram], February 23 1948, Centralia 1948, MHS-K; Kenny to Dear friends [Reverend and Mrs. Robert Hastings], May 26 1948, Centralia, Illinois, MHS-K; Dr. Kissel to Sister Kenny [telegram], [1948] Centralia, 1948, MHS-K; Harley Queen to Kenny [telegram], February 21 1948, Centralia 1948, MHS-K.

166. Kenny to Sir [Governor Dwight Green], June 4 1948.

167. Anthony Fleege "The 1947 Centralia Mine Disaster" *Journal of the Illinois State Historical Society* (2009) 102: 163–176. The governor's investigative commission exonerated Green but blamed officials of the mining company and poor attention by state inspectors.

168. "Sister Kenny Will Appeal to Governor Of Illinois for Certification of Polio Clinic" *Houston Chronicle* [August 1948], General Correspondence-K, MHS-K; "Only Kenny Clinic in Illinois Denied O.K. on Staff Setup" *Chicago Daily Tribune* July 22 1948.

169. Herbert J. Levine *I Knew Sister Kenny: A Story of a Great Lady and Little People* (Boston: Christopher Publishing House, 1954) 128–130, 137.

170. "Sister Kenny Will Fight State Ruling on Her Clinic Today" *Chicago Daily Tribune* August 6 1948; "Kenny Treatment Upheld" *New York Times* August 7 1948; John Chapman to Dear Sister Kenny, June 14 1948, Invited Physicians Letters, 1939–1949, MHS-K.

171. Levine *I Knew Sister Kenny*, 153, 162.

172. Herbert J. Levine to Dear Mr. Cohn, August 30 1972, Cohn Papers, MHS-K; Levine *I Knew Sister Kenny*, 203–206. Note that Huenkens later claimed that Matthews had had a stroke with paralysis in one leg which was called polio; [Cohn second interview with] E.J. Huenkens, June 3 1964, Cohn Papers, MHS-K.

173. "Centralia's Kenny Clinic Patients to Get Care in Chicago" *Chicago Daily Tribune* March 17 1949; Levine *I Knew Sister Kenny*, 173–174, 223.

174. "Polio Rises in Illinois" *New York Times* July 18 1949; Levine *I Knew Sister Kenny*, 222; B.K. Richardson *A History of The Illinois Department of Public Health 1927–1962* (Illinois: [Governor's Office] 1963), 85–87.

175. Kenny "For the Information of the Citizens of the State of Minnesota and the Citizens of the United States of American Concerning My Approaching Departure" [1947] Mayoralty Files 1945–1948, Box 10, Humphrey Papers, MHS.

176. "Scope of Kenny Clinics' Work Expanding in U.S." [Toowoomba newspaper, n.d.], Clippings, MHS-K; Margaret Opdahl Ernst, interview with Rogers, May 11 2001, St Paul, Minnesota; Kenny to Dear Mary [McCracken], May 7 1949, Kenny Collection, Fryer Library.

177. Kenny to Dear Mary and Stuart [December 1947], Kenny Collection, Fryer Library; Kenny to Dear Friends [November 1947], Personal Correspondence and Related Papers 1942–1951, MHS-K; Kenny to Mr. President, Mrs. Webber and Gentlemen, May 24 1948; Karen Peterson Butterworth *Mind over Muscle: Surviving Polio in New Zealand* (Palmerston North: Dunmore Press, 1994), 62; J.E. Caughey and D.S. Malcolm "Muscle Spasm in Poliomyelitis: A Study of a New Zealand Epidemic" *Archives of Disease in Childhood* (March 1950) 25: 15–17. For the intriguing suggestion that Bell began to "refine" Kenny's methods over the years see Butterworth *Mind over Muscle*, 64. The hospital was endowed by Thomas Duncan, a wealthy farmer and philanthropist.

178. Kenny to Dear Sir Norman [Nook], April 25 1949, Wilson Collection; Kenny to Dear Sir [W. Moore], March 24 1952, Wilson Collection; [Cohn interview with] Valerie Harvey, March 19 1953, Cohn Papers, MHS-K; [Cohn interview with] Pete Gazzola [Director of Public Relations, KF Eastern Area], August 25 1953, Cohn Papers, MHS-K; [Cohn interview with] Will O'Neill, May 20 1955.

179. Kenny to Dear Friend [Alejandro del Carril], June 24 1949, Argentina, MHS-K; Kenny to My Dear Mary and Stuart, September 24 1946, Mary Stewart Kenny, 1942–1947 MHS-K; Kenny to Dear Mary and Stuart, May 18 1947, Kenny Collection, Fryer Library; Kenny to Dear Mary, January 31 [n.d.], Kenny Collection, Fryer Library.

FURTHER READING

On medical politics in the late 1940s, see James G. Burrow *AMA: Voice of American Medicine* (Baltimore: Johns Hopkins University Press, 1963); Frank D. Campion *The AMA and U.S. Health Policy since 1940* (Chicago: Chicago Review Press, 1984); Jonathan Engel *Doctors and Reformers: Discussion and Debate over Health Policy 1925–1950* (Charleston: University of South Carolina Press, 2002); Elizabeth Fee and Theodore M. Brown eds. *Making Medical History: The Life and Times of Henry E. Sigerist* (Baltimore: Johns Hopkins University Press, 1997); Rickey Hendricks *A Model for National Health Care: The History of Kaiser Permanente* (New Brunswick, NJ: Rutgers University Press, 1993); Robert D. Johnston ed. *The Politics of Healing: Histories of Alternative Medicine in Twentieth-Century*

North America (New York: Routledge, 2004); Monte Poen *Harry S. Truman versus the Medical Lobby: The Genesis of Medicare* (Columbia: University of Missouri Press, 1979); Elton Rayak *Professional Power and American Medicine: The Economics of the American Medical Association* (Cleveland: World Publishing Company, 1967); Naomi Rogers *An Alternative Path: The Making and Remaking of Hahnemann Medical College and Hospital of Philadelphia* (New Brunswick: Rutgers University Press, 1998); Naomi Rogers "The Public Face of Homeopathy: Politics, the Public and Alternative Medicine in the United States 1900–1940" in Martin Dinges ed. *Patients in the History of Homeopathy* (Sheffield: European Association for the History of Medicine and Health Publications, ʔ002), 351–371; Paul Starr *The Social Transformation of American Medicine* (New York: Basic Books, 1982); Rosemary Stevens *In Sickness and in Wealth: American Hospitals in the Twentieth Century* (New York: Basic Books, 1989); Patricia Spain Ward "*United States versus American Medical Association et al.*: The Medical Anti-Trust Case of 1938–1943" *American Studies* (1989) 30: 123–153.

On medical science and research in the 1940s and 1950s see Toby A. Appel *Shaping Biology: The National Science Foundation and American Biological Research, 1945–1975* (Baltimore: Johns Hopkins University Press, 2000); Angela N. H. Creager *The Life of a Virus: Tobacco Mosaic Virus as an Experimental Model, 1930–1965* (Chicago: University of Chicago Press, 2002); Roger L. Geiger *Research and Relevant Knowledge: American Research Universities Since World War II* (New York: Oxford University Press, 1993); Bert Hansen *Picturing Medical Progress from Pasteur to Polio: A History of Mass Media Images and Popular Attitudes in America* (New Brunswick, NJ: Rutgers University Press, 2009); Victoria A. Harden *Inventing the NIH: Federal Biomedical Research Policy, 1887–1937* (Baltimore: Johns Hopkins University Press, 1986); Michael Kazin *The Populist Persuasion: An American History* (Ithaca, NY: Cornell University Press, 1995); Daniel J. Kevles "Foundations, Universities and Trends in Support of Physical and Biological Sciences, 1900–1992" *Daedalus* (1992) 121: 195–235; Gretchen Krueger *Hope and Suffering: Children, Cancer, and the Paradox of Experimental Medicine* (Baltimore: Johns Hopkins University Press, 2008); Harry M. Marks "Cortisone, 1949: A Year in the Political Life of a Drug" *Bulletin of the History of Medicine* (1992) 66: 429–432; Harry M. Marks *The Progress of Experiment: Science and Therapeutic Reform in the United States, 1900–1990* (Cambridge: Cambridge University Press, 1997); James T. Patterson *The Dread Disease: Cancer and Modern American Culture* (Cambridge: Harvard University Press, 1989); Steven P. Strickland *Politics, Science and Dread Disease: A Short History of United States Medical Research Policy* (Cambridge: Harvard University Press, 1972); James Harvey Young *The Medical Messiahs: A Social History of Health Quackery in Twentieth-Century America* (Princeton: Princeton University Press, 1967).

8

Fading Glory

KENNY HAD LONG argued that good medicine was global medicine. She boasted of her many international patients and especially the physicians from Canada, Europe, South America, Asia, and South Africa who came to study her work and then returned to establish it in their home countries. With the emerging Cold War divided nations sought to keep their scientists separated, and few countries dared to breach this gap. But for Kenny such Cold War global politics were of little importance. In her mind the totalitarian enemy was not the Soviet Union but the National Foundation for Infantile Paralysis (NFIP) and the American Medical Association (AMA), and she looked for places where their influence was muted. In the late 1940s as she sought to expand her work across the world, she ignored such Cold War boundaries as the Iron Curtain. In her view of global medical politics her work could connect the American public and sympathetic professionals with their counterparts around the world.

After the 1948 international conference organized by the NFIP, Kenny made much of the restriction of freedom of scientific speech that had left her unable to answer a question posed during the conference. Still, she recognized that the words of scientists carried more weight at such conferences than those of a nurse. While she continued to speak at small medical meetings organized by the Kenny Foundation (KF), she sought to enlist respected polio scientists, without the handicap of her gender and lack of training, to promote her ideas. The 1948 Congressional hearings had introduced Columbia University virologist Claus Jungeblut as a polio researcher opposed to the NFIP-funded scientific establishment and seeking to extend Kenny's theories. Jungeblut became a potent symbol for KF fundraising drives reinforcing the foundation's claim that it was raising money for both patient care and polio research.

Jungeblut's work sounded credible not only because he was a well-known virologist, but also because scientists were developing a new picture of polio. American postwar polio science had broken through the dead-end of the 1930s and early 1940s as recognition of distinctive viral strains of the disease had begun to allow laboratory researchers to focus on characteristics that had previously been dismissed as anomalous. Most significantly, in 1948 virologist John Enders and his team at the Boston Children's Hospital grew a strain of the polio virus in nonneurological tissue. A physiological and pathological picture of polio that no longer centered on the central nervous system sounded similar to Kenny's concept of polio as a "systemic" disease in which the virus could invade any part of the body, whether the central nervous system or peripheral structures. Strikingly, when Enders and his team published their findings in *Science*, they described experiments that demonstrated that the multiplication of the Lansing virus strain "occurred either in peripheral nerve processes or in cells not of nervous origin."[1]

These changes enabled a few scientists like Jungeblut to step outside the NFIP establishment and accept KF funding, while still being able to base their own work on the best science of their day. Researchers both in North America and in Europe, impressed by the well-publicized clinical results of Kenny's methods, began to pursue laboratory and clinical research based on—if not her exact theories—then ideas that sounded quite similar. As a result, Kenny at last had scientific evidence to support her claims that she had contributed not just to the best clinical practice but also to the best virological science.

To expand her nascent global network Kenny traveled frequently to Europe in the early Cold War years. She recognized that polio was becoming a global health issue and the subject of discussions by European health departments and by the new World Health Organization (WHO). Polio outbreaks also began to occur in Asia and Africa and were clearly a threat to both developed and developing nations.[2] In a letter to the KF board, Kenny claimed that a prominent WHO official had advised her that the KF should apply for WHO membership and that "he had every hope to keep this great organization free of politics."[3] Kenny went to Geneva to visit the WHO's new headquarters in 1950, and hoped that her meetings with officials there would "later bear fruit."[4] But although Kenny's network of sympathetic physicians and her celebrity reputation made it relatively easy to gain a hearing with a few influential WHO officials, these brief encounters did not create any formal alliance between the WHO and the KF.

By 1950, just as reporters found what she was saying not new, Kenny came to recognize that her health problems were more serious than she had admitted. At the end of the year she gave up her house in Minneapolis and moved back to Australia to make a new home amid family and old friends. But she kept returning to the United States, brimming with scientific news that she believed further confirmed her work. She sought to imprint a permanent legacy for her work and for herself, but by the time she died of a stroke in 1952 this was a failed project. The new science she had hailed was moving into a realm that would make polio's clinical care irrelevant. Emerging research on a polio vaccine made it easier for her enemies to depict her as a figure of a different age, no longer relevant or important.

THE STATE OF POLIO CARE

As polio outbreaks in Europe became more frequent after the war, European physicians began to seek out American expertise. In September 1950 Christopher Joseph McSweeney, an infectious disease specialist who was a Fellow of the Royal College of

Physicians of Ireland and the medical director of Dublin's infectious disease hospital, came to investigate polio care in the United States.[5] His observations give a good summary of the state of polio treatment.

A few months before he arrived McSweeney heard Frank Krusen at a medical meeting in Dublin compare the first 40 years of the twentieth century—"the years of immobilization"—to the 1940s in which the introduction of "the so-called Kenny concept" had led to the early treatment of muscle spasm. Krusen claimed "Kenny's contribution was little or nothing," but admitted that it was "extremely difficult" to define the modern treatment of polio as much of it was not new and some of it was "pure empiricism."[6] Not long after Krusen's talk McSweeney met Kenny in Dublin while she was visiting the city's infectious disease hospital where he practiced. She showed her film to an audience that included Noel Browne, Ireland's minister of health, and declared that she had had "no association" with Krusen for many years, and that "he had evidently forgotten what he had been taught." In Kenny's recollection, McSweeney boasted that 90 percent of his patients recovered, and she replied that "he was wasting his time going to America if that was so, as America should be going to him for information." When McSweeney remarked, "Why, you saw my recoveries," she replied "I saw many of your patients but there wasn't a recovery in the whole lot."[7] Such a flat dismissal intrigued McSweeney and led him to seek out proponents and critics of Kenny's work during his trip.

After visiting major polio centers in the United States, McSweeney concluded that physical medicine as a specialty was far more advanced in the United States than it was in Ireland. He also noted that polio patients were discharged from the hospital in as little as 3 or 4 weeks, a speed that surprised him. Polio treatment, he discovered, was "a field of controversy which is not yet finally resolved": most hospitals combined heat, hydrotherapy, muscle reeducation, and massage; avoided immobilization other than foot blocks and sand bags; and tried to postpone orthopedic surgery for as long as possible.[8]

While McSweeney deliberately sought out Kenny-oriented and anti-Kenny centers, he found every institution used some elements of her work. At the Willard Parker Hospital in New York Philip Stimson explained muscle spasm to him and showed him hot packs, which technicians applied twice or 3 times a day, along with body-length prone packs and hot baths. "Unlike packs," McSweeney noted, "hydrotherapy seemed to be liked and looked forward to by patients." In Minnesota he went to St. Mary's Hospital in Rochester where Mayo clinicians applied packs only twice a day and therapists told him they were "not sure that heat in any form is essential for the treatment of poliomyelitis." In Minneapolis Miland Knapp and Kenny technician Vivian Hannan showed him the Institute's practice, which relied on hot packs every hour or so during the acute phase and slightly less frequently thereafter. "There is no doubt that the application of these packs causes pain," McSweeney reported later, which could mean that "their routine employment in Europe might not be easy of attainment." "To pack or not to pack, that is the question," he concluded in his formal report of his trip. He and other Dublin physicians "think baths are better" and find that "the patients appreciate them much more."[9]

By the time of McSweeney's visit, pain seen as a serious symptom that required therapy was now at the heart of polio care in the United States. The use of heat was a central technique, with hot packs only one of many such therapies.[10] Doctors still debated the use of polio drugs (now termed "antispasmodic pharmaceuticals") such as curare and neostigmine in terms that could be "occasionally quite heated."[11] Proper care, physicians now argued, entailed the utilization of everything that could benefit a patient's progress "without concession to orthodoxy or dogma."[12] The fervor around Kenny's term mental alienation had also died down; even James Spence in *Modern Trends in Pediatrics* (1951) reflected that this concept had "caused the medical profession to think again about the management of patients with paralysis."[13] So widely accepted was the idea that both spasm and pain were important symptoms that one symposium held at the University of Colorado's School of Medicine was called "Pain and Spasm in Poliomyelitis."[14] A brochure handed out to the families of patients with polio who entered the Los Angeles County Hospital assured anxious relatives that muscle spasm and pain would be part of the patient's thorough clinical history. In language Kenny would have used, the brochure warned that muscle spasm could persist for weeks after fever abates and "may become more severe unless treated."[15]

Although it was not often acknowledged in print, Kenny's attack on muscle testing had also had an impact. Two California pediatricians urged that patients not be examined frequently for "early complete muscle tests cause unwarranted pain and fatigue to no good purpose."[16] Kenny's promotion of muscle exercises assumed a different view of the polio body, as Marjorie Lawrence had noted in her 1949 autobiography when she compared Kenny's methods to those of doctors and nurses in Mexico and Arkansas who "were forever cautious not to 'stretch' my muscles."[17] Physicians had "developed a saner view concerning the movement and handling of paralysed muscles [which] . . . are not the fragile structures they were once believed to be," agreed one British expert in 1950.[18] Even orthopedic operations were no longer seen as the automatic end to a process of rehabilitative polio care; surgery, argued a study in *Pediatrics*, was "formerly attempted with zeal which was perhaps mistaken."[19]

KENNY STEPS DOWN

Kenny had long protested modifications of her methods, although she accepted that the small number of technicians trained at her Institute could not alter care everywhere. Still, she was dissatisfied with the impact of her work. She spent as much time in New York City as she did in Minneapolis, and no longer worked as a clinician or teacher. She continued to raise money for the KF and tried to develop strategies to convince the American public that the modifications of her methods, which NFIP officials called "modern treatment," were not the proper Kenny method and could be harmful in their diluted form.[20]

Her methods were integrated in hospitals around North America, her ideas were widely publicized, and the Kenny technicians who graduated from the Institute were a prized group. The Institute remained her original center, and she proudly quoted from a survey by the American College of Surgeons that praised the Institute's efficient administration and the high caliber of its medical staff.[21] But the facility itself was under strain. Publicity had led to many applications, especially from neglected and seriously paralyzed patients. The Institute's wards were overcrowded, and without air-conditioning the use of hot packs created an almost unbearable level of heat and humidity.[22] The Kenny clinic in Centralia had closed for good after the summer epidemic in 1949, but clinics in Jersey City and Buffalo continued to prosper.[23] In any case, Kenny recognized, the expansion of her work could not depend on a single center. Instead of just raising money to pay for care provided by Kenny technicians, Kenny argued that the KF should become a major philanthropy, funding a network of Kenny clinics to provide technician training as well as patient care and to compete with the NFIP for the public's dimes and loyalty.

In April 1949 after a trip to Australia Kenny returned to the United States, telling reporters dramatically that she would go back "to her native land only if Australia calls for me," a remark, NFIP officials noted privately, that sounded "the same whether it's here or in Australia."[24] In Australia, she had discovered, she was no celebrity. Her work had few allies and the Australian technicians who had returned home were now immersed with their own lives. Her longstanding ally Charles Chuter had retired at the end of 1947 and died of a heart attack a month later.[25] Except for the clinic attached to the Brisbane General Hospital, her other Australian clinics had disappeared. There were no training facilities and, other than a small group in Brisbane, no interested physicians. Even the Brisbane clinic, one of her medical supporters admitted, was "just ticking over" and its patients were of such long standing that the treatment they were receiving probably had only psychological value.[26]

In her adopted home, too, Kenny had to face a weakening of her clout. On her return the KF board told her she was no longer the Institute's executive director, a position that would now be held by a physician. With bravado she told reporters that "my mission has been fulfilled" for scientific research "concerning the new concept of infantile paralysis and its treatment...now has been established." Yet her authority as the originator and interpreter of her work would, she hoped, remain. She had resigned only as the administrative head, she assured the public, and would continue "as a teacher and consultant."[27]

Behind the words and bluster, the Associated Press photograph that accompanied the story of her resignation caught a sense of her inner fears of mortality and irrelevance. Not only had the defection of her beloved ward Mary led to a great emotional crisis in her life, but death was in the air. While she was in Queensland her brother Henry had died, and then William died a few months later. It felt so strange, she told a niece, in one of the few personal letters that have survived, "to have no brother left after all these years. I felt as if the bottom had dropped out of the world when Mother died, and now I feel as if the world is not worth anything." Perhaps she reread these words and was uncomfortable with their tone, for she added, without much conviction, "but Time is a great healer."[28] Time, though, no longer felt so elastic. She was now aware that her own unsteady balance and shaking arm were signs of Parkinson's disease, a diagnosis she had not yet shared with anyone.[29] The AP photo shows her sitting stiffly, leaning back away from the physician who was replacing her as Institute director, her expression turned inward, almost in pain, and her eyes avoiding both the photographer and the physician beside her.[30] As one Brisbane friend remarked insightfully, "What will Queen Elizabeth do if she is not actively engaged in running her organisation!"[31]

The physician who replaced Kenny as the Institute's new executive director saw his role as mending bridges between the medical profession and the Institute. Now, announced pediatrician Edgar J. Huenkens, there would be "a change of atmosphere." Respected as a clinician with allies in the state legislature and the local medical community, he had accepted the position of medical director of the Institute in 1948, assured by the KF board that a more senior executive position would soon be his.[32] Huenkens began to say publicly and privately that the direction of the KF was now "entirely in the hands of members of the medical profession."[33] He composed a Dear Doctor letter inviting physicians "to visit

[the] Kenny Institute whenever you have occasion to be in this vicinity. The medical staff will welcome an opportunity to discuss the Kenny work with you."[34] Such language suggested that Kenny would not be involved in these discussions.

Huenkens also sought a more amicable relationship with the NFIP. He assured medical director Hart Van Riper that the KF was "making every effort to get Miss Kenny to return to Australia." Van Riper withheld judgment, noting in an internal memo "I believe that we should continue to be cooperative with Dr. Huenkens until he demonstrates that he, like Miss Kenny, cannot be trusted."[35] All medical meetings at the Institute, Huenkens told NFIP officials, would now focus on "actual demonstrations of the Kenny treatment to be followed by round table discussion in which each person who desires to be heard will be afforded an opportunity to present his views," another sign that Kenny's typical interruptions would not be tolerated.[36] Using the model of professional training set by the NFIP, the KF began to offer more technician training scholarships to nurses and physical therapists.[37] Huenkens also published a lukewarm assessment of Kenny's work in *Postgraduate Medicine* arguing that hot packs, while important, were "definitely of secondary value" compared to muscle exercises, and warning against the many "over[-]optimistic reports" about the results of Kenny treatment. He did, however, note that "it is possible that the virus attacks the muscle directly" and may not be "purely neurotropic but may invade the viscera and peripheral tissues."[38]

This emphasis on physician-directed meetings was a response to a wider discomfort among American doctors over the rising influence of physical therapists in polio care. Throughout the 1940s therapists, using their special knowledge of Kenny's work, had claimed clinical and professional power. Even at Queen Mary's Hospital, in England doctors complained that they were not going to take orders from therapists, leading to "one battle after another."[39] Patients and families, inspired by the hope of a nondisabled body that Kenny had publicized, felt that physical therapy was the answer, however long such care might take.

NFIP pressure had begun to alter hospital policy, opening the doors of voluntary and community hospitals previously resistant to polio patients and convincing administrators to shorten the official isolation period from the standard 3 weeks to around 1 week. Armed with new psychological arguments about the danger of psychic trauma in long periods of hospitalization, particularly for children, the NFIP began to encourage chapters to fund visiting nurse services, outpatient clinics, and new rehabilitation centers where patients "will receive intelligent care, and a chance to live again without complexes."[40]

But when NFIP officials tried to limit inpatient care they found that "unfortunately" the public and many physicians believed polio was "a disease requiring long periods of hospitalization."[41] In *JAMA* Hart Van Riper warned physicians and administrators not to rely "so heavily upon the guidance of physical therapists and nurses."[42] When physicians leave "the patient and therapist without direction or supervision," agreed another senior NFIP official, "overly zealous or inexperienced, medically abandoned therapists often may continue under such circumstances to treat the patient long beyond the need for hospitalization... [or] after any further practical benefits may be expected."[43]

Promotion of home care was part of an effort to deskill and deinstitutionalize polio therapy in ways that directly contradicted Kenny's reliance on properly trained technicians, even though she had taught mothers to use elements of her work before bringing their child to a hospital. It also reflected a broader cultural reliance on the availability of American women returning from wartime jobs to become domestic caregivers again. But during the 1940s polio had been significantly medicalized, the result of an effective campaign by the NFIP. Now many families sought out professional care in modern, expensive hospitals. Urging communities to rely on mothers seemed to undermine these changes, suggesting that polio care did not require the work of professionals in an institution.

Kenny's ouster as Institute director was followed by another upheaval—the defrocking of Morris Fishbein as AMA general secretary and *JAMA* editor. At the June 1949 annual meeting he was attacked again on the floor of the AMA's House of Delegates by members resentful at his opposition to group practice and perhaps envious of his celebrity reputation. His relationship with the National Physicians Committee, a right-wing lobby group, also left him vulnerable.[44] This time his enemies had the numbers. A professional advertising firm took over his AMA public relations work and the AMA's trustees pointedly announced that he must cease speaking on "controversial subjects." Basil O'Connor, Fishbein later recalled, was "fuming with anger" when he learned of the coup.[45] No longer *JAMA* editor, he continued to work as a consulting writer and editor for other medical journals, but his was no longer the single voice for American medicine and there was now no single powerful AMA censor looking over newspaper articles and radio and movie scripts.[46] It was the end of an era for America's organized profession.

CALIFORNIA CHAOS

During the war thousands of civilians migrated to California, and after the war the migration continued with the return of soldiers. Many families with young children lived in congested conditions, a good environment for the emergence of polio outbreaks. Polio continued to threaten every kind of family; even Governor Earl Warren's 17-year-old daughter Nina "Honey Bear" was paralyzed by polio in November 1950.[47]

By the late 1940s Kenny treatment was provided in most of the state's municipal and county infectious disease hospitals, and the KF was represented by 2 state chapters, the Northern and Southern. The expansion of the KF as an alternative philanthropy and the institutionalization of Kenny's work consistently faced 3 major problems: ensuring the cooperation of hospital staff, establishing congenial relations between the state chapters and the Minneapolis KF Board, and making certain that the chapters' campaigns were directed by honest men. Chaos ensued in 1949 as Kenny technicians protested that their patients who were to be transferred from Santa Monica's Harbor General Hospital to the Kabat Kaiser center would no longer receive proper Kenny treatment.[48] The technicians were fired for insubordination, but orthopedist Harvey Billig, who was a member of the Southern KF chapter and directed his own Kenny outpatient clinic, found them other positions.[49] The Minneapolis Board was frustrated by this sign of disloyalty, and tried unsuccessfully to rescind the Southern Chapter's charter.[50] Kenny had supported the technicians' decision to leave and decided to grant the original Southern KF chapter "self-government" with full power to campaign independently for "the promotion of my work."[51] Prominent Kenny proponents such as Billig and Superior Court Judge George Dockweiler retained their standing as KF representatives and ignored the Minneapolis Board's posturing.

Meanwhile, in San Francisco, members of the Northern KF chapter had long faced "personal dispute[s]" with KF executive director Marvin Kline and other Board members. As a result no Kenny clinics were ever established in northern California. Most disturbing were rumors of financial mismanagement by the chapter's executive director, Henry Von Morpurgo, a San Francisco public relations man. By the end of 1949 the chapter had collapsed, and Von Morpurgo had become the target of a fraud suit brought by the state of California for misappropriating $93,000.[52]

Kenny had initially tried act as conciliator but realizing this scandal threatened the reputation of both the KF and her own name, she argued that the Northern KF officers had "failed in their custody of public monies." When Von Morpurgo and his local defenders later approached her she refused to meet with them.[53] Her extensive network kept her well informed of public dissatisfaction with KF officials, and she began to keep a close watch on both foundations, especially "all foundations bearing my name."[54]

THE NURSE AND THE SCIENTIST

The mess in California threatened Kenny's hope of establishing a West Coast center to provide Kenny care. She was further frustrated to find that the KF Board was not enthusiastic about the efforts of other Kenny promoters.[55] Yet even with the backing of the KF Board, state and federal bureaucracy made KF expansion difficult. State Crippled Children's Bureaus set up during the New Deal had developed an extensive list of requirements for the formal approval of rehabilitative hospitals, and, piggybacking on this bureaucratic barrier, the NFIP adopted a policy in 1948 of refusing to pay for convalescent care provided in any facility not approved by a state's bureau.[56] These bureaus were usually directed by civic leaders or members of the state medical society who were friends of the governor, thereby transforming bureaucratic hurdles into political ones. The struggles around the Centralia clinic had demonstrated that even with the support of a mayor and a governor, the KF Board still had to find permanent specialists to staff its clinics.

The most powerful way to protect the KF from poor publicity and organizational chaos, Kenny came to believe, was to emphasize its commitment to funding research. Kenny noted frequently that the NFIP had spent 11 million dollars on scientific research without any "advance concerning the knowledge of the disease."[57] Meetings organized by the KF to showcase its contribution to the progress of polio science began to feature Kenny and virologist Claus Jungeblut, whom Kenny proudly called "our scientist."[58]

For Kenny these were opportunities to shore up her legacy, a goal made more pressing by her growing sense of mortality. She continued to pretend that she was in her early 60s rather than about to turn 70, but she did like to remind her allies of her heart condition, which had been identified many years earlier. "Contrary to my doctor's advice" and "at a great physical sacrifice," she told the KF Board, she had "endeavored to improve the financial situation of this Foundation upon many occasions."[59] Well aware that the Kenny method or some adaptation of it was used in hospitals and clinics across the nation, Kenny's complaints now focused on the lack of attention to her work as a scientific contribution. She warned that polio clinicians who denied or ignored the Kenny concept could not achieve proper efficacy of her methods, for if polio was treated "from the viewpoint of a central nervous system infection alone, only deformities develop in spite of best efforts."[60] News from her network of Kenny technicians had shown her the importance of working within a supportive hospital hierarchy; technicians without physician support were often left isolated and impotent. Teaching physicians to understand the ideas behind the method was critical for any hope of global expansion, especially with a number of international students training to be Kenny technicians at the Institute.[61]

Yet these arguments, Kenny found, did not alter hospital care or medical training policies. When she warned New York City officials that local hospitals "doing Kenny work" were not practicing the work "intelligently" for "the theory upon which the work is based is unknown," the city's commissioner of hospitals, she noted uneasily, "smiled and remarked: 'What odds about the theory so long as they get results?'" Surely, Kenny argued, it was impossible to teach a treatment "unless the theory upon which the treatment is based is understood." While the commissioner did not argue further, it was clear that for him and other officials a concern with theory and pedagogy was secondary to the provision of demonstrably efficacious clinical care.[62] The medical school deans at New York University and Columbia University were willing to allow her to lecture and show her technical film but these occasions did not alter the teaching of medical students.[63]

Kenny consistently hailed Jungeblut's work at all of these occasions. Jungeblut disliked Kenny's evangelical tone. Still, he acknowledged his KF grant had been "secured through Miss Kenny's personal efforts." He consistently asked that "there be no nonprofessional reports of these discussions, in the press or elsewhere," for only under such conditions could he "carry on my experimentation at Columbia." But these pleas were in vain. He was made central in KF publicity, and Kenny considered that his research had proven her concept of the disease.[64]

Jungeblut had established himself as a scientific outsider during the 1948 Congressional hearings and he was eager to show that his work was on the cutting edge. In June 1949, during an informal report of his work at a public meeting, he highlighted recent epidemiological and virological evidence that suggested that the polio virus produced "paralysis only as a complication, as complications occur in mumps or measles" and that, like these familiar infections, polio was also "a systemic disease." "It is possible," he speculated, that "we are dealing with a uniform disease which is essentially peripheral, with the early lesion involving only the peripheral muscles."[65] Jungeblut then cited what he called "a very classical experiment" by Boston virologist John Enders who had grown the Lansing strain of the virus in human embryo tissue. While some commentators disparaged this work, arguing that embryonic material was "not a good guide, that it has a different nervous and non-nervous tissue so the experiment was not of much importance," Jungeblut disagreed. He saw Enders' work and his own as providing "a clear demonstration that the poliomyelitis virus is not a neurotropic virus only."[66] It is likely that only Jungeblut, of all the participants at this and other KF meetings, had any inkling that these insights would become virological orthodoxy within the next couple of years and provide the intellectual and technical basis for the production of Jonas Salk's polio vaccine. In 1954 Enders and his Boston team received the Nobel Prize for just the experiments that Jungeblut was describing here.[67]

KF director Edgar Huenkens tried hard to rein Kenny in. He agreed that polio might indeed be "a peripheral disease as well as a central nervous system disease," but, he commented at a meeting in Jersey City after Kenny had spoken, "we should be awfully careful we do not make statements that are exaggerated and that cannot stand up." Hasty declarations made "a bad impression on physicians and scientific people," and statements by those not working in a laboratory might be seen as "proof [by]...a group of laymen [but not by]...a group of scientists." In his estimation, the KF should be concerned with "making the doctors believe...not in just making a bare announcement for the record."[68]

Never known for subtlety, Kenny retorted that "doctors are upbraiding me for not letting them know what I have discovered about this disease and what has been proven scientifically about this disease." She had heard all these arguments many times before, and in her experience, cautious presentations did not lead doctors to "believe." Evaluation, experimentation, proof—these were all obscurant techniques to delay expanding the scope of her work and her ideas. Thus, she declared dramatically, "if we wait for the finality of knowledge in all of these things, we will wait until thousands of children are crippled."[69] Like Huenkens, Jungeblut urged Kenny to accept that "the medical profession is a peculiar profession [which]...likes to see the improvements come from its own ranks."[70] Kenny was able to have the last word, though, when she described children screaming "because their poor inflamed muscles have been stretched instead of scientifically treated."[71] To these horrific pictures Huenkens and Jungeblut had no reply.

What Huenkens was able to do was to keep Kenny at a distance from the Institute. He refused Kenny's request for regular meetings with members of the medical staff "to present to them from time to time all my knowledge and material, and bring them up to the same standard as Doctor Pohl."[72] The Institute now rarely screened *The Kenny Concept of Infantile Paralysis* or its lay equivalent *The Value of a Life*.[73] Nor was Kenny able to place her technicians where she believed they should go. When she proposed that Ethel Burns, one of her original students, replace another technician, the KF board warned both technicians that if they moved positions they "would be fired from the Kenny Foundation, and so would any other technicians."[74] Huenkens also made sure that Kenny was no longer the major speaker at medical meetings and did not control their agenda. At one conference in Minneapolis, her participation was limited to 30 minutes on the first day and another hour on the second day.[75] To another, Kenny discovered, she was not even invited. This attempt by the KF "to forbid me communicating with the medical world," she complained to the head of the KF board, was "the exact replica of the National Foundation."[76]

Kenny's constant demands, no longer tempered by Mary Kenny, began to alienate her allies on the KF Board, especially Minneapolis businessman Donald Dayton and lawyer Henry Haverstock, whose loyalty she had captured by treating their sons. Both men began to hope that Kenny would go home to Australia and become a beloved, distant figurehead. She was becoming more impatient, more inflexible, and more domineering. "There wasn't any way to work with Sister Kenny as such, you worked for her, she was constantly imposing her will," one KF public relations man recalled.[77] In fact, although Kenny denied this, the organization was not hers, and even the Institute was slipping from her control.

But Kenny still had the power of the pen, the ear of newspaper reporters, and a network of allies. To buttress her argument that clinical care could not progress without a correct theoretical understanding of the disease, she organized a series of physician testimonials. Kenny's work had, orthopedists Robert Bingham and Alfred Deacon argued, "practically abolished the use of plaster casts and splints" and had significantly reduced "the amount of corrective surgery." They praised her "new concepts of the clinical picture and pathology of acute poliomyelitis" that had enabled doctors to diagnose many early and mild patients "previously unrecognized until deformities or paralysis developed."[78] Michigan physician Ethel Calhoun, who had been using the Kenny method at the infectious disease hospital in Pontiac since the early 1940s, praised Kenny's "amazing powers of observation" and the "remarkable improvement" she saw among her own patients.[79] Although Kenny tried to make much of the devastating impact on clinical practice when it was not informed by correct scientific theory, few of her testimonials mentioned this.

Kenny's claim that if laboratory research were not combined with a clinical understanding of polio in living human patients there could be no progress in polio science did not convince skeptical scientists. After a meeting with Australian virologist Francis MacFarlane Burnet, she noted that he believed "that the disease localized its activities to the central nervous system." Such a view of polio, Kenny was convinced, was the result of Burnet's limited clinical knowledge, for he "informed me he had seen very few, possibly only three, acute cases."[80] For his part Burnet, the director of the Walter and Eliza Hall Institute in Melbourne, found Kenny memorable but completely unconvincing. In his later autobiography Burnet recalled "a long two-hour interview" with Kenny, a "large white-haired, slow-moving woman dressed like old-fashioned royalty in purple with a large wide-brimmed hat." He found her ideas about polio's pathology and physiology "highly individual, heretical and, unless all reputable research men were grossly deceiving themselves, completely untenable," and was not impressed by her testimonials written by a "few not-very-well-known pathologists."[81]

When Kenny sought testimonials from laboratory scientists who did believe in her theory of polio, she had, as Burnet noted, few familiar names. Jungeblut sent her a Christmas letter in 1949, thanking her for her friendship and continued interest in his work, which had enabled his laboratory "to make a number of scientific contributions which provide direct evidence in favor of your concept of the peripheral origins of poliomyelitis." In words that Kenny subsequently quoted many times, Jungeblut said he firmly believed "that no intelligent approach to the control of poliomyelitis is thinkable without a clear understanding of these fundamental phenomena."[82] Neurologist Leon Laruelle, her major European ally, was, she reported, "completely convinced" that her concept was correct and the young British orthopedist Lancelot Walton, who had spent a few months at the Institute funded by the KF, similarly agreed "that the peripheral structures are primarily affected."[83] She also forced Huenkens to write a To Whom It May Concern letter stating that for the previous 8 years the medical staff of the Minneapolis General Hospital and the Kenny Institute had taught that polio "is a complex systemic disease, presenting many clinical manifestations, and that it attacks the peripheral system."[84]

THE HOPE OF EUROPE

As much as Kenny valued Jungeblut, she placed even greater faith in her European connections. She had come to see Europe as a promising site for leading clinical and research work that would be unfettered by the influence of the NFIP or the AMA. Although she had long spoken grandly of the Kenny treatment practiced around the world, before 1945 her work had been fully institutionalized only in the wards of the Queen Mary's Hospital in Carshalton by nurses and physical therapists she had trained in the 1930s. During the war doctors, nurses, and physical therapists from South America and Canada and a few from elsewhere had come to Minneapolis to study her methods and returned to their home countries, but such practice was individualized and fragmented. After the war prominent visitors included activist Krishna Nehru Hutheesing, the sister of India's first Prime Minister, who reminded Kenny that she had promised to send "a film for our Clinic in Bombay."[85] But a single Kenny technician accompanied by Kenny's technical film, even boosted by community goodwill, was unlikely to be able to transform polio care in a hospital or region, much less a nation.

At the end of the war as polio epidemics spread across Europe Kenny could see the possibility of expansion into communities where the NFIP did not reach and where scientists might be more willing to explore new ways of thinking. She began to travel regularly across the Atlantic with funding from the KF. Her reputation and her connections—as well as the RKO *Sister Kenny* film—opened doors for her.[86] Reflecting war-torn Europe's eagerness to "catch up" in medicine, science, and technology, and a wider gratitude toward Americans who had helped to win the war, Kenny was treated as an honored guest. When she stayed at the Hotel Metropole in Brussels, the Belgian flag was brought down and the Union Jack raised up. When she visited Prague and heard a band playing a song of welcome she wondered whether Stalin or some other Soviet leader had arrived. Realizing the band was honoring her, she "felt a little bit small and foolish but, however, it was nice of them to pay such homage to an alien."[87]

During these trips she tried to shore up medical respect and counter antagonistic publicity. Officials in Rome assured her they would be sending a doctor and 2 nurses to study at the Institute, but a skeptical Italian pediatric professor asked her why her procedures were not mentioned in an NFIP booklet. Kenny explained that the pamphlet "had been compiled in the very earliest days of my visit to America and was not authentic."[88] In Athens, the Minister of Hygiene thanked her for the film and pamphlets she had donated and said he would be grateful to learn of "further developments made in your Institute in the field of research and treatment of this disease."[89] In Spain the prominent orthopedic surgeon Vincente Sanchis-Olmos praised her for drawing attention to lesions in skin and cellular tissue and quoted virologist Julian Sanz Ibanez of the Ramon Y. Cajal Institute whose work showed that all problems in polio did not "result from lesions of the central nervous system." To her European audiences Kenny spoke freely of her battles with the NFIP and the AMA. "We know that there are political problems in America," Sanchis-Olmos declared in his own interpretation, "because this method is not American and Sister Kenny is not a doctor but a nurse." While the KF was trying to push Kenny aside, the board did reward these words of support with $3,000 to the Cajal Institute.[90]

A symbolic moment came in the summer of 1950 when Richard Metcalfe, the senior orthopedic consultant at the Queen Mary's Hospital, "shook my hand, congratulated me upon my great discovery and presented me with a copy of that very conservative medical journal, *The Lancet*, wherein it is stated that both my pathology and therapy had been proven correct." This "red letter day" reminded Kenny when, 13 years earlier, "in the very same ward, my theories were met with repudiation and rebuff."[91] Metcalfe had become a consultant at the hospital in the mid-1940s and had been impressed with its patients. Learning about Kenny's methods from the hospital's physical therapists, he had convinced other physicians to allow this work to continue. When he first met Kenny in 1948 she had struck him as "a battleship in full steam," but he had grown fond of her and championed her work.[92]

While Metcalfe may have spoken fulsomely to Kenny, in fact the *Lancet* reference was neither an editorial nor a research article, but a description of a recent symposium on polio held by the Society of Medical Officers of Health. Although the report was hardly an endorsement by the journal itself, it did show significant interest in her theories among English health officials. At this symposium Metcalfe had praised her ideas on pathology and therapy, pointing out that polio was not "the localized disease it was once thought to be" but in fact "involved not only nerves but also nerve end-plates, muscles, fascia and skin."[93] Without mentioning Kenny's name, one of Metcalfe's colleagues at Carshalton also praised the condition of patients who had received hot packs.[94] Kenny's treatment had first been condemned as of "no importance" and her "osteopathic" pathology dismissed, remarked another official. But now both her methods and her ideas were accepted.[95] Calling Kenny's ideas osteopathic reminded listeners that polio rehabilitation frequently attracted unorthodox practitioners, and such faint praise barely raised Kenny out of this despised crowd. Despite the cautious praise by individual European physicians, Kenny's work was never established as a fully institutionalized global enterprise. But there were 2 places where enterprising Kenny technicians were able to set down strong roots, at least for a time: Belgium and Czechoslovakia. The possibility for establishing a European center in Belgium came during a polio epidemic in the summer of 1945, when Kenny had visited a small Brussels polio clinic, which was part of a neurological institute directed by Leon Laruelle. Kenny and her technicians had treated some of the patients and she showed her technical film. Laruelle was impressed both with the clinical results and the film, which he compared to "a great interesting book which he could read many times."[96] He agreed to allow Dorothy Curtis and Nora Housden, Kenny technicians fluent in French, to work at the clinic from the summer of 1945 to February 1946.[97]

In 1948, Curtis and Housden, funded by the KF, returned to work with Laruelle to establish what Kenny believed would become a European training center and research institute. Like Kenny in her early years in Minneapolis, the technicians hoped that the bodies of their patients would stand as powerful evidence of the efficacy and validity of Kenny's work. At first they were allowed to treat only chronic patients, as local physicians were reluctant to allow them to care for patients in the acute stage "out of fear that the hot packs would strain the heart." The work was exhausting; the technicians had to do all the hot packing themselves "with very inadequate equipment." "The days are never long enough," they reported. But by the end of 1948 they were treating two-thirds of the clinic's patients and beginning to train 2 packers.[98]

Patients began to arrive from Israel, Spain, Turkey, North Africa, the Congo, France, Luxembourg, England, and Ireland.[99] By 1950 the technicians were teaching 5 students: nurses from France, Denmark, and Belgium, and a Romanian woman doctor. The Brussels clinic, a converted nursing home, was not large enough and its physical plant was awkward: 5 stories and no elevators, halls too narrow for carts, and bathrooms on stair landings. But it grew to 40 beds—most of them filled by private patients—and gained a significant reputation across Europe.[100]

Convincing Belgian physicians, even those who worked in the clinic, was, however, not easy. In November 1948, a Dr. Schwarz was appointed as the new medical supervisor of the polio wards. Although he had "hardly grasped the full Kenny concept," Curtis and Housden reported to Kenny, he appeared to be "favorably impressed by the results." He read the literature with interest and asked for more, "especially anything published in official medical journals."[101] Yet Curtis and Housden found that without their close supervision Kenny methods were easily modified. In the fall of 1949 Curtis left briefly to attend a private patient and Housden went to the Jersey City center for a working vacation. Although they had left explicit instructions as to how their patients should be treated, Housden was disturbed on her return to find her Brussels patients had been given "additional 'short wave' treatment" prescribed by Schwarz who "feels strongly the benefit of the increased blood supply to a limb, and is making charts to record his findings." She had a heart to heart talk with Laruelle, arguing that "our patients needed to have 'unmodified Kenny Treatment.'" Laruelle recognized that he was being called on to defend the technicians' sense of what was proper care against the interests of other members of staff. He responded quite well, Housden told Kenny, and agreed that "none of our new cases" would have this treatment. Housden had been "amicable about the matter," she assured her mentor, "but had to be amicably firm!" Schwarz, she added, "can do what he likes with his own old cases."[102]

Still, any gains in their efforts to disperse knowledge of Kenny's work around Europe remained precarious. Laruelle, for example, frequently lauded the Kenny treatment when he showed medical visitors through the clinic as a technique that was "physiologically rational, and has beneficial effects all its own." The method could show "its useful effects," he believed, only if it were applied "by technicians possessing a profound knowledge of anatomy,...the gift of observation, an innate intuition and a high moral conception of their mission."[103] But when the technicians asked him to let them teach local nurses, they were told either that no nurses were interested or that it was impossible to spare any.[104]

Laruelle was privately supportive of Kenny but he was not willing to make his views public. He gave Kenny a number of "micro-photographs and documentary papers" that she told reporters after returning to New York from a visit to Brussels in 1950, "prove what I have been teaching all these years."[105] But he refused to publish either clinical or pathological findings. His research laboratory studied "peripheral tissues" that he believed showed significant viral alteration, and also "peripheral lesions" in pigs, chickens, and cattle with a disease that clinically resembled human polio. He became convinced that Kenny's methods were "physiologically justified," and he praised the way her methods could reduce the intensity and duration of pain, improve circulation and the condition of the skin, and allow patients a remarkable ability to walk "in spite of marked muscle deficiency."[106] But these remarks appeared only in private reports to the KF, and he put off requests from other Belgium hospitals for Curtis and Housden to demonstrate their work.

"I have been disappointed in Dr. Laruelle," Curtis admitted to Kenny. "It seems to me he is definitely keeping the Kenny light under a bushel here."[107] Curtis became convinced that Laruelle's reticence was the result of a cautious proprietary stance. "If the Kenny treatment was good it was to be exclusively this doctor's," she concluded later, "and if it was not good, he was not going to be criticized by fellow doctors for endorsing it."[108] Laruelle did hope that the KF would enable him to establish a technician training school in "this European daughter-clinic of your Institute" that could mobilize its specially trained nurses to provide international aid for regions across Europe attacked by polio, "the necessity of which the World Health Organization has just confirmed."[109] This was exactly the model that Kenny herself envisioned. But Laruelle's small center was unable to play a major role in polio care, even in its immediate region, and the KF did not provide

any additional funds. By the early 1950s Belgium government officials faced with growing polio outbreaks put resources instead into building a new polio wing at the Hospital
Brugmann.[110]

Ironically in these fraught days of the early Cold War, the place that provided the most
promising site for expanding Kenny's work was Czechoslovakia, on the other side of the
Iron Curtain. In August 1949 Kenny had been invited to Prague by the Czech ministry of health, an invitation organized by Professor Marianna Vetterova-Pastrnkova, a
well-connected former teacher of English. Vetterova skillfully promoted Kenny's work by
aligning herself with František Pokorny, a physician who directed the well-known Janské
Lázně (Warm Springs) spa and had begun to use the Kenny method after a severe polio
epidemic in 1948. After meeting Kenny, Pokorny became an even more fervent proponent. He used the gray and red books Kenny left behind as the basis for treating his
patients and described his work in a local medical journal.[111] Vetterova urged Kenny to
send one of her technicians to Czechoslovakia to give lectures and clinical demonstrations, and the vice-minister of health promised that his officials would fit the film with
Czech subtitles and organize a 4-month course on the principles of the Kenny method
as long as Kenny sent an experienced teacher to direct the course.[112] The combination
of Vetterova, Pokorny, and the distinctive context of postwar Czechoslovakia led to an
unusual opportunity to institutionalize Kenny's work.

Dorothy Curtis was the obvious choice to lead the enterprise. As a graduate of Oberlin
College followed by a nursing degree from the University of Minnesota, she had a richer
academic background than most American nurses of her generation. During the war
she was a lieutenant in the Army Nurse Corps and then worked in public relations in
the Office of the Chief Surgeon of the European Theater of Operations.[113] After the war
Curtis, described by reporters as a "black-haired, energetic therapist," became a member
of Kenny's inner circle.[114] Frustrated by her work in Brussels, Curtis told Kenny she was
"intensely interested" in the opportunity "to further the distribution of your work" in
Czechoslovakia, whatever the "risks that may be incurred in fulfilling this request."[115] She
accompanied Kenny to Prague in 1949 and met Vetterova, whom Curtis identified as
a woman with "many prominent and influential friends [who was]…really the power
behind of this work here."[116]

Czechoslovakia had been reestablished as a republic immediately after the war, but
by 1948 it was under the control of the Soviet Union. The country had experienced its
first large polio epidemic in 1939, and during the 1940s Czech physicians had turned
to the latest medical technologies such as the convalescent serum and the preventive
nasal spray, and incorporated additional rehabilitation therapies such as hydrotherapy.[117]
When Curtis arrived in October 1949 Czech health officials offered Curtis the use of a
150-bed hospital in Prague that had been cleared of all patients other than patients with
polio. In addition to treating patients, Curtis gave courses in the Kenny method, which
were attended by more than 50 nurses and therapists. She also gave lectures and clinical
demonstrations to physicians, returning twice in 1950. One 2-week course was attended
by around 50 physicians, including the medical directors of 2 prominent thermal spas,
representatives from the national ministry of health, neurologists, pediatricians, and
members of the medical faculty of Charles and Plzen universities.[118]

Not only did Vetterova's influence open the doors of hospitals and spas, but Pokorvny's
professional enthusiasm also led senior physicians to let their junior associates attend

these courses. Emil Gutmann, a physiologist and senior anatomist at Charles University, allowed one of his assistants to give anatomy lectures to Curtis's students and made sure the assistant consulted with Curtis "to harmonize his lectures with mine." The assistant also invited Curtis and her students to view the university's anatomy department where he showed them the anatomy museum and then played a film of a "Muscle Man" who could contract any muscle of his body at will and make each stand out individually.[119] Her physicians' classes were too large, Curtis admitted, "but they learned enough to know how restoration of function is done" and what their nurses "are doing when they do it," and she was delighted when a senior neurologist supplied a "neurologic explanation and scientific support to K. concept."[120] After teaching a 2-week physicians' course in May 1950, Curtis spent 4 additional weeks lecturing to groups of doctors and nurses as she visited her former students, now loyal followers, in hospitals in Prague, Pardubice, Bratislava, and Kroc.[121]

Although Curtis praised Czech physicians as mostly open minded and eager to learn, they sometimes challenged her. At one meeting before an audience of 70, a physician who had not attended her course declared "I've read all the literature. Sister Kenny had not been accepted by Australia or America. Why should we go farther than they? Orthodox or Kenny treatment, the results are all the same." An orthopedic surgeon then warned the audience that "five years from now your K. patients will all be coming to me for operations." Nor, Curtis found, did her lectures about the concepts behind Kenny's work convince all members of her audience. Senior neurologists and other specialists told Curtis that "they wanted to see, not hear."[122] But even giving them a clinical demonstration was not enough. Curtis was only a therapist, and the doctors could not accept scientific explanations from someone who did not have their formal training. Sympathetic physicians pressed her to give them articles in recent medical journals "by virologists, epidemiologists, or other scientists advancing our knowledge of polio & supporting the Kenny concept."[123] But this material was difficult to come by. Kenny had been gathering this kind of material since the early 1940s, but the 1944 AMA report had led American physicians to publish further criticisms of her work. Despite the widespread acceptance of much of her work in the United States by the late 1940s, most American physicians who used her methods did so without fanfare.

Still, Curtis found that most of the physicians she met "treat me with a respect and deference that is touching (and almost embarrassing)." After she described the "rubbery symptom"—Kenny's early diagnostic sign that American physicians had largely ignored—she was asked to attend admission examinations at the Prague children's hospital. "This is a heavy and ticklish responsibility," she told Kenny. "I try hard not to overstep my position, and still give them the benefit of what I have been taught, and seen in experience." She was gratified to see the hospital physicians "try to see the signs as I point them out. In other words, the door is open for teaching; I am trying to do my best with the opportunity."[124] Curtis also proved open to constructive criticism. When her students complained that the film *The Kenny Concept* did not clearly show how to restore muscle function, she agreed to make another film showing the full treatment including points "not well covered in the documentary film." "I think myself it was skillfully done," she reported to Kenny about her new film. "I look fat and double chinned, but what matter if the work is correct."[125] She was especially pleased to learn that a pediatric professor had warned his students to ignore his own article on polio published in a local medical journal because it had been written the previous year, and "with what we are learning and seeing in the new treatment, we will have to revise all our thinking."[126]

By the time Kenny visited for the second time in June 1950, the Ministry of Health announced that every regional infectious disease hospital would be supplied with the appropriate equipment and personnel to treat all acute patients with the Kenny method, and that there would also be 4 special centers to provide Kenny treatment for up to 2 years. Kenny met many of Curtis's former students who praised their teacher as a "brilliant ambassador" and she was delighted when 2 professors told her that in the European medical press "she had been very much misrepresented, both personally and professionally."[127] In Czechoslovakia Kenny was, Curtis noted, "welcomed with deference and honor everywhere" and "cars and chauffeurs were always at hand." Most of all she was part of the discussions with senior physicians who asked her opinion about both theory and practice, and after her visit sent her an effusive letter of thanks. Her technical film, now translated into Czech, was shown during her visit. Officials talked with her about the use of the Kenny method for "spastic" patients and those with other muscular diseases. The Ministry of Health announced that orthopedic surgeons were "to hold off operations for two years."[128] Curtis kept a detailed record of Kenny's 1950 visit, but when Kenny turned the record into her Official Report she left out the times when she became ill or spent the afternoon resting.[129] This was not an image of herself that Kenny wanted to project.

Cold War politics, however, prevented Kenny from achieving her goal of cementing relations between these enthusiastic Czech professionals and her allies in Western Europe and the United States. She invited Pokorny, the spa director, to Minneapolis. But, although he was recommended by the American Consul in Prague, his application was rejected by the State Department as he was a member of the Communist Party, which, Curtis reminded Kenny in frustration, was the "road to advancement in government jobs here." Curtis was not surprised to find global medical progress undermined by Cold War politics. "This is really the best grounds and the best opening we have found in Europe," she reflected. "It is a pity that the Iron Curtain stands in the way of its [the Czech hospital] becoming *the* Kenny center for all Europe."[130] To try to enhance the institutionalization of her teaching, Curtis ordered a hundred copies of *Physical Medicine* (the gray book) to be sent to Czech medical libraries and to the 20 hospitals where her former students worked. Vetterova promised to translate selections from both the gray book and the red book and to add statements by prominent Czech doctors endorsing Kenny's method.[131]

Curtis had hoped that after she told Laruelle that the Czech doctors were writing up their clinical experiences it would "stimulate him to do something." "A word from him," she was convinced, "will really carry great weight in all the European medical world."[132] But prospects in Brussels seemed little improved, and she was disheartened but not surprised to hear from Helen Sare, the Kenny technician now based at the Brussels clinic, that patients had begun to develop "contractures and deformities."[133] Sare continued to train a small number of physical therapists but found that local physicians showed little interest in learning about the Kenny method. Satisfied that the results will be good, they "leave me alone to get on with it," she told Kenny's secretary, but "it would be SO much more satisfactory...to have them co-operate with me."[134]

Curtis's final opportunity to establish Kenny's work in Europe occurred when a German physician invited her to treat his acute patients at the Augsburg city hospital, and the head of the local children's hospital agreed she could work with patients there also.[135] Curtis became convinced that Kenny's work could expand in a country that was part of Western Europe rather than Eastern Europe. She allied herself with the newly established German Pfennig Parade, a kind of March of Dimes organized by the German-American Men's Club.[136] Using the KF's familiar promotional technique, Curtis made sure Kenny visited that summer and took part in a Pfennig Parade, held a clinical demonstration, and showed her film. Feted as a celebrity, presented with numerous bouquets, and serenaded by singing children, Kenny spoke delightedly of establishing a "training school...where all may share this knowledge," reminding her German audiences that "the Science of Medicine knows no frontiers."[137]

But while Curtis attracted eager patients and Kenny spoke to respectful medical audiences, many German physicians remained adamantly opposed to Kenny's work. Orthopedists frequently told Curtis that "America has rejected the Kenny treatment," comments which, Curtis was convinced, reflected the isolation of many European physicians from American medical journals during the early 1940s when Kenny's work was widely praised.[138] After 18 months Curtis had treated over 80 patients and trained one nurse thoroughly and 4 more with the basics of the method. Families from the region, from other German cities, and from Italy sought Curtis out.[139] But her position as a physical therapist made her efforts to win over doctors difficult. She described her efforts as being like "the Corporal trying to instruct Generals." Instead of being able to explain "the whole thing clearly and boldly" she could not speak to a doctor on his own professional level but instead had to "insinuate and suggest and slip in a word now and then." Still, her clinical results impressed individual pediatricians and internists.[140]

In Germany as in California, Kenny technicians only found opportunities to introduce the work possible in crowded city hospitals. Voluntary hospitals like Ausburg's orthopedic hospital were more resistant. Its medical staff refused to allow Curtis to train any of its nurses or to treat any patients. Her few medical allies were unable to institutionalize the work into the local health system, and by the time she left Germany no one had decided "who should employ or pay people who give the treatments." Well aware that her work was not yet a formal part of Ausburg's health bureaucracy, Curtis worried that the work might "die out after I leave."[141]

In 1953 Curtis returned to Minneapolis with a distinguished service medal she had received from the Bonn government for her work in Bavaria but little hope that her work there would leave a lasting mark.[142] She became convinced that to overcome the political, institutional, social, and medical barriers in Europe, there needed to be a model Kenny Institute and Teaching Center where American doctors—"sufficiently high in professional standing to command respect"—working with Kenny technicians could demonstrate, explain, and train, thereby inspiring other medical professionals throughout Europe. The location of such an institute would have to be in a country "where it would be welcome and... [where] the people would not take it as a substitution for their own efforts, or merely tolerate it because they could get some American money free."[143] To set up this kind of institution would require a physician or politician with significant clout, vision, and energy as well as financial resources. But while Kenny had collected many enthusiastic letters from European physicians and lay allies, nobody prominent or courageous enough emerged to set up such a center. Although polio epidemics continued to ravage Western and Eastern Europe in the early 1950s, the senior Kenny technicians left Europe and the KF retreated from the small efforts they had made at global expansion.

POLIO POLITICS

By 1950 the KF had become a nationally recognized philanthropy. Local KF groups joined the growing federated fundraising movement, which the NFIP continued to resist. The KF produced fundraising stamps, posters, pamphlets, and cans, all featuring a hopeful young child and the familiar figure of Kenny with her white hair. The KF Board in Minneapolis considered Kenny an inspiring figurehead, who could draw crowds and open wallets. But this figurehead did not just smile and wave; she gave fierce speeches that often left both NFIP and KF officials frustrated and defensive. She ignited antagonism

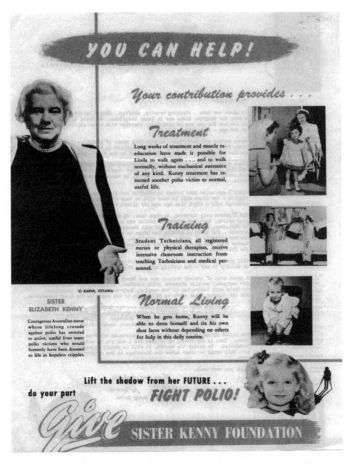

FIGURE 8.1 Part of the campaign brochure for the Kenny Foundation, showing the Yousuf Karsh portrait of Kenny and a blond girl with the shadow of a disabled figure on crutches behind her; Sister Kenny Foundation *You Can Help* [1950], Box 5, Elizabeth Kenny Papers, Minnesota Historical Society, St Paul.

between the 2 philanthropies and then added layers of disarray by pitting the national NFIP office against local and state chapters. Although Huenkens had begun to smooth ruffled feathers by establishing better relations among the KF, physicians, and the NFIP, Kenny's attacks made it hard to end the polio wars.

In a confusing mixture of pride and frustration Kenny simultaneously attacked the NFIP's neglect of her work and boasted of her centers' cooperation with local and state NFIP chapters. Mixed with this was her growing attack on the organization of the KF. Thus she compared the centers in Jersey City and Buffalo, which not only offered treatment that was "pure Kenny" but provided patient care funded through full cooperation with the NFIP, to clinics in Centralia, Yakima, and Chicago, which had "failed miserably" because the KF Board had refused to let them run as autonomous centers.[144] She also rejected any efforts by the Board to model the KF on the NFIP. KF chapters, she believed, should not have to send a proportion of their funds to the Minneapolis office, for the American public would become enthusiastic donors only when "the people understand that the money they contribute will be used in their own districts." When the KF Board directors made a "fuss over self-government," she warned one Board member, people say the Board members "are only squeaking because they could no longer share in the loot," adding "which I know is not the case."[145]

Although her speeches often angered KF officials, Kenny's imposing presence continued to be useful to ameliorate political obstacles. When the head of New York City's division of public charities tried to restrict "outdoor solicitations" by KF organizers Kenny pointed out that NFIP campaigners had used a loudspeaker at a recent football match to ask the crowd for donations and had passed around March of Dimes cans. "Mr. Sloane looked rather downcast at this statement," she recalled.[146] Kenny found it useful to point out NFIP fundraising strategies at the same time as she was denigrating the NFIP's leadership.

The struggle to expand the KF's support of patient care and technician training became caught up in domestic politics, including a renewed attention to civil rights. Until the late 1940s polio care, like most health care in America, was practiced in race-segregated institutions. Although some physicians continued to think of polio as a white disease, the growing visibility of black patients with polio led to demands for black specialists, and a wider awareness of philanthropic opportunities for black donors. The NFIP expanded its funding of the Tuskegee clinic, added funds for professional training for African American doctors and nurses, and hired an "Interracial Division" officer who traveled to black communities to organize March of Dimes events. The KF, similarly, began to pay attention to African American communities that might be sources of support for Kenny's work. As an emerging postwar civil rights movement began to target Jim Crow medicine, however, it was not clear how polio philanthropy was going to adapt.

By the late 1940s Kenny's Institute began to receive positive publicity from black newspapers like the *Pittsburgh Courier* for its "non-sectarian" training of black nurses alongside white nurses.[147] Marjorie Wells, a black Kenny technician studying at the Institute, came to New York City as a featured speaker at a campaign rally for the KF's Negro Committee.[148] Pruth McFarlin, a well-known disabled African American radio singer, raised money to "aid handicapped youth of all races" for the KF and was photographed beside Kenny in the *Chicago Defender*.[149]

In 1947 Jackie Robinson broke the color line in major league baseball and became a symbol of a new postwar world. In 1949, a few weeks after Robinson's well-publicized anticommunist testimony as a friendly witness before the House Un-American Activities Committee, KF officials, looking beyond the white society women in New York City who were Kenny's primary patrons, began to publicize Robinson as a KF celebrity. KF officials set up a fundraising drive to expand the Kenny clinic at the Jersey City Medical Center and named its new polio wing the Jackie Robinson Wing. Black Broadway and Hollywood stars, including Sarah Vaughan and Dizzy Gillespie, performed at a downtown cafe for a Jackie Robinson Night to raise money for the new wing.[150] The black press was delighted. "No greater tribute could be paid to any man than the naming of a healing ward after him," the *Atlanta Daily World* declared, and the *New York Amsterdam News* exulted that it was "the first such honor to be bestowed upon a Negro athlete."[151] During this campaign Kenny was pictured in the *New York Amsterdam News* seated amid the Jackie Robinson Wing Committee organizers.[152] This kind of philanthropic politics reflected a rising attention to black patients with polio and the hope that the KF, along with the NFIP, would be open to greater participation by African American celebrities.

KENNY AND THE INSTITUTE

Kenny may have resigned from her position as Institute director, but she did not, as Huenkens noted ruefully, "stay resigned."[153] Although she no longer spent much time in Minnesota she continued to act as if she were still in charge of the Institute. The Institute was supposed to stand as an emblem of what the Kenny treatment—properly applied by fully trained technicians—could achieve. Yet, Kenny warned the Institute's organizers, visitors noticed "procedures being carried out which are opposed to my theory" and "are not impressed with the results."[154]

When students at the Institute asked her for help in December 1949, she jumped easily into her role as clinical demonstrator to show them "that they were treating the wrong area in a certain case where a deformity had materialized, and that, with a correct knowledge of the disease, it was possible to correct this deformity in a few minutes." Some Institute patients, she discovered, had been treated for several weeks or months without any member of the staff explaining to students "the cause of the deformities and how to correct them." In Kenny's judgment, these problems were the result of Huenkens' decision to use physical medicine specialists who were less likely to allow her technicians to use her methods without modification than were orthopedist supervisors, and she complained about this during her visit. She organized a clinical exhibition, relying on 3 of her former patients from the early 1940s, including one young woman who had had an "apparently flail leg" and an "affected" torso, but was now married with children, looked after her own household, and earned her own living. "She walks very well without the aid of artificial supports," Kenny pointed out, and has "no bone shortening, no deformities."[155]

An angry Huenkens confronted Kenny and ordered her "in a very dictatorial manner" to take back her critical remarks about physical medical specialists, warning that otherwise Miland Knapp and the other Institute physicians "would leave the premises." Kenny refused and later talked to Knapp who did not walk out but instead arranged for her "to meet the medical staff and give my explanation of certain difficult problems they were met with."[156]

Knapp had learned to dodge confrontations with Kenny, an avoidance made easier by her frequent trips away from Minnesota. In the early 1940s he had been a prominent ally, but the rising prestige of physical medicine and his own prominence as the president of the American Congress of Physical Therapy had enabled him to ignore most local medical politics. He maintained a good working relationship with Huenkens and the KF Board and had expanded rehabilitation medicine at both the university hospital and the city hospital. Knapp had begun to articulate his discomfort with some of Kenny's theoretical claims around mental alienation and spasm as early as 1944, explaining to visitors to the Institute that his practice was "the best of Kenny mixed with the best of orthodox."[157] To try to avoid taking sides, however, he was willing to write a testimonial in 1949 stating that Kenny had "made a definite and important contribution of the field of poliomyelitis."[158] But he also began to prepare a follow-up study of patients treated under Kenny's direct supervision by her "well-trained therapists."[159] Knapp's amiable stance with Kenny personally may also have reflected his sympathy with her earlier battles and his growing recognition that she was not well and unlikely to fight back as fiercely as she once had.

Uncomfortable with the idea that medical knowledge was always unstable and tired of hearing about the need for additional research in order to confirm her ideas, Kenny began to lobby the KF for a Medical Council "consisting of the most outstanding orthopedic surgeons and neurologists in the world today." The Council's members would have studied her work, agreed that it was "satisfactory" and "the concept correct," and that "the confirmation of the theory abolishes the necessity for any further investigation concerning either treatment or theory." She also advocated a new institutional policy according to which each Kenny center would be self-governing and the KF would be run by a new board of directors representing each center. This new board would put in place fair and balanced policies so that no one center could rule the others.[160]

Not surprisingly, the KF Board rejected Kenny's effort to reimagine polio philanthropic politics. Her friend Henry Haverstock responded in March 1950 with complimentary bromides about her "tremendous constitution" and "the colossal task which you have performed, going hither and yon all over the world," all hints that it was time to retire. He did not agree that the KF needed a special medical council, and he warned of the dangers of fundraising campaigns not directed by the KF's national headquarters, lest "everybody who wants to run some racket on the strength of your reputation—race tracks, boxing benefits, all sorts of promotions—will feel free to go ahead and the work will disintegrate."[161] This was a warning that would, unfortunately, prove all too prescient.

HOPEFUL SIGNS

Amid these setbacks were signs that the American public saw Kenny as a treasured figure. In February 1950 Congress passed a bill authorizing Kenny visa-free passage across the borders of the United States. She became the first noncitizen to be honored in this way since General Lafayette.[162] "Now," announced Victor Cohn, science writer for the *Minneapolis Tribune*, "this 63-year-old gray-haired crusader...may come and go as she pleases."[163] The visa was approved a few weeks after a Gallup Poll asking "What woman living today in any part of the world, that you have heard or read about, do you admire the most?" had ranked Kenny second, after former First Lady Eleanor Roosevelt, who had led polls like this for most of the previous decade.[164] Another poll of over 200 women journalists conducted by *Pageant Magazine* rated Kenny as one of the nation's most influential women and praised "her courage against odds, her humanitarianism, and [her efforts at]...dramatizing the problem of polio and helping to solve it."[165] A special ceremony to highlight the *Pageant* awards was held at the temporary United Nations headquarters and featured Kenny, along with Eleanor Roosevelt, Emily Post, Dorothy Thompson, and others. In her "My Day" column the former First Lady noted that Kenny had "captured the imagination of a great many people because of her humanitarian work and her strong convictions," a careful distancing of Roosevelt's own unspoken views from those of the American public.[166]

The most promising sign during this period was the opening of a West Coast Kenny center in El Monte, California. Mrs. Ruth Kerr, a successful businesswoman who ran the Kerr Glass Company, offered Kenny the 15-acre facility in March 1950.[167] Run by the Pacific Coast Rescue Society, which financed institutions for disabled children in Oregon and California, the Ruth Home for Wayward Girls had been used since 1930 to treat and rehabilitate girls with "venereal problems," but that work was ending due to the advent of antibiotics. Kerr's offer was spurred, she explained to Kenny, by the institution's directors and staff who had "watched with great interest your very splendid work" and believed "thoroughly in your splendid program."[168]

The Ruth Home was formally opened as the Sister Kenny Polio Hospital in August 1950, after Kenny carefully organized her allies around the state in order to avoid another Centralia disaster. She met with the president of the Los Angeles County Medical Society, the state's public health director, and the director of the state's Bureau of Crippled Children, and showed them "evidence concerning the value of the work." The agencies gave the new Kenny center formal approval, thus ensuring good relations with local physicians and with local NFIP chapters. Kenny also convinced "several highly qualified doctors," including orthopedist Harvey Billig, to serve on the center's new medical board, and filled the board of directors with allies such as Rosalind Russell and executives of local corporations.[169]

At the opening ceremony Kenny spoke briefly about research from "a dozen different medical institutions around the world" that had confirmed that polio was "systemic" and thus proved "the concept for which I have been working to obtain recognition during the past 40 years." The *Los Angeles Times* accompanied this story with a typical picture of Kenny flanked by Russell, a nurse, and a child patient in a hospital bed. Although all her written reports in this period mentioned her delight at this new opportunity, the photo suggested signs of strain. Despite her familiar large black hat, corsage, and circle pin, Kenny was not at ease: she looked toward but not into the camera, her neck held stiffly, her mouth tight, a contrast to a relaxed and smiling Russell in a smart suit and hat.[170] An indication that some of her California friends recognized her growing physical infirmity came when she was presented with the keys to her own cottage on the El Monte site a few months later. "You've traveled constantly for the last 30 years and lived out of suitcases," the hospital's board chairman declared. "Put your belongings in this cottage and live here as much as you can...your cottage will always be waiting for you."[171] Kenny loved both her special cottage and the El Monte hospital, which, she believed, provided Kenny treatment the way she thought it should be given.[172]

Southern California remained a center of Kenny enthusiasm, but such support was not easily transferable. Buoyed by the El Monte success Kenny contacted a senior official at New York State's department of health, and offered to meet with representatives to discuss her knowledge of polio that would be "most valuable" to "the citizens of the state" and to demonstrate her work at the New York State Rehabilitation Hospital in West Haverstraw. Unlike the officials in California, however, the New York official dismissed her curtly. Kenny protested weakly that her work was "a service to the medical profession" and that the *Lancet* had stated she was "correct in both pathology and therapy." But the doors of this hospital remained closed, reflecting a wider sense among New York health officials that they had embraced as much of Kenny's work as they wanted.[173] She also contacted the deans of medical schools at Columbia University and New York University but with little success.[174] She continued to call press conferences in New York, and demand that KF organizers ensure that the major newspapers were represented, but one organizer later reflected, reporters would ask "what have you got that's new?" and it became "harder and harder to get them out for her."[175] In California her Hollywood friends and her status as a celebrity ensured a far more receptive response than in New York.

COLD WAR CELEBRITY POLITICS

Conscious of the need to demonstrate civic responsibility, nascent commercial television networks in the late 1940s used their studios to host charitable fundraising drives. These drives, known by 1949 as telethons, became a familiar fixture as celebrities from stage, screen, radio, and television appeared on the small screen to ask for donations. The first 2 major telethons centered on specific diseases, a focus that proved popular for many decades. In May 1949 comedian Milton Berle hosted a 16-hour effort on NBC that raised $100,000 for the Damon Runyon Memorial Cancer Fund, and in November a 14-hour drive raised money for the United Cerebral Palsy fund.[176]

The KF turned to its celebrity friends to host similar shows. Only a month after the first cerebral palsy telethon, the Dumont Television Network presented a 5-hour program hosted by comedian Morey Amsterdam to raise money for the KF; a gala KF benefit at the Shoreham Hotel in Washington, D.C., which drew top names from Washington society, was televised the following year.[177] Television enabled the KF to display its respectability and national prominence, especially as former KF campaign chair Bing Crosby had scaled back his involvement to participating in fundraising golf tournaments.

Kenny was as comfortable with this new medium as she had been with radio and newsreels.[178] She appeared on NBC's Vanity Fair program and as a guest on the Bigelow Show on KTVV, where the "famed mentalist" Joseph Dunninger tried to guess her thoughts while he was encased in a lead vault.[179] New York society commentator Ed Sullivan, who had publicly castigated O'Connor for his refusal to fund Kenny a few years earlier, invited her to be a guest on his television show "Toast of the Town." After her appearance spurred donations, which Sullivan and his producers sent on to Kenny, she thanked him saying "your life must be very satisfactory to comfort the sick and amuse the healthy."[180] "Sister has been on so many radio and Television programs lately," her secretary noted, that one of her visitors "suggested she should be known as 'Miss TV 1949.'"[181]

The highlight of Kenny's TV work was as the featured guest on "Meet the Press" on October 1 1950. "Meet the Press" had begun as a radio show in 1945 and was broadcast on television since 1947; American journalists and the public considered it the nation's feistiest news program. It had already won a Peabody award, and had attracted guests such as California governor and future chief justice Earl Warren, President Harry Truman, and Senator Joseph McCarthy. The format of "Meet the Press" was to invite a public figure without a script or prepared statements to face a panel of reporters to discuss contemporary issues. Journalist Martha Rountree, the program's moderator and co-producer who was memorably summed up by Mrs. William Randolph Hearst as "a diesel engine under a lace handkerchief," was a Kenny supporter and arranged that the show featuring Kenny would accept donations to the KF.[182]

Kenny was interviewed by 4 men: Edward Folliard of the *Washington Post*, Robert Riggs of the *Louisville Courier-Journal*, Frank McNaughton of *Time Magazine*, and Lawrence Spivak, the former editor of *American Mercury* and the show's other co-producer.[183] Although Rountree introduced Kenny as "one of the most controversial figures in medical history," the journalists treated her with jovial respect, raising familiar issues to which Kenny could give well-rehearsed answers that showed her more as a celebrity emeritus than a figure of current controversy. Asked why she did not submit "case studies" to physicians or medical journals she first said "That is not my job to do. That is [for] the medical director of my work," and then described detailed reports by Pohl, Laruelle, and Deacon. She attacked the NFIP's efforts to undermine her work and thereby "debar the patient from getting the very best," but she did agree that the KF and the NFIP should amalgamate, adding "I have been trying to get together with the National Foundation for ten years and haven't succeeded." Asked what kind of control she would want, Kenny replied "I'd like to be assured of the money that was collected in my name, for my work, that it was used for the purpose for which it was collected." The tone of the interview turned when Lawrence Spivak said provocatively that "a great many people who say they know you [say] that you are a very difficult person. Are you?" Unfazed, Kenny replied: "I am most difficult in anything that concerns the health and well-being of the children of America and the children of the world. I'd like to wipe every one off the face of the earth that stands in the way of their future health and happiness." Spivak said: "You must be able to do it when you get that look in your eye." In her effort to turn the discussion away from Kenny's character, Rountree commented archly that she was "sure the viewers of the program can ask Mr. Spivak the same question," and Spivak agreed "I am a very difficult person, too, Sister."[184]

This interview was a highpoint for Kenny, an opportunity to air familiar grievances in a reputable forum. Officials at the NFIP New York headquarters feared it might gain her views greater respectability and debated whether to continue their policy of not engaging in public debates with her. In internal memos the staff agreed that it would be unwise to take her on. "I don't think in the public's mind you can ever win an argument with a gray-haired, old lady, no matter what facts we presented," one official argued, for "the American public sides with the under-dog, which Miss Kenny has been shrewd enough to play upon."[185] The NFIP continued its policy of silence, but Kenny's fierce voice defending the children of the world reminded the public of her clinical skills and her humanitarian motivations.

By 1950 the NFIP had moved away from trying to decide which kind of polio therapy worked better than another. Indeed, the polio research it funded now centered on virology. With Harry Weaver as director of research the NFIP had begun organizing small conferences where laboratory researchers and clinicians could exchange ideas away from the bright lights of the media. The introduction of its poster child program, featuring young children in braces or struggling to rise from a wheelchair, highlighted the concrete, disabling effects of polio, rather than the ameliorating promise of physical therapy or orthopedic surgery. NFIP publicity featured male laboratory scientists in white coats to epitomize progress; in comparison, Kenny, a nurse and therapeutic innovator, seemed irrelevant and old-fashioned. Thus, NFIP publicist Roland Berg warned reporters not to compare the Kenny concept of polio with orthodox medical ideas. The medical viewpoint was not a concept "but a fact based on sufficient scientific evidence." In contrast, "Miss Kenny's concept of the disease is truly a 'concept'—a belief without any factual foundation as yet."[186] It was simply a fantasy, unlikely to lead to mastery over polio or to be useful in rethinking the way the polio virus caused paralysis or how it could be halted.

COLD WAR GLOBAL FEMINISM

The "Meet the Press" interview presented Kenny to a national audience just as she decided to return to live in Australia. Before leaving she positioned herself as a Cold War celebrity who could call on the support of a network of women, a version of global feminism that was emerging as part of a wider debate around women's role in global governance.

Women volunteers, whose power the NFIP had overlooked at its peril, could, Kenny believed, stand against corrupt and inept officials and misguided and unresponsive physicians. Long aware of the power of women as patrons and supporters, Kenny had basked in the gratitude of mothers, the camaraderie of her Kenny technicians, the loyalty and self-sacrifice of her secretaries and assistants, the glamorous attention of her Hollywood friends, and the admiration of members of women's clubs and other civic groups. Women allies in hospital auxiliaries, welfare agencies, and charities had provided her with an entry into medical and political circles. Margaret Webber, the first sponsor of her teaching in Minneapolis, remained a friend and patron. Ruth Kerr, the philanthropic businesswoman, was the driving force behind the transformation of the El Monte Ruth Home into a Kenny center. Marianna Vetterova had opened doors for Dorothy Curtis in Czechoslovakia, and physician Ethel Calhoun had made sure that the Pontiac infectious disease hospital and its local NFIP chapter stayed committed to Kenny's methods.

Kenny's supporters in women's clubs and rural women's groups immersed her more deeply in conservative politics. In 1949 Kenny spoke to 40,000 members of the Farm Women's Bureau in Lansing, Michigan and was heartened by the decision of the women of the Minnesota branch who appointed 5 members to meet with NFIP state chairmen to warn them to stop their opposition to KF drives. The Minnesota women also endorsed a state program for improving care for the mentally ill, blood tests before marriage, and to "clean up" movies, radio programs, literature, and comic books to help "correct" juvenile delinquency.[187] Such measures essentialized women's roles as wives, mothers, and daughters, and were intended to show women how to put their concern for the health of children and family ahead of parochial political loyalties. Many of these allies, as Kenny reminded the KF board, provided her with large donations that she turned over to the KF.[188]

The emerging role of women as global activists reflected a vision of the atomic age, which blurred distinctions between the public world of the battlefield and the private world of family and community. These women claimed a special role as global mediators, using words like friendship, a kind of gender-neutral equivalent to the "brotherhood of man." This version of global feminism was imbued with fervor but it could also frighten the unwary. In September 1950, for example, when Mrs. Henry Dodge, head of the Westchester county KF branch, paid for a plane to scatter 100,000 leaflets, some residents wondered if communists were distributing "subversive propaganda."[189]

Kenny eagerly embraced the concept of women as healers rather than destroyers. "Future humanitarian advancement must come from women," she declared during a visit to California in 1949, for "men are too busy talking wars and atomic bombs," a pithy comment that was reprinted widely.[190] At the *Pageant Magazine* award ceremony, Kenny announced that the women of the world had a great opportunity to work for peace "even in these difficult times." Her own efforts to expand her work across the globe, she declared, had established such a link. Thinking of her recent visit with Dorothy Curtis a few months earlier, she declared that when the "hundreds of little Czech children...grow up, they will remember that [an]...American girl went to their county" to teach therapists in "Moravia, Bohemia, [and] Slovakia how to let them walk again."[191] Implicit was the hope that her work could have a missionary effect, leading children on the other side of the Iron Curtain to see her work as another reason to reject their communist rulers.

Most of Kenny's new allies were conservative women. In New York she worked with wealthy patrons like Mona and Belle Fox, sisters of William Fox of Twentieth Century Fox Studios, and with the New York KF Women's Committee whose members included Ellen Tuck Astor, the former wife of John Jacob Astor IV. These women's social influence led Kenny to hope that her work could be maintained and her legacy assured through this kind of elite, informal female network. With funds from the 1949 Knickerbocker Ball and a series of fundraising luncheons, the Committee raised enough money to open the city's first outpatient Kenny clinic on Park Avenue in 1950.[192] Kenny and the Women's Committee saw this as a first step toward another major Kenny clinic. But KF officials disagreed. Relations between the Committee and Rex Williams, the salaried executive director of the KF's Eastern Division, disintegrated when he asked the Committee to pool the money they had collected with the KF's general New York fund. Deeply incensed at this request and arguing the Committee could be accused by the public of obtaining money "under false pretenses," Mrs. Edward Douglas Madden, the chair of the Committee who had raised funds from "members of the leading families of New York," resigned.[193] Using the model of Southern California, Kenny tried to heal the rupture by telling this "group of responsible citizens" to form a new board that she would personally charter. She knew that the Minneapolis board would dislike her acting like the sole KF executive, but, she haughtily informed KF officials, "it is my desire that the women of the world shall take a personal interest in this project," and as this New York group had been initiated "by me" she was confident that, unlike the "efforts of organizing secretaries and medical directors," it would not fail.[194] Kenny was no feminist, but she recognized that women could be more enthusiastic and perhaps also more reliable allies than men such as Rex Williams who were salaried officials. Her reliance on this older model of philanthropy based on wealthy women volunteers seemed to KF officials ill-suited to the modern postwar world of professional fundraising. Henry Haverstock and Marvin Kline thus informed her that the KF Board "had no intention of disposing of the services of Mr. Williams."[195]

FAREWELLS

In December 1950 Kenny said a series of farewells. In Minneapolis the mayor gave her the city's distinguished service award, and she tearfully thanked him and city aldermen for the beautiful home that had been "a haven of refuge" in "your beautiful city" for "ten very happy years." She also thanked the KF Board members "for their splendid help...unbiased attitude and generous nature."[196] "Wherever I am," she told New York reporters a few days later, "the American flag shall fly over my home." "My mission has been accomplished," she declared, with a touch of hyperbole, and she was returning "to my headquarters in Australia." Now, "the women of the world will take this matter up and support and further this great cause." "Of course," she added with her typical spark, "they will need help from the men."[197]

Behind the scenes, however, Kenny was neither sentimental nor content. In a heated conversation with Marvin Kline, preserved by a transcript, she said she had been "very, very disappointed" to find students at the Institute with almost no knowledge of her work. Her teaching was falling away and being replaced with "a lot of innovations that are of no value." She had heard that Huenkens had even said she was "mentally unbalanced," and she threatened to "take my name off this place" if Huenkens remained head of the Institute, warning "it will be very difficult to get money when I am not here."[198]

After her meeting with Kline, she wrote a fiery letter to the KF Board's new chairman, Minneapolis businessman George Crosby, warning that the KF needed a "thorough reorganization." Angry at being more and more marginalized by the KF board, she began to construct an unusually personalized defense, as she reflected on the reason many of the Minnesota "gentlemen" had initially joined the KF Board: her care of their children. Henry Haverstock Sr. "would still be carrying his son about in his arms, instead of seeing him an independent, useful citizen, happily married." Donald Dayton "would be looking at a very distressed young boy handicapped like his little wardmate...instead of a robust young footballer." Crosby himself "would be bothered about the readjustment of spinal supports on one or more of his three very delightful children, instead of watching them growing [in] health and strength and beauty."[199] But simply recalling clinical successes felt unsatisfying, like signs of an earlier golden era, which was, she feared, disappearing.

A KIND OF RETIREMENT

Kenny moved to a house in Toowoomba on the edge of the Darling Downs in southeastern Queensland where she had first worked as a bush nurse. Set "amongst the hills I love so well," her large picture windows gave "the most gorgeous panoramic view in the World, and I think I am qualified to say the World, for I have seen most of it." But despite this beauty and tranquility she missed "the girls at the old Institute, and my home at 24-46 Park Avenue."[200] Although she had said she was retiring, her celebrity reputation followed her, and she was asked, she claimed, to open hospitals and agricultural shows, receive debutants, patronize fashion parades, and even stand for Parliament. While she let it be known that she did not intend to take any part in public functions, she continued to promote her work. She hired a secretary, began writing another autobiography called *My Battle and Victory*, and made recordings on a special machine of "certain phases of my work, which are not clearly understood up-to-date." One Queensland reporter described her seated with her secretary at a table "strewn with documents and correspondence," and the *Minneapolis Sunday Tribune* featured "Sister Kenny At Home in Australia" with photographs of Kenny with her secretary Betty Brennan in the garden of her Australian home on the summit of the Toowoomba range, gathering letters sent her from many countries each morning, and tape-recording polio lectures as part of her daily routine.[201]

Henry Haverstock wrote hoping she was "having a good rest and not worrying too much about affairs over [here]."[202] But Haverstock knew better. Kenny continued to fight the same battles: trying to compel the Minneapolis Board to cooperate with other KF centers and to encourage those centers she felt best embodied her vision. She continued to play politics from afar, and distance made her memory sharper not fonder. Money and corruption were constantly on her mind, turning her memories of earlier days into horrific tales of conspiracy. For months when she was first in Minneapolis she had been "on the bread line," she reminded Haverstock, yet "when the National Foundation attempted to buy me . . . I refused to be bought." KF official Henry Von Morpurgo had tried to gain her support with the offer of $30,000 and a house in San Francisco, she went on, but "I informed him there was not enough money in the whole of the United State of America to buy me."[203]

To try to force the KF to adopt her own vision of polio philanthropy Kenny began to envision an International League of Universal Sisterhood, which would be organized on a volunteer basis and therefore "be non-political, non-racial, and non-sectarian."[204] In an article published in the *Woman's Home Companion* she urged readers to organize a Sisterhood of Service that would "show the world that democracy has more to offer than atomic bombs." Prejudice, she warned, had harmed the expansion of her work. The medical profession "regards each new claim, each new discovery, with a skeptical eye," an attitude, she admitted, that was "healthy in many respects" for it "sifts out much quackery." But her work had been blocked by "the often unfeigned hostility on the part of stiff-necked doctors who could not believe that any important contribution to medical science could possibly be made by a member of the lowly nursing profession." She assured American readers (perhaps too emphatically) that she had left with no sense of frustration or bitterness in her heart but "with a feeling of peace and contentment, the feeling that comes with a sense of accomplishment, of a mission fulfilled." She now forgave "those who set up obstacles along the path of help" and was passing the torch on "to the women of America and of the world, bound together by the universal love of children." In dramatic vignettes she used later for her second autobiography Kenny described Rita, a child she had saved, who became strong, grateful, and altruistic enough to return to the Institute as a nurse's aide to help patients during Minnesota's 1946 epidemic.[205] Four photographs accompanied this article: the famous 1943 image of Kenny with Roosevelt and O'Connor; a universalized picture of Kenny dressed in black next to a patient watched by nurses and technicians wearing white; a recent picture of Kenny with Rosalind Russell; and, as a reference to her continuing power as a fundraiser, a picture of her at a KF campaign drive in a black hat, black dress, and corsage along with the TV star Faye Emerson.[206]

Kenny sought to appeal to American women by combining gender, science, and healing, but this combination of attributes was rapidly becoming out of sync with the modern scientific medicine of the early 1950s. Jonas Salk, a young married man with medical training and scientific skills working in a laboratory, was about to become the nation's ideal scientific hero. The idea of an older woman, fighting bravely for the life and health of children, while frustrated by a lack of clinical and institutional support, was losing its cultural force in North America and elsewhere.

A NEW SISTERHOOD?

In Australia, her return home was not as triumphant as she had hoped. Many Australians, Kenny discovered, were not impressed by her American connections, especially her claim that without accepting her work Australian physicians could not properly help patients overcome polio paralysis. Kenny's fierce attitude also annoyed Australian reporters. When she held a press conference "she does the talking," a Sydney paper noted, while "reporters merely take notes." If a reporter had the temerity to ask a personal question, Kenny would pause, fix him "with a hostile glance," and continue to dictate what she considered "relevant news."[207]

Indeed, many Australians interpreted America's acceptance of Kenny and her work as a familiar pattern of American over exuberance. America claimed to have discovered her and was "unstinting in praise of her work," noted one blunt and undeferential article in a Sydney magazine, but in Australia she had not been given a single "official reception." The article made much of her temper, her eccentric behavior, and her tendency to belittle the work of doctors "when tact, discretion and good humor would have achieved more for her cause." A young Queensland socialite who had traveled extensively told the magazine: "A girl's poise hasn't really been put to the test until she meets Sister Kenny... being presented to the King and Queen is mere kindergarten stuff." As for her contribution to science, according to one physician, she "had served like an enzyme or ferment."[208]

On the other hand, Kenny's effort to construct a global sisterhood of service was taken up by her most active Australian supporters in the early 1950s: the Country Women's Association (CWA), a group Kenny had joined in the 1920s. Senior CWA officers had long considered her an underappreciated national treasure. In 1949 Pearl Baldock, the state president of Queensland's CWA, suggested that Elizabeth Sterne, the CWA's national president, contact the Prime Minister to show him the "scientific research [that had]... proven the long contested theory, put forth by Sister Kenny, to be correct."[209] Sterne does not seem to have followed Baldock's suggestion, but later became an enthusiastic Kenny supporter. In 1951 after she had retired from the CWA presidency, Sterne urged Queensland's premier and the federal minister for health to set up an independent investigation to "bring proof that Sister Kenny's work, accepted by such well known clinics as the famous Mayo Clinic, is all that the world, outside Australia, has acclaimed it."[210]

Connecting with the CWA allowed Kenny to imagine a wider link with a well-established women's organization with a global presence. In April 1951 Ruth Buxton Sayre, the president of the Associated Country Women of the World who was on a whirlwind tour of CWA branches in Asia and the Pacific, visited Kenny in Toowoomba. The organization was mainly concerned with the welfare of rural women rather than with broader public health issues, but its ideology fit well with the global activism Kenny had come to embrace. Like many women activists of the 1950s Sayre had urged hundreds of women during her lecture tour to "have a broader horizon and keep the international pot from boiling over just as she must look after the pot on the stove in her own home."[211] After meeting with Sayre Kenny grandly told friends that she was "handing the torch" to her. Sayre, she explained, would "assist in getting together the women's councils of the United Nations" so that Kenny could "meet them and present evidence."[212] Sayre, however, made no mention of Kenny either during her travels or back in America.[213]

A NEW FRAILTY

Charles Chuter's death in 1948 had left Kenny without a bureaucratic intermediary to convey her work to Queensland officials. But using her well-honed skills Kenny was able to link her CWA supporters with a group of new allies, mainly local physicians and hospital patrons of the Toowoomba General Hospital. She became a regular speaker at meetings of the hospital's board, and convinced the board to urge the Queensland government to "have Kenny's knowledge available to the people of the state." At one meeting Kenny read extracts from the *Lancet* and the Czech physicians' letter and then showed her technical film. Impressed, one board member said "the film spoke for itself"; another agreed that "if Sister Kenny had had a medical degree she would have been recognized by the medical profession"; and a third referred to "the battle that Louis Pasteur had to convince the medical world of the correctness of her theory relative to bacteria."[214]

The meetings of her Toowoomba allies grew larger. In August 1951, one meeting chaired by the city's mayor included 2 physicians from the hospital, local officials, a member of the women's caucus of the Sydney branch of the Australian Labor Party, and an organizer of a polio welfare society who was working to establish a Kenny clinic in Adelaide.[215] The group proposed a new international organization—the International Organisation for Combating Poliomyelitis—with Kenny as its "Patroness" and asked her to approach Eleanor Roosevelt to be its president.[216] Soon there were branch meetings in Warwick and Nobby, and 2 politicians praised Kenny's work in the state legislature.[217]

Such events confirmed Kenny's optimism that she could establish a lasting international organization, but nonetheless it was a hard fight. Not only was she far away from the enthusiasm of her American supporters, but she was now aware, or had allowed herself to become aware, that her hand tremors and balance problems were not just the result of age or fatigue but a specific neurological condition: Parkinson's disease. Still, she kept up a brave public façade, telling reporters who noted her trembling right hand that "I'm getting old. That's all that's wrong with me."[218] She blamed her growing infirmity on her struggles to have her work respected. Her inability to use her right arm, she told Henry Haverstock dramatically, was "a disability caused, so my doctors say, through agony of soul."[219] But to her intimate friends she acknowledged the specific diagnosis. Jarvis Nye urged her to rest. He agreed tactfully that she should be a consultant at some institution in Australia, for "your presence would attract the patients from far and wide," but he warned her to "never do any of the actual work—you have done more than your share of that."[220]

Perhaps it was this new awareness of her own body that led her to put new emphasis on the power of her work to prevent what she called "deformities." This was a change from her earlier emphasis on the bodies of her patients who she had hoped would achieve strength and functionality, even at the price of an ungainly appearance. Now she began to warn that polio's psychological effects, which could lead to anger and depression, made it especially crucial to adopt therapies that allowed the body to appear physically normal. "A deformed body in many cases induces animosity in the person deformed against mankind," she noted in a letter to the *Minneapolis Sunday Tribune*, even a person "who otherwise may be of the most friendly type." Knowledge of her work therefore had "social, economic and humane value."[221] Her attention to polio survivors' adjustment reflected a wider movement in polio care, but it also undermined the appeal of her work to many disabled survivors.

While Kenny recognized the limitations of her weakening body, she continued to believe in the power of personal appeals. Distance, she feared, was weakening the force of her message. Her letters to KF officials had unfortunately "found a home in the waste paper basket."[222] Only her physical presence, she was convinced, could sway the skeptical and the wavering. Her anger at the way her demands were being ignored by the KF directors was deepened by their refusal to provide her with the honorarium which, she had understood before leaving in 1950, was going to be given to her as a kind of philanthropic pension. Only after her Minnesota patron Margaret Webber died and left her a legacy did she feel financially confident enough to talk about placing a deposit on a piece of land to build a home "to meet life's sunset."[223]

COPENHAGEN: KENNY'S LAST CONFERENCE

As early as May 1951 Kenny had begun planning her next visit to the United States. After this plan was reported in the New York Times, NFIP officials told each other to "run for the hills."[224] The ostensible reason Kenny was traveling was in order to attend the Second International Polio Conference to be held in Copenhagen that September. "The situation in the world today is chaotic where Kenny treatment is being given or partially given," she argued in one of her many reports, so "it is imperative that I attend the International Conference being held in Copenhagen in order that I may present this knowledge."[225] She hoped that the European connections she had made over the past 6 years would enable her to play a far more active part than she had done in the 1948 conference, and she wanted to hear the latest polio research to assess how seriously her work was being taken. She had tried to get a formal invitation to the conference through Leon Laruelle but, perhaps to ensure his own good working relations with European polio organizers, he did not provide one for her. Her trip was not funded by the KF but by part of the bequest from Margaret Webber, and in Denmark she stayed at a hotel as the guest of Rosalind Russell's father-in-law Carl Brisson, a Danish movie star.[226]

She came to America in August 1951, a few weeks before the conference was to start. There she made the Parkinson's diagnosis public. Her illness became part of her new somber persona. "Sister Kenny Said To Be Incurably Ill" reported the New York Times. Reporters now remarked openly on her body's stance and gait as she gave interviews for what was supposedly her "last U.S. visit." She said she had plenty of pain, adding dramatically "only God knows how much longer I may live."[227] On what was now called her gray (rather than white) hair, reporters noted that she was wearing the same hat (a "wide-brimmed straw hat trimmed with cabbage roses") that she had worn in Los Angeles a year earlier. Instead of the jaunty celebrity who had boasted of collecting hats, a solemn Kenny now said that there were "too many things to be done [and]...too little time...to bother about hats." She said her trip was against doctor's orders, but with a glint of her earlier wit pointed out that 20 years earlier 4 doctors had given her only months to live and now "they all are dead."[228] Privately, however, she admitted to her friend James Henry that she felt like a "useless hulk."[229]

Before heading to Copenhagen Kenny spent time with her American friends. She was greeted at the airport by Russell and her husband and spent 5 days at the El Monte Kenny Hospital resting at her special cottage. On her flight from Australia to California she had traveled with Jack Hall, a Pan-American pilot who had spent 3 months in an iron lung in Melbourne. In a typically dramatic gesture she described Hall's experience and noted that he was now seeking proper care at El Monte.[230] In New York Kenny stayed at her favorite Delmonico Hotel and told reporters that a third volume on her work was necessary as she had not had "sufficient opportunities to explain her theories to medical men."[231]

While reporters in Los Angeles and New York still came to Kenny's press conferences and repeated her pronouncements, their reporting was now more dutiful than eager. Debates around Kenny's work no longer sparked professional fire and its newness had been tamed through 10 years of clinical adoption. Scientists still debated just how the polio virus traveled around the body, but despite the work of a few innovative virologists the scientific understanding of polio had not altered significantly. Although John Enders' 1948 work suggested that Kenny's insistence that scientists must look beyond damaged or destroyed neurons might not be so unscientific, the idea of polio as a non-neurological disease was largely ignored by most clinicians and laboratory researchers. Indeed Kenny's claim that polio was a muscle or skin disease sounded ridiculous. This was partly a reaction to Kenny as a nurse and an exaggerator but it also reflected a wider neglect of Enders' work. Until 1952 the ability to grow the polio virus in nonneurological tissue was considered by most of Enders' peers to be just another intriguing experimental finding.[232] A discussion of the pathogenesis of the polio virus in *Modern Trends in Pediatrics* (1951), for example, failed to mention Enders' work, and the author stated confidently that the virus multiplied in the walls of air passages and the alimentary canal and then "passes readily along the nerves to the central nervous system."[233] Nor did O'Connor refer to Enders' work in a fundraising appeal at the Waldorf-Astoria, although he did boast about other NFIP-funded research projects that had led to the isolation of at least 3 types of polio virus.[234]

In September 1951 the NFIP, in cooperation with the Danish National Foundation for Infantile Paralysis, held its second international conference in Copenhagen. Five hundred delegates from 38 countries attended the 5-day conference, which was jointly hosted by the Nobel Prize winning Danish physicist Niles Bohr and Basil O'Connor.[235] Along with 32 American polio experts sponsored by the NFIP, the conference also attracted a number of physical therapists who came to attend both the polio conference and the first World Confederation of Physical Therapy, which was meeting concurrently.[236]

University of Pittsburgh virologist Jonas Salk discussed not the vaccine experiments he was pursuing semicovertly, but the far less exciting conclusion of a 3-year NFIP project that established that there were only 3 distinct types of polio virus. Delegates were particularly interested in a report by virologists at the Rockefeller Institute about a new complement fixation test, which, although tested only on monkeys, held the potential to solve the problem of polio diagnosis.[237] John Enders gave a paper on "the multiplication and properties of poliomyelitis viruses in culture of human tissue," but science writers and other reporters did not see his work as especially remarkable. Dazzled by the modern abstract design of exhibits and by the closed circuit television programs that showed some of the presentations, delegates and reporters were far more intrigued by reports of a drug that might prevent the growth of polio virus in nerve cells and had been tested on patients with mumps and influenza.[238] Amid reports on pathology, physiology, and surgical techniques, there was some talk about a polio vaccine. O'Connor said publicly but vaguely, "I won't say when, but I believe a serum will be found against the polio virus during my lifetime."[239]

For Kenny the Copenhagen conference confirmed her sense that a few scientists were rethinking polio's pathology in the direction she had long propagated. She "had the pleasure of hearing my theory concerning the disease process in the human body once more confirmed in a paper read by Professor Enders," and, she later claimed, "it was my privilege to shake hands with this gentleman, who informed me that my discoveries had inspired his investigation."[240] In a courteous letter to Brisbane health official Abe Fryberg Enders later explained that he had not said this. His research had shown that the virus could propagate in "a variety of types of tissue from human beings." But "it would be hazardous…to draw conclusions from our observations that the virus attacks skin fascia in the living animal or in man."[241] When Kenny encountered O'Connor at a reception line at the conference he refused to greet her, a snub that both of them felt properly expressed their relationship.

Kenny returned to Los Angeles after the conference to dedicate a new wing at the El Monte hospital, and then traveled to Minneapolis where she celebrated her birthday (the chimes of city hall played her favorite song "Danny Boy") and took part in the dedication of a new 75-bed wing at the Institute. A few months earlier "souvenir-hunting crows" had jammed her former home at 24-46 Park Avenue, which had been put up for sale by the city.[242]

Her beloved Institute continued to harbor skeptics. A few physicians there said that they agreed "with my theories and practices," but overall she felt that the treatment and teaching were not "satisfactory." Wallace Cole, she learned, was no longer working as an Institute consultant and the 2 young orthopedic surgeons who had replaced him had "no knowledge of the concept of the disease."[243] John Pohl was also no longer connected with the KF or the Institute. Now a consultant to the Dowling School for Crippled Children he remained a strong supporter of Kenny and her work but had a new interest: children with cerebral palsy. His new textbook *Cerebral Palsy* (1950) represented a growing focus in postwar pediatrics and neurology, and his therapies sounded eerily like Kenny's polio methods, with descriptions of developing "voluntary control" of muscles and establishing muscle consciousness as specially trained therapists helped to direct "the thought of the patient to a specific area."[244] There had been a time when she was eager to see her work extended to the treatment of cerebral palsy, but now this was a topic in which Kenny was no longer especially interested.[245]

Other unsympathetic physicians remained influential. Huenkens continued to direct the Institute, and Miland Knapp, Kenny was "much disgusted" to hear, had received a KF grant of $1,000 for research in spinal deformity "when it was a well known fact that the only person with the knowledge concerning the materialization of spinal deformity was myself."[246] She enjoyed far more her brief stop in Centralia, where, although her clinic had been closed for more than 2 years, the mayor and the local medical society gave her a warm welcome, school children were given a half-day holiday, and streets were lined with thousands of people. That was the kind of reception she had become used to, but now it seemed bittersweet, as she was forced to rely on close friends to be able to walk steadily, and she kept her right arm and shoulder well covered to conceal their tremors.[247]

After Centralia Kenny traveled to New York City where she organized a meeting in New York with representatives from Kenny centers in Los Angeles, Pontiac, Jersey City, and the outpatient clinic in New York City. This was part of her effort to form a national KF Council, an idea KF officials had long discouraged. Although she hoped that the meeting would prevent the "jealousies and misunderstandings that unfortunately have become a part of [the] philanthropic movement," nothing came of it.[248] Kline was in New York but refused to attend. Nonetheless, he sought out her help: the New York City's Department of Welfare had denied the KF's application for a license to collect funds based on its "poor financial picture" and warned that KF "fund raising and operating expenses have been out of proportion to the amount of money spent for aid to polio patients," a problem city officials had noted for several years. The KF's legitimacy in New York was also contested by the group of influential women led by Mrs. Madden who claimed they had an exclusive right to raise funds under a charter granted by Kenny in 1950. Kline now asked Kenny to use her influence to try to get the application accepted.[249] Kenny had long been aware that Kline often tried to manipulate her, telling one friend that he had given her "a lot of palaver about what a wonderful person I was."[250] But this assessment of him could not overcome her joy at being appealed to as a power player. She convinced New York officials to issue a license allowing the KF to raise money in New York City, although, she warned the KF Board, she and the New York Women's Committee remained unsatisfied with the KF's financial dealings.[251]

Kenny flew back to Australia, planning to work on captions for a new film so that certain polio conditions could be "properly explained." This "new and important campaign film," she assured Kline, would soon be available for the KF "with very little expense."[252] Although tired and sick, she welcomed celebratory occasions that reminded her of America. She made a special trip to Townsville where the local press lauded the visit as "A Gracious Gesture by a Noble Woman." An impressive figure in a black dinner gown, she gave a public address at the Theatre Royal referring to specialists at universities in Vienna, Prague, and London who had described her treatment as a "splendid new weapon." Amid prolonged applause, her longstanding ally Tom Aikens praised her as "the noblest Australian woman of her generation." The city mayor, the head of the local CWA, and members of the Sister Kenny Memorial Committee showed her the playground named in her honor, which had been opened 2 years earlier, and she met many of her former patients from the clinic she had established in the town during the 1930s. At her request "Danny Boy" was played and sung at the end of the reception.[253] It was beginning to sound like a funeral song.

THE GRAYING WOMAN

In January 1952 a Gallup Poll asked American women "which of these famous women comes closest to your ideal of what, you, yourself, would like to be?" For the first time in a poll like this, Kenny was ranked first, above Eleanor Roosevelt. No other woman had been ranked above the former First Lady in a Gallup poll.[254] "Now, I'm really happy," Kenny supposedly told friends.[255]

Perhaps this unprecedented jump to first place was influenced by public knowledge of her serious illness. Still, Kenny's celebrity did not extend to her native country. Her name did not appear on Australia's annual Honours List, which recognizes outstanding service to humanity. Yet Kenny seemed content. She told Brisbane reporters she would decline an honor in any case, for she was as known "throughout the entire world as Sister Elizabeth Kenny [and]... the title of 'Sister' to the world is the one, in my opinion, that cannot be excelled."[256] Such a comment, despite its familiar tone of sentimental self-deprecation, had a new note. Kenny was beginning to recognize that despite her efforts during these last years of her life to shore up her legacy as a prescient scientific innovator, her international renown was based on her persona as a compassionate nurse-clinician. She was "Sister to the world," and all her angry outbursts could be feminized as the responses of someone who cared so profoundly that she could not help being frustrated at any efforts to hamper her work—just the tone she had successfully used during her "Meet the Press" interview in 1950.

The growing paralysis of her body gave her familiar story a new and poignant twist. She made her illness central in an article published by the Hearst newspaper Sunday supplement *American Weekly* with the arch title "Doctors, I Salute You." Kenny was shown looking through a window in her Australian home, saying "I'm a patient myself for a change." Parkinson's disease, Kenny explained carefully, was not fatal in itself but was "inclined to be rather abrupt with anyone who has a bad heart history." Her pride in her life's work enabled her to "help me forget the irony of becoming slowly incapacitated by a paralysis for which [there is]...no remedy." Doctors would one day find a cure, for "they're wonderful, wonderful men, most of them. I guess you have to fight them to appreciate them."[257] Here was a nurse who had once argued with physicians, demanding to be accepted on their level as both a clinician and as a scientific researcher. Now she was a woman, a nurse, and a patient, recalling former triumphs.

A NEW CONCEPT

In early 1952 a major turning point in polio science reinvigorated Kenny's sense that her ideas were leading scientists to victory over the disease. Although epidemiologists confidently used serological techniques to assess exposure to the polio virus, the bloodstream had not been considered important in explaining polio's pathology. When the NFIP's advisory committee decided to fund trials of gamma globulin (a protein fraction of blood plasma containing many antibodies) as a possible preventative in 1951, the decision was based on the older (although discarded) idea of passive immunization (which had supported the use of convalescent serum decades earlier) and on new evidence that antibodies concentrated in blood plasma could provide brief protection against polio.[258]

Suddenly blood captured the public and scientific imaginations in a new way. In April 1952 came the announcement by virologists Dorothy Horstmann of Yale and David Bodian of Johns Hopkins that they had identified the polio virus in the bloodstream of monkeys, suggesting there was a preliminary stage of "viremia" before the virus reached the nervous system.[259] This "surprising discovery," said the *New York Times*, which had "exploded" the "old theory" of polio suggested a "new concept of polio" that was now "generally accepted" by immunologists. Perhaps if antibodies are injected into a patient before the virus reaches the nervous system "we can kill the disease before it paralyzes its victims," the article opined. Conflating the gamma globulin trials with this announcement, the press reported that physicians would be testing "new polio theories on thousands of children" now that "it appears polio should be easily prevented by immunization."[260]

A polio discovery that "exploded" a mainstream theory delighted Kenny and her allies. Marvin Stevens, director of Kenny's Jersey City clinic, immediately told the press that Horstmann and Bodian's research was "scientific confirmation of Sister Kenny's deductions of many years ago." "We are on the verge of a great change in treatment," Stevens declared, that will end the "fanatical insistence in certain medical quarters" that polio was solely a disease of the central nervous system. Not only had Kenny's own clinical observations led her to conclude that polio is a systemic disease but KF-funded research-ers had "been reporting increasing evidence in the last four years that the polio virus is blood-borne."[261] The NFIP has "scoffed at the theory presented to the medical world by myself for the past 40 years that the primary invasion of the virus is not in the central nervous system," Kenny reiterated to reporters in Toowoomba. Now that this announce-ment had confirmed her theories, she expected to be returning to America "by invita-tion."[262] She wrote to the federal minister of health to draw his attention "to the complete somersault" made by the NFIP and other groups throughout the world as researchers at Yale and Hopkins had "exploded" the "old theory."[263]

In May, only a few weeks later, Kenny, accompanied by a companion, left for the United States although, she admitted to her friends, "the visit will be a tremendous physical effort on my part."[264] She joined the annual fundraising drive for the El Monte Kenny Hospital and took part in a parade. She also appeared as part of El Monte's TV campaign, which included an hour-long telethon hosted by character actor Eddie Albert as Kenny technicians explained how to become a Kenny therapist and demonstrated the Kenny treatment.[265]

In a new lecture on the "Cause and Prevention of Deformities in Poliomyelitis," which she also had printed as a 29-page pamphlet, Kenny used the announcement of Horstmann and Bodian's work to mock Roland Berg's 1948 claim that her treatment would have gained earlier and wider acceptance if she had not demanded that physicians accept her theories. Now, she said, "it has been acknowledged and published throughout the world that the orthodox theory has been exploded" and a contrasting theory of polio "which in all humility I can say I had the privilege of discovering forty-one years ago—does in truth exist."[266] This visit, she confided to Rosalind Russell a few weeks later, was "most profit-able in the interests of my work in the Country and abroad."[267]

Although sick and exhausted when she again returned home, Kenny was unable to keep away from the United States, where she could see the impact her work had made on clinical practice and American life. Polio epidemics were now a constant part of American life; indeed 1952 would be America's worst year since 1916.[268] At the end of June, only a few weeks later, Kenny appeared again looking, the *Los Angeles Times* remarked, "in bet-ter health."[269] This visit, like the previous ones, was filled with farewell dinners. She rested at her cottage in El Monte, and tried to monitor the hospital's standard of patient care. But while she was still quick to criticize, now she would often apologize, saying "I'm an old woman and I sometimes say things I don't mean." The physicians, nurses, and admin-istrators listened to her patiently and then continued their work.[270] She brought with her *Poliomyelitis A Systemic Disease*, a new lecture accompanied by a 15-page pamphlet, in which she reaffirmed the importance of Horstmann and Bodian's work in confirming her theory, and made a jibe at their refusal to believe that a KF-funded researcher had already made this discovery.[271] In an odd presentation of herself as a celebrity figure, she appeared on TV again, this time as the mystery guest on "What's My Line."[272]

In New York she met with Jungeblut and discussed plans for a European Poliomyelitis Research Laboratory, which Jungeblut believed would be supported by the new semi-official Western European polio organization headed by Leon Laruelle. Eager to be this laboratory's director, Jungeblut offered to leave his position at Columbia, but explained that he would need around $50,000 for an initial 3 years to cover salaries for himself and his assistants and for the purchase and maintenance of experimental animals.[273]

Kenny's wealthy women allies in New York assured her that $50,000 could be obtained for Jungeblut's "outstanding" work and listened sympathetically when Kenny repeated a story Jungeblut had told her about Horstmann and Bodian who had "ridiculed" his work at the Copenhagen conference and had "stooped to allow their photographs to appear in the papers as the scientists responsible for the viremia discovery."[274] Kenny hoped that this focus on polio's pathology would alter professional and public perceptions of her own contribution. But she was mistaken.

KENNY MODIFIED

With growing numbers of patients in this epidemic year both the *Medical Journal of Australia* and the *British Medical Journal* began discussing polio therapies, including Kenny's work. In an article on "Early Treatment of Poliomyelitis" a young Oxford orthopedist described efforts to ensure continuity of care for patients moving after 3 weeks in an infectious disease hospital to an orthopedic hospital. In a confusing mélange he warned against using muscle testing in the early stage but also against any "over-zealous application of hot packs," which would be mentally as well as physically exhausting for the patient and necessary only if there was "persistent muscular tenderness or pain" after the fever had subsided. Most children got great comfort from an ordinary hot bath, which "will usually overcome 'muscle spasm' and consequent deforming tendencies" by the time the patient left the infectious disease hospital.[275] Here were therapies to treat both pain and spasm, even if the latter still had textual quotation marks around it.

Even more enthusiastic about Kenny's methods were physicians at the Newcastle Hospital, around 95 miles north of Sydney. During Newcastle's polio epidemic of 1950–1951, as 2 of the hospital's physicians reported in the *Medical Journal of Australia*, patients at the hospital were treated without the use of any restraining splints; hot packs were given to as many patients as possible "especially those in whom the muscular spasm and pain were pronounced symptoms"; muscles were stretched although not "in a forcible manner"; and joints were put through their full range several times a day. After the acute stage, patients were given muscle reeducation without routine muscle testing. This treatment was coordinated by a trained physical therapist who "was receptive to the ideas prevailing in the clinic" and who taught this method to the hospital's nursing staff. Strikingly, the physicians agreed with Kenny that iron lungs were frequently unnecessary, even for bulbar patients. Their use of heat clearly relied on modes other than hot packs, and they suggested that during a polio epidemic "it would be of greater benefit to humanity to rush a water bath rather than a respirator."[276] In response, Melbourne orthopedist Jean Macnamara urged, as she had years earlier, that splinting be applied very early to ensure straight alignment. There was a school of thought, she noted, that questioned the utility of any splinting and she attributed this to Kenny's "teaching and influence." In her view Kenny had in fact used splints but pretended not to. Kenny's American staff was large enough to police the position of the patient and his limbs; in Australia "we have used more robot police staff called splints to attain the same objective."[277]

Away from the passion of the 1948 NFIP polio conference Oxford orthopedist Herbert Seddon had begun to offer a more mellow view of Kenny's contribution to polio care. In his *British Medical Journal* review of the 1951 edition of Kenny's autobiography he

described her theorizing as rash, but praised her attention to the harmfulness of immobilization—"so long a sacred tenet of the Liverpool school of orthopaedics"—as an important contribution to polio treatment.[278] Brisbane orthopedist John Lahz, a leader in
Australian physical medicine, was appalled to read Seddon's praise. In the *British Medical
Journal* Lahz protested that Kenny had not successfully challenged "the truth that a paralysed muscle is damaged by unopposed continuous gravitation pull." Lahz was convinced
that ignoring this "truth" could have "possibly caused many reversibly paralysed muscles
to go unsplinted and so have their weak fibres stretched and their paralyses prolonged."[279]
Orthopedist Lancelot Walton, in contrast, who had spent some months in the United
States observing Kenny's work, wrote to commend Seddon, but reminded him that
without a proper understanding of spasm many British physicians had left "hundreds
of patients" with unrelieved spasm and contributed to their "deformity."[280] Thus, British
and Australian physicians used Kenny's terms to disagree about polio care, especially the
pros and cons of splinting. They accepted parts of Kenny's work but managed to avoid
any acceptance of her conceptual understanding of the disease.

KENNY'S LAST MONTHS

In September 1952 Kenny returned to Australia. Once there she poured her energies
into completing a new autobiography, which she recognized would be her last book. In
My Battle and Victory (published a few years after her death) Kenny sought to defend
her awkward professional standing. She presented herself as an obscure contributor to
scientific progress who was nonetheless clinically skilled. Those "with mind and heart of
the true physician," she argued, do not "scorn...the offerings of the obscure" but seek "to
gather all proven truths and make the world of pain and crippling a little happier." She
also reflected on the possible conquest of polio, which some scientists said would occur
within this next decade and reduce polio "to the ashes of a memory."[281] The idea of a polio
vaccine had long fascinated Kenny, and in 1950 she had urged the KF Board "to obtain
a preventive vaccine" which would be "a crown of glory to the Kenny Foundation."[282] In
early 1952 she had been quick to notify MacFarlane Burnet when Yale virologist John
Paul was reported in the *Brisbane Courier Mail* commenting on the idea of a polio infection
"independent" of the central nervous system.[283] Now she proudly claimed that new vaccine research was based on the idea that "polio is a systemic disease attacking blood and
tissues," a statement that was reported by the *New York Times*.[284] But neither Jungeblut
nor her other scientific allies were working on such a topic and as NFIP-funded virologists moved closer to testing a vaccine Kenny's work seemed to have less and less to do
with science.

In Australia her flashes of temper and sharp tongue continued to abrade allies and
critics alike. After a sympathetic Labor Party physician urged the government to appoint
a "brilliant physiotherapist to investigate future claims by Sister Kenny" Kenny retorted
that the physical therapists at the Toowoomba General Hospital were brilliant and intelligent but nonetheless many symptoms and conditions were "unknown to them" and
"apparently unknown" to their medical supervisors.[285]

Kenny also failed to gain political support for institutionalizing her work in the
Australian hospital system. In 1951 the federal minister of health, Sir Earle Page, a

surgeon turned politician, had praised Kenny's "personal drive, magnetism and enthusiasm" in Parliament but noted that he had learned that her American clinics were closing because their patients were leaving to attend orthodox hospitals. In any case, he claimed, her methods of early movement had "now been adopted as policy throughout the whole medical profession."[286] Rebuffed by Page after her offer to meet him, Kenny began to rely on her local allies, particularly Pearl Baldock, who signed a series of letters sent to Page and the Prime Minister, which, officials noted, were "almost certainly written by Miss Kenny."[287] In early November 1952 Baldock finally received a formal response from the Prime Minister's office, stating that as the Director-General of Health had advised that as both systems of polio care were "in many particulars identical," the government "would not be justified in actively supporting the adoption of her curative treatment in preference to orthodox methods."[288]

Kenny continued to act as if she was a major player in global affairs and refused to see herself as the frail, monotonous, and defensive figure she had become. She urged KF officials to invite physicians from South Africa, India, and Egypt to the Institute, as therapists from these countries were studying at the Institute and "otherwise the training shall be lost and the opportunity of a further link of friendship also lost."[289] A group of polio survivors had founded a Kenny Association in England, and she was confident that this was a sign of further global expansion.[290] Feeling that the time was ripe for the KF to apply for WHO membership, she sent copies of her recent pamphlets to Anthony Payne, head of the WHO's Communicable Diseases Division, who thanked her and agreed diplomatically that there were "definite symptoms which lead one to suspect the presence of poliomyelitis, and that a wide dissemination of their nature is useful."[291]

In early November Kenny began to plan another visit to America "to straighten things out a bit" and make sure the WHO would help "get the book written."[292] She sensed a political turning point after the election of a Republican to the White House for the first time since 1928. She sent Dwight Eisenhower a congratulatory cable and was planning to have her personal representatives "make some approach to the new Government." It was time, she remarked to her friend James Henry, for "a policy change" in the NFIP as well.[293] Her Republican friends might well have organized some kind of formal recognition, but by the third week of November Kenny was too sick to travel.

Kenny declined precipitously. She had a stroke and fought what her doctor John Ogden described as "her last battle." Ogden and Betty Brennan, Kenny's secretary, issued regular bulletins, which were publicized across the United States in headlines such as "Sister Kenny Fights For Life" and "Sister Kenny's Condition Takes Turn for Worse."[294] There were a series of dramatic vignettes: Charles Carson, the American Vice-Consul, drove 85 miles from Brisbane to Toowoomba where Kenny managed her first smile in days for, according to Brennan, "hearing Carson's American accent was a real tonic for her." There was a telegram from Rosalind Russell saying "we hope our Waltzing Matilda will soon be up and at them again."[295] Then, with the flavor of a Hollywood drama, her physician contacted New York pathologist Irving Innerfield who had begun using trypsin, a pancreatic enzyme, as a blood-thinning drug, and a special parcel was rushed from New York across the Pacific. The plane was detoured from its normal Sydney landing to Brisbane's Eagle Farm airport, and the package was then sent by car under police escort for the 2-hour drive. The drug did not seem to make any difference but, Ogden told reporters, it had not had "a fair clinical trial" as Kenny's condition "had been too far advanced."[296] Kenny,

Ogden said, had "a very strong will to live" and "fought hard for her life. But it needs more than the will to live to beat this illness."[297]

On November 30, 1952 Elizabeth Kenny died, surrounded by a niece, 2 sisters, and Mary Kenny McCracken.[298] She was buried beside her mother at the Nobby Cemetery after a church service at Toowoomba's Neil Street Methodist Church. The church was full of people, many weeping openly. Charles Carson and his wife were there as were Kenny's Brisbane allies Abraham Fryberg, Aubrey Pye, Jarvis Nye, and Herbert Wilkinson. Even those who had disagreed with Kenny, the minister declared during the church service, which was broadcast by the Australian Broadcasting Commission, "nevertheless recognized the honesty and sincerity with which she pursued what was a God-given work." In what would become the first of many efforts to assess her significance, he declared that "the value of her work will become more apparent to future generations than it has been to men of our age."[299]

Her funeral was observed in celebrity fashion, which would have delighted her. Hundreds of people stood in silent groups along the funeral route as the 8-car funeral cortege traveled from the Toowoomba church to the cemetery. At the graveside her coffin was covered with the Union Jack (the British flag that traditionally covered the coffins of Australia's war dead) and the United States flag (the Australian Blue Ensign was not formally designated the national flag until 1953). There were wreaths of chrysanthemums, red roses, and other floral tributes around the coffin, including a wreath designed by Kenny's Toowoomba housekeeper in the shape of outstretched arms with a card that read "from your garden."[300] Pearl Baldock, who attended the funeral, sent a laurel wreath on behalf of the QCWA. Wreaths also came from the staff of the Jersey City clinic and from the Minneapolis Institute.[301] Members of the Returned Servicemen's League and the Australian Army laid poppies—the flower of remembrance that was used to raise money for veterans—at the graveside.[302] The *Brisbane Courier-Mail* had 3 photographs of the funeral: giant gum trees "as sentinels" above her grave surrounded by mourners, the British and American flags on her coffin, and children from Nobby State School in their summer uniforms standing in 2 lines as the hearse passed.[303] Her tombstone was inscribed with the false birth date she had popularized: 1886 instead of 1880.

Then the obituaries appeared. Some were short, like the one in *Newsweek*, which noted in only 8 lines that she had "fought many years to have the medical fraternity accept her method of treating polio" but that finally the Mayo Clinic and the University of Minnesota "gave her the support she needed."[304] Some were long. The *New York Times* began her obituary on its front page and continued for 2 more columns inside.[305] *JAMA* had 4 short lines but other medical journals allowed more space. The *Lancet* used two-thirds of a column, the *Medical Journal of Australia* used 2 columns, and the *British Medical Journal* devoted 2 pages.[306]

Most major Australian newspapers reported on her death. The *Sydney Morning Herald* retold her life and career, pointing out that, unlike America and Europe, Australia had never valued her properly.[307] Sir Arthur Fadden, the Acting Prime Minister, called her "a great Queenslander who had become a great Australian and a great international figure."[308] Health minister Earle Page, who had been a prominent opponent, awkwardly described his admiration for her "wonderful energy and enthusiasm" and her "extraordinary and dynamic character."[309] Abraham Fryberg, now Queensland's Director-General of Health, declared that during the past 16 years "though I have not always agreed with her views,

I have always respected her idealism and aims."[310] Less tactfully and with some bitterness, Pearl Baldock declared that "Australia has lost the greatest citizen that we have produced."[311]

In America Hollywood star Rosalind Russell said "I have lost a great friend and the world has lost a great, great benefactor," and she added dramatically that she "could not give up my Kenny work even if it means giving up my career."[312] In Minnesota obituaries and commemorations continued for some months. Whatever their differences, local papers reminded readers, American physicians recognized Kenny's contribution and there was universal acceptance today of the Kenny method or some modification of it. "The former Australian bush nurse was one of the great women of this century," according to the *Minneapolis Star*, and the *Minneapolis Tribune* praised her contributions to American medicine as "a revolutionary treatment" and "a new explanation of the way polio acts."[313]

Concrete forms of memorializing Kenny began that December. The Minneapolis Board of Education named a new million dollar elementary school after Kenny.[314] After a memorial service at El Monte attended by nurses, officials, employees, and around a hundred other supporters, the community began renovating her cottage, which opened in 1953 as the Sister Kenny Memorial Annex, expanding the number of inpatient beds.[315] Mary Kenny McCracken began planning a trip to California and Minnesota to present Kenny's medals and try to heal any institutional divisions.[316] But Kenny's legacy would prove much more fragile than any of her allies had anticipated.

NOTES

1. Paul *A History*, 373–381; Kenny "This Report Was Presented to The Honorable The Premier of the State of Queensland E. M. Hanlon, M.L.A. and to Doctors Pye, Nye, Lee, Arden, Wilkinson, and Fryberg of the City of Brisbane, Queensland, Australia Concerning the Disease Poliomyelitis [1950]," Kenny Collection, Box 1, Fryer Library, 3. See also John F. Enders, Thomas H. Weller, and Frederick C. Robbins "Cultivation of the Lansing Strain of Poliomyelitis Virus in Cultures of Various Human Embryonic Tissues" *Science* (January 28 1949) 109: 85–87.

2. On polio epidemics in Japan 1938–1942, Malta 1942–1943, El Salvador 1943, South Africa 1944–1945, Mauritius 1945, London 1947, and Berlin 1947 see Albert B. Sabin "Epidemiologic Patterns of Poliomyelitis in Different Parts of the World" in *Poliomyelitis: Papers and Discussions Presented at the First International Poliomyelitis Conference* (Philadelphia: J.B. Lippincott, 1949), 4–13.

3. Kenny to Mr. President, Mrs. Webber and Gentlemen, May 24 1948, Board of Directors, MHS-K.

4. Kenny "Report of My Activities In Switzerland" [1950], European Trip 1950, MHS-K; Kenny "Report of My Activities" [1950], Minnesota-Hospitals 1944–1961, Judd Papers, MHS.

5. C. J. McSweeney "A Visit to Poliomyelitis Centers in U.S.A." *Irish Journal of Medical Science* (February 1951) 302: 63–73. The hospital was known as the Cork Street Fever Hospital or the House of Recovery and Fever Hospital.

6. W. J. Treanor and F. H. Krusen "Poliomyelitis: Modern Treatment and Rehabilitation" *Irish Journal of Medical Science* (June 1950) 294: 257–269, 257. This paper was presented to the Medical Society of University College Dublin in May 1950. Kenny had heard that Krusen had told the audience that her contribution was "little or nothing"; Kenny "Report

of My Activities" [1950]; Kenny "Report of My Activities In Ireland" [1950], European Trip 1950, MHS-K.

7. Kenny "Report of My Activities" [1950]; Kenny "Report of My Activities In Ireland" [1950].

8. McSweeney "A Visit to Poliomyelitis Centers in U.S.A.," 70–72.

9. McSweeney "A Visit to Poliomyelitis Centers in U.S.A.," 65–71.

10. Walton Van Winkle, Jr. "Methods of Clinical Study and Evaluation of Therapeutic Agents in Poliomyelitis" *JAMA* (June 11 1949) 140: 534–539 see also [Board of Trustees] "Report of the Council on Pharmacy and Chemistry: Therapeutic Trials Committee" *JAMA* (November 5 1949) 141: 674.

11. "Pain and Spasm in Poliomyelitis: A Symposium" *American Journal of Physical Medicine* (August 1952) 31: 321–327; Edward B. Shaw and Hulda E. Thelander "Clinical Concept of Poliomyelitis" *Pediatrics* (1949) 4: 277–285.

12. Shaw and Thelander "Clinical Concept of Poliomyelitis," 277–285; see also Paul H. Sandifer "Neuropsychiatry: Anterior Poliomyelitis" in Francis Bach ed. *Recent Advances in Physical Medicine* (London: J. & A. Churchill, 1950), 218–221.

13. Sir James Spence "Poliomyelitis" in Sir Leonard Parsons ed. *Modern Trends in Pediatrics* (London: Butterworth and Co., 1951), 316.

14. "Pain and Spasm in Poliomyelitis," 316–345.

15. William P. Frank, Sam S. Woolington, and G. E. Rader "Diagnosis and Differential Diagnosis of Poliomyelitis: The Management of Patients in the Hospital Admitting Room" *California Medicine* (July 1950) 73: 30–32.

16. Shaw and Thelander "Clinical Concept of Poliomyelitis," 277–285.

17. Marjorie Lawrence *Interrupted Melody: An Autobiography* (New York: Appleton-Century Crofts, 1949), 194.

18. Sandifer "Neuropsychiatry," 221.

19. Shaw and Thelander "Clinical Concept of Poliomyelitis," 277–285.

20. Victor Cohn "Sister Kenny…Back in the Battle Again" *Minneapolis Sunday Tribune* March 26 1950.

21. Citing an unnamed 1951 survey, Kenny "Evidence Presented To The Honourable[sic] The Minister For Health, Sydney, New South Wales, Aust." [1952], Wilson Collection.

22. McSweeney "A Visit to Poliomyelitis Centers in U.S.A," 67.

23. "Fusion Fete Upset By Morris' Attack" *New York Times* October 5 1950; Kenny "Concerning the Extension of My Work in the State of California" [1949], Board of Directors, MHS-K.

24. "Sister Kenny Coming to U.S." *New York Times* April 6 1949; H. J. London to H. Van Riper Memorandum Re: Attached Clipping, April 6 1949, Public Relations, MOD-K.

25. Doug Tucker "Chuter, Charles Edward (1880 - 1948)" *Australian Dictionary of Biography*, Volume 13 (Melbourne: Melbourne University Press, 1993), 427–428.

26. Kenny "This Report Was Presented," 3–4; "Sister Kenny Won World Fame By Polio Treatment" *Sydney Morning Herald* December 1 1952; [Aubrey Pye] to Dear Cecil [Cecil I. N. Walters, Prince Henry Hospital, Sydney], October 16 [1951], Kenny Collection, Fryer Library; Chuter to Mr. Schneider [RKO Pictures, Brisbane] Memorandum: Re: Script of Picture "Sister Kenny" October 23 1945, OM 65-17, Box 3, Folder 12, Chuter Papers, Oxley-SLQ.

27. "Sister Kenny Yields Reins of Foundation" *New York Times* April 21 1949; "Doctor Heads Fund in Place of Sister Kenny" *New York Herald Tribune* April 21 1949; "Sister Kenny Will Continue Aid" *Los Angeles Examiner* April 21 1949; "Sister Kenny Denies Talk" *New York Times* May 4 1949; Marvin Kline to Dear Doctor Laruelle, April 22 1949, Dr. Leon Laruelle, 1945–1951, MHS-K.

28. Kenny to Dear Bessie, May 17 1949, Kenny Collection, Box 1, Fryer Library; see also Alexander *Maverick*, 178 who notes that Kenny had pneumonia during this Australian visit. For a similar letter and tone see Kenny to Dear Rosalind, May 25 1949, Rosalind Russell (Brisson), 1947–1952, MHS-K.

29. Note that she had commented on her "troublesome" arm and right hand to Mary and Stuart McCracken; see Kenny to My Dear Mary and Stuart, September 24 1946, Mary Stewart Kenny, 1942–1947, MHS-K; Kenny to Dear Mary and Stuart [December 1947], Kenny Collection, Fryer Library.

30. "Sister Kenny Will Continue Aid."

31. [Pye] to Dear Sister Kenny, June 6 1949, Kenny Collection, Fryer Library.

32. "Sister Kenny Ends Task" *Minneapolis Morning Tribune* April 21 1949; "Sister Kenny Quits U.S. Work" *Minneapolis Morning Tribune* April 21 1949; Victor Cohn "Sister Kenny Wins New Medical Praise" *Minneapolis Morning Tribune* October 4 1949; "Dr. E. J. Huenkens, Pediatrician, Dies" [unnamed newspaper] July 23 1970, Box 19, Folder 3, Myers Papers, UMN-ASC. Huenkens had his M.D. from the St. Louis University Medical School and had interned at the Minneapolis General Hospital; he taught at the University of Minnesota Medical School 1948–1953. Note that Huenkens became medical director of the Institute in 1948 after Pohl resigned; Alexander *Maverick*, 177.

33. "Sister Kenny Will Continue Aid"; E. J. Huenkens to My Dear Doctor Landauer, September 10 1949, Public Relations, MOD-K; "Doctor Heads Fund in Place of Sister Kenny."

34. E. J. Huenkens to Dear Doctor, September 1 1949, Public Relations, MOD-K.

35. Van Riper to Mr. Savage Memorandum Re: Visit from Dr. E. J. Huenkens, Kenny Foundation and Institute, January 7 1949, Public Relations, MOD-K.

36. E. J. Huenkens to My Dear Doctor Landauer, September 10 1949.

37. "Sister Kenny Foundation Offers Scholarships" *Washington Post* July 19 1949; "Kenny Scholarships Go to Four Illinois Nurses" *Chicago Daily Tribune* June 25 1949.

38. Edgar J. Huenkens "Diagnosis and Treatment of Infantile Paralysis" *Postgraduate Medicine* (February 1950) 7: 100–105.

39. [Cohn interview with] Amy Lindsey, May 19 1955, Cohn Papers, MHS-K. See also Jean Barclay *In Good Hands: The History of the Chartered Society of Physiotherapy, 1894–1994* (Oxford: Butterworth-Heinemann, 1994), 144; Sandifer "Neuropsychiatry," 219.

40. Basil O'Connor "The Fight Against Poliomyelitis: Everybody's Business" *Archives of Physical Medicine* (October 1952) 33: 594; Hart E. Van Riper "The Program of the National Foundation of Infantile Paralysis" *American Journal of Physical Medicine* (August 1952) 31: 311; Daniel Wilson "Psychological Trauma and Its Treatment in the Polio Epidemics" *Bulletin of the History of Medicine* (2008) 82: 848–877. See also Kenneth S. Landauer "The National Aspects In Providing Complete Medical Care in Poliomyelitis" [1950] [enclosed in] Landauer to Dear Dr. McCulloch, September 25 1950, Public Relations, American Academy of Pediatrics, MOD.

41. O'Connor "The Fight Against Poliomyelitis," 594; Howard A. Rusk and Eugene J. Taylor *New Hope for the Handicapped: The Rehabilitation of the Disabled from Bed to Job* (New York: Harper & Brothers, 1946, 1949), 163; Van Riper "The Program of the National Foundation," 311; Landauer "The National Aspects In Providing Complete Medical Care" [1950].

42. Hart Van Riper, letter to editor, *JAMA* (December 24 1949) 141: 1260.

43. Landauer "The National Aspects In Providing Complete Medical Care" [1950]. On the argument that the NFIP should not continue to support "prolonged and unnecessary hospitalization and physical therapy" see J. Albert Key in Question Period after "The Medical-Care Program of the National Foundation for Infantile Paralysis, Inc." *Journal of Bone and Joint Surgery* (January 1951) 33: 201.

44. "A.M.A. Board Orders Gagging of Dr. Fishbein" *Chicago Daily Tribune* June 7 1949; "Lightning Rod" *Time* (June 20 1949) 53: 50, 53; Frank D. Campion *The AMA and U.S. Health Policy since 1940* (Chicago: Chicago Review Press, 1984), 131–137.

45. "A.M.A. Board Orders Gagging of Dr. Fishbein"; for his version see Fishbein *Autobiography*, 298–313. On Fishbein's ouster see Milton Mayer "The Rise and Fall of Doctor Fishbein" *New York Times* June 8 1949; Patricia Spain Ward "*United States versus American Medical Association et al.:* The Medical Anti-Trust Case of 1938–1943" *American Studies* (1989) 30: 123–153; Campion *The AMA since 1940*, 113–125; Jonathan Engel *Doctors and Reformers: Discussion and Debate over Health Policy 1925–1950* (Charleston: University of South Carolina Press, 2002), 293–294.

46. "Morris Fishbein Quitting A.M.A. Journal Post" *Chicago Daily Tribune* November 24 1949; "Fishbein Tells Plans to Teach at U. of Illinois" *Chicago Daily Tribune* December 2 1949; "A.M.A. Journal Editor Is a Man of Many Words" *Chicago Daily Tribune* January 8 1950. See also John Burnham "American Medicine's Golden Age: What Happened to It?" *Science* (1982) 215: 1474–1479; Allan M. Brandt and Martha Gardner "The Golden Age of Medicine?" in Roger Cooter and John Pickstone eds, *Medicine in the Twentieth Century* (Amsterdam: Harwood Academic Publishers, 2000), 21–37

47. "Warren's Daughter Stricken by Polio" *Los Angeles Times* November 8 1950. It is not clear whether Nina received any Kenny treatment, but she did not join a KF campaign; by January 1952 she was featured as queen of a March of Dimes float in the Rose Parade; "Parade Launches U.S. Dimes Drive" *Los Angeles Times* January 1 1952.

48. Kenny "Concerning the Extension of My Work in the State of California" [1949]; [Cohn interview with] Robert Bingham May 19 1955, Cohn Papers, MHS-K.

49. Kenny "Concerning the Extension of My Work in the State of California" [1949]; "Doctor Claims Cure for Some Tissue Disease" *Washington Post* September 16 1949; Harvey E. Billig to Dear Sister Kenny, September 23 1949, Minnesota-Hospitals, 1944–1961, Sister Kenny Institute, Judd Papers, MHS; "Ex-Polio Patients Get Treatments" *Los Angeles Times* December 5 1949.

50. [Transcript] Telephone Conversation Between Dr. Van Riper and Dr. Huenkens From Los Angeles, California, April 12 1949, Public Relations, MOD-K; Kenny "Concerning the Extension of My Work in the State of California" [1949]; Huenkens to Dear Doctor Huddleston, April 22 1949, Public Relations, MOD-K; L. Dee Belveal [Southern California State Office NFIP] to Dr. Hart Van Riper Memorandum Re: Kenny Foundation Conflict, April 11 1949, Public Relations, MOD-K.

51. Kenny "Concerning the Extension of My Work in the State of California" [1949].

52. George D. Roberts "Activities of the Northern California Chapter," November 4 1949, San Francisco-Misc., MHS-K; "Kenny Polio Fund Diversion Charged" *Los Angeles Times* April 11 1950; "Bing Crosby Testifies In Mail Fraud Case" *Washington Post* April 11 1952; "Von Morpurgo Accused of Getting Money" *San Francisco News* April 10 1950; "$10,000 Bail Set in Sister Kenny Charge" *Los Angeles Mirror* August 31 1951; John J. Barnwell to Dear Sister Kenny, November 16 1949, John J. Barnwell, 1947–1950, MHS-K; "U.S. Accuses Publicist of Duping Sister Kenny" *Los Angeles Times* August 30 1951; "Convicted In Polio Fraud" *New York Times* April 27 1952; see also Cohn *Sister Kenny*, 239–240.

53. Kenny to Dear Mr. Barnwell, November 18 1949, John J. Barnwell, 1947–1950, MHS-K; Kenny to Dear Mr. Barnwell, January 16 1950, John J. Barnwell, 1947–1950, MHS-K; Kenny to Dear Mr. Kline, October 4 1951, Marvin L. Kline, 1942–1959, MHS-K; Kenny "Concerning the Extension of My Work in the State of California" [1949].

54. "Film Charity Group Gives $10,000 to Kenny Fund" *Los Angeles Times* March 14 1949; Kenny "Concerning the Extension of My Work in the State of California" [1949]; Kenny to Dear Mr. Henry, November 22 1949, James Henry, 1943–1951, MHS-K.

55. Thomas Angland, a physician in Yakima, Washington, had studied her work at the Institute during the war and then proposed a fundraising drive to expand his own small clinic into a Kenny center. The KF Board refused to help him and although Angland remained a proponent of the work, the opportunity to expand the KF organization in the Northwest faded; Kenny "Concerning the Extension of My Work in the State of California" [1949]; Thomas A. Angland to Dear Miss Kenny, September 21 1949, Minnesota-Hospitals, 1944–1961, Sister Kenny Institute, Judd Papers, MHS; see also "Statement by Dr. Thomas A. Angland, M.D. F.A.C.S., of Yakima, Washington, June 30, 1948," Washington 1942–1948, MHS-K.

56. Roland Berg to Dear Frank [Carey], April 26 1951, Public Relations, MOD-K; Van Riper to Dear Mr. [Charles B.] Sweatt, January 25 1949, Public Relations, MOD-K.

57. Kenny "This Report Was Presented," 7.

58. Kenny to Dear Miss Bridle, May 25 1949, Wilson Collection.

59. Kenny to Dear Mr. Dayton, January 31 1950, Donald C. Dayton, 1944–1951, MHS-K; Kenny "Report to the Board of the Directors of the Sister Elizabeth Kenny Foundation," September 1 1950, Board of Directors, MHS-K.

60. Cohn "Sister Kenny...Back in the Battle Again."

61. Kenny in "[Report] Poliomyelitis, Kenny Institute at Jersey City Medical Center, Jersey City, New Jersey, June 29 1949," Jersey City Medical Center, 1944–1950, MHS-K.

62. Kenny "Concerning the Extension of My Work in the State of California" [1949].

63. Kenny to Mr. President, Mrs. Webber and Gentlemen, February 24 1948; Kenny "Concerning the Extension of My Work in the State of California" [1949].

64. Jungeblut in "[Report] Poliomyelitis, Kenny Institute at Jersey City Medical Center, Jersey City, New Jersey, June 29 1949." By 1949 he was receiving $10,000 a year; [transcript], "Conversation Between Sister Kenny and Mr. Marvin Kline, November 29 1950," Marvin L. Kline, 1942–1959, MHS-K. For his growing prominence as a KF-funded researcher see Albert V. Szent-Gyorgyi to Dear Claus, December 4 1950, Box 2, St-Sz, Jungeblut Papers, NLM.

65. Jungeblut in "[Report] Poliomyelitis, Kenny Institute at Jersey City Medical Center, Jersey City, New Jersey, June 29 1949." For an example of research backing up Jungeblut's claim that the polio virus [or at least Jungeblut's SK virus] might affect muscle fibers see Robert Rustigan and Alwin M. Pappenheimer "Myositis in Mice Following Intramuscular Injection of Viruses of the Mouse Encephalitis Group and of Certain Other Neurotropic Viruses" *Journal of Experimental Medicine* (1949) 89: 69–92. Note that this paper was cited by Enders et al. in their 1949 *Science* article.

66. Jungeblut in "[Report] Poliomyelitis, Kenny Institute at Jersey City Medical Center, Jersey City, New Jersey, June 29 1949." He also suggested that researchers had used a misleading and incorrect strain of virus, which was cultured in the brains of experimental monkeys and then passed from laboratory to laboratory over the previous 3 decades.

67. Paul *A History*, 378–379. See also John Paul's comment that "I was stupidly unaware of the implications that this finding held. At least it did not appear to me as an electrifying piece of news...it hardly seemed to me a trick which could be put to any special or practical diagnostic use. How utterly mistaken was my preliminary judgment of this discovery!" in Paul *A History*, 373–374. For an example of the older concept see Roland H. Berg *Polio and Its Problems* (Philadelphia: J.B. Lippincott, 1948), 57.

68. Huenkens in "[Report] Poliomyelitis, Kenny Institute at Jersey City Medical Center, Jersey City, New Jersey, June 29 1949."

69. Kenny in "[Report] Poliomyelitis, Kenny Institute at Jersey City Medical Center, Jersey City, New Jersey, June 29 1949."

70. Jungeblut in "[Report] Poliomyelitis, Kenny Institute at Jersey City Medical Center, Jersey City, New Jersey, June 29 1949."

71. Kenny in "[Report] Poliomyelitis, Kenny Institute at Jersey City Medical Center, Jersey City, New Jersey, June 29 1949."

72. Kenny to the President And Members of the Board of Directors, December 15 1950, Board of Directors, MHS-K.

73. Kenny to Dear Mr. Henry, November 22 1949.

74. Kenny To The President And Members of the Board of Directors of the Elizabeth Kenny Institute, September 21 1950, Board of Directors, MHS-K.

75. [Program] "Medical Seminar on Infantile Paralysis Sponsored by Sister Elizabeth Kenny Foundation, October 3, 4, 5, 1949, Minneapolis, Minnesota," Kenny Collection, Fryer Library.

76. Kenny to Dear Mr. Haverstock, April 6 1951, Henry W. Haverstock, MHS-K.

77. [Cohn interview with] Pete Gazzola, August 25 1953, Cohn Papers, MHS-K.

78. Robert Bingham to Dear Sister Kenny, October 4 1949, Minnesota-Hospitals, 1944–1961, Sister Kenny Institute, Judd Papers, MHS; A. E. Deacon to Dear Sister Kenny, September 28 1949, Minnesota-Hospitals, 1944–1961, Sister Kenny Institute, Judd Papers, MHS.

79. Ethel Calhoun "A Report On The Use of The Sister Kenny Concept and Method of Treatment for Poliomyelitis Patients at Oakland County Contagious Hospital, 1944–1949" [1949], Minnesota-Hospitals, 1944–1961, Sister Kenny Institute, Judd Papers, MHS.

80. Kenny "This Report Was Presented," 7.

81. Francis MacFarlane Burnet *Changing Patterns: An Atypical Autobiography* (Melbourne: William Heinemann, 1968), 166–168; see also Paul *A History*, 225–229. He had published an influential paper co-written with Jean Macnamara in 1931 proposing that the strain of polio virus developed from patients in a local epidemic had properties distinctive from the Rockefeller Institute's MV strain.

82. C. W. Jungeblut to My Dear Miss Kenny, December 21 1949, Minnesota Hospitals, 1944–1961, Sister Kenny Institute, Judd Papers, MHS.

83. Walton [quoted in] Kenny "This Report Was Presented," 10; see also Lancelot H. F. Walton to Dear Sister Kenny, July 14 1950, Minnesota-Hospitals, 1944–1961, Judd Papers, MHS.

84. E. J. Huenkens To Whom It May Concern, June 30 1949, Dr. E. J. Huenkens, 1947–1949, MHS-K.

85. Mrs. Krishna Nehru Hutheesing to My Dear Sister Kenny, January 10 1950, India-Misc., 1943, 1949–1952, MHS-K.

86. Between 1945 and 1950 Kenny traveled to England, Ireland, Belgium, France, the Netherlands, Italy, the Soviet Union, Czechoslovakia, Switzerland, Spain, Denmark, Germany, Norway, Sweden, Greece, Australia, and New Zealand.

87. Kenny to Dear Sister, September 19 1949, Personal Correspondence and Related Papers, 1942–1951, MHS-K.

88. "Sister Kenny Here, Offers Polio Aid" *New York Times* August 20 1949; Kenny "Report Of My Activities In Rome, Italy" [1950], European Trip 1950, MHS-K; Kenny "Report of My Activities" [1950].

89. C. Rodopoulos to Madam [Kenny], July 27 1949, Home Secretary's Office, Special Batches, Kenny Clinics, 1941–1949, A/31753, QSA.

90. Dr. Sanchis-Olmos [statement], Minnesota-Hospitals, 1944–1961, Sister Kenny Institute, Judd Papers, MHS; see also J. Sanz Ibanez, Vincente Sanchis-Olmos, and A. Azpeitia to [Hubert Humphrey], July 14 1947, European Trip, 1947, MHS-K; Kenny to Dear Mr. [Rex] Williams, July 28 1950, General Correspondence-W, MHS-K.

91. Kenny "Report Of My Activities in England" [1950], European Trip, 1950, MHS-K; Kenny "Resume of Report Presented to Congressman Judd of Minnesota in Washington D.C. July 19 1950 for Transmission to the Honorable E. M. Hanlon, M.L.A., Premier of the State of Queensland, Australia," Minnesota-Hospitals, 1944–1961, Sister Kenny Institute, Judd Papers, MHS.

92. [Cohn interview with staff of Queen Mary's Hospital for Children, Carshalton] Richard Metcalfe, August 29 1955, Cohn Papers, MHS-K; [Cohn interview with] Amy Lindsey, May 19 1955.

93. "Medical Societies: Society of Medical Officers of Health; Poliomyelitis" Lancet (June 17 1950) 1: 1113–1115; R. H. Metcalfe in "Medical Societies: Society of Medical Officers of Health; Poliomyelitis" Lancet (June 17 1950) 1: 1114.

94. C. D. S. Agassiz in "Medical Societies: Society of Medical Officers of Health; Poliomyelitis" Lancet (June 17 1950) 1: 1114.

95. M. Mitman in "Medical Societies: Society of Medical Officers of Health; Poliomyelitis" Lancet (June 17 1950) 1: 1115.

96. Baron de Waha-Baillonville to Dear Sister Kenny, January 2 1946, Belgium, MHS-K; Laruelle to Dear Mr. President [of KF Board of Directors], August 10 1949, Home Secretary's Office, Special Batches, Kenny Clinics, 1941–1949, A/31753, QSA; Kenny to President and Members of the Board of Directors [Institute], September 10 1945, Public Relations, MOD-K; Kenny to Dear Doctor Bauwens, August 31 1945, Dr. Philip[pe] Bauwens, 1945–1947, MHS-K. On Laruelle's commitment to polio research and his founding of the Belgium League Against Poliomyelitis after the 1928 Belgium epidemic, see R. Ch. Behrend "Gedenwort fuer Leon Laruelle" Deutsche Zeitschrift fuer Nervenheilkunder (1962) 183: 305–306.

97. L. Laruelle "The Brussels Poliomyelitis Center: Report of the Activity of the Kenny Section" [enclosed in] Laruelle to Dear Mr. President [of KF Board of Directors], August 10 1949, Home Secretary's Office, Special Batches, Kenny Clinics, 1941–1949, A/31753, QSA.

98. Nora Housden and Dorothy Curtis to Dear Sister Kenny, [November 1948], Belgium— Nora Housden, 1948–1950, MHS-KL. Laruelle "The Brussels Poliomyelitis Center," August 10 1949; Housden to Dear Sister Kenny, December 14 1949, Belgium—Nora Housden, 1948–1950, MHS-K.

99. Curtis to Dear Miss Rizzotto [Mary Rizzotto, World Children's Foundation, Pasadena], March 4 1952, James Henry, 1943–1951, MHS-K.

100. Curtis to Dear Sister Kenny, May 2 1950, Dorothy Curtis, MHS-K. Most were private patients but as the institute was also funded by the Belgian National League against Poliomyelitis it may have accepted some public patients as well; Curtis to Dear Miss Rizzotto, March 4 1952.

101. Housden and Curtis to Dear Sister Kenny, [November 1948]; Curtis to Dear Sister Kenny, January 21 1949, Dorothy Curtis, MHS-K.

102. Housden to Dear Sister Kenny, December 14 1949.

103. Housden and Curtis to Dear Sister Kenny, [November 1948]; Laruelle "The Brussels Poliomyelitis Center," August 10 1949.

104. Curtis to Dear Miss Rizzotto, March 4 1952.

105. "Sister Kenny Says Photos Prove She's Right on Polio" *New York Journal-American* July 14 1950.

106. Laruelle "The Brussels Poliomyelitis Center," August 10 1949.

107. Curtis to Dear Sister Kenny, May 2 1950.

108. Curtis to Dear Miss Rizzotto, March 4 1952.

109. Laruelle "The Brussels Poliomyelitis Center," August 10 1949.

110. Housden to Dear Sister Kenny, September 28 1950, Belgium—Nora Housden, 1948–1950, MHS-K.

111. Curtis to Dear Miss Rizzotto, March 4 1952; Curtis to Dear Sister Kenny, November 27 1949, Czechoslovakia-Misc., 1949–1951, MHS-K. On the nationalization of all Czech spas in 1948 see Zdenek Stich *Czechoslovak Health Services* (Prague: Ministry of Health, Czechoslovak Socialist Republic, 1962), 62.

112. Hejlova [Prague Vice-Minister of Health] to Dear Sister Kenny, August 7 1949, Cohn Papers, MHS-K.

113. Walter Johnson "Therapist Returns From Iron Curtain" *Minneapolis Star* July 22 1953; Dorothy E. Curtis "Nurse, There's Typhus in Camp" *American Journal of Nursing* (September 1945) 45: 714; Dorothy E. Curtis "The Way It Was" *American Journal of Nursing* (October 1984) 84: 1254. She was supposedly the daughter of American missionaries.

114. Johnson "Therapist Returns From Iron Curtain"; Curtis to Dear Sister Kenny, July 15 1948, Dorothy Curtis, MHS-K.

115. Curtis to Dear Sister Kenny, August 27 1949, Belgium, MHS-K; Curtis to Dear Sister Kenny, April 14 1949, Belgium, MHS-K.

116. Curtis to Dear Sister Kenny, November 27 1949; Curtis to Dear Sister Kenny, August 27 1949; Curtis to Dear Sister Kenny, May 2 1950. See also Curtis "Sister Kenny's Visit to Czechoslovakia June 6–12, 1950," Czechoslovakia, Misc., 1949–1951, MHS-K.

117. D. Slonim, E. Svandova, P. Strnad, and C. Benes "A History of Poliomyelitis in the Czech Republic: Part II" *Central European Journal of Public Health* (1993) 2: 88–90.

118. Curtis to Dear Miss Rizzotto, March 4 1952; Johnson "Therapist Returns From Iron Curtain"; Hroch et al. to Dear Sister Kenny, March 4 1950, Kenny Collection, Fryer Library.

119. Curtis to Dear Sister Kenny, October 22 1949, Czechoslovakia-Misc., 1949–1951, MHS-K; see also "An Official Report of Sister Elizabeth Kenny's Activities in Czechoslovakia," Minnesota-Hospitals, 1944–1961, Sister Kenny Institute, Judd Papers, MHS; Curtis to Dear Sister Kenny, November 27 1949.

120. Curtis to Dear Sister Kenny, March 11 1949, Czechoslovakia-Misc., 1949–1951, MHS-K.

121. Curtis to Dear Sister Kenny, May 2 1950.

122. Curtis to Dear Sister Kenny, October 22 1949; Curtis to Dear Sister Kenny, March 11 1949; Curtis to Dear Sister Kenny, November 27 1949.

123. Curtis to Dear Sister Kenny, November 27 1949.

124. Curtis to Dear Sister Kenny, October 22 1949.

125. Curtis to Dear Sister Kenny, March 11 1949.

126. Curtis to Dear Sister Kenny, November 27 1949.

127. "An Official Report of Sister Elizabeth Kenny's Activities in Czechoslovakia"; see also M. Vetterova-Pastrnkova and Vera Flrcuskova [student representative] to Dear Sister Kenny, February 15 1950, Minnesota-Hospitals, 1944–1961, Judd Papers, MHS; and [graduation class] to Dear Sister Kenny, March 4 1950, Minnesota-Hospitals, 1944–1961, Judd Papers, MHS.

128. Curtis "Sister Kenny's Visit to Czechoslovakia June 6–12, 1950"; see also "An Official Report of Sister Elizabeth Kenny's Activities in Czechoslovakia."

129. Curtis "Sister Kenny's Visit to Czechoslovakia June 6–12, 1950"; compared to "An Official Report of Sister Elizabeth Kenny's Activities in Czechoslovakia."

130. Curtis to Dear Sister Kenny, November 27 1949; Curtis to Dear Sister Kenny, March 11 1949.

131. Curtis to Dear Sister Kenny, November 27 1949. While the impact of these efforts is difficult to assess, we do know that Alois Wokoun, a patient treated at Janské Lázně in the 1940s, became a wheelchair-bound Kenny therapist; see *SVETOBEZNIKEM SE SADISTKOU (Globetrotter with Sadist Polio)*; some of his experiences were published in the *Toomey j Gazette*; see Post Polio Health International "People We Know" post-polio.org/net/peo1.htm1, accessed 1/17/2013.

132. Curtis to Dear Sister Kenny, November 27 1949.

133. Curtis to Dear Miss Rizzotto, March 4 1952; Housden to Dear Sister Kenny, December 14 1949; Housden to Dear Sister Kenny, February 20 1950, Belgium—Nora Housden, 1948–1950, MHS-K. Helen Sare, a Kenny technician from England, had begun working with Nora Housden, but patient care and staff morale were disrupted when Housden developed ovarian cancer and died in late 1950; Naomi Rogers "'Silence Has Its Own Stories': Elizabeth Kenny, Polio and the Culture of Medicine" *Social History of Medicine* (2008) 21: 145–161. The KF had spent around $12,000 on funding Kenny work in Brussels, including Laruelle's research; Kenny to Dear Mr. [Rex] Williams, July 28 1950, General Correspondence-W, MHS-K.

134. Helen Sare to Dear Mrs. Rowe, May 25 1952, Belgium, MHS-K.

135. Curtis to Dear Miss Rizzotto, March 4 1952.

136. Curtis to Dear Dr. Bingham, April 17 1952, James Henry, 1943–1951, MHS-K; Johnson "Therapist Returns From Iron Curtain"; Curtis to Dear Miss Rizzotto, March 4 1952.

137. Kenny to Dear Mr. [Ralph] McBane, July 27 1950, General Correspondence–M, MHS-K; C. S. Wright [president, Munich German American Men's Club] Official Statement and Report on the Occasion of the Visit of Sister Elizabeth Kenny to Munich in Support of the 'Pfennig-Parade,' May 19–25, 1950, Minnesota-Hospitals, 1944–1961, Judd Papers, MHS.

138. Curtis to Dear Dr. Bingham, April 17 1952; Curtis to Dear Miss Rizzotto, March 4 1952. See also Max Stauffenegger "Poliomyelitis-Forschungen in USA, 1942–1946" *European Journal of Pediatrics* (January 1948) 65: 454–539 which noted Kenny's good results but warned that German pediatricians must keep their eyes open before accepting a new polio therapy that so clearly contradicted polio's pathology.

139. Curtis to Dear Miss Rizzotto, March 4 1952; Curtis to Dear Mr. Kline, April 17 1952, Marvin L. Kline, 1942–1959, MHS-K.

140. Curtis to Dear Miss Rizzotto, March 4 1952; Curtis to Dear Dr. Bingham, April 17 1952.

141. Curtis to Dear Miss Rizzotto, March 4 1952; Curtis to Dear Mr. Kline, April 17 1952.

142. Johnson "Therapist Returns From Iron Curtain."

143. Curtis to Dear Mr. Henry, April 17 1952, James Henry, 1943–1951, MHS-K; Curtis to Dear Miss Rizzotto, March 4 1952.

144. Kenny "Concerning the Extension of My Work in the State of California" [1949]; Kenny to Dear Mr. Haverstock, December 30 1950.

145. Kenny "Concerning the Extension of My Work in the State of California" [1949]; Kenny to Dear Mr. Henry, November 22 1949.

146. Kenny "Concerning the Extension of My Work in the State of California" [1949].

147. "Drive to Aid Sister Kenny" *Pittsburgh Courier* November 30 1946.

148. "Kenny Nurse Supports NY Polio Drive" *New York Amsterdam News* December 6 1947; see also "Kenny Technician" *Chicago Defender* July 10 1948; "The Defender News Reel" *Chicago Defender* March 20 1948.

149. "Polio Tenor Aids Victims Of All Races" *Atlanta Daily World* February 18 1948; "Pruth McFarlin..." *Chicago Defender* November 20 1948.

150. "Café Society Festivity" *New York Amsterdam News* August 6 1949; Allan McMillan "Allan's Alley" *New York Amsterdam News* July 30 1949. See also Ronald A. Smith "The Paul Robeson-Jackie Robinson Saga and a Political Collision" *Journal of Sport History* (Summer 1979) 6: 5–23; Martin Duberman *Paul Robeson: A Biography* (New York: New Press, 2005).

151. "Jackie Robinson Honored By Sister Kenny Institute" *Atlanta Daily World* August 13 1949; McMillan "Allan's Alley." This project was taken up by a group of influential Harlem women including Bessie Buchanan, a Cotton Club dancer and civil rights activist who a few years later became the first black woman in New York's state legislature; Allan McMillan "Allan's Alley" *New York Amsterdam News* September 24 1949; see also "Line Up Against Polio" *Philadelphia Tribune* August 20 1949.

152. "Sister Kenny in Harlem" *New York Amsterdam News* September 10 1949; Allan McMillan "Allan's Alley" *New York Amsterdam News* October 29 1949. See also "Stars of Stage, Screen Rally To Aid Jackie Robinson Ball" *New York Amsterdam News* September 17 1949; [advertisement] "Biggest Benefit Ball In The History of Harlem...Benefit Jackie Robinson Polio Fund of the Sister Kenny Institute" *New York Amsterdam News* September 17 1949; Allan McMillan "Allan's Alley" *New York Amsterdam News* October 8 1949. By December Harlem Citizens had established the Jackie Robinson Polio Fund for Sister Kenny and raised over $12,000; Allan McMillan "Allan's Alley" *New York Amsterdam News* December 31 1949.

153. [Cohn interview with] E. J. Huenkens, June 3 1964, Cohn Papers, MHS-K.

154. Kenny to Dear Doctor Huenkens, October 2 1951, New York City, 1942–1951, MHS-K; Kenny "Concerning the Extension of My Work in the State of California" [1949]; Kenny to Dear Mr. Dayton, May 8 1950, Donald C. Dayton, 1944–1951, MHS-K.

155. Kenny to Dear Mr. Dayton, December 27 1949, Donald C. Dayton, 1944–1951, MHS-K; Kenny to Dear Doctor Stevens, December 29 1950, Jersey City Medical Center, 1944–1950, MHS-K.

156. Kenny to Dear Mr. Dayton, December 27 1949.

157. Kenny "Concerning the Extension of My Work in the State of California" [1949]; Kenny to Dear Mr. Dayton, May 8 1950; Kenny to Dear Doctor Stevens, December 29 1950. Today the city hospital has a unit called the Miland E. Knapp Rehabilitation Center.

158. Miland E. Knapp To Whom It May Concern, October 27 1949, Dr. Miland Knapp, 1944–1945, 1949, MHS-K.

159. Miland E. Knapp, Lewis Sher, and Theodore S. Smith "Results of Kenny Treatment of Acute Poliomyelitis: Present Status of Three Hundred Ninety-One Patients Treated between 1940 and 1945" *JAMA* (January 10 1953) 151: 117–120.

160. Kenny to Henry Haverstock [telegram], February 5 1950, Henry W. Haverstock, 1942–1951, MHS-K; Kenny to Dear Mr. Crosby, November 30 1950, George C. Crosby, 1943–1951, MHS-K; Kenny to Dear Mr. Haverstock, March 15 1950, Henry W. Haverstock, 1942–1951, MHS-K; Kenny to Dear Mr. [E. J.] Rollings, May 3 1950, Michigan, Belgium, MHS-K.

161. Henry Haverstock to Dear Sister Kenny, March 18 1950, Henry W. Haverstock, 1942–1951, MHS-K.

162. "Bill Lets Sister Kenny Come and Go at Will" *Philadelphia Evening Bulletin* February 8 1950; Cohn "Sister Kenny... Back in the Battle Again;" "Sister Kenny Gets Privileges" *New York Times* February 12 1950. Kenny had organized a series of petitions asking the Secretary of State to give her such a visa months earlier, and gained the support of Minnesota Senator Democrat Hubert Humphrey and Congressman Republican Walter Judd; see "Humphrey Would Waive Visas for Sister Kenny" *Philadelphia Evening Bulletin* June 10 1949; "Gives Sister Kenny Key to U.S. Forever" *New York Journal-American* September 28 1949; E. J. Huenkens et al. to Dear Sir [Secretary of State], May 10 1949, Minnesota-Hospitals, 1944–1961, Sister Kenny Institute, Judd Papers, MHS.

163. Cohn "Sister Kenny... Back in the Battle Again."

164. Mildred Strunk "The Quarter's Polls" *Public Opinion Quarterly* (Summer 1950) 14: 380. Eleanor Roosevelt received 32%, Kenny 3%, Clare Booth Luce also 3%, and Helen Keller and Madame Chiang Kai-shek both 2%; George Gallup "Eleanor Roosevelt Is Voted The Most Admired Woman" [unnamed newspaper] January 25 1950, Misc. Collections, MHS-K.

165. Harris Shevelson [editor, *Pageant Magazine*] to Dear Sister Kenny, March 2 1950, General Correspondence-P, MHS-K; Mary Margaret McBride in [transcript] Radio Reports, Inc. "Sister Kenny Given Pageant Magazine Award," General Correspondence-P, MHS-K.

166. See Alexander *Maverick*, 181–182; Eleanor Roosevelt "My Day: March 13 1950" http://www.gwu.edu/~erpapers/myday/displaydoc.cfm?_y=1950&_f=md001538, accessed 6/20/2013.

167. "The Lord Helps Those..." *Time* (February 21 1949) 53: 96. The Kerr Glass Manufacturing Company was one of the top 3 manufacturers of canning jars in the 1940s.

168. Mrs. Alexander H. Kerr to Dear Sister Kenny, March 9 1950, Ruth Home, 1950, MHS-K; "Ruth Home Proposed as First Kenny Permanent Center for Polio in West" *Los Angeles Times* May 15 1950; Kenny "Ruth Home-Elizabeth Kenny Institute," October 25 1950, Ruth Home 1950, MHS-K; Kenny "Report to the Board of the Directors of the Sister Elizabeth Kenny Foundation," September 1 1950; [Cohn interview with] Ivar Anderson, May 19 1955, Cohn Papers, MHS-K; [Cohn another interview with] Harvey Billig, April 20 1955, Cohn Papers, MHS-K; "Kenny Hospital Drive Extended to June 17" *Los Angeles Times* June 4 1950.

169. "Hundreds See El Monte Polio Hospital Facility" *Los Angeles Times* May 21 1950; Kenny "Report to the Board of the Directors of the Sister Elizabeth Kenny Foundation," September 1 1950; Kenny "Ruth Home-Elizabeth Kenny Institute," October 25 1950; "Ruth Home Proposed as First Kenny Permanent Center for Polio in West."

170. "Sister Kenny Attends Polio Hospital Opening" *Los Angeles Times* August 25 1950.

171. "Sister Kenny Given Cottage at El Monte" *Los Angeles Times* October 9 1950; Hedda Hopper "Looking at Hollywood: Kaye Sought for Lead in Life of Famed Clown" *Chicago Daily Tribune* October 9 1950.

172. [Cohn interview with] Robert Bingham, May 19 1955, Cohn Papers, MHS-K; on the "ladies" of El Monte who had "worked day and night painting, scrubbing, making curtains, and decorating the home, just as they thought Sister Kenny would like it," see Hedda Hopper "Dickens' Clown Story Aimed at Danny Kaye" *Los Angeles Times* October 9 1950.

173. Kenny to Dear Sir [James W. Johnson], July 31 1950, General Correspondence-J, MHS-K; "Miss Kenny's Offer Declined by State" *New York Times* August 2 1950.

174. Kenny to Dear Doctor O'Hanlon, December 15 1950, Jersey City Medical Center, 1944–1950, MHS-K; Currier McEwen to Sister Elizabeth Kenny [telegram], May [1951], New York City, 1942–1951, MHS-K; Kenny to Dear Mr. Kline, October 19 1951, Marvin L. Kline, 1942–1959, MHS-K.

175. [Cohn interview with] Pete Gazzola, August 25 1953.

176. Willis Russell "Among the New Words" *American Speech* (December 1953) 28: 296; "Berle Cancer 'Telethon' May Produce $1,250,000" *Hartford Courant* April 11 1949. See also Frank Sturcken *Live Television: The Golden Age of 1946–1958 in New York* (Jefferson, NC: McFarland & Company, 1990), 46–61; "Cerebral Palsy Program of National Society for Crippled Summarized" *American Journal of Public Health* (October 1949) 39: 1353; "Palsy Association to Raise $1,034,000" *New York Times* October 16 1949; Richard Carter *The Gentle Legions* (Garden City, NY: Doubleday, 1961), 208.

177. "Kenny Fund Appeal Televised" *New York Times* December 26 1949; Marie McNair "Flaming Birthday Cake Surprises the Hostess At Alf Heiberg's Party" *Washington Post* September 25 1950. A 14-hour telecast "Celebrity Parade for Cerebral Palsy" with TV commentators from every network rotating as guest masters of ceremony was broadcast in December 1951, the same month as a similar program was broadcast from the Jersey City Armory to benefit the KF; both featured show business celebrities along with local and state politicians, physicians, and businessmen; Sidney Lohman "News and Notes of Television and Radio" *New York Times* December 2 1951.

178. [Cohn interview with] Mrs. Florence A. Rowe, August 26 1953, Cohn Papers, MHS-K. On the growing use of television by medical societies see "Television Broadcast" *New York State Journal of Medicine* (April 15 1950) 50: 1031; "Television Program in Color" *New York State Journal of Medicine* (April 1 1952) 52: 836.

179. "Television Highlights" *Washington Post* September 30 1950; D. Randall MacCarroll to Gentleman [National Broadcasting Co.], [n.d.], General Correspondence–M, MHS-K; "Sister Kenny" *Long Beach Independent* October 26 1949; Dorothy Doan to Dear Sister Kenny, July 19 1950, General Correspondence-C, MHS-K.

180. Kenny to Dear Mr. Sullivan, September 1 1949, General Correspondence—S, MHS-K. This was the second season of the show.

181. F. A. Rowe to Dear Miss Curtis, September 6 1949, Dorothy Curtis, MHS-K.

182. A Kenny fundraiser had featured an episode of Martha Rountree's show "Leave It to the Girls" that was televised "nationally"; McNair "Flaming Birthday Cake Surprises the Hostess At Alf Heiberg's Party"; see also She Made It: Martha Rountree, Paley Center for Media http://www.shemadeit.org/meet/biography.aspx?m=150, accessed June 12 2013.

183. Dorothy Ducas from KBA Memorandum Re: Kenny Broadcast, October 16 1950, Public Relations, MOD-K.

184. [Transcript] "Meet The Press—WNBT—Sunday, October 1 1950," Public Relations, MOD-K.

185. Dorothy Ducas from KBA Memorandum Re: Kenny Broadcast, October 16 1950.

186. Roland Berg to Dear Frank [Carey], April 26 1951.

187. "Farm Bureau Group Names Conciliators: Women Act To Heal Polio Discord" *St Paul Pioneer Press* January 18 1949; Kenny "Concerning the Extension of My Work in the State of California" [1949].

188. Kenny to Dear Mr. Dayton, March 14 1950, James Henry, 1943–1951, MHS-K. She referred to the transference of $80,000 from Mrs. Oberhoffer from herself to the KF.

189. "Leaflets Puzzle Area" *New York Times* September 7 1950.

190. "California Speaks" *[Perris, California] Progress* November 3 1949.

191. [Transcript] Radio Reports, Inc. "Sister Kenny Given Pageant Magazine Award," [1950], General Correspondence-P, MHS-K.

192. Mrs. Jean-Pierre Millon to Dear Sister Kenny, January 6 1949 [1950], Knickerbocker Ball, 1948–1950, MHS-K; "Resume [of Activities] October 13 1949," [enclosed with] Milton Hood Ward to Dear Sister, October 13 1949, Knickerbocker Ball 1948–1950, MHS-K.

193. "New Clinic Opened For Polio Victims" *New York Times* November 17 1950; Kenny to the President And Members of the Board of Directors, December 15 1950; Kenny To The National Board of the Elizabeth Kenny Foundation Memorandum Re: The Situation in the State of New York [1950], Board of Directors, MHS-K; "Kenny Benefit Ball Tonight" *New York Times* December 2 1950; "Ball Helps Sister Kenny Fund" *New York Times* December 2 1950; "Tells of $250,000 Drive For Kenny Institute Here" *New York Times* August 14 1950.

194. Kenny to Dear Mr. Crosby, November 30 1950; Kenny to Dear Mr. Shur, [Bertram Shur, Mrs. Madden's attorney], April 27 1951, James Henry, 1943–1951, MHS-K.

195. Kenny to the President And Members of the Board of Directors, December 15 1950.

196. John Nyberg "Sister Kenny Bids Adieu to Minneapolis" *Minneapolis Star* [December 1950], Public Relations, MOD-K; Kenny to Gentlemen [Mayor and Aldermen, City of Minneapolis], December 15 1950, Minneapolis, 1943–1950, MHS-K; "Sister Kenny Returning Home" *New York Times* December 6 1950; Kenny to the President And Members of the Board of Directors, December 15 1950.

197. "Sister Kenny Embarks For Native Australia" *Sunday Sun* December 17 1950, Public Relations, MOD-K; "Sister Kenny Departs" *New York Times* December 17 1950; Kenny to Dear Mr. Crosby, November 30 1950; Kenny to the President And Members of the Board of Directors, December 15 1950; John Nyberg "Sister Kenny Bids Adieu to Minneapolis" *Minneapolis Star* [December 1950], Public Relations, MOD-K.

198. [Transcript] "Conversation Between Sister Kenny and Mr. Marvin Kline, November 29 1950," Marvin L. Kline, 1942–1959, MHS-K.

199. Kenny to Dear Mr. Crosby, November 30 1950; Kenny to Dear Doctor Stevens, December 29 1950; Kenny to Dear Mr. Dayton, January 31 1950.

200. Kenny to Dear Mrs. Horton, April 28 1951, Henry Papers, MHS; "Sister Kenny in Australia" *New York Times* February 2 1951.

201. Kenny to Dear Mrs. Horton, April 28 1951; "Sister Kenny Sees Polio Patients" *Toowoomba Chronicle* March 17 1951; Kenny to Dear Mona and Belle, November 12 1951, James Henry, 1943–1951, MHS-K; "Sister Kenny At Home in Australia" *Minneapolis Sunday Tribune* August 26 1951.

202. Kenny to Dear Mr. Haverstock, May 17 1951, Henry W. Haverstock, MHS-K.

203. Kenny to Dear Mr. Haverstock, April 6 1951.

204. Kenny to Dear Mrs. Madden, January 1 1951, New York City, 1942–1951, MHS-K.

205. Kenny "Why I Left America" *Woman's Home Companion* (March 1951), 78: 38–39, 77–78, 80.

206. Kenny "Why I Left America," 38.

207. "Sister Kenny" *[Sydney] People Magazine* June 20 1951, 3.

208. "Sister Kenny," 3–4, 7.

209. Pearl Baldock (Mrs. R. G. Baldock) to Dear Mrs. Sterne, June 2 1949, General Correspondence-B, MHS-K.

210. "Establishment of Sister Kenny Clinics Long Overdue" *Warwick Daily News* July 13 1951, Wilson Collection; [Minutes] Public Meeting Held in the City Hall Theatre on Monday November 24 1952, at 8 p.m., Kenny Collection, Box 2, Fryer Library.

211. Sayre [1951] in Julie McDonald *Ruth Buxton Sayre: First Lady of the Farm* (Ames: Iowa State University Press, 1980), 118. Sayre was on a trip to 17 countries in 13 weeks, including New Zealand and Australia; McDonald *Ruth Buxton Sayre*, 115–118.

212. Kenny to Dear Mr. Shur, April 27 1951; Kenny to Dear Mrs. Madden, July 13 1951, James Henry, 1943–1951, MHS-K; Kenny to Dear Friend [Laruelle], May 30 1951, Dr. Leon Laruelle, 1945–1951, MHS-K.

213. McDonald *Ruth Buxton Sayre.*

214. "Sister Kenny Sees Polio Patients" *Toowoomba Chronicle* March 17 1951; "Request to Minister on Sister Kenny Concept" *Toowoomba Chronicle* June 13 1951.

215. "Minutes of Meeting Held Toowoomba: Conference Called by Sister Elizabeth Kenny at Request of Interested Groups and Individuals Throughout Australia and Elsewhere," August 4 1951, Kenny Collection, Box 2, Fryer Library. Sterne became the formal secretary of the new KF International Australia Branch; "Establishment of Sister Kenny Clinics Long Overdue"; "[Minutes] Public Meeting Held in the City Hall Theatre on Monday November 24 1952."

216. "Minutes of Meeting Held Toowoomba," August 4 1951. The group raised 200 pounds, which, they agreed, following Kenny's lead, would not be used to pay the salaries of any "paid officials."

217. "Minutes of Public Meeting Called By "International Organisation [sic] For Combating Poliomyelitis": Held October 24, 1951," Kenny Collection, Box 2, Fryer Library.

218. "Sister Kenny," 3; "Sister Kenny in Australia" *New York Times* February 2 1951.

219. Kenny to Dear Mr. Haverstock, April 6 1951.

220. J. J. Nye to Dear Sister Kenny, November 3 1951, Kenny Collection, Box 16, Fryer Library; Mrs. R. G. [Pearl] Baldock to Dear Dr. Pye, May 21 1951, Kenny Collection, Box 16, Fryer Library.

221. Kenny, letter to editor, "Sister Kenny Still Working, She Writes From Australia" *Minneapolis Sunday Tribune* April 8 1951.

222. Kenny to Dear Mr. Haverstock, May 17 1951.

223. Kenny to Dear Friend [Lloyd Johnson], July 17 1951, James Henry, 1943–1951, MHS-K.

224. Kenny to Dear Mr. Shur, April 27 1951; Kenny to Dear Mr. Haverstock, May 17 1951; Howard J. London To Dr. Van Riper Memorandum Re: Sister Kenny, May 3 1951, Public Relations, MOD-K.

225. Kenny "Evidence Presented Concerning the Kenny Concept and Treatment of the Disease Infantile Paralysis," [1951], Wilson Collection.

226. "Sister Kenny Departs From L.A. For Polio Meeting" *Los Angeles Herald Express* August 23 1951; Kenny to Dear Friend [Laruelle], May 30 1951; [Cohn second interview with] Rosalind Russell, August 18 1953, Cohn Papers, MHS-K.

227. "Sister Kenny Said To Be Incurably Ill" *New York Times* August 13 1951; "Nurse Who Ministered To Thousands, Now Ill" *Atlanta Daily World* August 14 1951; "Sister Kenny In Last U.S. Visit" *Atlanta Daily World* August 19 1951; "Sister Kenny, Incurably Ill, Arrives in L.A." *Los Angeles Times* August 18 1951; "Sister Kenny Off to Parley" *Los Angeles Times* August 23 1951; "Returns to U.S." *Chicago Daily Tribune* August 18 1951; "Sister Kenny Now in L.A.; Fights Pain" *Los Angeles Mirror* August 17 1951. Kenny's claim that she was dying and in great pain was squashed by John Sharpe, Rosalind Russell's personal physician, who reminded her that this way of dramatizing her story would scare many people who had Parkinson's, a disease which was "not as bad as she made it out to sound"; [Cohn interview with] Will O'Neill, [March 1955], Cohn Papers, MHS-K.

228. Elizabeth Coulson "Sister Kenny Races Death to Finish Her Work" *Pasadena Star News* August 20 1951; "Sister Kenny Off to Parley"; "Sister Kenny, Facing Death, Flies To U.S." *Santa Ana [California] Register* August 15 1951.

229. Kenny to Dear Mr. Henry, October 4 1951, Henry Papers, MHS. She was accompanied by Miss Ella Vigar from Toowoomba; "Sister Kenny Here" *New York Times* August 23 1951.

230. "Sister Kenny, Incurably Ill, Arrives in L.A."; "Sister Kenny Off to Parley."

231. "Sister Kenny Writes Data for 3D Volume" *New York Times* August 24 1951.

232. On the neglect of Enders' 1948 work see Aaron E. Klein *Trial By Fury: The Polio Vaccine Controversy* (New York: Charles Scribner's Sons, 1972), 58.

233. Spence "Poliomyelitis," 304–305.

234. "Polio Fund, in Debt, Seeking $50,000,000" *New York Times* November 14 1950.

235. "Polio Experts Assemble" *New York Times* September 2 1951; "Doctors Told of New Promise in Polio Fight, Way Is Found to Inject Drug in Nerve Cells" *Washington Post* September 4 1951; "President Informed of Progress On Polio" *New York Times* September 27 1951; *Poliomyelitis: Papers and Discussions Presented at the Second International Poliomyelitis Conference* (Philadelphia: J.B. Lippincott, 1952).

236. "Doctor To Discuss Polio-Like Virus" *New York Times* August 26 1951; "Rehabilitation Survey: Volunteer Worker Here to Study Methods in Europe" *New York Times* June 3 1951. A total of 150 physical therapists from 15 nations met to form a new World Confederation for Physical Therapy and Mildred Elson was elected as its first president; Howard A. Rusk "Major Gains Shown in Fight Against Infantile Paralysis" *New York Times* September 9 1951; "World Confederation for Physical Therapy" *Physical Therapy Review* (December 1951) 31: 525.

237. "Polio Test Reported" *New York Times* September 6 1951.

238. "Program: Second International Poliomyelitis Conference" September 2–7 1951, #1478, Series I, Box 74, Folder 1641, John Enders Papers, Yale University Library Manuscripts and Archives, New Haven; "Doctors Told of New Promise in Polio Fight, Way Is Found to Inject Drug in Nerve Cells" *Washington Post* September 4 1951; Howard A. Rusk "Major Gains Shown in Fight Against Infantile Paralysis" *New York Times* September 9 1951; W. C. Gibson "The Second International Poliomyelitis Conference: A Summary" *Canadian Medical Association Journal* (January 1952) 66: 69–71.

239. "Polio Serum Forecast at World Session" *Washington Post* September 2 1951.

240. Kenny to Dear Mr. Crosby, October 1 1951, George C. Crosby, 1945–1951, MHS-K; Kenny to Dear Mr. Kline, October 19 1951; "Move on Kenny Training Centre For Australia" *Toowoomba Chronicle* October 25 1951; Kenny *My Battle and Victory: History of the Discovery of Poliomyelitis as a Systemic Disease* (London: Robert Hale Limited, 1955), 104; Alexander *Maverick*, 185.

241. John F. Enders to Dear Doctor Fryberg, February 27 1952, Series I, Box 73, Folder 1637, Enders Papers. Fryberg responded that his answer "confirms what I have told Sister Kenny: that her concept is not proven"; A. Fryberg to Dear Professor Enders, March 6 1952, Series I, Box 73, Folder 1637, Enders Papers; see also A. Fryberg to Dear Professor Enders, January 10 1952, Series I, Box 73, Folder 1637, Enders Papers. When interviewed several years later, Enders confirmed that he had talked to Kenny at the conference and that she had asked whether his paper proved her theory that polio was not strictly neurotropic but also attacked peripheral tissue. He had replied that his work certainly did not disprove her theories, but the fact that the virus grew in a test tube did not mean it grew this way in the human body. He may have added, he recalled, "you may be right, of course... there may be something along these lines"; [Cohn phone interview with] John Enders, March 28 1955, Cohn Papers, MHS-K.

242. Richard Ulian "Sister Kenny Gets Sad Welcome on Final Visit" *Minneapolis Morning Tribune* September 17 1951. The house was sold by the city in July 1951.

243. Kenny to Dear Mr. Crosby, October 1 1951.

244. John F. Pohl *Cerebral Palsy* (Saint Paul: Bruce Publishing Company, 1950), 26–30; [Cohn interview with] William O'Neill, May 20 1955, Cohn Papers, MHS-K. According to

O'Neill Pohl's estrangement from the Institute was the result of a battle with Huenkens over the use of respirators during the 1946 epidemic.

245. There is no mention at all of this topic or Pohl's work in Kenny's final autobiography.

246. Kenny to Dear Mr. Kline, October 19 1951.

247. Kenny to Dear Mr. Crosby, October 1 1951; Herbert J. Levine *I Knew Sister Kenny: A Story of a Great Lady and Little People* (Boston: Christopher Publishing House, 1954), 225, 229–230.

248. Kenny to Dear Mr. Crosby, October 1 1951.

249. Philip Sokol [counsel, Department of Welfare, City of New York] to Gentlemen [KF], July 24 1951, General Correspondence-G, MHS-K; Peter Gazzola to Marvin Stevens, August 24 1951, General Correspondence-G, MHS-K; Kenny to Dear Mr. Crosby, October 1 1951.

250. Kenny to Dear Mr. Barnwell, November 18 1949, John J. Barnwell, 1947–1950, MHS-K. She had claimed that "this soft soap had no effect."

251. Kenny to Dear Mr. Crosby, October 1 1951.

252. Kenny to Dear Mr. Kline, October 4 1951; "Sister Kenny Departs By Air for Australia" *Washington Post* October 9 1951; "Sister Kenny in Southland for 'Last Visit'" *Los Angeles Mirror* September 27 1951.

253. "Sister Kenny's Work 'Not All Sadness'" *Townsville Daily Bulletin* [November 1951], Wilson Collection.

254. George Gallup "Sister Kenny Tops As Women's Ideal" [unnamed newspaper], January 1952, Wilson Collection. In February 1951 Kenny had been chosen second, below Eleanor Roosevelt; Kenny was followed by Madame Chiang Kai-Shek, Clare Luce, and Helen Keller; George Gallup "Nation Picks Mrs. Roosevelt As Woman Most Admired" *Philadelphia Evening Bulletin* February 4 1951.

255. [Cohn interview with] Pete Gazzola, August 25 1953.

256. "Sister Kenny Deserves to Be Included in Honours List" *Brisbane Courier-Mail* January 14 1952; "Sister Kenny Wants No Other Title" *Brisbane Courier-Mail* January 17 1952.

257. Kenny "Doctors, I Salute You" *American Weekly* March 2 1952, 19.

258. W. M. Hammon "Possibilities of Specific Prevention and Treatment of Poliomyelitis" *Pediatrics* (1950) 6: 696–705; "Utah Children Get Polio Serum Test" *New York Times* September 5 1951. Hammon's study of passive immunity to the polio virus was one of the first major double-blind, placebo-controlled clinical trials (Utah 1951, Houston and Sioux City, Iowa, 1952), which cost the NFIP $1 million; he presented the trial results at the American Public Health Association's annual meeting in Cleveland on October 22 1952; Charles R. Rinaldo, Jr. "Passive Immunization Against Poliomyelitis: The Hammon Gamma Globulin Field Trials, 1951–1953" *American Journal of Public Health* (2005) 95: 790–799; see also Stephen E. Mawdsley "Fighting Polio: Selling the Gamma Globulin Field Trials, 1950–1953" (Ph.D. dissertation, University of Cambridge, 2012).

259. "Two Reports Show Polio Can Be Beaten" *Washington Post* April 16 1952; see also Paul *A History*, 387–388. Note that Horstmann had reported these results at the 1951 Copenhagen conference.

260. Howard Blakeslee "Hope for Conquering Polio Seen; Scientists Find Its Origin in Blood" *New York Times* April 16 1952; "Prevention of the Crippling Form of Polio Believed Possible by Use of New Vaccine" *New York Times* April 16 1952. *JAMA* cautiously suggested the technique "may lead to the introduction of a successful chemotherapeutic agent;" "Immunization Against Poliomyelitis" *JAMA* (May 17 1952) 149: 278–279.

261. "Sister Kenny Upheld On Polio, Aide Insists" *New York Times* April 17 1952; "May Beat Polio by Vaccination" *Brisbane Courier-Mail* April 17 1952.

262. "Sister Kenny On Polio Report" *Toowoomba Chronicle* April 18 1952.

263. Kenny to Dear Sir [Earle Page], April 23 1952, Wilson Collection.

264. Kenny to Dear Friends [Henry, Mintener, and Johnson], May 3 1952, Henry Papers, MHS.

265. "Huntington Park Parade Honors Sister Kenny" *Los Angeles Times* May 11 1952; "Sister Kenny Returns to Aid Fight on Polio" *Los Angeles Times* May 10 1952; Amy Lindsey "A Welcome, A Surprise and A Television Review" *Kenny News* (May 1952) 2: 4–5; "Sister Kenny Flies East For More Medical Conferences" *Kenny News* (May 1952) 2: 1. So impressed was Kenny with this new technology that she hoped physicians would "record per medium of TV" her signs of early diagnosis; Kenny to Dear Dr. Payne, September 10 1952, Minnesota-Hospitals, 1944–1961, Sister Kenny Institute, Judd Papers, MHS. On the rising numbers of television stations and television sets during the late 1940s see Kathryn H. Fuller-Seeley "Learning to Live With Television: Technology, Gender, and America's Early TV Audiences" in Gary R. Edgerton ed. *The Columbia History of American Television* (New York: Columbia University Press, 2007), 101–105.

266. Kenny *Cause and Prevention of Deformities in Poliomyelitis: Presented to the Medical Staff of the Sister Kenny Polio Hospital, El Monte, California, Tuesday, May 20, 1952*, author's possession, 3–9, 11–14, 20–21, 26–28.

267. Kenny to Dear Rosalind and Freddie [Russell and Brisson], June 26 1952, Rosalind Russell (Brisson), 1947–1952, MHS-K.

268. On the 1952 polio epidemic see Julie Silver and Daniel Wilson *Polio Voices: An Oral History from the American Polio Epidemics and Worldwide Eradication Efforts* (Westport, CT: Praeger, 2007).

269. "Sister Kenny Arrives Here, Plans to Rest" *Los Angeles Times* July 16 1952.

270. [Cohn interview with] Ivar Anderson, May 19 1955, Cohn Papers, MHS-K.

271. Kenny *Poliomyelitis A Systemic Disease: Paper Read to the Advisory Medical Committee of the Sister Elizabeth Kenny Foundation at the Sister Kenny Treatment Center Buffalo, New York, July 14, 1952*, Box 1, Minneapolis-Hospitals, 1944–1961, Judd Papers, MHS, 2–6, 9–14.

272. Gil Fates *What's My Line? The Inside Story of TV's Most Famous Panel Show* (Englewood Cliffs NJ: Prentice-Hall, 1978), 221. Kenny was the mystery guest on June 29 1952, Episode #109.

273. Jungeblut to Dear Miss Kenny, July 5 1952, Box 2, Ke-Kn, Jungeblut Papers, NLM; and see Kenny *Poliomyelitis A Systemic Disease*, 6–7.

274. Kenny to Mesdames I. J. Fox and Albert Rosen, July 7 1952, General Correspondence-F, MHS-K; Kenny to Dear Friends [Mrs. I. J. Fox and Albert Rosen], July 9 1952, General Correspondence-F, MHS-K.

275. G. P. Mitchell "Early Treatment of Poliomyelitis" *British Medical Journal* (March 22 1952) 1: 649–650.

276. Ethel Byrne and Alan T. Roberts "The Poliomyelitis Epidemic of 1950–1951 in the Newcastle Area" *Medical Journal of Australia* (July 5 1952) 2: 10–13; see also H.J. Seddon "Treatment in the Convalescent Stage" *Journal of Bone and Joint Surgery* (August 1951) 33: 458; John M. Duggan and Peter I. A. Hendry "Royal Newcastle Hospital: The Passing of an Icon" *Medical Journal of Australia* (2005) 183: 642–645; R. G. Evans "A Professor 'Honorarius': An Australian Experiment in Medical Administration 1939–1964" *Health & History* (2003) 5: 115–138.

277. Jean Macnamara "The Prevention of Crippling Following Poliomyelitis" *Medical Journal of Australia* (July 5 1952) 2: 4–8.

278. H. J. Seddon [review of] "[Kenny] *And They Shall Walk*" *British Medical Journal* (April 12 1952) 1: 802–803.

279. J. R. S. Lahz, letter to editor, *British Medical Journal* (November 8 1952) 2: 1047.

280. Lancelot H.F. Walton, letter to editor, *British Medical Journal* (May 17 1952) 1: 1082.

281. Kenny *My Battle and Victory*, 11, 89.

282. Kenny "Report to the Board of the Directors of the Sister Elizabeth Kenny Foundation, Minneapolis, Minnesota," February 27 1950, Board of Directors, MHS-K; Kenny to Dear Mr. Dayton, March 14 1950, James Henry, 1943–1951, MHS-K.

283. Alexander *Maverick*, 186–187.

284. "Sister Kenny Sees Polio Beaten" *New York Times* September 9 1952.

285. "Move on Kenny Training Centre For Australia."

286. Extract of Page speech, in response to question from Mr. C. Morgan, October 16 1951, #707/9/A, Series A462, Australian Archives, AA-ACT; Kenny to Dear Mr. [Charles] Morgan, November 7 1951, Cohn Papers, MHS-K; "Move on Kenny Training Centre For Australia"; Kenny to Dear Mr. Kline, October 19 1951. Page had visited Europe and North America from July to September 1951. He was made Minister for Health in 1949 and held this post until 1956 when he retired to the backbench; see Carl Bridge "Page, Sir Earle Christmas Grafton (1880–1961)," *Australian Dictionary of Biography*, Australian National University, http://adb.anu.edu.au/biography/page-sir-earle-christmas-grafton-7941/text13821, accessed July 29 2012.

287. "Move on Kenny Training Centre For Australia"; A. J. Metcalfe to Secretary, Prime Minister's Department [A. S. Brown] Memorandum Re: 'Sister' Kenny and Poliomyelitis, October 27 1952, #707/9/A, Series A462, AA-ACT; see also Mrs. R. G. Baldock to Sir [Prime Minister], October 6 1952, #707/9/A, Series A462, AA-ACT; Mrs. R. G. Baldock to Dear Sir [Prime Minister], September 15 1952, #707/9/A, Series A462, AA-ACT.

288. A. S. Brown to Dear Mrs. Baldock, November 7 1952, #707/9/A, Series A462, AA-ACT. Baldock "will not accept any evidence that in any way contradicts the Kenny concept of polio-myelitis and the value of her methods of treatment" so that "any further evidence supplied would in all probability provoke further denial"; A. J. Metcalfe to Secretary, Prime Minister's Department [A. S. Brown] Memorandum Re: 'Sister' Kenny and Poliomyelitis, December 3 1952, #707/9/A, Series A462, AA-ACT. Note that Page also wrote to Sterne asking that his name not be associated with any of the "controversy" around Kenny; Page to Sterne, October 7 1952, cited in Alexander *Maverick*, 188.

289. Kenny to Dear Friend [George Crosby], September 29 1952, Henry Papers, MHS.

290. Kenny to Gentlemen [Nye, Arden, Pye, Lee, Wilkinson, and Fryberg], [September 1952], Wilson Collection; Kenny, letter to editor, *Toowoomba Chronicle* October 30 1952, Wilson Collection; Minutes, Executive Committee of the International Organisation for Combating Poliomyelitis, Held October 15 1952.

291. Kenny to Dear Doctor Judd, August 12 1952, Minnesota-Hospitals, 1944–1961, Sister Kenny Institute, Judd Papers, MHS; Judd to Dear Sister Kenny, August 15 1952, Box 2, Ke-Kn, Jungeblut Papers, NLM; Kenny to Dear Mr. Kline, October 19 1951; Kenny to Dear Dr. Payne, September 10 1952, Minnesota-Hospitals, 1944–1961, Sister Kenny Institute, Judd Papers, MHS; Payne to Dear Miss Kenny, September 30 1952, Minnesota-Hospitals, 1944–1961, Sister Kenny Institute, Judd Papers, MHS.

292. Kenny to Dear Friend [James Henry], November 13 1952, Henry Papers, MHS.

293. Ibid.

294. "Sister Kenney [sic] Fights For Life" *Atlanta Daily World* November 25 1952; "Sister Kenny's Condition Takes Turn for Worse" *Los Angeles Times* November 29 1952. Some of her first polio patients waited outside her house for the final bulletin announcing the death; "Sister Kenny Dies In Her Sleep at 66" *New York Times* November 30 1952.

295. "Sister Kenny Musters a Smile for America" *Minneapolis Star* November 25 1952; "Sister Kenney [sic] Fights For Life"; "Sister Kenny Resigned to Die Before She Lapsed Into Coma" *Philadelphia Evening Bulletin* November 30 1952; "Sister Kenny's Life Had Peaceful Close" *Toowoomba Chronicle* December 1 1952.

296. "Doctor Wires Advice To Help Sister Kenny" *Hartford Courant* November 27 1952; "Sister Kenny Resigned to Die Before She Lapsed Into Coma"; "Sister Kenny Dies In Her Sleep at 66"; "Sister Kenny's Life Had Peaceful Close"; "Sister Kenny Treated From N.Y. By Phone" *Chicago Daily Tribune* November 26 1952; "Sister Kenny Unconscious; Heart Weakens" *Chicago Daily Tribune* November 29 1952; Waldemar Kaempffert "Science in Review: Trypsin, Like That Flown to Australia for Sister Kenny, Dissolves Some Blood Clots" *New York Times* December 7 1952; "Sister Kenny's Condition Takes Turn for Worse"; "Sister Kenny, Polio Fighter, Critically Ill" *Washington Post* November 24 1952.

297. "Sister Kenny Resigned to Die Before She Lapsed Into Coma"; "Pneumonia Hastens Death of Polio Nurse" *Minneapolis Sunday Tribune* November 30 1952; "Sister Kenny's Life Had Peaceful Close."

298. "Sister Kenny's Life Had Peaceful Close"; "Sister Kenny's Services Held: Church Packed" *Chicago Daily Tribune* December 1 1952; "Sister Kenny Dies: Fought Polio 43 Years" *Chicago Daily Tribune* November 30 1952; "Sister Kenny, 66, Dies at Home in Australia" *Los Angeles Times* November 30 1952; Walter Johnson "Sister Kenny Fought Doctors to Win Battle Against Polio" *Minneapolis Star* December 1 1952.

299. "Sister Kenny Rites Held in Australia" *New York Times* December 1 1952; "Last Honor Paid to Sister Kenny" *Philadelphia Evening Bulletin* December 1 1952; "Sister Kenny's Services Held; Church Packed" *Chicago Daily Tribune* December 1 1952; "Town Will Watch Over Her Grave" *Brisbane Courier Mail* [1952], Kenny Collection, Box 18, Fryer Library; "Sister Kenny Rites To Be Held Today" *Hartford Courant* December 1 1952.

300. "Town Will Watch Over Her Grave"; "At Rest: Under the Gums" *Brisbane Courier-Mail* December 2 1952; "Last Honor Paid To Sister Kenny"; "Sister Kenny Rites Held in Australia."

301. "Last Honor Paid To Sister Kenny"; "Sister Kenny Rites Held in Australia"; "At Rest: Under the Gums"; "Town Will Watch Over Her Grave."

302. "Last Honor Paid To Sister Kenny"; "Sister Kenny Rites Held in Australia"; "At Rest: Under the Gums."

303. "At Rest: Under the Gums."

304. "Transition: Sister Elizabeth Kenny" *Newsweek* (December 8 1952) 40: 67.

305. "Sister Kenny Dies In Her Sleep at 66."

306. "Sister Kenny" *Lancet* (December 6 1952) 260: 1123; "Elizabeth Kenny" *Medical Journal of Australia* (January 17 1953) 1: 85; "Sister Kenny" *British Medical Journal* (December 6 1952) 2: 1262; "Sister Kenny: H. J. Seddon" *British Medical Journal* (December 6 1952) 2: 1262–1263; "Death of Sister Kenny" *JAMA* (January 3 1953) 151: 53.

307. "Sister Kenny Is Dead" *Sydney Morning Herald* December 2 1952, Wilson Collection.

308. "Many Pay Tribute to a 'Great Australian'" *Toowoomba Chronicle* December 1 1952; "Sister Kenny Is Dead."

309. "Many Pay Tribute to a 'Great Australian.'"

310. "Was A Great Influence" *Brisbane Courier-Mail* December 1 1952.

311. "Many Pay Tribute to a 'Great Australian.'"

312. "Actress Praises Sister Kenny" [unnamed newspaper], [December 1952], Clippings, MHS-K.

313. Johnson "Australian Nurse Is Dead"; Victor Cohn "Revolutionary Polio Treatment Sister Kenny Gift to U.S. Medicine" *Minneapolis Sunday Tribune* November 30 1952.

314. "Sister Kenny Honored" *Philadelphia Evening Bulletin* December 17 1952.

315. "Sister Kenny Memorial Conducted" *Los Angeles Times* December 3 1952; "History of the Sister Elizabeth Kenny Foundation of Southern California, Inc." [1955], Kenny Collection, Box 1, Fryer Library.

316. "Sister Kenny Awards Presented to Hospital" *Los Angeles Times* January 19 1956; "Rosalind Russell Gives Tiny Patient Welcome" *Los Angeles Times* January 29 1956.

FURTHER READING

On medicine, race and the Cold War see Mary L. Dudziak *Cold War Civil Rights: Race and the Image of American Democracy* (Princeton: Princeton University Press, 2000); Stephan E. Mawdsley "'Dancing on Eggs': Charles H. Bynum, Racial Politics, and the National Foundation for Infantile Paralysis, 1938–1954" *Bulletin of the History of Medicine* (2010) 84: 217–247; David M. Oshinsky *Polio: An American Story* (New York: Oxford University Press, 2005); Robert N. Proctor *The Nazi War on Cancer* (Princeton: Princeton University Press, 1999); Naomi Rogers "Race and the Politics of Polio: Warm Springs, Tuskegee and the March of Dimes" *American Journal of Public Health* (2007) 97: 2–13; Kevin Starr *Embattled Dreams: California in War and Peace, 1940–1950* (New York: Oxford University Press, 2002); Jessica Wang *American Science in an Age of Anxiety: Scientists, Anticommunism, and the Cold War* (Chapel Hill: University of North Carolina Press, 1999).

On gender and the Cold War see Mary C. Brennan *Wives, Mothers, and the Red Menace: Conservative Women and the Crusade Against Community* (Boulder: University Press of Colorado, 2008); Linda Eisenmann *Higher Education for Women in Postwar America, 1945–1965* (Baltimore: Johns Hopkins University Press, 2006); Helen Laville *Cold War Women: The International Activities of American Women's Organisations* (Manchester: Manchester University Press, 2002); Elaine Tyler May *Homeward Bound: American Families in the Cold War Era* (New York: Basic Books, 1988); Lisa McGirr *Suburban Warriors: The Origins of the New American Right* (Princeton: Princeton University Press, 2001); Joanne Meyerowitz ed. *Not June Cleaver: Women and Gender in Postwar America, 1945–1960* (Philadelphia: Temple University Press, 1994).

9

I Knew Sister Kenny

IN 1954 THE National Foundation for Infantile Paralysis (NFIP) sponsored the world's largest clinical trial and in 1955 the Salk polio vaccine became available to the public. With the widespread use of the vaccine during the late 1950s the clinical care of polio no longer seemed important. Fewer children were contracting polio and those who were had shorter hospital stays. Reflecting these changes the Baltimore Children's Hospital-School, where Florence and Henry Kendall still worked, was renamed the Children's Hospital in 1958; its NFIP-funded iron lung center had already closed a few years earlier.[1]

The Salk vaccine's victory over polio excited people across the globe, and Americans felt special pride as "it was their vaccine, ordered and paid for by them."[2] Elizabeth Kenny, a central character in the polio wars, was quickly—and, I think, not accidentally—forgotten. The story of how polio had been conquered was well crafted by the NFIP's publicity department and erased almost all previous debates in polio history, especially those around therapy. When, for example, Herbert Levine, a little known Illinois physician, tried to memorialize Kenny and the Centralia Kenny clinic, the NFIP quietly discouraged leading science reporters from reviewing his 1954 book *I Knew Sister Kenny: The Story of a Great Lady and Little People*. Kenny had been, Levine reminded readers, "a world-wide controversial figure [who had]...re-awakened and re-stimulated medical science to continue its research against this dreaded disease." Although the book was reviewed in regional papers like the *St. Louis Globe-Democrat* and the *Pittsburgh Sun-Telegraph* and received blurbs from Ed Sullivan and Hedda Hopper, it disappeared from sight. It was not enough, Levine discovered, to have known Kenny.[3] By comparison, in 1958 the NFIP used all of its media resources to highlight its organization of a special ceremony at Warm Springs to honor 17 polio heroes in a new Polio Hall of Fame. The NFIP chose to feature twentieth-century scientists whose NFIP-funded work had led to the polio vaccine, along with Roosevelt, O'Connor, and 3 nineteenth-century physicians.[4] There were

402

no modern orthopedists or physical medicine experts, much less any physical therapists or nurses.

These maneuvers helped to refocus the picture of polio away from the bedside to the laboratory. Boosted by NFIP publicity, a new symbol of the defeat of polio was emerging: not a woman surrounded by grateful child patients but a man in a white coat holding a test tube. During the 1950s and early 1960s polio's history was remade into the story of virus hunters; physical therapists, nurses, and even doctors, when they appeared, were portrayed as grateful for the insights of scientists who knew, as the authors of *Polio Pioneers* argued, "how to hunt a germ."[5] The forgetting of Sister Kenny reflected a wider cultural neglect of the pioneers of clinical care compared to the designers of preventive and curative techniques.

The NFIP encouraged science writers to see polio as a triumphant story of medical science, even when a batch of the Salk vaccine produced by the Cutter laboratory proved deadly and the federal government had to step in to monitor vaccine production more closely. By the late 1950s the making of a new vaccine by Albert Sabin similarly captured public attention, especially the purported rivalry between Sabin and Salk. The 2 polio vaccines, indeed, became the exemplar of Americans' ability to control disease, a high tech solution to a messy, frightening plague now gone forever. They were another emblem, like penicillin, of American medicine's Golden Age.[6] While the NFIP's publicity department continued to remind the public of the importance of making sure children received 3 separate injections of the Salk vaccine, the NFIP began to expand its mission beyond polio, focusing on "crippling" diseases such as arthritis before finally settling on birth defects. The term "infantile paralysis" had already lost its meaning; the organization renamed itself first the National Foundation (1958) and then the March of Dimes. In 1960 its poster child had spina bifida.[7]

SETTLING SCORES: GENDER, THEORY, AND CHARACTER

During her lifetime, admirers had placed Kenny in a pantheon of great scientists like Louis Pasteur, Paul Ehrlich, and Marie Curie—all subjects of Hollywood movies, which had depicted them as scientific figures who had battled conservative antagonists and had "shared their secrets with all mankind."[8] But most physicians were unwilling to go as far to put Kenny in the same category as double-Nobel-Prize-winner Marie Curie or another great contributor to medical science.

Kenny's gender, training, and claims to discovery were made central in the numerous obituaries published after her death where the act of memorializing offered an opportunity to settle scores. Kenny's story—bush nurse becomes medical celebrity—was too good not to retell. Indeed, the *Chicago Tribune* phrased her life much as the *Sister Kenny* movie had done, praising her "zeal" and arguing that it had prevented her from attaining a husband and family. Making it clear to readers that Kenny—a single woman and a crusading professional—had once had a sweetheart was especially important in an era in which American women were expected to embrace a life of marriage and domesticity.[9]

In a long unsympathetic obituary, the *New York Times* noted "the extraordinary character of Sister Kenny" whose "stubbornness" had allowed her "to revolutionize the methods of treating poliomyelitis" and to rise "from the status of an obscure Australian nurse to a personage of international importance in the medical world." Her personal characteristics were, however, "the primary cause of a deplorable conflict with physicians who disagreed with her concept of poliomyelitis." "Medical opinion has been against Sister Kenny for years" but physicians did acknowledge "her great service in introducing methods of treatment that are now standard." When her theories were "repudiated" she had lost the support of the NFIP, although it continued to fund the teaching of her techniques. Ignoring Kenny's argument that her work showed that the polio virus affected nonnervous tissues, the *Times* oversimplified her theory and said that Kenny saw polio not as a nervous disorder but as "an affliction of the muscles and skin," ideas that were the unsurprising result of one whose medical knowledge and grasp of anatomy "were those acquired by a nurse." By contrast, physicians who "had studied the damaged brains of monkeys that had been infected with polio and of fatal human cases...saw plainly that the nerves were affected, for all Sister Kenny's denials." "The technical arguments, the personal recriminations...are at an end," the *Times* concluded with relief, adding with an insincere-sounding reference to her patients, "there remains the figure of a strong-minded woman whose name will invoke blessings from thousands who would have been crippled for life had it not been for her courage, her forthrightness."[10]

This attack on Kenny's character and on her poor understanding of polio's pathology outraged Columbia University virologist Claus Jungeblut who wrote an angry letter to the *Times*. The *Times* obituary, Jungeblut complained to KF head Marvin Kline, had probably been written "some two or more years ago...in readiness for this occasion." Its accusations would make it difficult to organize an effective KF campaign, for now KF promoters would have to try "to memorialize someone whose work was made to appear professionally unsound and whose claim to honor was a stubborn courage and an unshaken but unshared belief in her own ideas."[11]

Jungeblut's letter to the *Times* protesting the portrayal of Kenny's scientific contribution was passed on to Waldemar Kaempffert, the paper's science editor. Jungeblut argued that the obituary failed "to do justice to the meaning of the 'Kenny concept' and [had confused]...existing scientific facts." A new viewpoint, Jungeblut pointed out, showed that the polio virus traveled through the bloodstream and could perhaps cause "a widespread involvement of peripheral areas, including skeletal and cardiac muscles."[12] Kaempffert wrote back to Jungeblut, defending the obituary as written "only after we had consulted clinicians and virologists whose opinion we respect."[13] But Jungeblut replied firmly that his claims were "based on recorded facts and not on personal opinion" and cited specific research studies, including Dorothy Horstmann's viremia studies and work by John Enders showing that the polio virus could grow in nonneurological tissue. "Many of the earlier differences of opinion have been resolved," he wrote, and "at last a concept of the systemic nature of the disease emerges on which there is general agreement."[14]

Jungeblut's own career spiraled downward. He continued for a few years to seek evidence of a genetic factor to explain susceptibility to paralytic polio, but his research plans were rejected by the National Institutes of Health.[15] His reputation as an idiosyncratic scientist who had rejected the NFIP was recognized by other neglected researchers who hoped that his support by the KF could help break up "this Polio Foundation Control System."[16] Appearing before Congress in 1953, he reiterated his belief that the paralytic process in polio was both central and "peripheral" and that his Columbia team had been "some of the first ones to sponsor the viewpoint that the bloodstream was one way of disseminating the virus."[17] Jungeblut retired from Columbia in 1962 and died in 1976. In his *New York Times* obituary he was described as a bacteriologist who was well known for his research on transferring the polio virus from monkeys to mice, which led to a "changed virus that protected monkeys and prevented their paralysis if used in time."[18] The obituary made no mention of his support by the KF or his alliance with Kenny.

Kenny's death also offered physicians the opportunity to get in the last word on her contributions. In a pointed juxtaposition *JAMA* paired its 4 line obituary with a 4 page study of follow-up examinations of 346 Kenny-treated patients from the Minneapolis General Hospital written by Miland Knapp and 2 younger physicians from Minneapolis. Knapp's study found that 69.1% of the patients were now "essentially normal" and that early treatment decreased "the necessity for operation and the incidence of scoliosis" but also detailed the various orthopedic operations and apparatus 8.3% of the patients required. The *Journal*'s "Poliomyelitis" items in its subject index for the first 3 months of 1953 had only 20% on treatment and around 35% on preventive research such as gamma globulin and immunization.[19] In contrast, the *British Medical Journal* published 2 separate full obituaries. The first noted that the controversy over Kenny's unorthodox methods had filled "many pages of this and other journals." In a character assessment that probably pleased neither her allies nor her critics, the *Journal* called her "a shrewd, combative woman, intolerant of opinions which conflicted with her own [but also]... a woman of deep compassion and one who sought no great reward for herself."[20] In an unusual separate obituary in the same issue, Oxford orthopedist Herbert Seddon argued that Kenny had gone astray when she had elevated muscle spasm "into an important aspect of the pathology of the disease." The hot packs used to ameliorate "this so-called spasm" were too often used in "a drill... that was elaborate, extensive, and tiresome." Her theory of mental alienation, further, was just a new name for a variety of functional disorders, which, despite her protests, had no "permanent influence in the designing of remedial exercises." In Seddon's view Kenny's "initial small store of knowledge" had been expanded as the result of "increasing contact with able medical people." Had she been content "to talk about treatment without embarking on speculations about pathology" and "had she been a little kindlier [sic] and more tolerant," Seddon concluded, "she might now be regarded as the Florence Nightingale of orthopaedics, or at any rate of that part of it concerned with poliomyelitis."[21]

Seddon's reference to "the Florence Nightingale of orthopaedics" reflected a consciously gendered notion of what made an appropriate female contribution to medical science. Seddon had elsewhere compared Kenny unfavorably to 2 "other great humane women of our time" Dame Agnes Hunt and Lady Marjory Allen. Hunt, a disabled nurse, had collaborated with British orthopedist Sir Robert Jones and worked with tubercular children and disabled veterans; Allen, a landscape architect, had founded an international organization for early childhood education and was working with UNICEF and UNESCO. These 2 women, Seddon believed, were "every bit as tenacious, every bit as impatient of red tape and professional complacency" as Kenny had been. But they had finally got their way by "cheerful persistence and by inspiring that greatest of all reforming forces— affection." Kenny, in contrast, was never content to let an idea "sink in and do its work." She "hammered everybody with the whole powerful apparatus of modern propaganda" and, worse, claimed "she never made a mistake."[22] It was Kenny's stubborn demand for scientific legitimacy, Seddon believed, that had alienated potential male allies who preferred insightful women contemporaries who were cheerful, patient, and humble.

Kenny's stubbornness and impatience were highlighted in many obituaries. "She never won for her methods or theories the unconditional approval that she and her many supporters believed them to deserve," the *Lancet* pointed out, and "she did not realize that her own enthusiasm could go against her." Still she had whipped up a global interest in polio treatment, and her ideas "aroused discussion and controversy all over the world."[23] In the *Medical Journal of Australia* Kenny's antagonist Jean Macnamara argued that progress in medicine came from the efforts of 2 types of people: those who "patiently observe and record" like physical therapists Florence and Henry Kendall and others who "battle for the application of knowledge to the individual patient." Kenny's "forceful personality" may have helped to destroy complacency but, Macnamara believed, her contribution would have been greater if she had shared "her gifts of patience, pertinacity and attention to detail" with those working for the same objectives. Still, Macnamara was not surprised Kenny had chosen the path of a celebrity. "Fame, travel, press interviews, her book, the film controversy were her choice, and perhaps suited her temperament better." Macnamara conceded that publicity around Kenny's work had led to a welcome "loosening of purse strings" for physical therapy and rehabilitation facilities. As for her contribution to polio science, Kenny had "provided a stimulus to research workers to abandon the servile adherence to the theory of essential neurotropism of the virus."[24]

Kenny's clinical skills as well as her sense of humor were featured in the few obituaries that defined her primarily as a nurse. The *British Journal of Nursing* praised her as one of nursing's "most brilliant colleagues."[25] Mildred Elson's obituary of Kenny in the *Physical Therapy Review* was pointedly upbeat, giving a sense that Elson had known Kenny as a person as well as a clinician. Kenny had been "a very warm person [with]...a delightful and, at times, mischievous sense of humor." Elson was sure that "the controversy and furor" that Kenny had aroused would be forgotten. In any case it had "stimulated everyone to do a better job and the patient [had] benefited." Her visit to Minneapolis, along with the Kendalls and other therapists in January 1941, had been "thought provoking." True, there were differences of opinion, but it was just the "good give-and-take which is enjoyed between professional colleagues." The therapists had found Kenny "a charming and dedicated person" and had been intrigued by her hats. For Elson the central issue was patient care and patient perspective. Patients loved Kenny, she recalled, and appreciated "her kindness, reassuring manner, and skillful hands." "Her name will continue to be associated with the treatment of polio throughout the world [and]...for her courage and devotion to the polio patient."[26] Few of the physicians who memorialized Kenny after her death commented on patients at all, but for physical therapists the changes that Kenny's work had made to the routine care of patients were impressive and worth remembering. What Elson could not imagine in 1953 was that attention to polio's clinical care would almost totally disappear for at least 3 decades.[27]

FADED CELEBRITY

Kenny's status as a celebrity, admired and feted by movie stars, largely disappeared with her death as well. Buffeted by the disruption of the Hollywood studio system and the growing popularity of television, movie attendance dropped significantly.[28] McCarthyism also convulsed the Hollywood community with attacks on politically and sexually suspect people. As allegiances made decades earlier were used to insinuate political suspicions, movie stars were wary of the controversy surrounding Kenny and her work. Thus, screenwriter Mary McCarthy assured a journalist in 1953 that while Kenny had been a liberal and supported the Labor Party in Australia she had always "hated Communism."[29]

During the 1950s Rosalind Russell was still a member of the KF board, but a second stage of her career in which she moved from Hollywood to Broadway allowed her to move away from Kenny-related activities.[30] Although Russell spoke of Kenny's importance to American and global medicine immediately after Kenny's death, she waited until the end of her life to discuss her own support of Kenny's work in any detail. Her autobiography *Life Is a Banquet* appeared in 1977, a year after her death from breast cancer. In a brief but not apologetic section on Kenny, Russell fondly recalled meeting her for the first time at an airport in California as she "stepped off that plane wearing that Aussie hat and a sad-looking black dress, which was half of her wardrobe." Russell had never forgotten the ways that some jealous and suspicious doctors had tried to trick her, although, she maintained, "good doctors liked Sister Kenny." Like the other commentators in this period Russell linked Kenny to the Salk vaccine: "If she hadn't gone stamping through the world, stirring people up, we'd have been a whole lot longer getting the Salk vaccine."[31]

KENNY AS A CHILDREN'S HERO

Fittingly, Kenny's legacy fared best in the literature of the group she devoted herself to most: children. "Just before she died she prayed...first, that her treatment might spread throughout the world; and second, that someone might find a vaccine to abolish polio forever," wrote the author of *Lives to Remember* (1958), a children's series that included Louis Pasteur and Helen Keller.[32] She lived on in other children's books as well. In *The Girl Book of Modern Adventures* as "The Nurse from Australia" Kenny proudly recalls the moment when President Roosevelt (still the most celebrated polio survivor) invited her to lunch at the White House and thinks "If only I could have treated him...he need never have suffered!"[33] Her oddity as not exactly a nurse meant that some children's writers ignored her. *Nurses Who Led the Way* (1957) featured Edith Cavell, Mary Breckenridge, and Lillian Wald, but not Kenny.[34] But she stayed visible in books such as *Six Great Nurses* (1962) and *Heroic Nurses* (1966) in which she appeared along with Florence Nightingale, Mary Breckenridge, Clara Barton, and Edith Cavell.[35]

TRUTH SEEKING: WHO WAS KENNY?

A few years after Kenny's death, science writer Victor Cohn, who had covered Kenny's story many times when she lived in Minneapolis, decided that he would write a book about her. A 1941 graduate of the University of Minnesota and a war veteran fascinated by science and its possibilities, Cohn felt that he knew her story well. In 1953 he wrote "Angry Angel," a series about Kenny for the *Minneapolis Tribune*, which was widely syndicated.[36] Then, like other science writers of his time, Cohn got caught up in one of the biggest science stories of the 1950s: the Salk polio vaccine. In 1955 he wrote a series of articles on the March of Dimes leading to its funding of the Salk vaccine. The *Tribune* published the series under the title *Four Billion Dimes*.[37] The response to both series convinced Cohn that a full-length study of Kenny would engage a wide audience.

Cohn had already interviewed 2 of the leading figures in this story: Morris Fishbein and Basil O'Connor. Fishbein, no longer the general secretary of the American Medical Association (AMA) or the editor of *JAMA*, had become a productive editor, writer, and lecturer. He was eager to put Kenny in her proper place as a fraud. One of his file cabinets, he wrote in a letter to O'Connor with whom he remained friends, had "a big fat special folder dealing only with Sister Kenny."[38] Fishbein told Cohn that most of Kenny's claims were "pure poppycock." Her methods had been given "a thorough trial" and been rejected. Fishbein had long experience fighting antivivisectionists, cancer entrepreneurs, and left-wing physicians who promoted government health insurance. Women, in Fishbein's view, were the worst of these: sentimental about animals and children, dramatic in their horror of the routine work of the laboratory and the clinic, and hysterical enough to be able to sway public opinion for patently false causes. Thus, he dismissed Kenny as having "the drive and the enthusiasm of a woman like [Christian Science founder] Mary Baker Eddy," an analogy he considered a serious insult.[39]

O'Connor bluntly described Kenny to Cohn as a publicity seeker. In his opinion, "she had no more use for the crippled children than for a broken-down elephant." Her constant use of the term Sister, he believed, had created the impression that she was a Catholic. And her gender had fooled otherwise hard-boiled commentators. Early on, O'Connor recalled, he had asked Basil "Stuffy" Walters, the executive editor of the *Minneapolis Tribune*, why he was so easy on her. In the earthy slang of a newspaper man, Walters had replied that "she's a skirt and we're afraid of a skirt." In the 1940s the March of Dimes had tried in vain to evaluate her method; now, O'Connor said, "we know not to evaluate anybody's method." Asked whether he had snubbed Kenny at a reception at the 1951 Copenhagen polio conference, O'Connor admitted he had and added "and I'm proud of it."[40]

Cohn took a leave of absence from the *Tribune* in 1955 to give himself time, as he told potential informants, "to be set straight on any points that were wrong in my previous articles."[41] He first traveled to California where he talked to lay supporters and sympathetic physicians who had established the El Monte Kenny Hospital. Orthopedist Robert Bingham assured Cohn that he had always accepted Kenny's theory that polio was a systemic disease and that the virus "affected all tissues." Bingham had "never known a physician anywhere in the world" who had understood polio so thoroughly. With her keen observation Kenny could tell just by watching a child breathe how much paralysis there would be in the chest wall and how much in the neck and throat. She could predict whether a child would recover without use of an iron lung and was "very, very seldom wrong." She had "a tremendous native intelligence" and was independent and resourceful. Her ideas, Bingham stressed, had been based on what was "probably the most careful examination" of patients in the history of polio.[42] While Cohn was somewhat interested in clinical issues he was already convinced that Kenny had made no sense scientifically. He confirmed his belief by conducting a phone interview with John Enders who assured Cohn that no researcher had shown that the polio virus attacked the muscles or had "any local action of any sort." Enders also denied that he had been influenced by

Kenny's theories, declaring that her statements "certainly had no effect on the work in my laboratory."[43]

John Pohl, whom Cohn considered "strong looking" with a Yankee face and "deep good manners," tried to place his own loyalty to Kenny in a wider medical and cultural context. Her concept of polio, he told Cohn, made sense to her and to physicians in Minneapolis, but she "just couldn't get it across to anyone else." There was much she did not know, he conceded; when she said that spasm came from the spinal cord, "that was wrong." Cohn tried to push his argument that Kenny was not properly trained, but Pohl was not convinced. He agreed Kenny had probably not been a graduate nurse, reflecting that when she talked about her past she "never got down to cases" and never talked about her training "as a nurse will." But, Pohl stressed, the most crucial issue was her clinical acumen: Kenny "saw the spasm, the doctors did not." She was a fine diagnostician, clever enough to see whether a muscle "was or [was] not in spasm." If she could see a little movement in a muscle she could get a child to use his or her belly muscles and sit up, which Pohl felt was how she had first impressed Miland Knapp.[44]

Then Cohn organized a 5-week trip to Australia. With an eye to history he warned Mary and Stuart McCracken that the topic of Kenny might soon lose public interest for "polio, as a disease, is on the way out." While he did not mean to minimize the current problems with paralyzed children, in his opinion "the next few years is the time when the history of polio is going to be written."[45]

Cohn's "Angry Angel" series had alienated Julia Farquarson, one of Kenny's sisters, who warned Cohn that she had advised her relatives not to cooperate with him.[46] In vain did Cohn protest that he believed Kenny "was a *great* woman" who had made a great contribution. When he tried to convince Farquarson that his "impartial" investigation would show the "human" side of Kenny in contrast to the *Sister Kenny* movie "which presented only the sugar-coated side," he found himself in another morass.[47] The movie, Farquarson retorted, had "very truthfully portrayed the Sister Kenny of those earlier years," and neither Cohn nor any other American had "the slightest knowledge of . . . [the] charming personality of the Sister Kenny of those days," for she had been "loved and trusted by all whom she ministered for."[48]

Farquarson and her side of the family remained uncooperative, but other relatives and friends in Australia agreed to be interviewed. A number of Australian physicians who had known Kenny were eager to set the record straight.[49] Cohn's typed summaries of all of these interviews are in the Minnesota Historical Society. To each summary Cohn added his own comments, relating each informant to a type familiar to him from his newspaper work. Just as he asked each man and woman to assess Kenny's character, so he judged their own character and tried to assess the extent of their bitterness, nostalgia, and honesty.

Many of his Australian informants defended Australia's tepid reception of Kenny as the result of Australian reserve. Some praised the appropriately conservative attitude of the Australian medical profession. Nonetheless, Cohn discovered, almost every physician claimed that he had played a major role in Kenny's career. An exception was University of Queensland pathologist James Duhig who called Kenny "a liar and impostor" compared to "really great" innovators such as Marie Curie and Florence Nightingale who were "scrupulously honest."[50] But in Cohn's assessment, Duhig was "a very vindictive and unreliable man, given to broad unscientific statements." Cohn had also heard from others that he was temperamental, a communist sympathizer, and had been arrested for drunk driving.[51]

Already knowledgeable about Raphael Cilento's past support of fascism, Cohn listened skeptically when Cilento claimed to have given Kenny her hot-packing and muscle exercises in the 1930s and to have suggested that she go to America in 1940. Cilento, Cohn concluded, "is rather a sad character these days—can't get a good job and is above a small one" and "nobody trusts him."[52] Brisbane physician Jarvis Nye, whom Cohn found a "lovely gentleman," said he had suggested that Kenny go to America, and Cohn was "much more inclined to trust him."[53] James Guinane, who had helped to write Kenny's first textbook, now felt that Kenny had not been "absolutely honest" and had known nothing about pathology. Although Cohn's book later reiterated both these points, Cohn disliked Guinane whom he saw as an "aging Irishman with dirty nails" who had "gone downhill."[54]

While Cohn kept the notes of all of his interviews, his project was twice seriously interrupted: first in 1960 when the Kenny Foundation was rocked by scandal and again in 1968 when he moved to Washington to become science editor of the *Washington Post*. The book did not come out until the mid-1970s.

THE KF AFTER KENNY

In 1958 Marvin Kline went on a nationwide tour with Al Capp, creator of "Li'l Abner" and the KF's new featured celebrity. As part of its role as a research philanthropy, the KF awarded 19 research grants to American scientists to study neuromuscular diseases including arthritis, amputation, and cerebral palsy.[55] In 1959, in a strange bookending moment, *Reader's Digest* published an article by Kline describing Kenny as the most unforgettable character he had ever met. Illustrated by a sketch based on Yousuf Karsh's photograph of Kenny in pearls and a cape, Kline placed her firmly in the past. In an "imperious feminine voice" she had demanded he and other city officials open wards for her child patients and then had brow-beaten doctors until they agreed to move their patients into her Institute. Her assertive attitude was the result of the "vast misfortune of being both a woman and a non-doctor who had discovered a vital medical truth." He also praised her as a healer who "knew that she had a sublime gift, and that crippled children needed her." Kline noted almost casually that there was no solid evidence that Kenny had "ever graduated from a formal nursing course." This did not mean she was not well informed or without professional standing, however: she had attended nursing school and for many years had "studied medical books voraciously and sought out doctors in their free moments to ask them questions." The KF had been established, he claimed, to deal with the financial problem of so many patients coming to the Institute and in response to Kenny's declaration that she would "not permit anyone to pay for this treatment." The Kenny method—"one of the most effective treatments for polio"— was still flourishing, Kline continued, and both clinical and vaccine research were part of the KF's ongoing program. Indeed, the KF had helped to finance testing of a new live-virus vaccine that "may eradicate polio once and for all." In a tone of self-sacrifice, perhaps reminiscent of Kenny's own, Kline described devoting himself to this cause. He had "rid myself of my remaining business interests, to devote all my energies [to the KF] . . . remembering her, I could not do otherwise."[56] Within a year of his *Reader's Digest* paean, however, the legacy that Kenny had tried so fiercely to shore up and Kline's own reputation were in tatters.

In the early 1950s Kline had become involved with Empire Industries of Chicago, a professional fundraising company owned by Abraham and David Koolish. Board member James Henry, Kenny's friend, suspected that Kline had been using KF funds to pay for his own golf club memberships and vacations and noticed that some of the Koolishes' solicitation appeals had not been approved by the board. When Henry spoke up he was asked to leave the board.[57] The Koolishes were indicted for mail fraud in 1955, but Kline assured the board (falsely) that New Century, the company with which the KF now worked, was not run by the Koolishes.

Kline also had the board approve substantial raises for himself: his salary during the 1950s increased from $25,000 to $48,000. As rumors of fiscal improprieties intensified, Minnesota's attorney general Miles Lord began to investigate Kline and the KF, and when Lord became U.S. district attorney the investigation was taken over by Walter Mondale, the state's new attorney general.[58]

When the investigation became public in March 1960 Kline resigned and was replaced by Edgar Huenkens, formerly the KF's medical director.[59] Local citizens began to protest this "betrayal of public confidence and debauchery by trusted officials" and argued that claims by KF board members that they did not know what was going on were no excuse.[60] In vain did an editorial in the *Minneapolis Tribune* remind the public of the KF's "vastly important and beneficial work."[61] Soon the story was appearing in the Chicago press and then the *New York Times*.[62] Kline was indicted for grand larceny by a local jury who recommended that all KF board members resign as they had been neglectful and shown "a grave lack of responsibility."[63]

The scandal continued to reverberate through the local and national press. With headlines like "Kline Gets 10 Years In Kenny Fund Fraud," Kenny's name was linked to signs of greed and corruption. Each time reporters noted the "lavish gifts" that KF officials had accepted—including paid trips to the World Series, fishing vacations, television sets, and luggage—the implication was clear that these officials had deprived disabled children and adults of medical care and betrayed the trust of patients and the public.[64] District and federal judges spoke harshly of KF board directors' neglect and indifference, and the issue became part of a wider debate about voluntary health and welfare agencies that duplicated services and fundraising.[65] As a result of the scandal, the Minnesota legislature required charities to make full annual reports to the state's attorney general.

In September 1960 the KF board announced a further reorganization with the appointment of a new KF head: Frank Krusen, now senior consultant at the Mayo Clinic.[66] Taking a leave of absence from the Mayo Clinic, Krusen closed down the KF offices in the Foshay tower and hired a respected accounting firm to audit the KF books. His success in shoring up the KF's reputation was demonstrated in December 1961 when the federal Office of Vocational Rehabilitation located one of the nation's first federally funded rehabilitation centers at the Institute.[67]

After 3 years Krusen retired.[68] His successor was Paul M. Ellwood, Jr. who had been appointed head of the Institute's inpatient services in 1953. Ellwood was eager to help turn the Institute from a polio hospital into a rehabilitation center. In his view Kenny's work had been "too much a cult," and he had particularly disliked the Kenny technicians' resistance against the use of tracheotomies and iron lungs. When the "Blue Girls" went home in the evening, he recalled, the interns gave some patients tracheotomies and placed others in iron lungs.[69] In 1965 the KF changed its name to the American Rehabilitation Foundation, and the remnants of Kenny's connection to it were sloughed off. Ellwood assured reporters that the 1960 scandal had figured only partly in the name change. If KF officials had changed the name in 1960, he explained, "it might have appeared we were doing nothing more than putting a false front on the old structure."[70]

KENNY REMEMBERED

During the late 1960s a few memoirs mentioned Kenny. In his 1969 autobiography Morris Fishbein pointed out that Kenny had no formal education and had never become "what is called a registered or graduate nurse," although she had tried domestic work and had worked as a governess. She had been unable to establish her ideas in Australia, he claimed, and speculated that perhaps this was due to her personality or perhaps her "disregard for medical custom." Her work, Fishbein admitted vaguely, led to further intensive studies of polio's "pathological changes." He did not mention any of Kenny's theories; in his view she was an untrained empiric who "knew nothing really of anatomy, physiology, pathology or any other of the basic sciences on which scientific medicine rests." "Confronted with an emergency... she tried what she thought would help, and it did, but she never did know why it helped." He made much of her character and body. She was a big woman who wore a 3-cornered hat and "came to luncheons and dinners invariably late so as to make a grand entrance." Fishbein made himself a central figure in Kenny's career. Kenny had stopped to see him any time she passed through Chicago and never hesitated to call him long distance "at whatever time of the day or night, to recount her resentment at some actual or fancied slight or difference of opinion." Unlike his statement to Cohn in 1953, Fishbein now felt that her work had *not* been properly evaluated. Repeating a widely held belief among many physicians about the hysteria around polio epidemics, Fishbein argued that "the psychological effects of those so burdened by emotion were such as to make further controlled evaluation of her techniques difficult if not impossible." As a medical popularizer who no longer had the power to control the portrayal of medical professionals in any media, Fishbein blamed both Kenny and the press for the adulation around her. Her celebrity reputation in the 1940s was a typical example of how "most of the press liked to portray... another unprofessional investigator and discoverer being denied and overwhelmed by medical authority."[71]

In 1967, historian Saul Benison published a study of virologist Thomas Rivers, a book that was honored with the American Association for the History of Medicine's William Welch medal the following year.[72] Rivers, who had died in 1962, was a leading virologist at the Rockefeller Institute for Medical Research. He had been an NFIP advisor since the late 1930s, and was later the foundation's medical director and then Vice President for Medical Affairs. He was also one of the 1958 Polio Hall of Fame scientists.[73] Rivers was uncompromising in his assessment of Kenny, whom he saw as an ignorant woman who pretended to understand complex medical science. He admitted to Benison, "I couldn't stand her... She had no notion of the nature of poliomyelitis as a virus disease and certainly knew nothing about its pathology. For example, she thought it was a disease of the muscle. The kindest thing I can say about her ideas of physiology and anatomy is that they best be forgotten." Rivers had lived through America's polio epidemics and knew he had to say something about the efficacy of her methods. Reluctantly he told Benison "there is no denying, however, that she got effects, and I think that on the whole she did some good."[74]

In his 1968 autobiography Melbourne virologist Francis MacFarlane Burnet recalled that "being an Australian I had heard much of Sister Elizabeth Kenny." He had met Kenny about a year before her death and he described the tremor in her right arm and her "heavy-fleshed Irish face" that had looked tired. Kenny was now almost forgotten by the world, Burnet admitted, but "there was an air of greatness about her and I shall never forget that meeting." She had been "strong-willed and persuasive enough" to have many of her ideas adopted in a Queensland hospital; in the United States she "became an increasingly influential figure ... as well as a gadfly to the medical profession ... removing medical apathy and defeatism about the residual effects of polio." Her most important contributions, Burnet wrote, had been to show paralyzed children how to make the best use of what functional muscles they had, to demonstrate to their parents that something active was being done, and to destroy "the orthodox superstition of immobilization by splinting." He had disliked her extreme claims, recalling that she had told him that a primary site of viral infection could be the skin and offering the example of a patient who she had known would die within 48 hours as his skin was "contracting all over."[75]

John Pohl did not write about Kenny after her death. During the 1960s he was interviewed by Victor Cohn a number of times and also read and commented on a draft of Cohn's manuscript. Pohl called one draft "a superb piece of work" and praised Cohn for capturing what he saw as the main theme: that "this was a battle of concepts: The Kenny vs. the orthodox." After all, he reminded Cohn, Kenny had "frankly stated she did not know the cause of spasm." In a letter to Cohn in 1967 Pohl claimed that Kenny had got the idea of peripheral disease from himself. While her hope of "scientific interest or investigation" had been sincere, when none had developed "she knew she was doomed."[76] This was a strange rethinking of the fierce debates around Kenny's ideas, but perhaps Pohl could tell that Cohn had already made up his mind about the scientific validity of Kenny's ideas.

Yale epidemiologist John Paul's *A History of Poliomyelitis* was published in 1971, the year he died. Paul's Yale Polio Unit, funded by the NFIP since the 1930s, had produced crucial serological studies of polio, and like Rivers, Paul was one of the NFIP's Hall of Fame scientists. His *History* dealt awkwardly with polio's clinical care, ignoring the work of nurses and physical therapists.[77] Primarily a virology researcher, Paul believed that most orthopedic care—splints, braces, corrective surgery, and electrical treatments— lacked "real efficacy" and impressed patients mainly "from a psychological point of view." Kenny was fortunately able to break through the "the slough into which it [polio care] had sunk in the 1930s," he said. Paul described the 1944 AMA report as an attempt by "prominent American orthopedic surgeons ... to discredit Miss Kenny's reputation—almost, it would seem, out of professional jealousy."[78]

Kenny, Paul noted sadly, had attracted fanatic allies among "both lay and professional people" who believed "there was something magical in her personality as well as in her treatment." Kenny herself had exacerbated this situation, for the aggressive way she had presented her ideas had been "calculated to antagonize physicians." She had also forsaken her appropriate role as nurse and clinical assistant: "instead of sticking to her daily work in the hospital wards, caring for and rehabilitating her patients, work for which she was eminently qualified, she became busy with all the paraphernalia of public campaigns and press agents, who, needless to say, loved a fight." Uncomfortable with the way the NFIP had forced scientists to participate in its propaganda efforts, Paul argued that the reputation of physicians was apt to become tarnished when they engaged in "medical polemics"; thus, he concluded, "how much more tarnished is the image of a nurse who, forsaking her natural duties, becomes similarly embroiled."[79]

Physical medicine physicians also sought to lay Kenny to rest. In a special 1969 commemorative issue of the *Archives of Physical Medicine and Rehabilitation* entitled "Our Experience With Poliomyelitis," Robert Bennett recalled "this controversial woman, [who] through the sheer force of her personality and her words, made us defend and reconsider methods of treatment popular at that time and, by so doing, changed some of our ideas regarding early care." Bennett was convinced, however, that "the 'Kenny method'... reflected more the effect of our clinicians upon Sister Kenny than her effect upon them," especially the influence of the physiatrist Miland Knapp.[80] Bennett's article was followed by a reprint of a 1932 article by Walter Galland, a little known orthopedist. Galland, the journal's editor noted, had used terms like "spasm" and warned that treating spasm with splints would increase a patient's pain "tremendously." Thus, the editor pointed out delightedly, "long before Sister Elizabeth Kenny arrived in America... and began espousing the ideas which created quite a national uproar, Dr. Walter Galland's enlightened views... appeared in our journal."[81]

The *Archives* also reprinted 2 more articles: the AMA committee's "Evaluation of the Kenny Treatment of Infantile Paralysis" from *JAMA* in 1944 and Knapp's article "The Contribution of Sister Elizabeth Kenny to the Treatment of Poliomyelitis," which had been first published in the *Archives* in 1955. Knapp sought to establish the proper distance between Kenny's work (and his own early enthusiasm for it) and the view of a reputable physical medicine expert. Kenny's "background in pathology and medical training left much to be desired," Knapp acknowledged, but "she was an excellent clinical observer with keen perception and... an intimate knowledge of muscle function." He praised her "well thought-out logical and physiological treatment" that had been appropriate "for the symptoms as she saw them." The enthusiasm of the general public had been spurred by her zeal, but her efforts to convert the medical profession to her way of thinking had been "a difficult and often an impossible task." She loved a fight—probably as a result of "her Irish temperament"—and she could not see "any point of view other than her own." Unfortunately, Knapp continued, newspapers had reported many of these arguments. Kenny had remained frustrated by what she saw as "her snail-like progress," but Knapp felt that "very few medical ideas have gained such rapid momentum and prestige and have affected the general treatment of a disease as completely as did hers."[82]

Finally, Kenny was remembered and commemorated in Congress. In the early 1970s Minnesota Senator Walter Mondale chaired congressional hearings on the mismanagement of charities and formally commemorated Kenny's birthday in the *Senate Record* praising "a very great lady of this century" who at first had been "dismissed rather coldly by our medical leaders, but then won them over and became an international heroine." Kenny deserved to be remembered, he told Congress: she was "a dynamic backwoods nurse" and her "spirit and philosophy" lived on at the Institute in Minneapolis, which, he added, was one of nation's leading rehabilitation centers.[83]

COHN'S CRUSADER

Cohn's book *Sister Kenny: The Woman Who Challenged the Doctors* finally appeared in 1975. Published by the University of Minnesota, *Sister Kenny* was a well-produced book, with 260 pages of text, many photographs, endnotes, and a 6 page bibliography. It was no feminist text. While its focus on a woman protagonist was distinctive, Cohn's portrayal fell into familiar tropes. Kenny had grown up in a matriarchy and her father had been quiet and dreamy. Irritatingly, Cohn chose to call Kenny "Liza" throughout (a name that he claimed her relatives used and she disliked), although he admitted that her closest friends and relatives had called her "Sister."[84]

Cohn recognized that many of his readers would no longer remember Kenny from popular magazines or the rarely shown movie. He tried to convey how impressive she had been: "in her prime...overpowering...five feet, eight inches tall, about 170 solid pounds...large, open brown eyes and a direct gaze that could turn to sharp steel." It was not only her physical appearance that had made her such an effective crusader. She had modeled herself, he believed, on "a sort of turn-of-the-century combination of Emmeline Pankhurst, Sarah Bernhardt, and Joan of Arc." The combination of a suffragist, a celebrated actor, and a religious crusader who had been burnt to death suggested a confusing mélange of feminist advocacy, dramatized acting, and evangelical fervor. She battled with men and enjoyed it, he wrote, and quoted her as saying "I won't let any man boss me."[85]

Cohn made much of what he thought of as his own great discovery: the fact that Kenny had lied about having graduated from a nursing school. This fact, Cohn claimed (incorrectly), was never uncovered by "even her worst enemies in the United States." It explained what he identified as a deep seated insecurity, leading Kenny to move "through life with the air of a duchess, half-cloaking the uncertainty of a self-trained outback nurse." While he considered her an innovator whose "one-woman revolution [had] helped start modern medical rehabilitation," he noted that her "honeymoon with the doctors" had been brief. In part this had been her fault, for, despite their making great changes in polio treatment, she had "demanded more change, in some cases justifiably, in some not." "In her own way," he argued, she was "a questioner like a Kepler or a Freud, a rebel whose life casts light on all times," and she "helped turn medicine toward a new aggressive approach to all injury."[86] Cohn remained unsure about how to explain the heights of adulation and the depths of hatred that Kenny inspired. He decided, finally, that a combination of her gender and her personality was the answer.

Cohn's *Sister Kenny* was reviewed in the national press, in history journals, and in *JAMA*. Audrey Davis, historian and curator at the Smithsonian, enjoyed Cohn's depiction of the controversial figure who had been "a celebrity of the highest rank" and suggested that Kenny's reception by the medical community "reveals much about the standards of American medicine in the 20th century." Davis wished Cohn had reflected more on the sources of clinical change and the role of scientific theory. "Empiricism," she argued, could not have been "sufficient to change medical procedures." Physicians would have expected "a theory to explain the results," but when Kenny's "theoretical rationale was unsatisfactory, the practice was shunned as unacceptable." Only Kenny's "incessant appeal[s]," according to Davis, had led her methods to be "incorporated into modern medical practice."[87]

In the mid-1970s women's history was only just emerging as a separate discipline. Another woman historian, Glenda Riley, praised Cohn's book as well researched and pleasantly written but complained that nowhere did Cohn "demonstrate that Kenny understood or advocated the philosophy of feminism." She felt that Cohn lacked "a feminist perspective," noting his "vaguely patronizing tone" and his use of "Liza" rather than "Kenny."[88]

The medical and popular press acclaimed Cohn's stories of Kenny and, like history journals, chose women to review it. "Today, her name is seldom mentioned," Marjorie Mehan, the *JAMA* reviewer, noted, but because "the emotions she aroused [had]...subsided...a relatively unbiased biography and evaluation is possible." Her method had directly opposed standard treatment, and her explanations "conflicted with accepted beliefs." But the American public was "panicky" and therefore "enthusiastic for any approach that offered new hope" and most physicians "gradually...modified their therapy to resemble hers."[89]

In the *Washington Post* Sonya Rudikoff argued that Kenny's "revolutionary treatment of polio [had] conquered medical skepticism." The reviewer compared the modern post-vaccine era to the years before antisepsis, antibiotics, modern surgery, and vaccines when what mattered were speed, proper nursing, diagnostic skill, and "exact obedience to prescribed regimens." A lack of formal training had not been crucial in such an old-fashioned era, and Kenny had learned to help patients with "intuition, swift care and meager knowledge." After the polio vaccines were developed Kenny's methods "and their inventor's dedication became antediluvian." Rudikoff was shocked by Cohn's description of the "incredible indifference, resistance and even active opposition to her methods by the medical establishment of her day." Such "cruelty, suspicion and hostility" among physicians, she concluded, had been "extreme and unworthy."[90]

Kenny's harshest critics saw Cohn's book as too mild. Jay Myers, for example, who had retired from the University of Minnesota in 1957 after over 40 years on the faculty, had written a "little review of the Kenny episode" that by 1971 had become a manuscript of around 70 pages. But after the publication of Cohn's book Myers grew discouraged, as he admitted to his friend and colleague Maurice Visscher.[91] During the KF scandal in 1960 he had gleefully offered a talk to his local medical society entitled "How Could It Happen" to explain how his and Visscher's "investigation" had revealed that Kenny was not a nurse and did not deserve the title Sister.[92] But the directors of the Hennepin County medical society had declined his offer, and although Myers was convinced that the KF's new board should learn that Kenny was "an impostor pure and simple," no local paper was willing to publish his material.[93] In Myers' longer manuscript, which he continued to work on during the 1970s, he castigated "the uninformed and misinformed public" that had been impressed by Kenny's propaganda. He remained frustrated by the limited impact of his and Visscher's anti-Kenny campaign, which he defended by explaining that he and his colleagues had sought to understand why Kenny "manifested no understanding of the mechanism" of polio and why she lacked the "knowledge, finesse and other well known qualities of a graduate nurse."[94]

In 1977 Myers sent a short version of his manuscript to Leonard Wilson, an historian of medicine at the University of Minnesota who was the editor of the *Journal of the History of Medicine and Allied Sciences*. He doubted whether Wilson and his editorial board would accept it, "especially after reading Vic Cohn's book," but hoped that if it was rejected perhaps the *Journal of Bone and Joint Surgery* might accept it.[95] Neither journal published his work, but Visscher continued to encourage Myers, reminding him that his material on "the Sister Kenny episode [must] be preserved for future scholars" and urging him to hold onto Wilson's letter of rejection to illustrate "the difficulty in getting matter like this published." Visscher suspected that timing might be another reason that this topic had not yet intrigued historians, telling Myers "I doubt that present day medical historians are as interested in the Kenny story as some may be a hundred years from now."[96] Myers died in 1978.[97] His Kenny manuscript was never published.

FORGOTTEN

By the time Cohn's book appeared, Kenny, as the author had suspected, was fully forgotten. The RKO movie was shown only occasionally on late night TV. Because the Salk and Sabin vaccines had dramatically decreased the number of America's polio cases, the El Monte Kenny hospital, among others, had closed.[98] When the disease was discussed at all, it was mainly as an historical artifact. In 1973 the second season of the TV show "The Waltons," which dramatized the life of a family in Virginia during the Great Depression, opened with a special 2-hour episode in which Olivia, the mother, was paralyzed by polio. Her children sought out an alternative therapy to help her walk again, in this case the Kenny method, which was presented as a kind of folk remedy promoted by a doctor, or as the *New York Times* described it in its review of the episode, "unorthodox treatments developed by a Sister Kenny in Australia."[99] In this episode, the paper noted, "polio is defanged, an occasion for family solidarity as the children, grandparents and father work together to bring hot packs to the bedridden mother."[100]

Aaron Klein's *Trial By Fury: The Polio Vaccine Controversy* (1972) did not discuss the care of polio patients at all. His chapter on "The End of Orthodoxy" was a study not of polio therapies but of polio science. The work of insightful epidemiologists and pathologists, Klein argued, should have overthrown some of the dearly cherished polio orthodoxies but was initially unsuccessful because "orthodoxies have a way of growing long roots." Klein also pointed out that during the 1940s "the 'significant breakthroughs' upon which the foundation fundraisers relied to inspire the public to greater giving were non-existent."[101]

The story of polio as a vaccine victory was solidified with the death of Basil O'Connor in 1972. The *Washington Post* depicted him as the man who had made the polio vaccines possible, and the *New York Times* called him "a singleminded and ingenious fund-raiser."[102] O'Connor, who remained head of the March of Dimes after the Salk and Sabin vaccines were developed, was still considered a shrewd philanthropic organizer, but after the death of Roosevelt and the rise of the Republican Party during the 1950s he was no longer a power broker. In 1965, his claim to have sacrificed his potential earnings as a Wall Street lawyer to take on the voluntary March of Dimes position as director was undermined when the *New York Times* revealed that since 1959 he had been receiving a salary of around $50,000, plus expenses, for the job.[103] His memorial service was attended by leading polio scientists; Jonas Salk declared that O'Connor had "made history happen."[104] But his legacy as a sacrificial administrator continued to be buffeted by reports of his love of the good life. Only a few months after his death a *Washington Post* commentator described O'Connor as "a dapper man who lived lavishly at his charity's expense and dealt lavishly with other people's money."[105]

GETTING THE LAST WORD: KENNY IN THE RECENT PAST

Florence Kendall never forgot Kenny. She and her husband Henry remained the bulwark of the anti-Kenny movement, and in 1956 Kristian Hansson praised them for having "opposed Sister Kenny's questionable idea of the pathology and the therapeutics of polio-myelitis."[106] Their textbooks *Muscles: Testing and Function* (1949) and *Posture and Pain* (1952) became the gold standard for musculoskeletal evaluation and treatment. The books were translated into many languages and were in print through 5 editions into the early twenty-first century.[107] After Henry died in 1979, Florence became a promi-nent lecturer and received 4 honorary doctorates. In 2002 she was chosen as a member of the Maryland Women's Hall of Fame, and the Maryland American Physical Therapy Association chapter named her "Physical Therapist of the Century."[108] She had always been suspicious of Kenny's bold claims and her florid style of self-promotion. Florence, by contrast, was known as "a drill sergeant [and]...perfectionist," quick to say "if you weren't taking the time to do it correctly, you were wasting your time—and the patient's time."[109]

In 1997 Kendall took the opportunity as the John Stanley Coulter Lecturer at the American Congress of Rehabilitation Medicine's annual meeting to revisit Kenny. The search for the best polio treatment, Kendall declared, had been hampered by politics and by the press. Recalling the 1941 meeting with Kenny in Minneapolis, Kendall did not mention the critical report she and her husband had written or the notes she had carefully taken at the end of each day, saying simply that "Henry and I had a brief, not uneventful, personal meeting with her." During the 1940s, which Kendall termed the Kenny Era, the press had praised Kenny lavishly, ignoring many problems with her work as well as more promising conservative work by orthopedic surgeons and physical therapists in Boston, Baltimore, Los Angeles, and Warm Springs. Her hot packs, for example, were usually so hot that a nurse or therapist needed tongs to pick them up. Although "adverse reactions" were seldom discussed, Kendall knew of a boy with a temperature of 108 who had been hot packed regardless and had "succumbed" (probably a reference to the patient described by Hansson in 1942). As Kenny condemned muscle testing there were no proper statistics to be able to assess her work, but a few studies had shown that her much vaulted recovery rates were no different from those of orthodox care. Kendall compared Kenny's work to that of her husband and herself who had "made continuous efforts to keep records that would provide meaningful information." Their therapy, sometimes called "traditional, conventional, or orthodox," had included the use of "moist foments" but also heat lamps, warm baths, half-shell (bivalve) plaster casts, foot boards, sand bags, pillows, rolled blan-kets, massage "used judiciously," and immobilization "in rare instances." "The combined power of politics, the press, and public passion that enveloped the controversy over Sister Kenny and her theories...nearly succeeded in blinding the truth," Kendall concluded, for "reason, perspective, and judgment can be sidetracked by the hysteria, helplessness, fear and anxiety caused by a devastating disease such as polio." After all, she reminded her audience of physical medicine experts, "we must hold fast to the sound principles that have been developed through years of scientific research."[110] In an era when polio care was barely remembered Kendall sought to turn Kenny into a misguided, unscientific innovator whose methods had fortunately been abandoned.

POLIO SURVIVORS REEMERGE

By the early 1980s polio epidemics in the United States were a thing of the past. Polio survivors had largely accepted the idea that their individualized physical therapy had enabled them to "conquer" polio or at least that their remaining disabilities would not get worse. Most specialized polio centers had closed, and physical medicine specialists now worked with conditions such as multiple sclerosis and cerebral palsy. Some adult survivors in visible apparatus such as wheelchairs or iron lungs published institutional newsletters, which satirized rehabilitation institutions and berated the "A.B." (able-bodied) world, advocating for full access to public facilities.[111] But outside of these few newsletters, polio survivors tended not to identify as a community.

Only in the mid-1980s, with the emergence of Post-Polio Syndrome (PPS), did polio gain a new cultural prominence. Frustrated at the growing weakness in muscles they had "normalized" through hard work—along with other symptoms such as joint pain, sensitivity to cold, and extreme fatigue—survivors began to seek medical advice. Physicians, they discovered, had rarely if ever treated a case of polio and did not see these symptoms as indicating anything other than the familiar signs of aging. Identifying this emerging syndrome and fighting for its proper diagnosis and treatment brought together polio survivors who had rarely thought of themselves as a distinctive community before. Dissatisfied survivors created a new specialty with a new set of experts, a few of them polio survivors themselves such as rehabilitation physician Lauro Halstead who organized the first international PPS conference at Warm Springs in 1984.[112] Survivors also began to develop a counternarrative about their previous polio care. The lessons taught by nurses, physical therapists, and physicians during the epidemic years, PPS activists now argued, had been counterproductive, for "pushing through" did not, as promised, bring stable physical achievements. New medical research suggested that polio survivors may have originally recovered muscle function through a process of branching or regeneration whereby surviving nerve cells developed extra branches (axonal sprouts) that reattached themselves to orphaned muscle fibers. Survivors developed PPS because these branches had been under heavy usage for some years and therefore were likely to age especially rapidly.[113] It was a devastating new science of muscle physiology.

As weakness forced many PPS survivors to move to crutches and wheelchairs, some became disability rights activists. Survivors turned newsletters into activist organizing tools. One, the *Toomeyville j. Gazette*, was named after a critic and rival of Kenny's. Ideas such as rights and citizenship buoyed this community whose members had previously been isolated not in institutions but in the self-perception of being "cured."[114] Polio survivors were key lobbyists for the Americans with Disability Act of 1990 and joined other activists to protest the proposed 1997 Roosevelt memorial that gave no indication of his disability, leading National Park Service officials to agree reluctantly to add a statue of Roosevelt seated in his wheelchair.[115]

As stories of Kenny resurfaced in PPS newsletters and memoirs, a newly harsh memorialization emerged. Survivors remembered the messiness and pain of hot packs and the careless and brutal way they had sometimes been applied. As one survivor recalled, "two times every day the therapists took hot packs out of the boiling water. The wool was too hot for them to touch so they used tongs. Every time they threw them on my bare legs I screamed." Others reported "they still feel fear when they smell wet wool."[116] In his memoir, Robert Hall, who had been a patient in an Omaha county hospital in 1949, described how the treatment cart, a shiny cylinder for heating the hot packs, emitted steam with such "an acrid, nauseating smell" that he had gagged. The packs were greased with a "jelly like substance, to keep you from burning" and then the "steaming and stinking" flannel pieces were placed on the skin. In his memory "the packs sapped my strength more than my polio did."[117] Dorothea Nudelman recalled other children on her polio ward screaming during hot pack treatment, and when she herself was burned she "sobbed out loud, wore myself out with it. The shock was as bad as the pain. I knew it could happen again."[118]

Although Kenny claimed to take pain seriously as a crucial symptom that must be relieved, pain was a constant part of polio therapy, whatever method was used, even Kenny's. Robert Hall's memory of pain came with the use of a footboard, which the Kenny method used to anchor the patients' feet, stretch the leg muscles, and "re-establish and...stimulate the normal standing reflexes."[119] "My hamstrings hurt more and more the tighter they became," Hall recalled. Kenny had instructed her technicians not to use the footboard until the leg muscles were no longer in spasm, but the distance between Kenny's prescriptive directions and routine hospital practice can be seen by the horrific example Hall reported of 2 men in his hospital ward who writhed in pain "back and forth across their beds with their feet anchored to their footboards."[120]

In 2002 psychophysiologist Richard Bruno published *The Polio Paradox*, which sought to explain why polio survivors had been reluctant to link their new symptoms to their former experience with polio. Among other factors, Bruno drew attention to examples of abusive care suffered by survivors years earlier. In shocking vignettes he quoted survivors who recalled nurses who slapped them and turned off an iron lung to punish them for crying and physical therapists who lay on a patient's knee to stretch the muscles in the leg while the patient screamed and who hit patients with rubber truncheons to make them stand up in their braces.[121] Not all mistreatment, of course, took place on wards using the Kenny method, but some was a specific result of her treatment.

According to Bruno, some of Kenny's techniques "to identify alienated muscles and...to get polio patients to 'take up their beds and walk' were painful, terrifying, and also dangerous." On occasion polio survivors recalled Kenny herself as one of the abusers; in one recollection in Bruno's book Kenny "slapped me on the face several times as a means of 'defining my reflex response.'"[122] This sounds quite different from the frequent descriptions of Kenny's gentle hands and her reminders to technicians that "the handling of the patient should always be so gentle that pain is never caused as this arouses fear in the mind of the patient and defeats efforts to get his cooperation."[123]

GLOBAL LEGACIES

In Australia in the 1980s both PPS communities and feminist scholars rediscovered Kenny. In 1983 feminist writers added Kenny to their list of Significant Australian

Women, drawing with relish a picture of a "boastful and tactless" nurse who "rebelled against so-called respectability" and sought acceptance "on her own terms." Her lack of formal education and her limited knowledge of anatomy had meant that some of her claims were "untrue and based on ignorance," and she antagonized the medical profession "by exaggerating her success." Unlike Australian physicians who had treated her with hostility, American physicians had "followed the lead of this self-taught, elderly nurse from outback Queensland," and as a result "polio treatment in the United States changed almost overnight." She had invented "a 'respectable' education and nurses' training course," but she had also "persevered against great odds to prove that 'experts' are not always right" and "brought about a revolution in medical treatment and relief and hope to people all over the world."[124] The authors also quoted Hollywood star Alan Alda who tried to make Kenny a feminist example, telling an Australian women's magazine in 1980 about his experience as a boy paralyzed by polio: "If it weren't for an Australian woman, Sister Kenny, I might not have lived... I got the Sister Kenny treatment—it was a very rough treatment with hot packs, but it kept me from becoming crippled. I might not have lived if Sister Kenny had not been inventive, creative and exploratory—all those things that men are supposed to be." What this interview did not mention, but appeared in his later memoirs, was that this Kenny treatment had been designed and practiced by his mother who had been inspired by Kenny's work as it was described in newspaper and magazine articles.[125] In 1995, writing as a nurse activist and a historical sociologist, John Wilson provided a scholarly examination of Kenny's work, arguing that many of her clinical insights were crucial for today's nurses.[126]

In 2004, drawing on material provided by a polio survivor, a biographer, a psychologist, a cultural historian, and Mary Kenny McCracken, the Australian Broadcasting Commission produced a radio show entitled "Sister Kenny: Saint or Charlatan?" Hers was "a name that rings few bells these days" historian Michelle Arrow acknowledged. She was "a self-trained Aussie bush nurse" who "claimed she had the answer to polio, and Americans believed her." On one side Betty Newell, daughter of Charles Thelander (chair of the 1938 Queensland Royal Commission), unsympathetically declared that "Kenny's egotism was incredible... I think she actually believed her own propaganda to a huge degree." Kenny had once sat at her father's dinner table, Newell recounted, and told the family "I put my hands on the little withered limb and I feel my power going into it," a statement that was followed by "silence at the dinner table." In a quite different tone Mary McCracken recalled that Kenny would say "Oh, it's useless to try and convince these blockheads," and Mavis Bosswell, a former patient at the Townsville clinic, praised Kenny's work, while admitting that in her case her muscles were too badly damaged to allow her to able to walk again. McCracken's effort to defend Kenny's significance could not overcome Arrow's presentation of Kenny as part charlatan, part messiah, and a "great self-publicist." University of Sydney psychologist Mary Westbrook, a polio survivor who had studied PPS, claimed that Kenny's theory of polio "was just medically, anatomically, physiologically so unsound." But like Cohn, Arrow was not interested in debating the scientific issues. She noted that while Kenny had never found a "cure" she had given patients "hope."[127]

Despite her dream of a lasting legacy Kenny has only a few memorials in Australia or the United States. In Warialda, her birthplace, the local Baptist church has a memorial stained glass window that was a gift from the KF. In Townsville, where she had her first government clinic, there is an Elizabeth Kenny playground and also a memorial sundial.

In Nobby, where she lived and later died, the town council and the Nobby branch of the Queensland Country Women's Association established a memorial park, and the house where she lived with her mother and Mary has been opened as a museum with a Kenny mural nearby.[128] To honor the fiftieth anniversary of her death, donors to the Australian Sister Kenny Memorial Fund, which has provided scholarships to nursing students with an interest in remote and rural nursing, established the Sister Elizabeth Kenny Chair in Rural and Remote Nursing at the University of Southern Queensland.[129]

There is no special museum in Minneapolis, although Kenny is still important for the city. In 1986 the Kenny Institute celebrated Kenny's 100th birthday, discovering too late her true 1880 birth date. During the celebration Institute employees wore "Kenny" clothes as they showed children an iron lung, an odd choice considering Kenny's long-standing dislike of that technology. Institute medical director Richard Owen, a polio survivor, recalled the time in the 1940s when Kenny had visited the Indiana hospital where he had been a teenage patient; she was "an awesome lady, large physically and in aura." Her ideas about early mobility and reeducation were still part of current therapies for spinal cord and head injuries, Owen said. While "she did not know the technical language of medical doctors" she made accurate observations, which others had missed, "that were totally correct."[130] Kenny's place in the region's history was cemented in 1989 when Leonard Wilson, who had rejected Myers' article on Kenny for the *Journal of the History of Medicine and Allied Sciences* in the late 1970s, devoted 8 pages to her in his book on the history of the University of Minnesota's medical school. Wilson portrayed Minnesota faculty members as hospitable and open-minded, especially dean Harold Diehl, who was "remarkably open to new ideas" and "a perceptive judge of character." In Wilson's assessment, "although her training was that of a nurse, Sister Kenny acted toward poliomyelitis as a Hippocratic physician" and university physicians "gave Elizabeth Kenny's methods a full and fair trial when no one else would, to the immeasurable benefit of poliomyelitis patients during the fifteen years or so before the introduction of polio vaccines." While noting that "many medical men were never reconciled to Sister Kenny, and attacked her repeatedly," he did not name Visscher or Myers.[131] *Healing Warrior*, a children's book about Kenny published in Minneapolis at the same time, defended Kenny's invention of professional credentials because she believed "doctors wouldn't listen to her if they knew she was not an educated, certified nurse."[132]

In 1992, Owen and other administrators organized a celebration of the 50th Anniversary of the Institute, calling on former patients and their families to offer their memories and honor "a pioneer in changing the way the world viewed polio treatment." The Institute featured an exhibit on Kenny, a portrait of Kenny at the Institute was restored, students at the city's Kenny School studied the Kenny story, and the state's governor declared December 17 Sister Kenny Day. The city hosted an Indoor Wheelchair Tennis Tournament along with the International Art Show by Disabled Artists, an annual event partly sponsored by the Institute.[133] In a local newspaper Henry Haverstock, Kenny's former patient, reminded readers that "doctors could never quite understand or accept her theories, but they could not dispute the evidence of their own eyes."[134]

It was during this anniversary that I first came to the Twin Cities to begin my research on Kenny. Like most Australians born in the late 1950s, I had not heard of her while I was growing up in Melbourne, but as a doctoral student in the United States working on the history of polio I became intrigued by the story of a woman from Australia who made her mark in America. In 1992 I had begun an academic position at Monash University in Melbourne and become committed to this project after a friend told me that Mary Kenny McCracken was alive, living in Queensland, and willing to be interviewed. I went up to see Mary and her husband Stuart and found them hospitable, a bit wary, and willing to show me papers and photographs that they had not yet given to the University of Queensland. The 5 years Mary had spent in the United States had left a profound impression on her; my dual background (born and raised in Australia but trained in American history in the United States) intrigued her.[135] Other informants such as Richard Owen and Margaret Opdahl Ernst, Kenny's first secretary in Minnesota, invited me to attend the Institute's celebrations. I was asked to interview the former patients who spoke warmly of their memories of being treated by Kenny and her technicians and described in matter-of-fact ways their experiences of living with PPS.

As the Twin Cities reclaimed Kenny as part of their heritage I became part of a small group of scholars and informants. I was interviewed in 2002 by Minnesota Public Radio for a program on Kenny in which Richard Owen, now retired from the Institute, remembered being horrified when Kenny undid the strings of his loin cloth in front of reporters.[136]

Civic boosters in Minnesota also found a place for Kenny. A 2007 pamphlet celebrating the state's 150th year anniversary described Kenny as "a force to be reckoned with— a statuesque woman with snow-white hair who did not suffer fools gladly" but also as someone whose "ideas are still in use around the world and in Minneapolis at the Sister Kenny Institute."[137] A special issue of *Daedalus* on Minnesota described Kenny as "one of the most prominent and popular people in Minnesota in the 1940s." "She invented her nursing credentials along with her nurse's costume," one commentator noted casually, and "affected an intimidating public presence, dramatic hats and all." "She was not a Minnesotan...but we claim her as partly ours."[138]

In 2010 Minnesota's History Theater put on the world premiere of "Sister Kenny's Children," sponsored partly by the Institute. Playwright Doris Baizley based her play on patient letters from the Minnesota Historical Society as well as Cohn's biography and Kenny's autobiography. Reviewers found the play inspiring and touching, but wondered about Kenny's fame: "Was she a publicity hound, or a private person who reluctantly used her celebrity status to further the cause of her treatment centers?"[139]

FINAL THOUGHTS

In her final autobiography *My Battle and Victory*, Kenny suggested that "in the history of medicine...it is not always the great scientist or the learned doctor who goes forward to discover new fields, new avenues, new ideas"; rather progress was sometimes sparked by God's "weakest minister."[140] Her contemporaries knew that she did not see herself this way at all. She wanted to be remembered as a major contributor to medical progress, as a world renowned scientist like Marie Curie. But by and large, that was a failed project. She was always an outsider with an exotic background, an Australian bush nurse who became an American celebrity. As an unmarried, middle-aged woman who fought unapologetically with male physicians and hospital administrators, Kenny did not fit neatly into any available cultural scripts. After her death, as in her life, she was often evaluated harshly, and she was largely written out of polio history along with disabled patients and clinical care. When she was remembered by polio survivors who experienced a reappearance of their symptoms, it was often with bitterness.

I have sought to present Kenny not as a heroic figure but as someone worth remembering. I hope this book adds another layer to the stories about Kenny: as a woman, a nurse, a clinician, and a scientific innovator. When historians seek to highlight a forgotten figure they are frequently accused of hagiography. I am uncomfortable with the notion of a commemorative biography, which tends to eschew ambiguity and to present the past from a single committed perspective.

This retelling of the story of Kenny and her work is framed as a way of understanding how American medicine was practiced in the 1940s and 1950s. Kenny's struggle to gain respect forced both professionals and the public to debate how to assess clinical practices and medical evidence. Clinical authority, the public knew, was considered a matter of social status and institutional affiliation. Yet Kenny loomed large, in every way. She demanded an upheaval of polio care and the gendered power relations in medical practice and its institutional structure. She insisted that her distinctive understanding of polio was the result of clinical research, a field she saw as the integration of clinical observations with laboratory evidence. She borrowed scientific terms she heard around her and peppered her lectures with them. But she cared little for nuance. Her skill was as an integrative thinker rather than as a theorist. She developed her theories in a kind of collage, where the pattern as a whole was more important than the intricate strands; she did not try to assess their intellectual coherency. Battered by skepticism and patronizing dismissal, she developed a professional persona in which the distinctions between her work and medical orthodoxy were crucial. She heard remarks that similarities between the old and the new implied a lack of originality, perhaps even the result of borrowing of others' ideas. Her defense of her work was sometimes illogical, but her arguments—irrational-sounding or not—were always placed behind the supple, strong bodies of her patients.

She also claimed a distinct way of assessing efficacy that threatened standard techniques. Thus, while orthodox practitioners saw muscle testing as a way to measure her patients' improvements and assess her claims of recovery, Kenny saw such testing as inaccurate and harmful to the patient. In a time before modern evidence-based medicine, she called for fair comparisons of her work with the methods of others, yet she rejected standard testing techniques in favor of demonstrations and testimonials and warned that she would not allow a single child to be subjected to the pain and suffering that the poor care of a controlled test would surely bring.

She demanded formal recognition for the changes she brought to the workings of polio institutions, and trained her technicians to see themselves as special experts deserving popular and professional respect. As one popular work in 1958 argued, in some hospitals the Kenny method "entered with a flourish through the front doors and with the official sanction of the board of governors"; in others her work was "admitted surreptitiously through the service door...in the rear, and the governing staff pretend[ed] to have no official knowledge of it."[141] Kenny's work helped to ensure that clinical care captured the public imagination—at least until the NFIP was finally able in the late 1950s to turn the polio story into a new story of men in white coats, saving children through carefully prepared scientific vaccines—and the American public demanded her methods be used to treat their children, and were not satisfied when physicians claimed to have "improved" it. In short, her legacy was complex at best and at times completely paradoxical.

Like her colleagues, patients, and critics Kenny shared a deep respect for the power and prestige of medical science. She relied on the expanding government investment in biomedical institutions; indeed she sometimes tried to redirect such investments when she believed they were made incorrectly. Yet she also found she was not alone when she excoriated antagonistic and patronizing physicians and attacked the ways that disabled patients were dismissed as troubling or clinically uninteresting and therefore as proper subjects for institutionalization. Kenny was no microbe hunter but she claimed insight into polio science through her understanding of the bodies of her patients. Bodies were central to her work and central to the extraordinary publicity around it. Until the Salk polio vaccine, images of a Kenny-treated fully recovered child overshadowed NFIP posters depicting children awkwardly leaving their crutches or wheelchairs.

It is difficult but I think crucial to explore the experience of polio in an era before the polio vaccines. Kenny's successes and failures tell us much about what was supposed to constitute good science and medical expertise in the 1940s and 1950s. The touching of bodies, the healing of pain, and the softening of twisted limbs were all elements in a familiar picture: a female clinician whose special nurturing skills enable her to devise methods to rehabilitate a suffering patient. But Kenny claimed professional authority in a distinctive vision of medical science where clinical observation could lead to scientific insight. Thus, she said she could look inside the paralyzed body and recognize the path of a deadly virus. No virologist considered these claims scientific. Yet in unclear and unacknowledged ways her claim that polio was not a neurotropic but a "systemic" disease became part of a complicated new picture of polio that emerged in the early 1950s and provided the foundation for the production of safe and effective polio vaccines. With the polio virus now understood as traveling through the bloodstream and lingering in the intestines, other versions of polio science have faded and with them the memory of the fierce battles over how this disease had been understood and why it had mattered.

Before the 1950s the care of disabled patients was seen as extraneous to the daily workings of most health facilities, other than "crippled children's homes." Children and adults with disabling conditions were often neglected or given orthopedic operations and then returned home to domestic supervision or sometimes to alternative healers. If their condition worsened it was usually blamed on careless or apathetic parents or on meddling therapists who practiced outside the orthodox profession. Kenny's attack on elite professionals and harmful medical therapies resonated with patients and families long suspicious of the standard care of polio and other disabling conditions, especially the sometimes horrific results of orthopedic surgery. Her refusal to fear what was considered the "infectious" acute stage or to avoid touching and trying to heal polio patients helped to ease the stigma of people with the disease. For children with birth injuries or cerebral palsy her work offered a source of hope, one that disappeared as she faded from American memory.

Finally, the story of Sister Kenny illustrates the fragility of memory. Forgetting is sometimes seen as a passive process rather than as an active one, but both remembering and forgetting are responses to the present. Recent studies of memorials have shown that communities were convinced that the choice of the moment to be memorialized must be informed by a moral message. The continuing popularity of documentaries, memoirs, and truth commissions evidences an unabated public interest in the production of memorials. Yet Kenny's legacy in many ways has been one of forgetting rather than memorializing. The scattered memorials to Kenny in Australia appear in small rural towns: Toowoomba, Townsville, and Nobby, not in Brisbane or Melbourne. In North America there are a few signs in Minneapolis, but not in Winnipeg, Los Angeles, New York City, or Washington, D.C. There was never a federal Kenny clinic, directed by a board of Kenny-inspired professionals and former patients, as Senator William Langer had envisioned.

Polio is an old person's disease now in North America; only in parts of the developing world, in countries with inadequate or disrupted vaccine programs, are children paralyzed today. How they are treated for their paralysis is simply not news. The eradication of polio in the Western world has served to make Kenny's contributions largely irrelevant to modern practitioners.

Exploring the history of clinical care has meant addressing the tricky issue of efficacy. I have often been asked if Kenny was right or wrong.[142] The many ways in which her story was continually reinvented by herself and others make it impossible to answer this question. In the story I tell here I emphasize the ways clinical practice has been pushed to the side, especially in histories of polio; the vaccine story has rendered disabled polio survivors and clinical therapy almost invisible. Clinical practices and clinical research, especially during the twentieth century, have not attracted many historians.[143] Without a comfortable niche and with the help of her many enemies Kenny has slipped out of public memory.

It was perhaps in response to his sense that this was happening that in October 1953 at a Congressional hearing on "causes, control, and remedies of the principal diseases of mankind," Charles Wolverton, still the powerful chair of the House Committee on Interstate and Foreign Commerce, returned to the issue of Kenny and her work. Wolverton assumed that most other Congressmen would remember her as he did from her appearance before his committee in 1948 where she had "made an indelible impression on all who were present...both as to her sincerity and her conviction and her ability." She was, Wolverton added, "a great character [who deserved]...all the honors that have been paid to her."[144]

Others, including epidemiologist Gaylord Anderson who was the dean of the University of Minnesota's recently established School of Public Health, were more critical. Anderson made clear in his testimony before Wolverton's committee that he did not "accept her explanation as to why it worked and [did]...not think many people today accept her explanation." And he brought up all the old arguments that nothing about her technique was really new. But, in conclusion, he spoke as a father, not a doctor: "If my daughter had polio, she would have the Kenny treatment."[145] It was the kind of conclusion Kenny would have liked.

NOTES

1. Mavis Kenny "The Children's Hospital," June 1 1960, [enclosed in] Joseph E. Shaner to Dear Board Member [1960], George E. Bennett Papers, #503122, Alan Mason Chesney Medical Archives, Johns Hopkins University, Baltimore.

2. Richard Carter *The Gentle Legions* (Garden City, NY: Doubleday, 1961), 92, 96.

3. "*I Knew Sister Kenny: The Story of a Great Lady and Little People* by Herbert J. Levine, M.D." [announcement] Christopher Publishing House, Cohn Papers, MHS-K; Herbert J. Levine *I Knew Sister Kenny: The Story of a Great Lady and Little People* (Boston: Christopher Publishing House, 1954).

4. Jacob von Heine, Oskar Medin, Ivar Wickman, Karl Landsteiner, Jonas Salk, Thomas Rivers, Charles Armstrong, John Paul, Albert Sabin, Thomas Francis, Joseph Melnick, Isabel Morgan, Howard Howe, David Bodian, John Enders, Franklin Roosevelt, Basil O'Connor; "Leaders in Campaign Against Polio Are Honored at Warm Springs" *New York Times* January 3 1958.

5. Dorothy and Philip Sterling *Polio Pioneers: The Story of the Fight Against Polio* (Garden City, NY: Doubleday, 1955), 47, 76.

6. Richard Carter *Breakthrough: The Saga of Jonas Salk* (New York: Pocket Books, 1967); John Rowland *The Polio Man: The Story of Dr. Jonas Salk* (New York: Roy Publishers, 1961); John Rowan Wilson *Margin of Safety: The Story of the Poliomyelitis Vaccine* (London: Collins, 1963); Greer Williams *Virus Hunters* (New York: Knopf, 1959); Robert Coughlan *The Coming Victory over Polio* (New York: Simon & Schuster, 1954).

7. "Polio Fund Plans Arthritis Drive" *New York Times* July 13 1958; "March of Dimes Picks Poster Child" *New York Times* November 5 1959; David Rose "March of Dimes Poster Children/ National Ambassadors Personal Medical Conditions" October 4, 2005, MOD.

8. Vivian R. Humphrey "Your Journal and Mine" *California Journal of Physical Therapy* (September 1948) 4: 3; see also Humanitarian, letter to editor, *Toowoomba Chronicle* December 2 1952.

9. "Sister Kenny Dies; Fought Polio 43 Years" *Chicago Daily Tribune* November 30 1952.

10. "Sister Kenny" *New York Times* December 1 1952.

11. Jungeblut to Dear Mr. Kline, December 2 1952, Box 2, Ke-Kn, Jungeblut Papers, NLM.

12. Jungeblut to Dear Sir [Editor, *New York Times*], December 2 1952, Box 2, N, Jungeblut Papers, NLM.

13. Waldemar Kaempffert to Dear Dr. Jungeblut, December 4 1952, Box 2, Ka, Jungeblut Papers, NLM.

14. Jungeblut to Dear Mr. Kaempffert, December 19 1952, Box 2, Ka, Jungeblut Papers, NLM. On KF funding of Jungeblut's research at Columbia see Marvin Kline in *Health Inquiry (Poliomyelitis): Hearings before the Committee on Interstate and Foreign Commerce House of Representatives Eight-Third Congress First Session on The Causes, Control, and Remedies of the Principal Disease on Mankind* [Part 3 October 6 1953] (Washington, DC: Government Printing Office, 1953), 609–610.

15. Claus Jungeblut to Dear Mr. Kline, December 2 1953, Box 2, Se-Sm, Jungeblut Papers, NLM; Franz J. Kallmann to Dear Claus [Jungeblut], June 21 1954, Box 2, Ka, Jungeblut Papers, NLM.

16. Fred R. Klenner to Dear Dr. Jungeblut, June 1 1954, Box 2, Ke-Kn, Jungeblut Papers, NLM.

17. Claus Jungeblut in *Health Inquiry (Poliomyelitis)* [Part 3 October 6 1953], 634–638; see also Claus W. Jungeblut and Gonzalo Bautista Jr. "Further Experiments on the Selective Susceptibility of Spider Monkeys to Poliomyelitis Infection" *Journal of Infectious Diseases* (1956) 99: 103–107.

18. "Claus Jungeblut, Bacteriologist, 78" *New York Times* February 2 1976. In the early twenty-first century his 1930s research on polio and vitamin C was rediscovered by a new group of alternative healers who claimed him as a forgotten heroic nutrition researcher; see

A. W. Saul "Taking the Cure: Claus Washington Jungeblut, M.D.: Polio Pioneers, Ascorbate Advocate" *Journal of Orthomolecular Medicine* (2006) 21: 102–106.

19. "Death of Sister Kenny" *JAMA* (January 3 1953) 151: 53; Miland E. Knapp, Lewis Sher and Theodore S. Smith "Results of Kenny Treatment of Acute Poliomyelitis: Present Status of Three Hundred Ninety-One Patients Treatment Between 1940 an d 1945" *JAMA* (January 10 1953) 151: 117–120; "Subject Index: Poliomyelitis" *JAMA* (April 25 1953) 151: 1570–1571.

20. "Sister Kenny" *British Medical Journal* (December 6 1952) 2: 1262.

21. "Sister Kenny: H. J. Seddon" *British Medical Journal* (December 6 1952) 2: 1262–1263.

22. H. J. Seddon [review of] "[Kenny] *And They Shall Walk*" *British Medical Journal* (April 12 1952) 1: 802–803.

23. "Sister Kenny" *Lancet* (December 6 1952) 260: 1123.

24. Jean Macnamara "Elizabeth Kenny" *Medical Journal of Australia* (February 17 1953) 1: 85. Macnamara herself was moving away from the field of polio care. While she remained an orthopedic consultant at the Royal Children's Hospital in Melbourne, by the late 1940s she was caught up in a heated newspaper exchange about the use of the myxoma virus to control Australian rabbits. The debate led to further testing in Victoria and success when the virus became epizootic in 1951, leading to significant savings for initially skeptical wool-growers and Macnamara's renewed reputation as a virus expert; Ann G. Smith "Macnamara, Dame Annie Jean (1899–1968)" *Australian Dictionary of Biography*, Vol. 10 (Melbourne: Melbourne University Press, 1986), 345–347; Brian Coman *Tooth and Nail: The Story of the Rabbit in Australia* (Melbourne: Text Publishing, 1999), 128–135.

25. "The Passing of Sister Elizabeth Kenny" *British Journal of Nursing* (January 1953) 101: 3.

26. [Mildred Elson, Editorial] "Sister Elizabeth Kenny" *Physical Therapy Review* (February 1953) 33: 81.

27. Marilyn Moffat "The History of Physical Therapy Practice in the United States" *Journal of Physical Therapy Education* (2003) 17: 15–25.

28. Gregory D. Black *The Catholic Crusade Against the Movies, 1940–1975* (Cambridge: Cambridge University Press, 1997), 67–71.

29. [Cohn interview with] Mary McCarthy, April 4 1953, Cohn Papers, MHS-K. On McCarthyism see Ellen Schrecker *Many Are the Crimes: McCarthyism in America* (Boston: Little, Brown & Company, 1998); David M. Oshinsky *A Conspiracy So Immense: The World of Joe McCarthy* (New York: The Free Press, 1983); David K. Johnson *The Lavender Menace: The Cold War Persecution of Gays and Lesbians in the Federal Government* (Chicago: University of Chicago Press, 2004).

30. "Sister Kenny Awards Presented to Hospital" *Los Angeles Times* January 19 1956; "Rosalind Russell Gives Tiny Patient Welcome" *Los Angeles Times* January 29 1956; see also Hedda Hopper "Betrothal Party for Bette Davis' Daughter" *Chicago Tribune* June 28 1963. In the early 1950s Russell toured with the comedy "Bell, Book and Candle" and then began a successful Broadway career, earning a Tony Award in 1953 for her portrayal of Ruth in the Broadway show "Wonderful Town," a musical based on her 1942 film *My Sister Eileen*. Russell's great success was the lead role in "Auntie Mame" for which she received a Tony nomination in 1957 and an Academy Award nomination and a Golden Globe award as the star in the 1958 movie version. During the 1960s Russell's movie career expanded with roles as an older still feisty woman in films such as *Gypsy* (1962) and *The Trouble with Angels* (1966); Bernard F. Dick *Forever Mame: The Life of Rosalind Russell* (Jackson: University Press of Mississippi, 2006), 224–230.

31. Rosalind Russell and Chris Chase *Life Is a Banquet* (New York: Random House, 1977), 143–144.

32. Henry Thomas *Lives to Remember: Sister Kenny* (London: Adam and Charles Black, 1958), 95. Other *Lives to Remember* volumes included Oliver Cromwell, Louis Pasteur, Helen Keller, Isaac Newton, and Elizabeth Garret Anderson.

33. Alan Jenkins "Adventure in Perseverance: The Nurse from Australia" in Alan Jenkins ed. *The Girl Book of Modern Adventures* (London: Hulton Press, 1952), 81.

34. Adele de Leeuw and Cateau de Leeuw *Nurses Who Led the Way* (Racine, WI: Whitman Publishing Co., 1957).

35. Frances Wilkins *Six Great Nurses: Louise de Marillac, Florence Nightingale, Clara Barton, Dorothy Patterson, Edith Cavell, Elizabeth Kenny* (London: Hamilton, 1962); Robin McKown *Heroic Nurses* (New York: G.P. Putnam's Sons, 1966).

36. James Stacey "Victor Cohn, Dean of Science Writers, Dies at 80," www.medscape.com/viewarticle/408047, accessed on 7/15/2011; "Science Writer Victor Cohn Dies" *Minneapolis Star-Tribune* February 15 2000; see also Lucy Y. Her "Victor Cohn, 80, Science, Medicine Writer" *Minneapolis Star-Tribune* February 14 2000, www.startribune.com/templates/11598646, 7/15/2011; Cohn "Angry Angel" *Minneapolis Tribune* October 29–November 18, 1953.

37. Cohn *Four Billion Dimes* (Minneapolis: Minneapolis Star and Tribune, 1955).

38. Morris [Fishbein] to Dear Basil [O'Connor], January 26 1953, Public History, MOD.

39. [Cohn interview with] Morris Fishbein, November 16 1953, Cohn Papers, MHS-K.

40. [Cohn interview with] Basil O'Connor, June 20 1955, Cohn Papers, MHS-K.

41. Cohn to Mrs. Julia Farquarson, June 8 1955, Cohn Papers, MHS-K. He was arriving entrusted with a new task: the Minnesota Historical Society had asked him to "secure her files and papers now in Toowoomba" and authorized him "to make an offer."

42. [Cohn interview with] Robert Bingham, May 19 1955, Cohn Papers, MHS-K.

43. [Cohn phone interview with] John Enders, March 28 1955, Cohn Papers, MHS.

44. [Cohn interview with] John Pohl and Betty Pohl, May 12 1953, Cohn Papers, MHS-K; [Cohn second interview with] John Pohl, October 2 1953, Cohn Papers, MHS-K.

45. Cohn to Dear Stuart and Mary [McCracken], July 22 1955, Kenny Collection, Box 2, Fryer Library.

46. Julia Farquarson to Cohn, October 10 1954, Cohn Papers, MHS-K. She had especially disliked his assumption that Kenny had considered Mary Kenny McCracken as her "adopted daughter." Kenny, Farquarson told Cohn, had seen Mary only as her adopted ward, and Mary had called her by "Sister" not "Mother," which "surely...speaks for itself."

47. Cohn to Mrs. Julia Farquarson, June 16 1953, Cohn Papers, MHS-K.

48. Julia Farquarson to Cohn, May 23 1953, Cohn Papers, MHS-K; Julia Farquarson to Cohn, October 10 1954, Cohn Papers, MHS-K.

49. Cohn to Harry Summers, January 24 1956, Cohn Papers, MHS-K. He met physicians, friends, and relatives, one of Chuter's former assistants, a *Women's Weekly* reporter, and looked at files in government archives and at Queensland and Sydney newspapers.

50. Duhig to Cohn, November 16 1955, Cohn Papers, MHS-K. Duhig pointed out that her belief "that a hot pack could alter the lesion in the spinal cord" would be analogous "to treating the headache of a brain tumor with aspirin."

51. [Cohn interview with] J. V. Duhig, November 14 1955, Cohn Papers, MHS-K.

52. [Cohn interview with] Sir Raphael Cilento, November 16 1955, Cohn Papers, MHS-K; Cohn to Summers, January 24 1956; see also Douglas Gordon "Sir Raphael West Cilento" *Medical Journal of Australia* (1985) 143: 259–260.

53. Cohn to Summers, January 24 1956.

54. [Cohn interview with] James Guinane, November 23 1955, Cohn Papers, MHS-K.

55. Howard A. Rusk "Kenny Fund Expansion" *New York Times* August 24 1958; "$735,459 Awarded As Research Grants" *Washington Post and Times Herald* May 15 1958.

56. Marvin L. Kline "The Most Unforgettable Character I've Met" *Reader's Digest* (August 1959) 75: 203–208; see also Rusk "Kenny Fund Expansion." The KF had funded trials of the Lederle oral vaccine in the late 1950s, under Dr. Martins da Silva, a University of Minnesota pediatrician from Brazil; Paul *A History*, 344–345.

57. Cohn *Sister Kenny*, 240–247; "Challenges Expenses of Kenny Fund" *Chicago Tribune* April 2 1960.

58. Larry Fitzmaurice "Mayo Doctor to Head Kenny" *Minneapolis Star* September 9 1960. See also a rumor that an El Monte board member had pocketed funds; Alexander *Maverick*, 204.

59. "Kline Resigns as Director of Kenny Group" *Minneapolis Tribune* March 29 1960.

60. D.W. Frear, "The Good Name of Sister Kenny" letter to editor, *Minneapolis Star* July 7 1960; "Irregularities Are Charged In Sister Kenny Fund Drive" *Philadelphia Evening Bulletin* June 27 1960; "Challenges Expenses of Kenny Fund."

61. "Keeping Perspective" *Minneapolis Tribune* April 6 1960.

62. "Challenges Expenses of Kenny Fund"; "Questionable Drives for 'Charity'" *Chicago Tribune* April 6 1960; "Irregularities Are Charged In Sister Kenny Fund Drive"; "Kenny Fund Accused of Misusing Money" *Chicago Tribune* June 28 1960; "Funds for Polio Found Diverted" *New York Times* June 28 1960. B. C. Gamble, a local businessman, was chosen as KF president along with 6 new directors; Huenkens was not invited to the directors' meeting to discuss the report.

63. Cohn *Sister Kenny*, 245–246; "The Kenny Report" *Chicago Tribune* July 6 1960; "Ex-Kenny Fund Official Faces Theft Charges" *Chicago Tribune* July 30 1960; "Kenny Fund Sues 2 Former Aides" *New York Times* August 12 1960; "Suit Filed to Recover Millions in Kenny Funds" *Chicago Tribune* August 12 1960.

64. "4 Chicagoans Indicted for Kenny Fraud" *Chicago Tribune* January 31 1962; "3 Kenny Foundation Ex-Officials Indicted" *Washington Post* January 31 1962; "Convict 5 in Kenny Fraud" *Chicago Tribune* May 30 1963; "5 Convicted of Defrauding Sister Kenny Foundation" *New York Times* May 30 1963; "Kline Gets 10 Years In Kenny Fund Fraud" *Washington Post* April 6 1961; "Settlement Taken By Kenny Fund" *Washington Post* October 11 1963; "Kenny Suit Settled for 1 Million Dollars" *Chicago Tribune* January 8 1966.

65. Robert H. Hamlin *Voluntary Health and Welfare Agencies in the United States: An Exploratory Study* (New York: Schoolmaster's Press, 1961); Emma Harrison "Ribicoff Advises Charity Agencies" *New York Times* September 15 1961.

66. Local reporters published Krusen's salary; at the KF he was making $35,000 a year; at the Mayo Clinic he had made $34,600 in 1958 and $34,700 in 1959; "Dr. Krusen Reviews Kenny Plans" *Minneapolis Star* November 10 1960; Daniel J. Hafrey "He's Rehabilitating the Rehabilitators" *Minneapolis Sunday Tribune* October 23 1961.

67. "Krusen to Head Kenny Institute" *[Rochester, MN] Post-Bulletin* September 9 1960; Bob Murphy "Doctor Honored by 37 Awards" *Minneapolis Star* August 18 1960; "Dr. Frank Krusen of Mayo Clinic, 75" *New York Times* September 18 1973; G. Keith Stillwell "In Memoriam: Frank H. Krusen, M.D. 1898–1973" *Archives of Physical Medicine and Rehabilitation* (1973) 54: 493–495. Krusen, who had become head of the Minnesota State Board of Health, had just returned from Washington, D.C. where he had assisted the federal Office of Vocational Rehabilitation.

68. Cohn *Sister Kenny*, 251–252; "Dr. Krusen Given Distinguished Service Award" *JAMA* (July 5 1958) 167: 1250; "Dr. Frank Krusen Dies at Cape Cod Home" *JAMA* (October 29 1973) 226: 523–524. He died in 1973.

69. Cohn *Sister Kenny*, 251–252; Paul Elwood in *Health Inquiry (Poliomyelitis)* [Part 3 October 6 1953], 638–642; see also "Paul M. Ellwood, Jr., MD. In First Person: An Oral History" interviewed by Anthony R. Kovner, September 16 2010, Hospital Administration Oral History Collection (Chicago: Health Research and Educational Trust, 2011); http://www.aha.org/aha/resource-center/Center-for-Hospital-and-Health-Administration-History/Ellwood%20-%20FINAL%20-%20205311.pdf, accessed 8/6/2011.

70. "Sister Kenny Foundation Changes Name" *Chicago Tribune* January 29 1965.

71. Morris Fishbein *Morris Fishbein, M.D.: An Autobiography* (New York: Doubleday, 1969), 229–234.

72. John K. Alexander "Saul Benison" *[AHA] Perspectives* (October 2007) http://www.historians.org/perspectives/issues/2007/0710/0710mem1.cfm, accessed 11/25/2012; "In Memorandum: Saul Benison (1920–2006)" *Bulletin of the History of Medicine* (2008) 82: 42–423; Saul Benison "Reflections on Oral History" *American Archivist* (1965) 28: 71–77. Benison had worked as an oral historian at Columbia University and then accepted a position in the history department of the University of Cincinnati.

73. F. L. Horsfall "Thomas Milton Rivers, September 3, 1888–May 12, 1962" *Biographical Memoirs National Academy of Sciences* (1965) 38: 263–94; see also Saul Benison "The History of Polio Research in the United States: Appraisal and Lessons" in Gerald Holton ed. *The Twentieth-Century Sciences: Studies in the Biography of Ideas* (New York: W.W. Norton and Co., 1972), 308–343.

74. Saul Benison *Tom Rivers: Reflections on a Life in Medicine and Science* (Cambridge: MIT Press, 1967), 282–284.

75. Francis MacFarlane Burnet *Changing Patterns: An Atypical Autobiography* (Melbourne: William Heinemann, 1968), 165–168.

76. [Cohn fourth interview with] John Pohl, August 27 1963, Cohn Papers, MHS-K; John Pohl to Dear Vic [Cohn], July 29 1967, Cohn Papers, MHS-K.

77. There is a brief reference to the Kendalls' PHS bulletin, described as an effort "on the part of the U.S. Public Health Service" to combat the widespread tendency of splinting limbs "to excess"; Paul *A History*, 338.

78. Paul *A History*, 336, 342–343.

79. Paul *A History*, 340–344.

80. Editorial [Robert Bennett] "The Contribution to Physical Medicine of Our Experience With Poliomyelitis" *Archives of Physical Medicine and Rehabilitation* (September 1969) 50: 524.

81. Editor's Note, Walter I. Galland "The Post-Paralytic Treatment of Poliomyelitis From the Orthopedic Standpoint" [abridged from] *Archives of Physical Therapy* (1932), [reprinted in] *Archives of Physical Medicine and Rehabilitation* (September 1969) 50: 525.

82. Ghormley et al. "Evaluation of the Kenny Treatment of Infantile Paralysis" [abridged from] *JAMA* (June 17 1944) [reprinted in] *Archives of Physical Medicine and Rehabilitation* (September 1969) 50: 531–535; Miland E. Knapp "The Contribution of Sister Elizabeth Kenny to the Treatment of Poliomyelitis" [abridged from] *Archives of Physical Medicine* (August 1955), [reprinted in] *Archives of Physical Medicine and Rehabilitation* (September 1969) 50: 535–542.

83. Cohn *Sister Kenny*, 247–250; Mr. Mondale "Sister Kenny" *Congressional Record—Senate* August 7 1972, S12907, Biographical Data, MHS-K.

84. Cohn *Sister Kenny*, 20–23.

85. Cohn *Sister Kenny*, 10, 30, 100.

86. Cohn *Sister Kenny*, 3, 7–8, 36.

87. Audrey B. Davis "[review] *Sister Kenny*" *Clio Medica* (1976) 11: 206.

88. Glenda Riley "[review *Sister Kenny*]" *South Dakota History* (fall 1976) 6: 482–483, Cohn Papers, MHS-K.

89. Marjorie C. Meehan "Sister Kenny [review *Sister Kenny*]" *JAMA* (May 31 1976) 235: 2435.

90. Sonya Rudikoff "Using Her Intuition in A Crusade Against Polio" [review *Sister Kenny*] *Washington Post* March 4 1976.

91. J. A. Myers to Dear Maurice [Visscher], May 6 1971, Box 19, Folder 1, Myers Papers, UMN-ASC; see Meyers "Poliomyelitis (Infantile Paralysis) in Minnesota Including the Elizabeth Kenny Episode," Box 19, Sister Kenny Institute 1938–1946, Myers Papers, UMN-ASC.

92. Myers to Dear Harold [Miller], September 8 1960, Box 19, Folder 1, Myers Papers, UMN-ASC.

93. "[Report of] Board of Directors Meeting" *Bulletin of the Hennepin County Medical Society* (December 1960) 31: 532; Thomas P. Cook to Dear Doctor Miller, November 23 1960, Box 19, Folder 1, Myers Papers, UMN-ASC; Myers to Dear Maurice [Visscher], June 29 1960, Box 19, Folder 1, Myers Papers, UMN-ASC.

94. Myers "Poliomyelitis (Infantile Paralysis) in Minnesota Including the Elizabeth Kenny Episode," 24–25, 28, 45.

95. Myers to Dear John [Moe], December 8 1977, Box 19, Folder 3, Myers Papers, UMN-ASC.

96. Maurice [Visscher] to Dear Jay [Myers], April 21 1977, Box 21, Myers Papers, UMN-ASC.

97. Harold S. Diehl "Jay Arthur Myers: Teacher, Colleague, Friend" *Diseases of the Chest* (1968) 53: 666; "Deaths: Jay Arthur Myers, World-Renowned Tuberculosis Expert" *American Journal of Public Health* (1979) 69: 190.

98. "Sister Kenny Hospital for Polio Patients Closes" *Chicago Tribune* December 26 1957.

99. "TV: C.B.S. Turns 'Waltons' Into 'Easter Story'" *New York Times* April 19 1973; "Today's Best Bets" *Los Angeles Times* April 19 1973.

100. Anne Roiphe "The Waltons: Ma and Pa and John-Boy in Mythic America" *New York Times* November 18 1973.

101. Aaron E. Klein *Trial By Fury: The Polio Vaccine Controversy* (New York: Charles Scribner's Sons, 1972), 43–45.

102. "Basil O'Connor, Polio Fighter, Dies" *Washington Post* March 10 1972; Alden Whitman "Basil O'Connor, Polio Crusader, Died" *New York Times* March 10 1972.

103. McCandlish Phillips "March of Dimes Is Now Paying Basil O'Connor for His Services" *New York Times* February 12 1965.

104. "Memorial for Basil O'Connor Is Attended by 200" *New York Times* March 14 1972; "Basil O'Connor, Polio Fighter, Dies."

105. Harvey Katz "The Cool Hand of Charity" *Washington Post/Times Herald* December 24 1972.

106. Rebecca L. Craik "Editor's Postscript: Florence P. Kendall, PT" *Physical Therapy* (March 2006) 26: 336; K. G. Hansson "[Review] Henry O. Kendall, Florence P. Kendall, and Dorothy A. Boynton *Posture and Pain* (Baltimore: The Williams & Wilkins Co., 1952)" in *Journal of Bone and Joint Surgery* (April 1956) 38: 473.

107. Lucie P. Lawrence "Florence Kendall: What a Wonderful Journey" *PT Magazine of Physical Therapy* (2000) 8: 42. See also [advertisement] Kendall et al.: *Posture And Pain* [in] *American Journal of Physical Medicine* (December 1961) 40: n.p., Kendall Collection.

108. Lawrence "Florence Kendall: What a Wonderful Journey," 45. She died in 2006; Matt Schudel "[Obituary] Physical Therapist Florence P. Kendall" *Washington Post* February 5 2006.

109. Michele Wojciechowski "Remembering Florence Kendall" *Proficio* (2006) 15: 3.

110. Florence P. Kendall "Sister Elizabeth Kenny Revisited" *Archives of Physical Medicine and Rehabilitation* (1998) 79: 361–365. According to Kendall, Kenny's theory of mental alienation "gave false hope to many victims." I contacted Kendall after this article appeared and interviewed her in her home in Silver Springs, Maryland where she showed me these sources and spoke clearly and antagonistically about Kenny; Kendall, interviews with Rogers, April 26 and April 27 1999, Silver Springs, Maryland.

111. For a nuanced reading of polio publications such as the [Warm Springs] *Wheelchair Review* and the [Cleveland] *Toomey j. Gazette* see Jacqueline Foertsch *Bracing Accounts: The Literature and Culture of Polio in Postwar America* (Madison, NJ: Fairleigh Dickinson University Press, 2008).

112. Oshinksy *Polio*, 282–285; see also Victor Cohn "Recurrent Polio Strikes Victims of Epidemics" *Washington Post* May 26 1984.

113. Daniel J. Wilson *Living with Polio: The Epidemic and Its Survivors* (Chicago: University of Chicago Press, 2005); Richard L. Bruno *The Polio Paradox: Understanding and Treating 'Post-Polio Syndrome' and Chronic Fatigue* (New York: Warner Books, 2002); Lauro Halstead *Managing Post Polio: A Guide to Living And Aging Well with Post-Polio Syndrome* (Washington, DC: National Rehabilitation Hospital Press, 2006); Julie K. Silver *Post-Polio: A Guide for Polio Survivors and Their Families* (New Haven: Yale University Press, 2011).

114. John Toomey had disliked Kenny and felt her work overshadowed his own, but, reflecting Toomey's eminence in his home town, after he died in 1950 the polio rehabilitation center connected to Cleveland's infectious disease hospital was renamed the Toomey Rehabilitation Pavilion. His name gained lasting recognition when Gini Laurie founded the *Toomeyville j. Gazette* in 1955, a newsletter that linked together polio survivors and became one of the nodes of the postwar disability rights movement.

115. Rosemarie Garland Thomson "Imaging FDR: Separate Still" *Ragged Edge Online* (2001) issue 2; http://www.ragged-edge-mag.com/0301/0301ft3.htm, accessed 8/17/2011; Oshinksy *Polio*, 284–285; Rosemarie Garland Thomson "The FDR Memorial: Who Speaks From the Wheelchair?" *Chronicle of Higher Education* January 26 2001; Kim E. Nielsen "Memorializing FDR" *OAH Magazine of History* (2013) 27: 23–26.

116. Bruno *The Polio Paradox*, 73.

117. Robert F. Hall *Through the Storm: A Polio Story* (St. Cloud, MN: North Star Press, 1990), 6–7.

118. Nudelman and Willingham *Healing the Blues* (1997) quoted in Wilson *Living with Polio*, 56–57.

119. Pohl and Kenny, *The Kenny Concept of Infantile Paralysis*, 87–94.

120. Hall *Through the Storm*, 8.

121. Bruno *The Polio Paradox*; Wilson *Living with Polio*. On sexual abuse by doctors and by orderlies, see Bruno *The Polio Paradox*, 76–77.

122. Bruno *The Polio Paradox*, 74. Bruno argued that "Kenny's preeminence and her own dogmatism blotted out at least equally effective and more humane treatments for polio, such

as the procedures developed by the Kendalls a decade earlier," a view that probably came from his reading of Kendall "Sister Elizabeth Kenny Revisited," 361–365.

123. Pohl and Kenny *The Kenny Concept of Infantile Paralysis*, 175.

124. Suzane Fabian and Morag Loh "Elizabeth Kenny 1880–1952: Nurse, Pioneer Therapist, Inventor" in *The Change[-]makers: Ten Significant Australian Women* (Milton, Queensland: Jacaranda Press, 1983), 131–142. See also George Blaikie "Sister Elizabeth Kenny: A Bold Crusader Against Polio" *Australian Women's Weekly* (November 1984) 52: 346–347; Jim Bowditch "Bush Nurse's Magnificent Obsession: Sister Kenny a Polio Angel" *Sunday Sun [Magazine]* October 16 1988, 2, Kenny Collection, Box 18, Fryer Library; George Blaikie "Sister Elizabeth Kenny: Controversial Crusader Against Polio" in *Great Women of History* (Broadway, New South Wales: John Fairfax Marketing, 1984), 117–118. For examples of the lack of attention to Kenny see Helen Gregory *A Tradition of Care: A History of Nursing at the Royal Brisbane Hospital* (Brisbane: Boolarong Publication, 1988); it has no discussion of Kenny in the text but does include a photograph of her; Elizabeth Burchill *Australian Nurses since Nightingale 1860–1990* (Richmond: Spectrum Publications, 1992) has no mention of Kenny.

125. Alan Alda in *Woman's Day* March 13 1980, quoted in Fabian and Loh "Elizabeth Kenny 1880–1952: Nurse, Pioneer Therapist, Inventor," 131–142; see for example Alan Alda *Never Have Your Dog Stuffed: And Other Things I've Learned* (New York: Random House, 2005), 19–20.

126. John R. Wilson *Through Kenny's Eyes: An Exploration of Sister Elizabeth Kenny's Views about Nursing* (Townsville: Royal College of Nursing Australia, 1995).

127. Rewind ABC-TV "Sister Kenny: Saint or Charlatan?" August 29 2004; abc.net.au/tv/rewind/txt/s1184925.htm, accessed 9/29/2005.

128. "Memorial to Sister Kenny" *Melbourne Age* September 20 1961; http://www.post-polionetwork.org.au/particles/part13.pdf, accessed 1/10/2013; Toowoomba Sundial http://jhwagner.com.au/sister-kenny-memorial.php, accessed 1/10/2013.

129. http://www.post-polionetwork.org.au/particles/part13.pdf, accessed 1/10/2013.

130. "Sister Kenny Recalled on '100th' Birthday—and Again Famous Founder Has Upper Hand" *Minneapolis Star* September 20 1986.

131. Leonard G. Wilson *Medical Revolution in Minnesota: A History of the University of Minnesota* (St. Paul: Midewiwin Press, 1989), 357–365.

132. Emily Crofford *Healing Warrior: A Story about Sister Elizabeth Kenny* (Minneapolis: Carolrhoda Books, 1989), 50.

133. Nancy Rehkamp to Dear Friend of Sister Kenny Institute, February 18 1992, Chris Sharpe Collection, in author's possession; "Major 1992 PR Activities in Conjunction with 50th Anniversary," Chris Sharpe Collection, in author's possession. On the Institute's merger with Abbott-Northwestern Hospital and then the Allina hospital system see http://www.allina.com/ahs/ski.nsf/page/aboutus, accessed 1/10/2013; B. Lee Ligon "Sister Elizabeth Kenny: A Controversial Participant in the War against Polio" *Seminars in Pediatric Infectious Diseases* (October 2000) 11: 287–291, 290. It is now the Sister Kenny Rehabilitative Institute.

134. Henry W. Haverstock, letter to editor, "Russia and Sister Kenny" [Minneapolis newspaper], August 10 1993, Cohn Papers, MHS-K.

135. Mary and Stuart McCracken, interviews with Rogers, November 1992, Caloundra, Queensland.

136. "Fighting Polio with 'Gentle Hands'" by Dan Olson, Minnesota Public Radio, August 22, 2002; http://news.minnesota.publicradio.org/features/200208/22_olsond_sisterkinney/part4.shtml, accessed 9/22/2011.

137. Kate Roberts *Minnesota 150: The People, Places, and Things That Shape Our State* (St: Paul: Minnesota Historical Society Press, 2007), 96–97.

138. Annette Atkins "Facing Minnesota" *Daedalus: Minnesota: A Different America?* (2000) 129: 45–46.

139. Minnesota History Theatre "Sister Kenny's Children," http://www.historytheatre.com/shows/2009-2010/sister_kenny.asp, accessed 9/22/11; see also Bev Wolfe "Claudia Wilkens Gives a Commanding Performance in 'Sister Kenny's Children'" *Twin Cities Daily Planet* January 28 2010. The Play Guide listed Cohn's biography, the ABC and the MPR broadcasts, Kenny's 2 autobiographies, and one of her textbooks.

140. Kenny *My Battle and Victory: History of the Discovery of Poliomyelitis as a Systemic Disease* (London: Robert Hale, 1955), 10. The correct quotation is "He that of greatest works is finisher/Oft does them by the weakest minister"; William Shakespeare *All's Well That Ends Well*, Act 2, Scene i.

141. A. L. Baron *Man Against Germs* (London: Scientific Book Club, 1958), 126–129.

142. For one effort at addressing some aspects of this issue see Rogers "The Debate Considered" *Australian Historical Studies* (2000) 31: 163–166.

143. One major exception to this is the history of drugs; see Elizabeth Siegel Watkins and Andrea Tone eds. *Medicating Modern America: Prescription Drugs in History* (New York: New York University Press, 2007); Jeremy A. Greene *Prescribing By Numbers: Drugs and the Definition of Disease* (Baltimore: Johns Hopkins University Press, 2007); Robert Bud *Penicillin: Triumph and Tragedy* (Oxford: Oxford University Press, 2007); John E. Lesch *The First Miracle Drugs: How the Sulfa Drugs Transformed Medicine* (Oxford: Oxford University Press, 2007).

144. Charles A. Wolverton in *Health Inquiry (Poliomyelitis)* [Part 3 October 6 1953], 608.

145. Gaylord Anderson in *Health Inquiry (Poliomyelitis)* [Part 3 October 6 1953], 611–621.

FURTHER READING

For polio after 1945 see Richard L. Bruno *The Polio Paradox: Understanding and Treating 'Post-Polio Syndrome' and Chronic Fatigue* (New York: Warner Books, 2002); Nancy Baldwin Carter *Snapshots: Polio Survivors Remember* (Omaha: NPSA Press, 2002); Thomas M. Daniel and Frederick C. Robbins eds. *Polio* (Rochester, NY: University of Rochester Press, 1997); Jacqueline Foertsch *Bracing Accounts: The Literature and Culture of Polio in Postwar America* (Madison, NJ: Fairleigh Dickinson University Press, 2008); Lauro Halstead *Managing Post Polio: A Guide to Living And Aging Well with Post-Polio Syndrome* (Washington, DC: National Rehabilitation Hospital Press, 2006); Lauro Halstead and Gunnar Grimby *Post-Polio Syndrome* (Philadelphia: Hanley and Belfus, 1995); Edmund J. Sass ed. *Polio's Legacy: An Oral History* (New York: University Press of America, Inc., 1996); Richard K. Scotch *From Good Will to Civil Rights: Transforming Disability Policy* (Philadelphia: Temple University Press, 1984); Richard K. Scotch "Politics and Policy in the History of the Disability Rights Movement" *Milbank Quarterly* (1989) (supplement part 2) 67: 380–400; Nina Gilden Seavey, Jane S. Smith, and Paul Wagner *A Paralyzing Fear: The Triumph Over Polio in America* (New York: TV Books, 1998); Marc Shell *Polio and Its Aftermath: The Paralysis of Culture* (Cambridge: Harvard University Press, 2005); Julie K. Silver *Post-Polio: A Guide for Polio Survivors and Their Families* (New Haven: Yale University Press, 2011); Daniel J. Wilson "Braces, Wheelchairs, and Iron Lungs: The Paralyzed Body and the Machinery of Rehabilitation in the Polio Epidemics" *Journal of Medical Humanities* (2005) 26: 188–190; Daniel J. Wilson *Living with Polio: The Epidemic and Its Survivors* (Chicago: University of Chicago Press, 2005).

On history and remembering and forgetting see Pascal Boyer and James V. Wertsch eds. *Memory in Mind and Culture* (Cambridge: Cambridge University Press, 2009); Maria G. Cattell, Jacob J. Climo, and Maria G. Cattell eds. *Social Memory and History: Anthropological Perspectives* (Walnut Creek, CA: Altamira Press, 2002); Mark Crinson ed. *Urban Memory: History and Amnesia in the Modern City* (London: Routledge, 2005); Katharine Hodgkin and Susannah Radstone eds. *Contesting Pasts: The Politics of Memory* (London: Routledge, 2003); Andreas Kitzmann, Conny Mithander, and John Sundholm eds. *Memory Work: The Theory and Practice of Memory* (Frankfurt am Main: Peter Lang, 2005); Norman M. Klein *The History of Forgetting: Los Angeles and the Erasure of Memory* (London: Verso, 1997); Seth Koven "Remembering and Dismemberment: Crippled Children, Wounded Soldiers, and the Great War in Great Britain" *American Historical Review* (1994) 99: 1167–1202; Selma Leydesdorff, Luisa Passerini, and Paul Thompson eds. *Gender and Memory: International Yearbook of Oral History and Life Stories,* Vol. IV (New York: Oxford University Press, 1996); Susan R. Suleiman *Crises of Memory and the Second World War* (Cambridge: Harvard University Press, 2006); David Thelan ed. *Memory and American History* (Bloomington: Indiana University Press, 1989); Jay Winter *Sites of Memory, Sites of Mourning: The Great War in European Cultural History* (Cambridge: Cambridge University Press, 1995); Barbie Zelizer *Remembering To Forget: Holocaust Memory through the Camera's Eye* (Chicago: Chicago University Press, 1998).

INDEX

Note: Page numbers followed by *f* indicate material found in Figures; page numbers followed by *n* indicate material found in Notes